Special Medication Precautions

DRUGS ASSOCIATED WITH SERIOUS ADVERSE EFFECTS

HEPATOTOXIC DRUGS

acetaminophen
4-aminoquinoline
amiodarone
Anabolic steroid agents
Antithyroid agents
asparaginase
azlocillin
carbamazepine
carmustine
Contraceptives (estrogen)
dantrolene
daunorubicin
disulfiram
divalproex
erythromycin
estrogen, conjugated
etretinate
gold compounds
halothane
isoniazid
ketoconazole
mercaptopurine
methotrexate
methyldopa
mezlocillin
naltrexone
phenothiazine
phenytoin
piperacillin
plicamycin
rifampin
sulfonamides
tetracycline
valproic acid

NEPHROTOXIC DRUGS

acyclovir
aminoglycoside antibiotics
amphotericin B
analgesic combinations
capreomycin
captopril
cisplatin
cyclosporine
demeclocycline
edetate calcium disodium
enalapril
gold compounds
lithium
methotrexate
methoxyflurane
neomycin
NSAIDs
penicillamine
pentamidine
plicamycin
rifampin
streptozocin
sulfonamides
tetracycline
Vancomycin

OTHER TOXICITIES

Anaphylaxis: penicillins, heparin, aspirin, parenteral iron, dextran
Asthma: aspirin, ibuprofen
Blood dyscrasias: chloramphenicol, anticonvulsants, penicillins, hydralazine, sulfonamides, anticancer drugs
Damage to eighth cranial nerve: furosemide, aspirin and other salicylates, Vibramycin, gentamicin
Eye damage: topical corticosteroids, ethambutol, Thorazine, chloroquine
Peripheral neuritis: isoniazid, vincristine, hydralazine, ethambutol

NSAIDs, Nonsteroidal antiinflammatory drugs.
Data from McKenry LM, et al. Mosby's pharmacology in nursing, ed 22, St Louis, 2006, Mosby; Hardman JG, Limbird LW et al, editors: Goodman and Gilman's pharmacological basis of therapeutics, ed 10, New York, 2001, McGraw-Hill; and Katzung BG: Basic and clinical pharmacology, ed 8, Norwalk, Conn, 2000, Appleton & Lange.

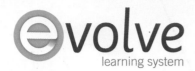
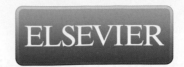
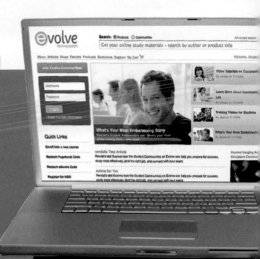

Introduction to Clinical Pharmacology

Marilyn Winterton Edmunds, PhD, ANP/GNP
Adjunct Faculty
Johns Hopkins University
School of Nursing
Baltimore, Maryland

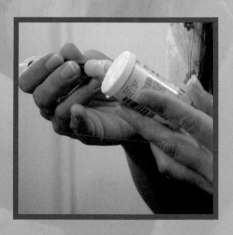

Seventh Edition

ELSEVIER

3251 Riverport Lane
St. Louis, Missouri 63043

Introduction to Clinical Pharmacology   ISBN: 978-0-323-07398-1
Seventh Edition
Copyright © 2013 by Mosby, an imprint of Elsevier Inc.
Copyright © 2010, 2006, 2003, 2000, 1995, 1991 by Mosby Inc., an affiliate of Elsevier Inc.

Notices

The content and procedures in this book are based on information currently available. They were reviewed by instructors and practicing professionals in various regions of the United States. However, agency policies and procedures may vary from the information and procedures in this book. In addition, research and new information may require changes in standards and practices.

Standards and guidelines from the Centers for Disease Control and Prevention (CDC) and the Occupational Safety and Health Administration (OSHA) may change as new information becomes available. Other federal and state agencies also may issue new standards and guidelines. So may accrediting agencies and national organizations.

You are responsible for following the policies and procedures of your employer and the most current standards, practices, and guidelines as they relate to the safety of your work.

To the fullest extent of the law, neither the Publisher nor the authors or editors assume any liability for any injury and/or damage to persons or property as a matter of products liability, negligence or otherwise, or from any use or operation of any methods, products, instructions, or ideas contained in the material herein.

Previous editions copyrighted 2010, 2006, 2003, 2000, 1995, 1991

Library of Congress Cataloging-in-Publication Data

Edmunds, Marilyn W.
  Introduction to clinical pharmacology / Marilyn Winterton Edmunds.—7th ed.
      p. ; cm.
  Includes bibliographical references and index.
  ISBN 978-0-323-07398-1 (pbk. : alk. paper)
  I. Title.
  [DNLM: 1. Pharmacology, Clinical—Nurses' Instruction.   2. Drug Therapy—Nurses' Instruction.   QV 38]

  615.5'8—dc23
                                                                2011045077

Executive Content Strategist: Teri Hines Burnham
Associate Content Development Specialist: Heather Rippetoe
Publishing Services Managers: Deborah Vogel and Hemamalini Rajendrababu
Project Managers: Bridget Healy and Janaki Srinivasan Kumar
Designer: Karen Pauls

Printed in China

Last digit is the print number: 9 8 7 6 5 4 3 2 1

Acknowledgments

Writing a pharmacology text is like running a race that never ends. There are always new drugs arriving on the market and new information available about old products. The available information is endless, and it is a real challenge to try to acquire enough knowledge to be a safe practitioner. But wisely and safely administering drugs is an important part of the nursing role.

I wish to acknowledge my personal stimulation from the many students who have asked challenging questions throughout my years as a teacher, and the support of my professional colleagues. I am grateful for the help of the Elsevier editorial, production, marketing, and design staff. Teri Hines Burnham, executive editor; Heather Rippetoe, associate developmental editor; and Jennifer Shropshire, associate developmental editor at Elsevier, provided ongoing editorial guidance and support, and were wonderful advocates for adding new features, color, and content. Bridget Healy, project manager, smoothly directed the the fine details and numerous facets of a complex manuscript through the production process. Karen Pauls, book designer, created a beautiful new full-color design for this edition. Vinod Kothaparamtath, multimedia producer, helped enhance the companion Evolve website. Todd McKenzie and Danielle LeCompte, marketing managers, applied creative ideas to promote the book and announce its presence to students and instructors.

My sincere thanks to the following people for their hard work and dedication in preparing a terrific ancillary package for the textbook: Allison Terry for the interactive review questions for the NCLEX-PN® Examination; Bill Olson and Laura Kanavy for the ExamView test bank; Dan Matusiak for the Open-Book Quizzes; Allison Muller for the PowerPoint presentations; and Donna Hubbard for the TEACH lesson plans.

I'd also like to acknowledge several educators who have lent their knowledge and expertise to this textbook over many editions: Karen Odle Ippolito, Linda Fluharty, Raquel Braithwaite, and Elaine Princevalli.

As always, I owe a special debt of gratitude to my family, who is so important in my life and who supports me in all the things in which I get involved. Much gratitude is expressed to my long suffering husband, Cliff, who over many years, jobs, children and countries, has always been there. Special appreciation is also expressed in memory of Alice (Ali) Parke Edmunds who will always be in our hearts.

MARILYN WINTERTON EDMUNDS, RN, PhD

Contributor and Reviewers

CONTRIBUTOR

Travis Sonnett, PharmD, FASCP
Clinical Assistant Professor
Washington State University
College of Pharmacy
Spokane, Washington

REVIEWERS

Karen Amsden, RN, BSN, MSHA
CNA Program Coordinator/
Professor
Jefferson College
Hillsboro, Missouri

Terry Bischel, RN, BSN
Coordinator of Practical Nursing
Program
Moberly Area Community College
Moberly, Missouri

Michelle Blackmer, MSN, RN
Manager, Education
Trinity Medical Center
Rock Island, Illinois
Adjunct Faculty
Trinity College of Nursing and
Health Sciences
Rock Island, Illinois

Chris Bridgers, PharmD, RPh
Clinical Pharmacist
Operations Manager, Pharmacy
Services
Saint Joseph's Hospital
Atlanta, Georgia

Drew Case, RN, MSN, APRN
Instructor
Southeast Community College
Lincoln, Nebraska

Deborah Clarkston, RN, MSN
Associate Professor of Nursing
Virginia Appalachian Tricollege
Nursing Program
Mountain Empire Community
College
Big Stone Gap, Virginia

Irene Coons, MSN, RN, CNE
Professor
Department of Nursing
College of Southern Nevada
Las Vegas, Nevada

Diane Daddario, MSN, ACNS-BC, RN, BC, CMSRN
Urology Nurse Specialist
Geisinger Medical Center
Danville, Pennsylvania

Sally Flesch, PhD, RN
Professor
Practical Nursing Program
Black Hawk College
Moline, Illinois

Cheryl Goretti, MA, MT(ASCP), CMA (AAMA)
Professor and Coordinator
Medical Assisting and Allied
Health Programs
Quinebaug Valley Community
College
Danielson, Connecticut

Laura Higgs, RN-BC, MSN, MEd
Associate Professor of Nursing
Chesapeake College
Wye Mills, Maryland

Diane M. Kemper, MSN, CCRN-CMC, ANCP-BC, CNE
Assistant Professor
Harrisburg Area Community
College
Gettysburg, Pennsylvania

Renee Lewis, RN, MS
Program Director
Practical Nursing
Francis Turtle Technology Center
Oklahoma City, Oklahoma

Michele Matthews, PharmD
Assistant Professor of Pharmacy
Practice
Massachusetts College of Pharmacy
and Health Sciences
Boston, Massachusetts

Sandra Meeker, RN, MSN
Assistant Professor
University of Mary Hardin Baylor
Belton, Texas

Jean Mendoza, RN, BS, MSN
Assistant Professor of Nursing
Heritage University
Toppenish, Washington

Joshua Neumiller, PharmD, CDE, CGP, FASCP
Assistant Professor
Department of Pharmacotherapy
Washington State University
College of Pharmacy
Pullman, Washington

Sallie Noto, RN, MS, MSN
Director
Career Technology Center
School of Practical Nursing
Scranton, Pennsylvania

Sue Parker, DNP, RN, APN, FNP-BC
Assistant Professor
College of Nursing
University of Arkansas
Fort Smith, Arkansas

Kendra Seiler, MSN, RN
Associate Professor
Rio Hondo College
Whittier, California

Cassie Shaw, BSN, RN
Instructor
Vernon College
Vernon, Texas

Mary Stassi, RN, BC
Health Occupation Coordinator
St. Charles Community College
St. Peters, Missouri

Eileen Stork, RN, BSN, MS, RNC, OB
Instructor
Great Oaks School of Practical
Nursing
Cincinnati, Ohio

Laura Travis, MSN, BSN, RN
Health Careers Coordinator
Tennessee Center at Dickinson
Dickinson, Tennessee

Sarah E. Whitaker, DNS, RN
Nursing Program Director
Concorde Career College
Memphis, Tennessee

Erin Yesenosky, RN, BSN, MSN
LPN Instructor
Excelsior College
Albany, New York
Chamberlain College
DeVry, Illinois

LPN Threads and Advisory Board

LPN THREADS

Standard LPN Threads series features incorporated into *Introduction to Clinical Pharmacology*, Seventh Edition, make it easy for students to move from one book to the next in the fast-paced and demanding LPN/LVN curriculum. The following features are included in the LPN Threads:

- A **reading level evaluation** is performed on all LPN texts to increase the consistency among chapters and ensure the text is easy to understand.
- **Full-color design, cover, photos,** and **illustrations** that are visually appealing and pedagogically useful.
- **Objectives** (numbered) begin each chapter, provide a framework for content and are important in providing the structure for the TEACH Lesson Plans for the textbook.
- **Key Terms** with phonetic pronunciations and page number references are listed at the beginning of each chapter. Key terms appear in color in the chapter and are defined briefly, with full definitions in the **Glossary.** The goal is to help the student reader with limited proficiency in English to develop a greater command of the pronunciation of scientific and non-scientific English terminology.
- A wide variety of **special features** relate to critical thinking, clinical practice, care of the pediatric patient and older adult, health promotion, safety, complementary and alternative therapies, communication, and more. Refer to the To the Student section of this introduction on page x for descriptions and examples of features from the pages of this textbook.
- **NCLEX Review Questions, Case Studies, Drug Calculation Review Questions,** and **Critical Thinking Questions** presented at the end of chapters give students opportunities to practice critical thinking and clinical decision-making skills with realistic patient scenarios.
- **Key Points** at the end of each chapter correlate to the objectives and serve as a useful chapter review.
- A full suite of **Instructor Resources** including TEACH Lesson Plans, Lecture Outlines, and Power-Point Slides, Test Bank, Image Collection, and Open-Book Quizzes.
- In addition to consistent content, design, and support resources, these textbooks benefit from the advice and input of the **Elsevier LPN/LVN Advisory Board.**

LPN ADVISORY BOARD

Marjorie L. (Gie) Archer, MS, RN, CNE
Dean, Health Sciences
North Central Texas College
Gainesville, Texas

Patricia A. Castaldi, RN, BSN, MSN
Union County College
Plainfield, New Jersey

Mary Ann Cosgarea, RN, BSN
PN Coordinator/Health Coordinator
Portage Lakes Career Center
Green, Ohio

Dolores Ann Cotton, RN, BSN, MS
Meridian Technology Center
Stillwater, Oklahoma

Ruth Ann Eckenstein, RN, BS, MEd
Oklahoma Department of Career and Technology Education
Stillwater, Oklahoma

Gail Ann Hamilton Finney, RN, MSN
Nursing Education Specialist
Concorde Career Colleges, Inc.
Mission, Kansas

Pam Hinckley, RN, MSN
Redlands Adult School
Redlands, California

Patty Knecht, MSN, RN
Nursing Program Director
Center for Arts & Technology
Brandywine Campus
Coatesville, Pennsylvania

Lieutenant Colonel (RET) Teresa Y. McPherson, RN, BSN, MSN
LVN Program Director
Nursing Education
St. Philip's College
San Antonio, Texas

Frances Neu-Shull, MS, BSN, RN
Supervisor, Adult Ed Health
Butler Technology and Career Development Schools
Fairfield Township, Ohio

Sister Ann Wiesen, RN, MRA
Erwin Technical Center
Tampa, Florida

Preface

Introduction to Clinical Pharmacology, Seventh Edition, provides just the right level and depth of pharmacology content for LPN/LVN students. Pharmacology content quickly becomes outdated, and the past three years have brought unprecedented changes in drugs available. Many of the drugs that have been on the market for three to four decades are gradually being removed from the market as newer products take their places. Many more drugs have become available in generic form or over the counter. Direct-to-consumer advertising has led many patients to believe that they can self-diagnose and self-treat. All of these changes mean that there has never been a time when nursing knowledge about drugs has been more important.

This new edition of *Introduction to Clinical Pharmacology* reflects these changes in ways that will assist students in learning what they need to know. Up-to-date information on many new drugs, procedures, regulations, and issues provides a strong foundation of essential knowledge for the safe, effective administration of drugs. Every effort has been made in this edition to incorporate the excellent suggestions of instructors, students, and practicing nurses who have used and evaluated the text. One major change made in response to faculty suggestions is that the dosing information for medications has been removed from the book. Faculty suggested that students use current drug handbooks for this information and felt this content was not required here. Several chapters have been revised, refocused, and updated to keep them current with latest developments and guidelines. Some additional content only taught in a few LPN/LVN programs, such as dimensional analysis, has now been moved to the Evolve website.

ORGANIZATION AND FEATURES

Pharmacology is a science; in it there are both right answers and wrong answers. Accuracy, safety, and precision are therefore extremely important, and nurses are legally responsible and accountable for how they administer drugs. The science of medication administration for nurses is outlined in **Unit One: General Principles of Pharmacology.** This unit stresses the nursing process, the importance of working with patients to assess medication needs and actions, and the differences among many types of medications. It also discusses establishing patient trust, teaching the patient or family about drugs and how to take them appropriately, and evaluating patient responses to drugs.

Chapter 1: Pharmacology and the Nursing Process in LPN Practice, has been revised and refocused for the Seventh Edition to include information on unique aspects of the contemporary LPN/LVN practice environment, including increased levels of responsibility, increasing resource constraints, safety, and common cultural misunderstandings. **Chapter 2: Patient Teaching and Health Literacy** and **Chapter 5: Lifespan and Cultural Modifications** have been refocused to emphasize pharmacology rather than disease processes.

Some reviewers have felt that including information about using common household measures, drug calculations, and administration of medications seems outdated. And for LPNs/LVNs who practice in hospitals that have computers, bar scan coding of medications and patient identification bracelets, and sophisticated medication dispensing systems or individual packs of medicine, that may seem true. But many LPNs/LVNs continue to practice in nursing homes, assisted-living centers, occupational health clinics, and daycare or school health centers, where none of these high-tech systems may be available. LPNs/LVNs must therefore have the basic mathematical and drug calculation skills to work safely in whatever environment they find themselves.

The United States has had a huge effect on the world through education, research, and drug development. This book itself has been translated into several different languages and has been used in many different countries. As I have traveled throughout the world, I have found both local nurses and RNs and LPNs/LVNs from the United States practicing, many in less than modern conditions. The foundational knowledge about drugs, how to calculate dosages, and how to correctly administer drugs has been essential to the types of nursing care they were asked to deliver. Those nurses who expect and are familiar only with high-tech environments will face stiff challenges in such settings.

To this end, we continue to include **Unit Two: Principles of Medication Administration,** which provides students with a review of the mathematical concepts necessary for administering drugs safely. This unit concludes with coverage of the essentials of medication administration, providing step-by-step **Procedure** boxes with clear instructions and illustrations for various routes of drug administration. **Drug Calculation Review** questions in Chapter 9 and in every chapter in Unit Three provide additional practice. *Answers to these questions are provided in Appendix B.*

Unit Three: Drug Groups provides essential information on 14 specific groups of medications. Its consistent, practical format helps the student to develop critical thinking skills in preparing and administering medications. A brief review of anatomy and physiology is provided at the beginning of each drug chapter. Drugs are then grouped by their therapeutic class within body system chapters, allowing students to learn quickly about individual drugs by understanding their drug class. The narrative content in the text focuses on major drug groups, and coverage of specific drugs appears in reference tables. This edition features the addition of many new drugs. Each drug class is presented in a consistent format with a separate **Nursing Implications and Patient Teaching** section. As faculty have indicated that LPN/LVNs who are using the book also refer to drug formularies for specific information about each drug when administering it, this edition has omitted specific drug dosages. A chapter-ending **Case Study** requires the student to use information not only from the present chapter but also from previous chapters. *Suggested answers to the Case Studies are provided online in the TEACH Instructor Resources on Evolve at http://evolve.elsevier.com/Edmunds/LPN/.*

Chapter 12: Antiinfective Medications has been updated to include coverage of MRSA and other drug-resistant organisms. **Chapter 21: Hormones and Steroids** reflects the increasing health priority of reducing obesity, as well as the latest developments in drug therapy for diabetes mellitus. It also equips LPN/LVN students to promote healthy lifestyles that reduce the risk of diabetes, heart disease, and related "lifestyle diseases."

TEACHING AND LEARNING PACKAGE FOR THE INSTRUCTOR

TEACH INSTRUCTOR RESOURCES

TEACH Instructor Resources on Evolve, available at http://evolve.elsevier.com/Edmunds/LPN/, provide a wealth of material to help you make your pharmacology instruction a success. In addition to all of the Student Resources, the following are provided for faculty:

- **ExamView Test Bank** contains approximately 450 multiple-choice and alternate-format questions for the NCLEX-PN® Examination. Each question is coded for correct answer, rationale, page reference, Nursing Process Step, NCLEX Client Needs Category, and Cognitive Level.
- **TEACH Lesson Plans,** based on textbook chapter Learning Objectives, serve as ready-made, modifiable lesson plans and a complete roadmap to link all parts of the educational package. These concise and straightforward lesson plans can be modified or combined to meet your particular scheduling and teaching needs.
- **PowerPoint Presentations** with incorporated **Audience Response Questions** provide approximately 578 text and image slides for classroom or online presentations.
- **Open-Book Quizzes** for each chapter in the textbook help ensure that your students are reading and comprehending their textbook reading assignments.
- **Image Collection** includes all the illustrations and photos from the textbook.
- **Bonus Animations,** many in 3-D, help you enhance classroom and online presentations.
- **Suggestions for Working with Students Who Speak English as a Second Language** help you promote the success of ESL learners.
- **Answer Keys** to the Critical Thinking Questions, Case Studies, and Study Guide activities and exercises are available for your own use or for distribution to your students.

FOR THE STUDENT

- **Evolve Student Resources,** available at http://evolve.elsevier.com/Edmunds/LPN/, include more than 400 interactive **Review Questions for the NCLEX-PN® Examination, Animations, Video Clips,** an **Audio Glossary** with pronunciations for more than 150 Key Terms, 12 **Interactive Drug Dosage Calculators,** new proposed FDA Guidelines on Pregnancy and Lactation, and links to updated information on the Top 200 Prescription Drugs.
- A comprehensive **Study Guide,** available separately, includes Worksheets and Review Sheets with an enhanced focus on critical thinking, prioritizing, care of older adults, and cultural considerations. The exercises focus on promoting medication safety and prevention of drug errors.

In working with patients, the nursing student will quickly learn that giving medications is one of the most challenging parts of the nursing role. A nurse who develops the knowledge and skills needed to correctly give medications will be noticed and recognized with respect by both patients and colleagues in the health care system. Both the responsibilities and the personal rewards are great.

MARILYN WINTERTON EDMUNDS, RN, PhD

To the Student

READING AND REVIEW TOOLS

Objectives introduce the chapter topics.

Key Terms are listed with page number references, and difficult medical, nursing, or scientific terms are accompanied by simple phonetic pronunciations. Key terms are considered essential to understanding chapter content and are defined within the chapter. Key terms are in color the first time they appear in the narrative and are briefly defined in the text, with complete definitions in the Glossary.

Each chapter ends with a **Get Ready for the NCLEX® Examination!** section that includes (1) **Key Points** that reiterate the chapter objectives and serve as a useful review of concepts, (2) a list of **Additional Resources**, (3) an extensive set of **Review Questions for the NCLEX® Examination** with answers located in Appendix A, (4) **Case Studies** with answers located on the Evolve site, (5) **Drug Calculation Review Questions** with answers located in Appendix B, and (6) **Critical Thinking Questions** with answers located on the Evolve site.

A complete **Bibliography and Reader References** in the back of the text cite evidence-based information and provide resources for enhancing knowledge.

CHAPTER FEATURES

Procedures are presented in a logical format with defined *purpose*, relevant *illustrations*, and clearly defined and numbered nursing *steps*. Each Procedure includes icons that serve as reminder to perform the basic steps applicable to *all* nursing interventions:

 • Check orders.

 • Gather necessary equipment and supplies.

 • Introduce yourself.

 • Check patient's identification.

 • Provide privacy.

 • Explain the procedure/intervention.

 • Perform hand hygiene.

 • Don gloves (if applicable).

 Memory Jogger boxes restate key points from anatomy, physiology, or pharmacology that are important for the nurse to remember and that provide foundational information for drug use. In the math chapters, they remind the student of basic principles or reinforce what has just been learned.

 Clinical Goldmine boxes identify the important knowledge that will aid nurses in giving particular drugs.

 Clinical Pitfall boxes point to critical information, warnings, or adverse effects that nurses must know if they are to safely administer drugs or monitor drug therapy.

 Complementary and Alternative Therapies boxes highlight special considerations for herbal therapies, including drug interactions.

 Lifespan Considerations boxes draw attention to information that would be especially important to remember in giving a specific drug to a child or an older adult.

★ **Must-Know Drugs** indicated in the tables highlight the 35 drugs that most prescribers use on a daily basis. This helps students focus their study on the specific drugs that they will see most often in clinical practice.

✦ **Canadian Drugs** indicated within the tables point out brands available only in Canada.

 Video Clips and **Animation Icons** located in the margins of the text indicate available relevant videos located on the Evolve site.

Contents

Pharmacology and the Nursing Process in LPN Practice

Objectives

1. List how LPNs are involved in the five steps of the nursing process.
2. Identify subjective and objective data.
3. Discuss how LPNs use the nursing process in administering medications.
4. List specific nursing activities related to assessing, diagnosing, planning, implementing, and evaluating the patient's response to medications.

Key Terms

assessment (ă-SĔS-mĕnt, p. 2)
auscultation (ăw-skŭl-TĀ-shŭn, p. 3)
database (DĀT-ă-bās, p. 2)
diagnosis (dĭ-ăg-NŌ-sĭs, p. 4)
evaluation (ĭ-văl-ū-Ā-shŭn, p. 7)
implementation (ĭm-plĕ-mĕnTĀ-shŭn, p. 5)
inspection (ĭn-SPĔK-shŭn, p. 3)
nursing process (NŬR-sĭng PRŎ-sĕs, p. 1)

objective data (ŏb-JĔK-tĭv DĀT-ă, p. 3)
palpation (păl-PĀ-shŭn, p. 3)
percussion (pĕr-KŬ-shŭn, p. 3)
six "rights" of medication administration
   (mĕd-ĭ-KĀ-shŭn ăd-mĭn-ĭ-STRĀ-shŭn, p. 5)
subjective data (sŭb-JĔK-tĭv DĀT-ă, p. 3)
therapeutic effects (thĕr-ă-PŬ-tĭk, p. 8)

THE LPN'S TASKS AND THE NURSING PROCESS

Licensed Practical or Vocational Nurses (LPNs/LVNs) play an important role in giving nursing care, and their responsibilities are predicted to grow. There are many factors that will increase the future demand for nurses: many more people are retiring, older people are living longer, chronic diseases are affecting more people, and the incidence of problems like obesity and dementia are increasing. At the same time, more registered nurses (RNs) are retiring and leaving the workforce and fewer RNs are being trained to replace them.

The LPNs/LVNs of the future will have more responsibility in this changed environment. More tasks of the RN will be delegated to the LPN/LVN. There will be a growing need for LPNs/LVNs in most places where health care is being offered. The patients in today's hospitals are often very ill and require close attention. There may be many new types of technicians and technology to dispense unit-dose medications in large city hospitals, but in nursing homes or small community hospitals, there may be few nurses and little equipment. Nurses may copy medications orders from a patient's chart and carry the medicine in paper souffle cups to the patient. LPN/LVNs will be increasingly employed in these areas. Caregivers and patients may come from different cultural backgrounds, and there may be co-workers from several different cultures. All these changes in the health care workplace may lead to stress, cultural conflicts, misinterpretation, or confusion unless these factors are recognized and addressed.

Although most LPNs/LVNs are familiar with the nursing process, it is likely there will be fewer RNs in the future, and LPNs/LVNs should understand clearly how to proceed in an organized way as they plan care for patients. LPNs/LVNs will find work in some of the most technically complex and challenging aspects of health care, as well as working in facilities both in the United States and abroad, where they may be the health care leader and there are no fancy machines, testing equipment, or treatment plans. LPNs/LVNs will learn to use the latest equipment to provide care or to calculate drug dosages with a paper and pencil.

Nursing care is often complex. Nursing actions are specific behaviors that are carefully planned. The well-known process that helps guide the nurse's work in logical steps is known as the **nursing process**. The nursing process consists of the following five major steps:

1. Assessment
2. Diagnosis

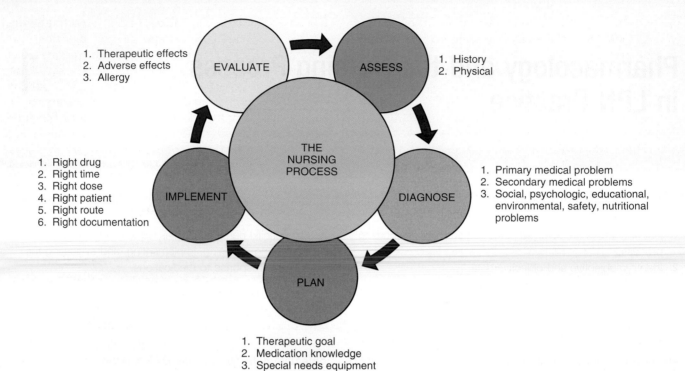

1. Therapeutic effects
2. Adverse effects
3. Allergy

EVALUATE

ASSESS

1. History
2. Physical

THE NURSING PROCESS

1. Right drug
2. Right time
3. Right dose
4. Right patient
5. Right route
6. Right documentation

IMPLEMENT

DIAGNOSE

1. Primary medical problem
2. Secondary medical problems
3. Social, psychologic, educational, environmental, safety, nutritional problems

PLAN

1. Therapeutic goal
2. Medication knowledge
3. Special needs equipment
4. Teaching needs

FIGURE 1-1 The nursing process.

3. Planning
4. Implementation
5. Evaluation

All of these steps are followed when you are giving medications to patients. The nursing process is shown in Figure 1-1.

RNs have both the knowledge and the authority they need to carry out all the steps of the nursing process. Their nursing actions do not require a legal order, so the RNs are acting independently. LPNs/LVNs do not have the same type of authority when they work with patients. Although LPNs/LVNs may need to rely on the RNs they work with in the planning and evaluation steps of the nursing process, they may be more independent as they collect data (assessment step) or help with the care of the patient (implementation step). For example, RNs interview the patient and do a physical examination of the patient, while LPNs/LVNs also learn information as they work with patients. It is usually the LPN/LVN who takes vital signs, checks response to medications and treatments, and monitors symptoms the patient is having. RNs and LPNs/LVNs work together to carry out medication or treatment orders written by health care providers. (Physicians are not the only ones who write orders. You may work with nurse practitioners, physician assistants, or other types of health care providers who may legally write orders.)

As you grow in the LPN/LVN role and gain experience, you will learn more complex skills that help with the nursing process. LPNs/LVNs are often given greater responsibility as they show they can do the work. In nursing homes and extended-care facilities, you may have opportunities to be a charge nurse and to manage patient care under the supervision of the RN. So it is important to master all parts of the nursing process. Experienced LPNs/LVNs will also assume more responsibility if no RN is directly available.

ASSESSMENT

An RN is legally assigned as the staff member who must perform the initial assessment for each patient. However, the LPN/LVN is often asked to assist with this task.

Assessment involves looking and listening carefully. It is a process that helps you get information about the patient, the patient's problem, and anything that may influence the choice of drug to be given to the patient. This step of the nursing process is important because it gives you initial information as you begin to make a **database**, or record, from which all other nursing-process plans grow. Assessment means getting information by talking to the patient, looking at old records, or reviewing materials that the patient may bring. When the patient is admitted to the hospital, ask carefully about any current health problems, as well as any history of illnesses, surgery, and medications taken both now and in the past. This information is important for all team members to know and helps everyone plan the patient's care. Information in the patient's history often directs the nurse and the physician to look for certain physical signs of illness that may be present.

Information you gather through assessment falls into two groups: subjective data and objective data. **Subjective data**, or information given by the patient or family, includes the concerns or symptoms felt by the patient. Examples of subjective data include:

- The chief problem of the patient (in the patient's own words)
- The detailed history of the present illness
- The medical history of the patient
- The family medical history
- Social information: the patient's job, education level, and cultural background
- A review of problems found in different body systems

Some patient problems are more subjective than others. For example, if a patient reports pain in the abdomen, you must accept the patient's word that the pain is present. The nurse cannot see, hear, or feel the patient's abdominal pain—that is why it is subjective. A patient may state that he or she has trouble breathing. Although you may observe rapid breathing, the degree of difficulty cannot be measured. Information is subjective if you have to rely on the patient's words or if the symptoms cannot be felt by anyone other than the patient. In such cases, you would report, "The patient states that. . . ."

Objective data is obtained when the health care provider gives the patient a physical examination. It also comes from documents that patients bring with them, such as old laboratory results, electrocardiogram (ECG) printouts, or x-rays, and from information you gather during the physical examination. Patients may even bring their medicines with them to the hospital or clinic. Objective data are gathered through assessment of vital signs (respiratory rate, pulse, blood pressure, weight, height, temperature); physical findings you can see during careful **inspection** (close observation), **palpation** (feeling), **percussion** (feeling differences in vibrations through the skin), and **auscultation** (listening with the stethoscope); and the results of recent laboratory tests and diagnostic procedures.

It is especially important to get subjective and objective assessment data when the patient is first seen or on admission to the hospital. This provides initial, or baseline, information that can be used to determine how ill the patient may be. Assessment is then done throughout the period of care to see if the patient is getting better with the treatment ordered.

The nurse may not always be the one gathering the subjective and objective data; however, the nurse and everyone else on the health care team should learn whatever information they can from the chart, the physician, the family, or other team members, and use that information to plan the patient's care. Understanding the difference between subjective and objective information will help you in reporting, or charting, the information. For example, if the patient reports pain (subjective information), your notes should say, "The patient complains of pain" rather than "The patient has pain," because you do not know if what the patient is feeling is actually pain or only discomfort. Much of your job in assessing will be reporting data you collect to the RN. As you learn more skills, or work in places such as nursing homes where you may have more responsibility, you will play a larger role in assessing the patient. How big a part you play in assessing the patient is defined by your state nurse practice act, which lists what LPNs/LVNs may and may not do.

Factors to Consider in Assessing the Patient

Certain information is very helpful in planning drug therapy. The nursing assessment at the time of the patient's admission to the hospital should take special note of the drug history. You must talk to the patient, who is the first or primary source, but sometimes you also have to talk to a patient's relatives or get old medical records, ECG results, or laboratory reports (secondary sources). Sometimes your nursing books or the Internet (tertiary sources) may also provide helpful information about a specific disease, medication, or procedure.

When asking about the patient's drug history, the nurse makes assessments in the following areas:

1. Symptoms, signs, or diseases that explain the patient's need for medication (such as high blood glucose levels, high blood pressure, or pain)
2. Current (and sometimes past) use of all medications and drugs:
   - All prescription medications (patients often forget to mention birth control pills in this category)
   - Over-the-counter medications such as aspirin, vitamins, laxatives, cold and sinus preparations, and antacids
   - Alcohol or street drugs used for recreational purposes (such as marijuana or cocaine)
   - Alternative therapies such as herbal medicines or aromatherapy
3. Any problems with drug therapy:
   - Allergies: What is the patient's response to a medicine he or she believes he or she is allergic to? Does it represent a true allergy? An adverse effect? A common side effect?
   - Diseases that may prohibit or limit use of some medications (such as sickle cell anemia, glucose-6-phosphate dehydrogenase deficiency, migraine headaches, or angina)

You will also be assessing changes in patient condition or status that may influence drug therapy during the time the patient is in the hospital. This is how you will know if the medication is helping the patient or not.

Memory Jogger

Nursing Assessment

Assessment means learning as much as you can about your patients and their problems.

DIAGNOSIS

Once the assessment information has been collected, the LPN/LVN and other health care team members must make a diagnosis (a conclusion about the patient's problem). The physician will decide the medical diagnoses. The RN will identify the nursing diagnoses. The hospital where you work may use the formal nursing diagnosis system developed by the North American Nursing Diagnosis Association–International that allows RNs to share a common language and a common way of describing a patient's condition. However, many hospitals do not recognize or use this system. In either case, after talking to the patient, you will come to some decisions about how sick the patient is and how carefully you need to watch them. You will make your own decisions about some of the following questions:

- What are the major problems of this patient? (Think about the problem that led to the patient's coming to the hospital.)
- How sick is this patient?
- What procedures or medications will this patient require?
- What special knowledge or equipment is required in giving these medications?
- What special concerns or cultural beliefs does the patient have?
- How much does this patient understand about the treatment and medicine prescribed?

The answers to these questions will (1) help you set the goals of nursing care, (2) affect how closely you need to work with the patient, and (3) tell you what type of patient education will be needed. Getting accurate answers to these questions may be harder with children, older adult patients, or people whose language or culture is different from yours. However, just as a physician must have the correct diagnosis to prescribe the right treatment, the nurse must find the correct answers to these questions to be able to plan the best care for the patient.

PLANNING

Based on the data you help collect, the medical and nursing diagnoses are made, goals are set, and care plans are written. As a member of the health care team, the LPN/LVN will be able to assist with the planning step. As you help the RN plan the care for each patient, the plan will become easier to write. Nursing plans involve two groups of people: the nurses and the patients. Patient goals help the patient learn about a medication and how to use it properly. Nursing goals help the nurse plan what equipment or procedures are needed to give the medication. Using the information gathered in the assessment about the patient's history, medical and social problems, risk factors, and how ill the patient may be, both types of plans can be prepared. The patient-focused care plan will include any medications that will be given on either a short-term or a long-term basis. For example, goals may be written regarding the application of ointments or patches or for showing the patient how to self-administer an aerosol nebulizer treatment. Nursing goals may include deciding how to rotate the injection site for drugs that require repeated injections (such as insulin), or teaching the patient about specific side effects of medications that might develop and when they should be reported.

As you write a list of the patient's problems, you may find that problems are related. For example, a patient who cannot see very well may have a risk of tripping and falling in an unfamiliar hospital setting. The importance of problems may also shift as the patient's condition changes. For this reason, what you do for the patient may change according to the patient's changing needs.

Factors to Think About in Planning to Give a Medication

Planning to give a medication involves four steps:

1. Decide the reason or goal for each medication to be given. (That is, what is this drug supposed to do for the patient?)
2. Learn specific information about the medication:
   - The desired action of the drug
   - Side effects that may develop
   - The usual dosage, route, and frequency
   - Situations in which the drug should not be given (contraindications)
   - Drug interactions (What is the influence of another drug given at the same time?)
3. Plan for special storage or procedures, techniques, or equipment needs.
4. Develop a teaching plan for the patient, including:
   - What the patient needs to know about the medication's action and side effects
   - What the patient needs to know about the administration of the medication
   - What the patient needs to report to the nurse or physician about the medication and his or her response

The most important step in planning is to collect and use information about the patient (physical condition, cultural background, and expectations) and the medication. This step requires knowledge of the patient and the drug prescribed, plus your common sense and professional judgment.

In today's hospitals and clinics, not only doctors order medications. Nurse practitioners, nurse mid-wives, nurse anesthetists, and physician assistants may all write some types of medication orders. Large hospitals may have a staff hospitalist—a physician who is always available in the hospital to oversee care for all patients. Teaching hospitals may have resident doctors who are still in educational programs. These individuals may write legal medication orders.

Once the medication is ordered, the nurse must verify that the order is accurate. This is usually done by checking the medication chart, medication card, medication administration record, or computer medication record with the original order. You will need to learn and follow the procedures of the agency where you work when checking medications. LPNs/LVNs will work in some of the most sophisticated health care settings with new equipment, computers, and many resources. They may also work in facilities in which there is no technology used, and following institutional procedures, the nurse will carry the medication on a tray, watch while the patient takes it, and then record this in the patient's chart. No matter the process, this step of checking must be done each time the medication is given. In this way, errors resulting from changes can be avoided.

The nurse must also apply knowledge about the drug to the specific drug order to determine whether the drug and the dosage ordered seem correct. No part of the order or the reason for giving the medication should be unclear. Any questions about whether a drug is appropriate or safe for that patient should be answered before the medication is given. Use good judgment in carrying out the medication order. If you decide that (1) any part of the order is incorrect or unclear, (2) the patient's condition would be made worse by the medication, (3) the physician may not have had all the information needed about the patient when drug therapy was planned, or (4) there has been a change in the patient's condition and a question has arisen about whether the medication should be given, the medication should be withheld (not be given) until the question can be answered and the physician called. If you believe there is a problem with the medication order and the physician cannot be contacted or does not change the order under question, notify the charge nurse and the nursing supervisor as soon as possible. Most hospitals have clear policies about whom to contact, how to report this problem, and what to do next.

Memory Jogger

Medication Orders

Make certain you understand each part of the medication order.

The planning step of the nursing process is also the time to do the following:

1. Get any special equipment you need to give the medication (such as intravenous [IV] infusion bottles, IV poles, or nebulizers).
2. Review any special procedures you will need to give the medicine (such as the Z-track injection technique or the IV-push policy).
3. Decide what you will need to tell the patient.

All this information can be written on the nursing care plan or in the Kardex file or entered into the computer so that other team members can see the plan.

IMPLEMENTATION

Implementation involves following the care plan and giving the medicine accurately to the patient. This step of the nursing process requires that the nurse use the information learned about each patient and about each drug ordered. It is your job to understand why each medication is ordered, to know about the drug's actions, and to know how to safely administer it. For example, if you add an antibiotic solution to an IV line, you need to know about the proper equipment, aseptic technique, rate of flow, and reactions with the drugs already in the IV solution, as well as how to flush the line after therapy has ended. Implementation also may require you to do specific nursing tasks before giving the medication. For example, you will take the patient's pulse before giving digitalis to make sure it may be given safely. Implementation also means that you will watch for any changes in the patient's condition that may make it unwise to give the medication. For example, if a patient receiving antibiotics says she has an itchy rash on her chest and arms, you will withhold the next dose of the antibiotic until you have called the patient's physician to report the rash. Once the medication is given, this needs to be recorded in the patient's chart.

There are **six "rights" of medication administration** the nurse must always keep in mind. You must give the right drug, at the right time, in the right dose, to the right patient, by the right route, and use the right documentation to record that the dose has been given.

Memory Jogger

The Six "Rights" of Administering a Medication

1. The right drug
2. The right time
3. The right dose
4. The right patient
5. The right route
6. The right documentation

The Right Drug

Many drug names are hard to remember and difficult to read. Also, many drugs have names that sound or look nearly the same as the names of other drugs. It is important to carefully check the spelling of the name and the dose of each medication before any drug is given. For example, NovoLog and Novolin are both insulin products used for diabetics, but they are quite different in dosage and duration of action. It is also easy to get confused when a medication is ordered by a trade name (such as Valium), but the pharmacy sends up the medication labeled with the generic name (diazepam). Do not assume that the correct medication has been sent without checking a reliable source or calling the pharmacy.

The drug may come in a unit-dose-system package, locked cabinet for the patient, as a prescription filled for one person, or the medication may be taken from a unit's stock. Sometimes the medication dose has a barcode that is scanned by a computer. However it comes, you must read the drug label at least three times:

1. Before taking the drug from the unit-dose cart or shelf
2. Before preparing or measuring the prescribed dose of medication
3. Before putting the medication back on the shelf or just before opening the medication at the time you give it to the patient

The Right Time

The drug order should say when the medication is to be given. Hospitals have policies that tell you what time drugs will be given when they are ordered (such as "every 4 hours"). You must be familiar with hospital policy and use only standard abbreviations in recording the drugs given (see Chapter 3 for information on standard abbreviations). To be effective, many drugs must be given exactly on schedule day and night to keep the level of medication constant in the body. Other medications may only need to be given during the day.

You will also need to plan around other patient activities when you give medications. For example, if a patient is taking an anticoagulant to thin the blood and decrease the risk of blood clots, the medication must be given at the same time every day. Patients with infections need to have specimens taken for culture before starting antibiotic therapy. Patients undergoing evaluation of thyroid function need to have blood tests for those functions done before having gallbladder x-ray studies, which involve the use of chemicals that may confuse thyroid function study results or make them inaccurate.

Medications are usually given when there is the best chance for the body to absorb it and the least risk for side effects. This may mean that some medications should be given when the patient's stomach is empty, and others should be given with food. Some medications require that the patient not eat certain foods. Others do not mix well with alcohol. When a patient

is taking several medications, check to make sure the drugs do not interfere with each other. (For example, some antibiotics interfere with the action of birth control pills, so a woman taking both could get pregnant if she does not use another form of contraception.)

Finally, one-time-only, as-needed (prn), or emergency medications are especially important to check. The nurse must be certain that no one else has already given the medication or that it is the appropriate time to give the drug. Narcotics are often ordered as "stat" (given within a few minutes of the order) or prn medications. Note on the patient's record as soon as possible that you have given a narcotic so that it is clear the patient has been given the medication.

Box 1-1 lists the main factors to remember in giving medication at the right time.

The Right Dose

The amount of medicine to be given is usually ordered for the "average" patient. A patient who is old, who has severe weight loss as a result of illness, or who is small or very obese may require changes in the usual dosages. Pediatric patients have doses ordered depending on how much they weigh. Geriatric, or older adult, patients may be very sensitive to many medications and may require a change in dosage. If patients have other diseases or poor liver or kidney function, this may make changes in dosage necessary. Patients who have nausea or vomiting may be unable to take oral medications. Also, the physician may order the correct dosage of the medication when treatment begins, but changes in the patient's condition may require that you go back to the physician to have the dose altered.

Giving the correct dosage of a medication also requires that you use the proper equipment (for example, insulin must be measured in an insulin syringe), the proper drug form (oral or rectal, water or oil base, scored tablets or coated capsules), and the proper concentration (0.25 mg or 2.5 mg) and that you accurately calculate the right drug dosage. Most

Box 1-1	Factors to Think About in Giving Medication at the Right Time

- Understand and follow the rules of your hospital regarding the times to give scheduled drugs.
- Follow drug treatment guides to achieve the best drug absorption and to limit chances for drug interactions with other drugs. Give medications as ordered to help keep blood levels constant.
- Plan drug therapy keeping in mind other diagnostic and laboratory testing plans.
- Be especially careful in giving prn or stat medications to avoid the risk of overdosing the patient (giving too much medicine).

hospitals and clinics have rules that require two nurses to check any medication dosage that must be calculated, particularly for medications such as narcotics, heparin, insulin, or IV medications.

The Right Patient

Typically, hospital procedure requires that we ask the patient for their name and birth date and also confirm their identify by examining the wrist band. Although it seems like common sense to make certain the right patient gets the medication, errors may occur on a busy hospital unit. Several groups of patients are most at risk for errors: the pediatric patient, the geriatric patient, the non–English-speaking patient, and the very confused or critically ill patient. The common factor among these four groups is that it might be hard for them to tell the nurse who they are. They also may not understand what you are asking or that a drug is being given to them. The identification bracelets (name bands) that some patients wear may have been removed for tests or when blood was drawn. Be especially careful with children, because they enjoy hiding, changing beds, answering to another name, and so on. Ask for the name as you check the patient's identification bracelet or scan their name tag to confirm it is the correct patient. In a hospital, medications should never be given to a patient who is not wearing an identification bracelet. Nursing homes may present a special challenge for a nurse who does not know the patients well, because these patients may not wear identification bracelets, and they may be confused or unable to answer to their name. When available, the use of computers to scan the patient's identification bracelet and the drug itself are helpful in making sure the correct patient gets the drug.

The Right Route

The drug order should state how the drug should be given (route of drug administration). The nurse must never change routes without getting a new order. Although many drugs may be given by different routes, the dose is often different for each route.

The oral route is the preferred route if the patient is oriented (awake and able to understand). In some cases, faster delivery or a higher blood level of a drug is needed, so the medication may be given intravenously or intramuscularly. There may be special precautions for medications given through these routes (such as how fast they can be given or in what dosage). Some injections should be given into the subcutaneous tissue rather than intramuscularly. Because of these differences, you need to know how to give an injection in several different places on the body. Also, some drugs are very painful if given intramuscularly, so giving them intravenously is preferable.

When drugs to help breathing are ordered, you need to find out whether the aerosol nebulizer is to be used through the nose or the mouth. Teach the patient the correct way to use the nebulizer so that the medication goes all the way into the lungs. Teach patients how to correctly use their eye drops, eardrops, ointments, lotions, shampoos, and rectal or vaginal medications.

The Right Documentation (Record Keeping)

Increasingly, electronic charting systems are being introduced into medical settings. Whether the nurse records medication administration and patient observations by hand or using an electronic chart, the basics are the same. A note about how and when you gave the drug should be made on the patient's chart as soon as possible after the drug is given. In an emergency or when a drug is only used once or twice, this is very important. Rules at your agency may require that the chart note of intramuscular medications also include where on the body you gave the injection and any complaints made by the patient at the time of the injection. The chart note should always list the drug given, the dose, and the time it was actually given (not the time it was supposed to be given). In some offices or clinics where immunizations are given, the policy may require that the lot number listed on the bottle be recorded in the patient's chart. Progress notes should include a note about the patient's response to the medication. Any complaints or adverse effects should be noted in the chart and reported to the head nurse and the physician. When you make notes in the patient's chart about medications, never record medications that were not given or record them before they are given. If a patient does not receive the medication, for any reason, notify the nurse in charge or the person who wrote the order.

It must be stressed that *you must never give medication prepared by another nurse.* Even when you are very busy, when there is an emergency, or when you are interrupted, you cannot assume that all the "rights" are followed unless the person who prepares the medication is the one who gives the medication. Sometimes a physician will ask you to prepare the medication for the physician to give. You may then prepare the medication, but go with the physician to see that the medication is given as ordered and write in the notes that the physician gave the medication.

Following the rules of your hospital, using common sense, and being accurate and ethical will reduce the risk of medication error. Should an error be made, talking about it honestly and taking quick action to correct any damage are especially important to protect the patient from harm.

EVALUATION

Evaluation is the process of looking at what happens when the care plan is put into action. Evaluation requires the nurse to watch for the patient's response to a drug, noting both expected and unexpected findings. When antipyretic medications (drugs that reduce fever) are given, take the patient's temperature to see if the medication lowered the fever. When medications are given to make the patient's heartbeat more regular, taking the pulse will help show how the patient responded to the medication.

Evaluation of what happens when you administer a drug helps the health care team decide whether to continue the same drug or make a change. Gathering such information is also a part of the continuing assessment of a patient during care that the nurse will record in the patient's chart. Thus the nursing process may be seen as a circle (see Figure 1-1). For example, taking the patient's temperature is part of the evaluation step of the nursing process, but it may also be part of the assessment step when you notice that the patient's temperature is still high, indicating the patient needs more medication, a cooling bath, or some other treatment.

 Memory Jogger

Evaluate Response to Medication

It is important to watch the patient and look for any adverse reactions, side effects, or allergic responses.

Factors to Think About in Evaluating Response to Medication

The nurse checks for two types of responses to drug therapy: therapeutic effects and adverse effects.

Therapeutic effects are seen when the drug does what it was supposed to do. If you understand why the medication is being given (the therapeutic goal of the drug), you will be able to decide whether or not that goal is being met. For example, if the patient's blood glucose is high and regular insulin is given, you should see a lower blood glucose level when the test is repeated in 1 to 2 hours.

Adverse or side effects are seen when patients do not respond to their medications in the way they should or develop new signs or symptoms. For example, a patient with pneumonia may be given penicillin. Although this antibiotic may be working to control the infection, the patient may develop shortness of breath, which may be an allergic reaction to the medicine, and the penicillin must be stopped. A patient getting an anticoagulant to thin the blood must be closely watched for signs of bleeding or bruising that would indicate overdosage or overresponse to the medication. Sometimes, side effects such as nausea or vomiting may be stopped by decreasing the dosage or by giving the medication with food. Telling the physician about whether the side effects are mild or severe helps the physician decide whether the patient should keep taking the drug or it should be stopped.

The nurse is the health care worker most often with the patient and is in an important position to notice the patient's response to drug therapy. Carefully and repeatedly evaluating the patient and writing down the findings in the patient's chart are especially important in the care of the hospitalized patient.

 Clinical Goldmine

Critical Decision Points in Administering Drugs

- Assess the patient and clearly understand why the patient is getting that medication.
- Prepare the medication to be given (for example, check labels, prepare injections, observe proper aseptic technique with needles and syringes).
- Accurately calculate dosages.
- Administer the medication (with proper injection technique, aids to help swallowing, materials needed for topical creams).
- Record the medications given.
- Watch the patient's reaction and evaluate the response.
- Educate the patient about medications.

Get Ready for the NCLEX® Examination!

Key Points

- The nursing process is a logical plan that helps you give good care to the patient and avoid making mistakes.
- The nursing process involves assessing the patient, making a nursing decision or diagnosis about what is required, planning to give medications, doing the correct procedures, and evaluating the patient's response. These steps will become more automatic as you gain greater skill and experience.
- For new nurses, the nursing process gives you a safe and clear way to do things when you are learning many new and important skills.

Additional Learning Resources

SG Go to your Study Guide for additional learning activities to help you master this chapter content.

evolve Go to your Evolve website (http://evolve.elsevier.com/ Edmunds/LPN/) for additional online resources.

Get Ready for the NCLEX® Examination!

Review Questions for the NCLEX® Examination

1. The most important time to obtain assessment data on the patient is:
   1. any time care is administered by the nurse
   2. when the patient is first admitted to the hospital
   3. when the patient's condition changes significantly
   4. any time additional objective data is required

2. The nurse assesses the patient's drug history with the knowledge that the prescription medication frequently overlooked by patients in providing information for a drug history is:
   1. laxatives
   2. antacids
   3. birth control pills
   4. aspirin

3. The nurse is considering various factors in planning to give a medication. The highest priority step in the planning process is:
   1. collect and use information about the patient and the medication
   2. develop a teaching plan for the patient
   3. decide on a reason for the administration of the medication
   4. plan for special equipment that will be needed

4. Which patient is most at risk to experience a medication error?
   1. a 38-year-old male patient admitted for repair of a fractured femur
   2. a 14-year-old female patient who is experiencing a urinary tract infection
   3. a 52-year-old female presurgical patient who speaks English as a second language
   4. an 82-year-old male who is experiencing a cardiac arrhythmia

5. The most appropriate way to evaluate the result of the administration of an antipyretic medication is:
   1. measure the patient's blood pressure
   2. measure the patient's respiratory rate
   3. measure the patient's temperature
   4. measure the patient's radial pulse

Critical Thinking Questions

1. Identify each of the following as either objective (O) or subjective (S) information:
   a. The patient complains of pain in the abdomen.
   b. The nurse takes the patient's blood pressure and determines that it is too high.
   c. The nurse counts rapid respirations and deep movements of the chest, notices blueness of the skin, and decides that the patient is short of breath.
   d. After feeling the patient's abdomen, the nurse reports that the patient says it is tender to the touch.
   e. The patient complains of being "too fat."
   f. Four-year-old Sean's thermometer registers a temperature of 102° F.
   g. After weighing Mr. Tracy this morning, the nurse reports that he has gained 2 pounds in 6 days.
   h. Ms. Jackson says that almost every day she has trouble breathing or "catching" her breath.
   i. A 50-year-old female patient asks for aspirin, saying she is getting "hot flashes."
   j. Mr. Clark tells the nurse, "My heart is really pounding!"
2. You are assigned to give medications to eight different patients this morning. Write a paragraph describing the step-by-step procedure you would use to make sure that you are observing the six rights of drug administration.
3. Describe four things that would fall under the category of *assessment* that a nurse might do for a patient taking morphine.
4. What is the difference between *planning* and *evaluating* in drug administration? Are they sometimes the same thing? Give examples of each.
5. What would you do if one of your patients refused a medication that was ordered?
6. Why does the nurse have to keep doing assessment of the patient receiving medications?
7. Identify three areas of assessment necessary in completing a patient's drug history.

Patient Teaching and Health Literacy

Objectives

1. Identify the common causes of patient medication errors.
2. List some of the problems patients have when they cannot read or understand health instructions.
3. Describe the process of teaching patients about medications.

Key Terms

compliant (kŏm-PLĪ-ănt, p. 10)
concordance (kŭn-KŌR-dăns, p. 10)
health disparity (dĭs-PĂR-ĭ-tē, p. 11)

health literacy (LĬT-ĕr-ă-sē, p. 11)
literacy (LĬT-ĕr-ă-sē, p. 11)
noncompliant (NŎN-kŏm-plĭ-ănt, p. 10)

OVERVIEW

One of the basic parts of the nursing role is teaching patients. If patients are to have successful results with medications, they must learn all they can about the drugs and how to take them properly. The nurse must learn how to speak clearly as they teach. This can be very difficult when patients do not speak English or have poor reading or writing abilities. It is also hard if patients are not ready to learn.

The reason we teach patients about their diseases, their drugs, and what to expect when they take the drugs is to help them improve their health. Patients who do not clearly understand basic health information have less ability to carry out the treatment plan. Patients who are unable to carry out the treatment plan, for whatever reason, are at greater risk for having problems or not getting well.

COMPLIANCE, NONCOMPLIANCE, AND CONCORDANCE

Often a patient is said to be **compliant** when a plan of care is followed and **noncompliant** when it is not. A better term to use, one that does not judge the patient, is **concordance**. *Concordance* or agreement might be defined as the nurse, patient, family, physician, and pharmacist working together as a team to implement the treatment plan.

There are two basic reasons a patient has difficulty meeting treatment goals:

1. The patient does not understand what to do.
2. The patient understands what should be done but fails to do it, because he or she:

- may not believe the plan needs to be carried out.
- may believe something should be done but fails to carry out the plan.
- may believe something should be done but does not have money, time, or ability to do it.

In teaching the patient, focus on helping the patient make informed decisions about taking medications. (See Chapter 5 for other factors that might make it difficult for patients to follow treatment plans, including cultural and life span considerations.)

COMMUNICATING WITH THE PATIENT

In the busy health care setting, it may be difficult to find time to talk with patients. In addition, many of our patients are from different countries or cultures and have different languages and beliefs that affect their ability to understand or talk about their health. Many nurses also are from different countries and cultures. This means that beliefs about what is important or harmful may not be the same. Even words used by both patient and nurse might have different meanings to each. A growing number of patients are older adults, with their own challenges to hearing, understanding, and acceptance of suggestions.

Although speaking clearly to patients is important, much of the teaching that patients need will be given in writing. Thus what is written and how it is written is very important if we wish to send the right message.

In the U.S. (per house style), we say that people are *literate* when they have the ability to read, write, and speak in English, to do math, and to solve problems at the level necessary to function on the job and in society. During the last 20 years, research has shown that many people in the United States do not have the basic level of **literacy** to allow them to do these tasks. In 2003, the latest National Assessment of Adult Literacy reported that 30 million Americans scored at *Below Basic* level of literacy, the lowest of four levels, and another 63 million were at *Basic* level of literacy, the second lowest level. People are placed in these two lowest levels if they have trouble finding pieces of information or numbers in a long text, putting many pieces of information together into one story, or finding two or more numbers in a chart and doing a math problem. These levels are roughly equal to being able to read at about the fifth-grade level.

While general literacy is a problem, we have also learned that many patients do not have high levels of **health literacy**—the ability to understand and use information that is important in keeping them healthy. Low literacy limits a person's ability to deal with the health care setting, which has become more complex and uses written materials even more difficult to understand than those used in everyday life. This may mean patients cannot read a prescription to learn how many pills they should take, cannot figure out when their next appointment is, or cannot read a map to help them find a pharmacy or get where they need to go for their appointment. It often means they cannot read the information nurses or physicians send home with them explaining their disease, the medicines they are taking, and important things they need to know. Thus they often do not have the information they need to help them get well or stay well.

Even patients who read at college level have been found to prefer medical information written at the seventh-grade level. Recent research suggests that written information given to most patients should be written at a fifth- to seventh-grade level if we wish to make it more likely patients will understand it. This will be a challenge.

Although there may be large numbers of people in the United States with low literacy, research has documented that certain groups may have more problems than others. People who are older, are from minority races or ethnic backgrounds where English is not the dominant language, live in certain areas of the country, have a low income level, or are in prison tend to have lower literacy levels. Research about the reasons for these disparities has shown that frequently these individuals have not been able to stay in school and get an education.

It makes sense that people who have low literacy levels often have poor health outcomes. Because they cannot read or write they are at higher risk for disease and disability. This situation is called **health disparity**. Unfortunately, such individuals often die from a disease several years earlier than someone with higher literacy simply because of this difference in ability to read and write.

Because of these factors, there is no more important teaching than that given by the nurse to the patient about the patient's disease and its drug treatment. This teaching is a big factor in whether the drug therapy ordered will be effective. When patients don't understand and so cannot follow the treatment plan, there are often limitations in what the patient can do to take care of themselves. Accurate, careful teaching of the patient by the nurses involved in their care should help reduce such problems. This is very true when medications are involved, because drug information is usually complex and thus is often given in writing.

THE PROCESS OF PATIENT EDUCATION

ASSESSMENT OF PATIENT EDUCATION NEEDS

The fact that a nurse *knows* a patient should have information does not mean the patient is aware of that need or, in fact, expects to learn from the nurse. Patient education has to involve both teacher and learner and cannot be forced. Patients may show one of four types of behavior when seeking drug information, as shown in Table 2-1. Patients will go to the person they feel is the best source of information or with whom they feel most comfortable.

Table 2-1 Behaviors of People Seeking Drug Information

CLASSIFICATION	PERCENTAGE	CHARACTERISTICS
Uninformed	34%	This group tended to be older, was less likely to have received written or verbal counseling from a provider or pharmacist, and did not seem to recognize the results of improper drug use.
Rely on physician	40%	This group took information as given from the physician and was most likely to get prescriptions filled at chain pharmacies.
Rely on pharmacist	19%	This was the youngest group; they got information at the pharmacy and saw few barriers to getting information.
Questioners	7%	This group included those who were more likely to receive information from books or magazines. They required clear information about specific questions and appeared to be the most difficult group to satisfy.

Modified from Morris LA, et al: A segmentational analysis of prescription drug information seeking, *Med Care* 25:953-64, 1987.

There may be some differences between the information clinicians see as important and the information patients want. For example, it may be hard to discuss some of the serious side effects that might be caused by a drug. Nurses may not want to talk about some of these problems for fear of scaring patients to the point they won't take the drugs. However, research has shown just the opposite result with many patients. Patients who are given more information feel more comfortable taking their drugs and can correctly recognize side effects, should they occur.

More emphasis is being placed on the use of computers, both in learning the needs of patients and in meeting those needs. In some situations, computers are even helpful in teaching patients with low literacy skills. Computers may be used for health surveys and have been shown to result in more honest reports of certain health behaviors. A few years ago, a study found that patients might actually be more comfortable revealing personal information on a computer than to a human being—even though they know the information will be seen later by health care workers.

The registered nurse has primary responsibility for patient teaching, but all nurses caring for the patient play a role. The important items to include in the patient-teaching process are the following:

1. *Assess the patient's specific needs to learn.* Often the nurse may wish to provide information about a new treatment plan or medication, or the patient may ask direct questions. Teaching materials should then be written that take into account the specific needs of the patient, including knowledge, reading ability, beliefs, and experiences.
2. *Assess the patient's willingness to learn.* This requires getting to know patients and talking with them about their interest in learning. Patients must see a need for the patient education they receive.
3. *Decide what needs to be taught.* The patient and nurse decide this together. This information should be written down as objectives that can be measured (that is, you can determine when they are met). For example, the objective "Learn about adverse reactions of the medication" is not measurable. The objective "List five possible adverse reactions" is measurable.
4. *Select a teaching method.* This may include verbal instructions, written materials, audiovisual materials, or a combination of methods. The method and pace of the teaching must be designed for each patient, recognizing differences in the ways people learn and the rate at which they learn. Plan for repetition. Different teaching skills may be needed at different times for the same patient. Teaching should be provided in small amounts over several meetings.
5. *Determine how well the material has been learned.* Have the patient repeat the information given, repeat a demonstration they have been shown, or follow through on a behavior. Giving feedback allows the patient to realize what has been learned or identify areas in which help is still needed. Giving verbal praise, being excited about good compliance, or showing support for a change in behavior may be the most effective types of feedback for patients. Negative or fear-arousing comments may also be effective, but must be used rarely and cautiously. Ask questions to learn reasons for noncompliance and address that need. For example, giving the patient special pill containers, making changes in the time medicines are taken (to fit in with the patient's activities), or getting the patient drug samples or coupons to reduce costs.
6. *Remember to use a variety of teaching methods.* This is more effective than using one single teaching method.

PREPARING A TEACHING PLAN

The patient's need for information is based on the patient's disease, the treatment plan, and the patient-nurse relationship. When a patient is first diagnosed with a problem, education must start with what has gone wrong in the body and what is likely to happen next. To consider what to do to return to good health, the patient must first understand what has led to illness in very general terms. The nurse teaches in simple terms and in line with their own understanding.

As patients begin any therapy, there is a good deal of information that needs to be shared: what they think, what they expect, and any choices they might have. For example, starting the patient on a new medication requires a lot of teaching. It is clearly not possible to provide all the information a patient might need in one teaching session. Instead, you need to have a plan in mind for the things that need to be covered, and this plan needs to be shared with the patient (Box 2-1). Additional teaching will be required when drugs are changed, when the dosage or schedule is altered, or when changes in patient condition warrant further adjustment in therapy. Therefore, teaching becomes specific to what the patient requires, but it is always given in quantities that the patient can handle.

Informed consent is something we assume in the process of giving a medication to a patient. The nurse shares a legal obligation with other health care providers to make certain that the patient understands the condition, the treatment, and the risks and benefits of treatment plans. The law requires that the amount and type of information provided to the patient be "reasonable." It is up to the nurse who is given the task of teaching the patient to determine what is reasonable for a specific patient to understand; the nurse may be held legally responsible for failure to teach the patient this information.

In the clinic or hospital, teaching often happens in response to a patient's question, and the nurse may

Box 2-1	Key Information for Patients Receiving Medications

- Drug name (generic and brand)
- Intended use and expected action
- Route, dosage form, dosage, and schedule (hours of day to take)
- Special directions for storage or preparation of medication
- Special directions for taking the medication
- Common side effects
- What the patient should do if there are side effects
- Possible drug-drug, drug-food, or drug-alcohol interactions
- Information about getting a prescription refilled
- Action to take if the patient misses taking a dose
- Special precautions when taking medication (driving, actions requiring alertness)
- Other information particular to the patient or drug
- When to return to the health care provider
- How the patient will know that the drug is doing what it should do

Data from Katzung B, Masters S, and Trevor A, *Basic and clinical pharmacology*, ed 11, New York, 2009, McGraw-Hill Medical, and McPhee, Papadakis, M, and Rabow MW, *Current medical diagnosis and treatment 2011*, ed 50, New York, 2010, McGraw-Hill Medical.

need to respond quickly without time to prepare, plan, or consider overall what the patient needs to know. Using scientific or nursing language or jargon, giving too much technical detail, or being vague does not provide clear information. It is impossible to avoid answering questions, even if they take you by surprise—just do your best to answer. It is also important for there to be a written plan that covers what will be taught, how it will be taught, and how you will know when the patient has learned the material. This plan can be changed if necessary or if it makes sense to present some information earlier based on patient questions.

The plan developed by the nursing staff for teaching the patient should have specific objectives to guide teaching. The objectives must state the new behaviors that will occur because of changes in the patient's thinking or understanding. The best objectives are clearly stated by describing the desired outcome and what makes it acceptable. Specific goals help clarify for patients what they are to do. For example, "Blood pressure will drop to diastolic reading less than 90 mm Hg within 3 months" is a specific, measurable goal based on national guidelines. As patients and nurses create objectives together, the nurse has a chance to evaluate the patient's knowledge, understanding, and general desire to change behavior.

IMPLEMENTING THE TEACHING PLAN

Both the content of patient education and the process of patient education are important to think about in planning the specific teaching-learning objectives. Many patients are fearful when they first learn their diagnosis. Stress and anxiety increase the confusion they often feel and interfere with their ability to learn.

Teaching needs to be offered in a systematic manner to decrease stress. It needs to be provided in a timely way and in a quiet and unhurried setting that gives the patient a chance to ask questions. It is hard to find a setting like that in today's busy health care system. Research has suggested that people are able to remember three major things they are taught in any one session. Also, they generally remember those three things in the order in which they are presented. If you keep this in mind when developing a teaching plan, you can set aside small periods to use for teaching a few very specific things. At future visits, you can review the information presented in an earlier session to find out how much the patient remembers before you move on to the next phase of teaching.

To help the patient accept what is taught, the nurse may use a variety of ways to give patients information about their medications. Some of these methods include telling patients the necessary information, reviewing written instructions with them, and using audiovisual aids such as audiotapes, videotapes, CD-ROMs, or computer teaching systems that may use animation, color, music, and action figures to help the patient learn the information.

Verbal Education

Verbal education is often direct teaching, with the nurse telling the patient information and then giving the patient a chance to ask questions. Patients who have extensive needs for teaching may also be brought together in small groups for part of their teaching experiences; these might be patients with chronic diseases such as diabetes or hypertension.

Written Information

Written information can include special labels for prescription bottles, materials inserted in the drug package, or specially prepared materials or booklets that accompany the medicine. Preprinted instructions about medicines are available from manufacturers, pharmacy associations or some medical associations, and private companies. This information is often written and a high school or college level. Written information may also be created by the nurse, hospital, clinic, or may come from a professional group such as the Arthritis Foundation or the Asthma and Allergy Foundation of America. Increasingly, professional materials are written at a lower education level and may even be marked as to grade level.

Many books and preprinted patient information materials are already available from commercial sources (Box 2-2). With the growing use of the Internet, information about new products is widely available and often may be downloaded by the nurse to create high-quality handouts that may be changed as

Box 2-2 Patient Teaching Resources

Many of the best texts in this area are very old but are still currently available through commercial sources:

Andrus MR, Roth MT: Health literacy: a review. *Pharmacotherapy* 22(3):282-302, 2002.

Baker DW, Gazmararian JA, Sudano J, et al: Health literacy and performance on the Mini-Mental State Examination, *Aging Ment Health* 6(1):22-9, 2002.

Bennett IM, Chen J, Soroui JS, White S: The contribution of health literacy to disparities in self-rated health status and preventative health behaviors in older adults, *Ann Fam Med* 7(3):204-11, 2009.

Bosworth HB, Oddone EZ, Weinberger M: *Patient treatment adherence: concepts, interventions, and measurement,* ed 1, New York, 2005, Lawrence Erlbaum.

Canobbio MM: *Mosby's handbook of patient teaching,* ed 3, St Louis, 2005, Mosby.

Coles ME, Coleman SL: Barriers to treatment seeking for anxiety disorders: initial data on the role of mental health literacy, *Depress Anxiety* 27(1):63-71, 2010.

Davis TC, Wolf MS, Bass PF 3rd, et al: Low literacy impairs comprehension of prescription drug warning labels, *J Gen Intern Med* 21(8):847-51, 2006.

DeWalt DA, Hink A: Health literacy and child health outcomes: a systematic review of the literature, *Pediatrics* 124 Suppl 3:S265-74, 2009.

Doak CC, Doak LG, Root JH: *Teaching patients with low literacy skills,* ed 2, Philadelphia, 1996, JB Lippincott.

Falovo DR: *Effective patient education: a guide to increased compliance,* ed 3, New York, 2004, Jones & Bartlett.

Gausman Benson J, Forman WB: Comprehension of written health care information in an affluent geriatric retirement community: use of the Test of Functional Health Literacy, *Gerontology* 48(2):93-7, 2002.

Lokker N, Sanders L, Perrin EM, et al: Parental misinterpretations of over-the-counter pediatric cough and cold medication labels, *Pediatrics* 123(6):1464-71, 2009.

Moore SW: *Griffith's instructions for patients,* ed 7, Philadelphia, 2005, WB Saunders.

Murtagh J: *Patient education,* ed 3, New York, 2001, McGraw-Hill.

Pomeranz AJ, O'Brien T: *Nelson's instructions for pediatric patients,* Philadelphia, 2007, Saunders.

Rankin SH, Stallings KD, London F: *Patient education in health and illness,* ed 5, Philadelphia, 2005, Lippincott Williams & Wilkins.

Redman BK: *The practice of patient education,* ed 10, St Louis, 2006, Mosby.

Rothman RL, Housam R, Weiss H, et al: Patient understanding of food labels: the role of literacy and numeracy, *Am J Prev Med* 31(5):391-8, 2006.

Sackett DL, Haynes RB, Guyatt GH, Tugwell P: Helping patients follow the treatments you prescribe. In *Clinical epidemiology: a basic science for clinical medicine,* Boston, 1991, Little, Brown.

Sentell TL, Halpin HA: Importance of adult literacy in understanding health disparities, *J Gen Intern Med* 21(8):862-6, 2006.

Sodeman W, Sodeman T: *Instructions for geriatric patients,* ed 3, Philadelphia, 2005, WB Saunders.

Springhouse: *Patient teaching reference manual,* ed 2, Philadelphia, 2001, Lippincott Williams & Wilkins.

Teaching patients with acute conditions, Springhouse, Philadelphia, 1992, Springhouse.

Teaching patients with chronic conditions, Springhouse, Philadelphia, 1992, Springhouse.

Turner T, Cull WL, Bayldon B, et al: Pediatricians and health literacy: descriptive results from a national survey, *Pediatrics* 124 Suppl 3:S299-305, 2009.

U.S. Pharmacopeial Convention: *Advice for the patient in lay language* (USP DI Vol II), Rockville, Maryland, 2002.

Yin HS, Johnson M, Mendelsohn AL, et al: The health literacy of parents in the United States: a nationally representative study, *Pediatrics* 124 Suppl 3:S289-98, 2009.

Wolf MS, Davis TC, Bass PF, et al: Improving prescription drug warnings to promote patient comprehension, *Arch Intern Med* 170(1):50-6, 2010.

necessary for specific patients. In fact, the problem is not in finding patient teaching materials, but in evaluating their quality and how they may be used. Many materials are written at a high grade reading level and thus are not very helpful to those with reading difficulties.

To see if published handouts would be helpful for your patients, keep the following in mind:

- Be sure the goals of the teaching are stated.
- Limit content to one or two objectives and state what the patient will learn or do after reading the information.
- Focus on the behavior they should have rather than the medical facts.
- Have clear headings and lots of white space on the page; use photographs or realistic illustrations to attract the patient's attention and tell the message.
- Use common or familiar words and not medical words.
- Involve the patients by asking them to do, write, say, or show something to confirm their understanding.
- Clear communication should use short, simple sentences without complex grammar.
- The handout is more likely to be read when the information is on no more than one page, front and back.
- When possible, the material should be written in lists rather than in paragraphs. Key items or warnings should be highlighted with bullets or symbols.
- The print size should be fairly large (at least 14 points) if elderly patients will use the material.
- If only one handout will be used for all patients receiving a drug, short sentences and simple words result in materials at a more basic reading level.
- Whenever possible, the readability should be below the eighth-grade level—preferably at the fifth-grade level. Grade level of English documents written in Word may be assessed on the computer by going to

Tools, and then clicking on Word Count. Each readability score bases its rating on the average number of syllables per word and words per sentence.
- In some settings, handouts may be needed in several languages

Audiovisual Resources

Audiovisual programs such as slide-tape programs, videocassettes, and CD-ROMs are also available for patient teaching. Some patients will be able to use the Internet, and this allows patients to select what they want and download it for future reference.

Television ads that are created by drug companies for patients are called *direct-to-consumer advertising.* Patients may have many questions or inaccurate information because they have seen these ads. When patients raise questions because of these ads, this is a good opportunity for you to assess what they know and provide correct information.

Talking to patients and giving them written information, or talking to the patient along with showing audiovisual aids, is usually better than only giving the patient things to read. This is very important for patients with new prescriptions.

Nurse and Patient Use of the Internet

One of the biggest challenges for health care workers is finding up-to-date information to use in teaching. Textbooks and journal articles may be years or months old before being printed. New information is available every day, so it is essential to provide patients with the latest information. This task is easier than it has been in the past because of the Internet. The Internet is becoming a source of up-to-date health information, not only for nurses, but for patients as well. Many Internet sites meet the needs of both. A number of sites offer directions for using the Internet. They range from those which focus on the basics, to more advanced Internet courses (Table 2-2).

Although many business websites have accurate information, others may be more interested in selling something. Commercial or business sites use "com" near the end of their web addresses. They often scatter ads throughout their web pages, charge fees or dues, or talk about things to buy. The letters "org" identify a nonprofit group, "gov" a government agency, and "edu" an educational site.

EVALUATION OF LEARNING

Patient education occurs to help change patient behavior and increase satisfaction. When objectives are written for each patient, the behavior change sought is clearly stated. Thus it should be simple to determine if learning has taken place. When blood sugar levels do not come down and stay down to the desired level, when blood pressure remains high, or when weight is not lost, there is failure somewhere

Table 2-2	Websites that Offer Information for Navigating the Web
WEBSITE	**URL ADDRESS**
The Help Web	www.imagescape.com/helpweb
The Internet Learning Tree	www.walthowe.com/navnet/
Internet Web Text Index	www.december.com/web/text
Navigating the Web	http://digitalenterprise.org/navigation/nav.html
Navigating the Web: Using Search Tools	http://healthlinks.Washington.edu/howto/navigating/
Navigating the Web— Library Services	http://lib.mnsu.edu/research/navwebtext.html

in the education process. Sometimes the process breaks down when a patient does not understand what to do, cannot afford the treatment plan, or loses confidence in being able to change. Whatever the problem, the nurse must attempt to discover where the process went wrong.

You, as a licensed practical or vocational nurse, may be the teacher, or may just observe the teaching process. Active questioning and discussion helps the learner remember what was taught. You may follow up a more formal teaching session with your own comments and questions. As you have a chance to work with the patient you can provide active teaching with sensory involvement (like handling things, hearing things, eating something, and so forth) that will reinforce what the patient has learned in class and allows more effective learning to take place.

Throughout the teaching process, it is important for the nurse to summarize, repeat, and keep it simple. Check for understanding as the teaching continues by having the patient repeat back the important points. It is important not to create fear or stress when quizzing patients on information that has been discussed. Note in the patient's record what has been taught—the important topics covered, what material was given to the patient, and your view of the patient's level of understanding. List anything you believe shows the patient's willingness to carry out the treatment plan.

Other factors that improve the success of drug treatment plans for most patients include developing plans that have frequent nurse-patient contacts, using reminder cards, giving blood tests for drug levels, making the plan fit the patient's needs and culture, giving feedback and encouragement, and encouraging the patient to be actively involved in things like taking blood pressures at home or having a behavior contract with the nurse. Build these things into the written objectives.

Get Ready for the NCLEX® Examination!

Key Points

- Research suggests that patient education is an important activity for the nurse.
- Today, more than ever, it is important to teach patients well.
- Giving patient education allows patients the chance to help in making and meeting their own health care goals.

Additional Learning Resources

SG Go to your Study Guide for additional learning activities to help you master this chapter content.

evolve Go to your Evolve website (http://evolve.elsevier.com/ Edmunds/LPN/) for additional online resources.

Review Questions for the NCLEX® Examination

1. The nurse is caring for an older adult female whose only income is a small pension. A treatment goal for the patient is to lose 25 pounds, which may help reduce her blood pressure. The nurse finds that although the patient is eager to lose weight, she didn't buy the recommended food because it was too expensive. The main reason this patient is not meeting her treatment goal is:
   1. she did not understand what to do
   2. she does not believe the plan should be carried out
   3. she believes something should be done, but does not implement the plan
   4. she believes something should be done, but does not have money to do it

2. The nurse is preparing to develop objectives for a teaching session. The highest priority action regarding the development of objectives is:
   1. make the objectives broad enough to be easily achieved
   2. do not involve the patient in the planning process
   3. ensure that the objectives are specific and measureable
   4. make certain that the objectives only involve one teaching model

3. The nurse has been teaching the patient how to self-administer injections. The most appropriate way to determine how well the material has been learned is:
   1. have the patient demonstrate the procedure for administration of an injection
   2. ask the patient to complete a written evaluation of the teaching material
   3. ask the patient if he feels comfortable administering the injection to himself
   4. have the patient repeat information about the administration of injections

4. The nurse is developing handouts for an older adult patient. The highest priority nursing action will be:
   1. include content from at least six objectives
   2. use a font size of at least 14 points
   3. present information in paragraph style
   4. avoid using photographs or illustrations

5. The patient has questions related to a television ad for a drug company's product. This is an opportunity for the nurse to accurately assess:
   1. the patient's reading level
   2. the patient's motivation for learning
   3. the patient's need for a variety of teaching methods
   4. the patient's information about the medication

Critical Thinking Questions

1. What would be most important to do first if you needed to develop a teaching plan for Mr. Brown, who is newly diagnosed with type 1 diabetes?
2. Give some examples of ways in which the nurse's skill in talking and teaching can affect outcomes of patient teaching.
3. Giving information in a teaching plan is necessary for patient understanding and compliance. How might the following sentences be changed to provider better patient understanding?
   a. "Take this tablet twice a day."
   b. "You can have three pieces of bread a day on your new diet."
   c. "A dish of macaroni equals one serving."
   d. "You need to drink at least three glasses of water a day."
   e. "It might be a good idea to cut down to two cups of coffee a day."

Legal Aspects Affecting the Administration of Medications

Objectives

1. List the names of major federal laws about drugs and drug use.
2. Explain what is meant by "scheduled drugs" or "controlled substances," and give examples of drugs in the different schedules.
3. Describe the differences between authority, responsibility, and accountability.
4. List rules of states and agencies that affect how nurses give drugs.
5. Explain how the nurse is responsible for controlled substances.
6. List what information is included in a medication order or prescription.
7. Define and give examples of the four different types of medication orders.
8. List what you need to do if you make a medication error.

Key Terms

controlled substances (kŏn-TRŌLD SŬB-stăn-sĕz, p. 17)
delegation (dĕl-ĕ-GĀ-shŭn, p. 21)
engineering controls (ĕn-jĭn-ĒR-ĭng, p. 29)
legal responsibility (LĒ-gŭl, p. 21)
nurse practice act (p. 21)
over-the-counter (OTC) medications (mĕd-ĭ-KĀ-shŭnz, p. 17)

physical dependence (FĬZ-ĭ-kăl, p. 18)
prescription, or legend, drugs (prĭ-SKRĬP-shŭn, p. 17)
problem-oriented medical record (POMR) (p. 23)
professional responsibility (p. 21)
psychologic dependence (sĭ-kō-LŎJ-ĭk, p. 18)
scheduled drugs (SKĔD-jūld, p. 17)

PHARMACOLOGY AND REGULATIONS

Nurses who give medications have three levels of rules they must follow:

1. Federal laws, which describe rules that control how certain drugs may be given
2. State laws and regulations, or rules, which say who may prescribe, dispense (give a supply), and administer, or give, medications and the process to be used
3. Individual hospital or agency rules, which may use other guidelines or policies about how and when drugs are given and the records that must be kept to record drug treatment

FEDERAL LAWS

Laws passed by Congress try to make medications as safe as possible for patients to take and to make sure that the drug does what it claims to do (effectiveness). Congress created the Food and Drug Administration (FDA) to monitor or watch the testing, approval, and marketing of new drugs. These regulations are very strict and so U.S. drugs are some of the most pure and protected drugs in the world. Many laws have been passed to control drugs that might easily be abused and are dangerous. Table 3-1 lists some of the major federal drug laws that have been passed.

Federal laws created three drug categories in the United States:

1. **Controlled substances**, which include major pain killers (narcotics) and some sedatives or tranquilizers that can be ordered only by someone with a special license
2. **Prescription, or legend, drugs** such as antibiotics and oral contraceptives
3. **Over-the-counter (OTC) medications**, which patients may buy without a prescription

Controlled Substances

Most regulations are written for controlled substances, because they are often abused both by patients and people using them illegally. After the Controlled Substances Act of 1970 classed these medications into five "schedules," they became known as **scheduled drugs**. The degree of control, the record keeping required, the order forms, and other regulations are different for each of these five classes. Table 3-2 describes the five drug schedules, with examples of medications in each category. Sometimes the drugs are moved from one

Table 3-1   Summary of Major Federal Drug Legislation

TITLE OF LEGISLATION	YEAR	DESCRIPTION OF LEGISLATION
Harrison Narcotic Act	1914	Limited the indiscriminate use of addictive drugs. Regulated the importation, manufacture, sale, and use of opium, cocaine, and their compounds and derivatives. Amended many times and finally repealed and replaced by the Controlled Substances Act in 1970.
Federal Food, Drug, and Cosmetic Act	1938	Authorized the Food and Drug Administration of the Department of Health and Human Services to determine the safety of drugs before marketing, to determine labeling specifications, and to ensure that advertising claims are met.
Durham-Humphrey Amendment	1951	Restricts the number of prescriptions that can be refilled.
Kefauver-Harris Amendments	1962	Provides greater control and surveillance of clinical testing and distribution of investigational drugs. A product must be proven to be both safe and effective before it may be released for sale.
Comprehensive Drug Abuse Prevention and Control Act (Controlled Substances Act)	1970	Composite law that repealed almost 50 other laws. Designed to improve the administration and regulation of manufacturing, distributing, and dispensing of controlled drugs. The Drug Enforcement Administration was created to enforce the Controlled Substances Act, gather intelligence, train investigators, and conduct research on potentially dangerous drugs and drug abuse.
Needlestick Safety and Prevention Act	2001	Requires hospitals to have programs to prevent needlestick injuries, document them when they occur, and purchase safe equipment regardless of cost.

Table 3-2   Controlled Substance Schedule

SCHEDULE	POTENTIAL FOR ABUSE	COMMENTS AND EXAMPLES
I	High	No currently accepted medical use in the United States. Lack of accepted safety for use under medical supervision. Examples: hashish, heroin, lysergic acid diethylamide, marijuana, peyote, 2,5-demethoxy-4-methamphetamine.
II	High	Abuse potential that may lead to severe psychologic or physical dependence. Examples: amphetamines, meperidine, methadone, methaqualone, morphine, pentobarbital, oxycodone (Percocet), secobarbital.
III	High, but less than I or II	Abuse potential that may lead to moderate or low physical dependence or high psychologic dependence. Examples: glutethimide, aspirin with codeine (Empirin with codeine), aspirin with butalbital and caffeine (Fiorinal), methyprylon, paregoric, acetaminophen with codeine (Tylenol with codeine).
IV	Low compared with III	Abuse potential that may lead to limited physical or psychologic dependence. Examples: lorazepam (Ativan), diazepam (Valium).
V	Low compared with IV	Abuse potential that may lead to limited physical or psychologic dependence. Examples: diphenoxylate with atropine sulfate (Lomotil), guaifenesin with codeine sulfate antitussives.

class to another if it becomes clear they are being abused.

Federal and state laws make it a crime for anyone to have controlled substances without a prescription. Each state has a practice act that lists which health care providers may dispense or write prescriptions for controlled substances. Pharmacists usually dispense the medications; physicians, dentists, osteopaths, nurse practitioners, physician assistants, and sometimes

 Clinical Goldmine

Dependence

Physical dependence refers to the physiologic need for a medication to relieve shaking, pain, or other symptoms. **Psychologic dependence**, on the other hand, refers to anxiety, stress, or tension that is felt if the patient does not have the medication. One type of dependency often leads to the other; they are often found together in the same individual.

nurse midwives may write prescriptions. Licensed practical nurses (LPNs) or licensed vocational nurses (LVNs) may give controlled substances to a patient only under the direction of a health care provider who is licensed to administer or prescribe these drugs. Mediation aides or technicians are also used by some hospitals to administer drugs. Student nurses work under the delegated authority of the registered nurse (RN). The RN is responsible for any errors that might be made by these individuals.

Nurses may not have controlled substances in their possession unless one of the following conditions is met:

- The nurse is giving them to the patient for whom they are ordered.
- The nurse is the person in charge of the supply of medications of a ward or department.
- The nurse is the patient for whom a physician has prescribed the medication.

LPNs/LVNs work in some of the most sophisticated areas of medicine with high technology as well as some of the least sophisticated areas where they may be the health care worker with the most training and relatively no technology available. They must be prepared to practice within this large range of settings. Each state and health care agency has rules that cover the ordering, receiving, storing, and record keeping of controlled substances. Narcotics are a scheduled drug and they must all be counted every shift. Records must be kept for every dose administered. Agency policy will decide which nurses will be held responsible for handing over the control of these medications from one shift to the next and for how medications will be counted and checked. All controlled substances ordered for a patient but not used during their hospital stay go back to the pharmacy when the patient is discharged.

Nurses may not borrow medicine ordered for one patient to use for another patient or for themselves. In a time when drug abuse is so common, the nurse who has responsibility for the controlled substances must remain alert. Abuse is not limited to patients. Some health care professionals may not be able to resist such a large supply of medication and will seek to hide their theft of a patient's medication. Things that should arouse suspicion might include a pattern in which medication is frequently "dropped" or "spilled" or records that show a patient got large or frequent doses of medications on certain shifts but the patient reports no pain relief. In these cases, perhaps the patients are not really getting their medication.

 Memory Jogger

Federal Regulations

The nurse must know the federal, state, and agency rules about giving medications.

The rules that govern controlled substances are very clear and very strict. Breaking the rules is very serious. If it is found that the nurse has violated the Controlled Substance laws, the nurse may be punished by a fine, a prison sentence, or both. Nurses with proven drug abuse problems will lose their license to practice and may have a hard time getting it back. Nurses who do not report their suspicion that other nurses may be breaking the rules risk their own jobs. In most states, the state nursing association has a program to help nurses who have drug abuse or other problems that affect their ability to carry out their nursing duties.

Prescription, or Legend, Drugs

The FDA has decided that many drugs are dangerous and their use must be carefully controlled. Access to these drugs is provided by a few health care professionals (physicians, dentists, and nurse practitioners). This control is through a written prescription or order that must be written before the drug may be given. Prescription drugs make up most of the medications the nurse gives to patients in a hospital. Prescription drugs are carefully tested before they are put on the market. The drugs have been shown to be safe and effective. However, even though much may be known about a particular medication, each patient is different and may have a somewhat different reaction to the drug. Pediatric patients, older adult patients, and critically ill patients may be weak and more likely to have problems taking a drug. The nurse must be alert and watch for signs that the drug is working the way it should, as well as for adverse reactions that may develop. Because the patient often gets several drugs at the same time, the interaction among the drugs may make it hard to tell how each drug affects the patient. Although a lot of research about drugs has been done, many drugs are not FDA approved as safe and effective for children or pregnant women. Geriatric patients are at high risk for problems with prescriptions drugs, because they may not take the drug properly because of poor eyesight, memory, or coordination; they may take many drugs that interact with each other; or they may have chronic diseases that interfere with how the drug works.

The Omnibus Budget Reconciliation Acts of 1989, 1990, and 1991 placed further controls on drugs for Medicare or older patients. More and more, insurance or government groups who pay for drugs limit the types and numbers of drugs that may be ordered to those on a preferred drug list. The preferred drug list may require the use of cheaper generic drugs to control costs because new or brand-name drugs usually cost more.

Over-the-Counter Medications

The FDA has also found that many drugs are quite safe and do not need a prescription. These drugs may easily be purchased at a drugstore or pharmacy. These drugs often come in a low dosage, and they have low risk for abuse. Warning labels and special information supplied with these drugs make them safe for the average buyer. They are used to treat many common human illnesses: colds, allergies, headaches, burns, constipation, upset stomach, and so on. These drugs are often the first thing patients try before they go to the doctor. Although OTC medications are widely available, they are not without risk. Like all drugs, some may produce adverse effects in some patients. They may also have "hidden" chemicals such as caffeine or stimulants that may produce problems if taken with other drugs. Confusion by parents over the correct dosage of common cold preparations led to many accidental overdoses in children, so these drugs have been removed from the market. Other cold products that contain dextromethorphan and might be abused are now stored behind the pharmacy counter. Talking to patients about the use of OTC medications is very important for patients who are already taking many prescription drugs. New federal laws for labeling of these products will make more information available about the drug and make it easier for the patient to understand.

OTC drugs are also given in the hospital for minor problems patients may have. Although these medications do not require a prescription for purchase, a physician's order is required before they may be given in the hospital. In fact, without an order, hospitalized patients cannot take even their own OTC medicines brought along to the hospital. This policy is necessary for safety reasons. If patients could take their own medicines in addition to those medicines given by hospital staff, it could result in an overdose of medicine.

In recent years, many people have become interested in herbal products. Research shows that most people will try an herbal product at some time in their lives. Health food stores, grocery stores, and pharmacies all carry some of these products. Some people take these herbal products instead of their prescription drugs, and some use them along with their prescription drugs. Although research may someday find that these products are safe and effective, at present these herbal products are not regulated, standardized, or tested for safety and effectiveness. Because the federal government considers herbal products to be nutritional supplements rather than drugs, there are no regulations to control how they are made. There is no way to know if one leaf that is ground up and made into a pill will work the same as another leaf that is ground up. Also, the nurse cannot easily tell how much of the herbal product is in each pill, or even if each pill in a bottle contains the same amount of the product. Because research on these products is only beginning, little is known about side effects, and it is hard to tell if some of them actually have the intended effect. Finally, adverse effects may occur when a patient takes herbal products and prescription drugs at the same time.

Because of the high cost of drugs in the United States, some patients try to buy drugs from other countries where they both cost less and are easier to buy—usually in Mexico or Canada. Although low-cost drugs can be good for patients, in some cases there is a risk the drugs may not be pure, may not be the drugs patients believe they are buying, or may even be dangerous. Drugs that originate in China or India often look like real drugs but may be fake. It is hard to know if the drugs sold in other countries or over the Internet are real. At this time, buying drugs in other countries and bringing them into the United States is not legal. The FDA is opposed to patients being able to get drugs that cannot be proven to meet high U.S. standards.

Because U.S. drug companies often sell their drugs to other countries at a cheaper rate than in the United States, there is growing interest by many groups in buying some of these drugs, particularly from Canada. Many nurses and patients in Canada or along the U.S.-Canadian border must deal with Canadian drug regulations and classifications that are different from those in the United States; some specific information is provided in the next section.

CANADIAN DRUG LEGISLATION

The Canadian Health Protection Branch of the Department of National Health and Welfare is like our FDA of the U.S. Department of Health and Human Services. This branch is responsible for the administration and enforcement of federal legislation such as the Food and Drugs Act, the Proprietary or Patent Medicine Act, and the Controlled Drugs and Substances Act. These acts, together with provincial acts and regulations that cover the sale of poisons and drugs and those that cover the health care professions, are designed to protect the Canadian consumer from health hazards; misleading ads about drugs, cosmetics, and devices; and impure food and drugs. The Canadian Food and Drugs Act divides drugs into various categories. Regulations covering the various categories or schedules of drugs differ from those in the United States. There are three major classes of drugs under the Food and Drugs Act: nonprescription drugs, prescription drugs, and restricted drugs.

The laws within the Canadian Food and Drugs Act allow the government to withdraw from the market drugs found to be toxic. New drugs put on the market must be shown in human clinical studies to be effective and safe to the satisfaction of the manufacturer and the government.*

---

*For more specific information, the nurse can obtain a copy of *Health Protection and Drug Laws* from Supply and Services Canada, Canadian Government Publishing, Ottawa, Canada, K1A 0S9.

The Proprietary or Patent Medicine Act provides for a class of products that may be sold to the general public by anyone. The drug formula is not found in the official drug manuals or printed on the label. The formulas for all such proprietary (trade secret) non-pharmacologic drugs must be registered and have a license under the Proprietary or Patent Medicine Act. The nurse needs to be aware of this act in the case of possible drug interactions.

The Canadian Controlled Drugs and Substances Act covers the possession, sale, manufacture, production, and distribution of narcotics in Canada. Only authorized persons may have narcotics in their possession. All persons authorized to be in possession of a narcotic must keep a record of the names and quantities of all narcotics dispensed, and they must ensure the safekeeping of all narcotics. The law covering this act is enforced by the Royal Canadian Mounted Police. Nurses are in violation of this act if they are guilty of illegal possession of narcotics.

OTC drugs are regulated in Canada by the Canadian Food and Drugs Act. These drugs can be purchased without a prescription, but there are rules about the package, label, and dispensing of the drug. The nurse needs to be aware of the risks these medications have and watch for possible adverse effects and interactions with other drugs. OTC drugs available in Canada differ from those available in the United States.

STATE LAW AND HEALTH CARE AGENCY POLICIES

Although many regulations about giving medications come from federal laws, the details about who may give medications are set by each state. This authority is spelled out for nurses in the **nurse practice act** of each state, which describes who can be called a *nurse* and what they can and cannot do. These rules vary from state to state and have changed over the years to reflect the increased responsibility many nurses have for giving medications. The authority to administer medications is clearly specified for LPNs/LVNs, RNs, and nurse practitioners in the state nurse practice act. Giving medicines is a task reserved for those nurses who are named by law to administer medications and who can document their educational preparation to do so. These nurses must also show they are willing to accept **professional responsibility** for administering drugs correctly, ethically, and to the best of their ability. This means they also accept **legal responsibility** for good judgment and their actions while doing these professional tasks.

Differences in practice from state to state make it essential that each nurse learn what is legal with regard to medications and make sure they and others follow all the rules. Because people in our society tend to move from state to state, nurses must know exactly what is in the nurse practice act of the state where they are now working. Using computers for ordering drugs, record keeping, and even advising patients (telemedicine) makes it possible for doctors and nurses in one state to be involved in health care for patients in different states. Today, nurses frequently move between jobs, and some states recognize the nursing license of another state through an agreement called the *Nurse Licensure Compact*. There is a growing list of states that participate in the *Compact* (available at www.ncsbn.org). Because of the differences among states in what is allowed, a national nursing license may one day be granted.

 Memory Jogger

State Nurse Practice Act

Understand how your state nurse practice act describes your drug administration responsibilities.

State rules about nursing practice often list the basic or minimum standards of practice. Therefore, agency or institutional policies and guidelines may be more specific or restrictive than state nurse practice acts. Agency employers should provide:
1. Written policy statements regarding:
   - educational preparation of nurses administering medications
   - agency or institutional policies nurses must follow
2. Orientation to particular policies, procedures, and record-keeping rules

When the nurse accepts a job, it implies he or she is willing to obey the policies or procedures of that institution. Sometimes the nurse must meet very formal rules in order to give medications. It may be an agency's policy to require employment for a certain period, completion of special orientation and training sessions, and passing a probation period before permission is given to administer medications. Even when the nurse may have the legal authority to give medications, they can do so only when the nurse has a valid medication order signed by an authorized prescriber.

All nurses have legal responsibility for what they do. As stated before, what they are and are not permitted to do is listed in the nurse practice act of the state. Some RNs with advanced training like nurse practitioners have expanded their clinical practice to include tasks that only doctors did in the past, and LPNs/LVNs in some settings perform tasks that were once done only by RNs. These trends are likely to continue because of efforts to cut overall health care costs. The changes in who does what are legally linked to the term *delegation*.

Delegation is when the responsibility for doing a task is passed from one person to another, but the accountability for what happens, or the outcome, remains with the original person. The person who delegates a task to someone else must have the authority to do so, and the person to whom it is delegated must also have the authority to perform that task. RNs now often delegate many of their tasks, including giving medications, to an LPN/LVN. For example, if the LPN/LVN has the educational preparation, clinical experience, and agency authority to give medications, then the RN may delegate this task to her or him. The RN still retains accountability for making sure that the LPN/LVN is able to perform the task correctly, whereas the LPN/LVN is responsible for what she or he does. In some settings, an LPN/LVN may direct the work of other LPNs/LVNs or unlicensed personnel such as nurse's aides. The LPN/LVN in this situation remains accountable and responsible for assigning tasks to the nurse's aide or other LPN/LVN, and the aide or other LPN/LVN is responsible for the care that is actually delivered. This principle is also true for the student nurse. The student in an RN or LPN/LVN program is held to the same standard of practice as the graduate. The student works under delegated responsibility from the RN, but the RN maintains accountability.

Although there are many formal regulations for giving medications, there are also some requirements of medication administration that are less formal and rely on the judgment and knowledge of the nurse. The agency expects the nurse to carry out the steps of the nursing process and, in fact, holds the nurse responsible for good assessment, diagnosis, planning, implementation, and evaluation of the patient when medication is given. The nurse will be held responsible for failure to perform any of these steps well.

The nursing process is a helpful system to be used when giving medications. There is a professional and an implied legal requirement that nurses use this process. *The nurse must understand information about the patient:* symptoms, diagnosis, and why the medication is to be given. The nurse also learns other information about the patient's past medical history, allergies, risk factors, and reaction to medications or any information that contraindicates (forbids) giving the drug. *Nurses learn about the medication itself:* the dosage, the route of administration, the expected response, and adverse reactions. Knowledge about other medications is also mandatory, because nurses must watch for possible drug interactions. *The nurses understands and follows the medication procedure:* how, when, and where the medication is to be given and equipment or special techniques needed. *The nurse also acts to monitor the patient's response after the medication is given,* record the information about the drug that was given, and report promptly to the RN or physician any unexpected results. Finally, the nurse uses every chance they have to teach the patient and the family the information they need to know for continued and safe administration of this medication.

Patient Charts

The patient's chart, whether it is paper or electronic, is a legal record. It is the major source of information about the patient and the care received while in the hospital. It provides a central place where members of the health care team record information about the patient and all treatment. The physician or other health care provider describes the patient's condition on admission, determines the diagnosis, and provides orders to identify or resolve the patient's problems. The nurse records the assessment of the patient's condition, the implementation of basic nursing procedures, the patient's response, and the progress in completing the diagnostic and therapeutic plans. While the patient might request a copy of the chart, the chart belongs to the hospital. It is not the property of the patient, the nurse, or the physician. It is the legal record of the patient's stay in the hospital. It is kept after the patient has been discharged, and it is often used for billing, insurance, and auditing activities; in medical or nursing research; and to provide information if the patient should be admitted again. In cases of court action or lawsuits, the chart may be used by lawyers as evidence. It is especially important that nurses write meaningful and accurate information in a complete and readable manner. Using electronic medical records and data entry systems helps nurses do this.

 Memory Jogger

The Patient's Chart

In every organization the patient will have a chart, but the chart may differ in content and format depending on the type of health care organization.

Health care is delivered in many different places in this country and around the world. Some agencies and countries have few resources, and care is very limited. Others have the latest computers and treatment systems. Throughout the nurses career, they will probably work in places with different resources. For example, a nurse may work in an agency that has the latest computerized medication system installed in each patient's room or in a nursing home that has no medication recording system. If the nurse has the chance to practice in another country, they might find that although the tasks nurses perform for patients are often the same, there may be different ways of carrying out nursing activities. Nurses learn the basics about nursing activities related to giving medications, and then adjust that knowledge to the setting in which they practice. Some of the basics include the following:

- The nurse is responsible for checking that the medication order is correct. This may mean you need to

Box 3-1 Parts of the Problem-Oriented Medical Record Patient Chart

SUMMARY SHEET

The summary sheet is the standard hospital information form that gives basic information about the patient: name, address, date of birth, sex, marital status, nearest relative, employer, insurance carrier or payment arrangements, religion, date and time of admission, admission diagnoses, and attending physician. It may also contain information about allergies, past diagnoses or admissions, and the patient's occupation. A summary of surgeries, diagnoses, and the date and time of discharge may also be added when the patient leaves.

HISTORY AND PHYSICAL EXAMINATION

On admission, a total history and a physical examination are completed by the physician. The nurse admitting the patient may also conduct a nursing history and a physical examination to supplement the physician's report. All findings are listed, and the problem list is constructed from this information.

PROBLEM LIST

The problem list contains all the symptoms, signs, problems, and diagnoses that have been identified. New problems are added as indicated. The list is numbered, and dates are given for when each problem began and when it was detected. All further entries in the chart that relate to a given problem would use the problem number.

PHYSICIAN'S ORDERS

All procedures and treatments are ordered on the physician's order form. These orders include general care (activity level, diet, vital signs), diagnostic and laboratory tests (blood work, x-ray studies), and medications and treatments (hot packs, dressings, physical therapy).

PROGRESS NOTES

The progress notes section contains observations made by health care workers about the patient. Physicians' and nurses' notes are written in a SOAP format: **S**ubjective information, **O**bjective findings, **A**ssessment of problem, and **P**lan of care. (Some hospitals put physicians' and nurses' notes into separate sections.) These may be handwritten or entered into an electronic medical chart.

GRAPHIC RECORD

The graphic record section contains forms for recording vital signs, fluid intake and output, and treatments. In some hospitals, medications are also recorded in this section. In other hospitals, medications are kept in a separate medication Kardex and are not part of the chart until the patient is discharged.

LABORATORY TESTS

All laboratory test results are recorded either on a single sheet as separate entries as they are received by the unit or as sequential entries or summaries updated by computers. (If a patient is critically ill, charts may be developed to show all laboratory test results in one place so any changes can be easily seen.) These are often called *flow charts*. Results of electrocardiograms, electroencephalograms, x-ray studies, or other tests are usually placed here.

CONSULTATIONS

When other specialists are asked to see the patient, the summary of their examination and suggestions are placed here.

---

check the order you have (in a medication Kardex or drug system or on the computerized medication record) against the original order in the patient's chart.

- The nurse must record the drug administration information. Every agency has its own order sheets and recording forms for the patient's chart. Agency policy will tell you what information is to be placed in each section. Although there are a variety of forms, certain things are traditionally part of every chart. These parts are listed in Box 3-1. There is growing use of computers and electronic record keeping. Many hospitals take computers to the bedside, scan all medication barcodes as they are given to the patient, and the information is recorded electronically in the patient's record. These systems help prevent errors.
- Many hospitals use the chart format called the **problem-oriented medical record (POMR)**. The POMR uses a list of numbered patient problems as an index to the chart. The way the notes are written in the chart also helps make information easy to find.

Kardex

The Kardex is a flip-file card system used for many years that has important information from the patient summary form and the physician's orders. It is regularly updated and changed to reflect current orders. This format keeps important information about the patient easily available for all team members. In the past, all tests, medications, and treatment orders were listed here, along with the nursing care plan. Some agencies still require use of a medication card for each drug to be given to the patient (Figure 3-1). More commonly, when a unit-dose system is used, individual medication cards are not needed, because all medications are listed in the Kardex or medication profile sheet (Figure 3-2). Some computerized dispensing systems create their own separate patient medication forms as drugs are dispensed. The Kardex card is thrown away when the patient is discharged. It is not a legal document and serves no further purpose. Some settings may not use this Kardex system but will use an electronic order entry system and charting system. This prevents illegible prescriber handwriting. Many systems are designed to indicate if the dose ordered is out of the acceptable range, would interact with another ordered medicine, or other dosing errors. LPNs/LVNs may find that they often work in health care settings that continue to use the older, low-cost information systems, so they need to be comfortable in either setting.

Drug Distribution Systems

Each agency has its own way of ordering and administering medications. There are four commonly used systems to distribute medications to the nurse:

Name ____________ Room ______

Drug ____________________

Dosage __________________

Time ____________________

Date ____________ Initials ______

FIGURE 3-1 Example of a medication card.

1. The floor or ward stock system
2. The individual prescription order system
3. The unit-dose system
4. The computerized or automated dispensing system

These four systems are described in Box 3-2.

Both the unit-dose system and the computerized or automated dispensing systems currently in use in the U.S. may link a barcode on the medication to a barcode on the patient to help reduce medication errors. Scanning the barcode helps get the right drug to the right patient.

Narcotics Control Systems

Both federal and state laws, as well as agency policies, are very clear about how controlled substances are handled in the hospital. These procedures are nearly identical from hospital to hospital. The primary goal of all regulations and policies is to verify and account for all controlled substances. When controlled substances, particularly narcotics, are ordered from the pharmacy, they come in single-dose unit or prefilled syringes and are attached to a special inventory sheet. The nurse receiving the order from the pharmacy must

MEDICATION KARDEX

PRN MEDICATIONS

Order date initials	Expir. date	Medication dose/frequency/route	Doses given	
			Date	
			Time	
			Initials	
			Date	
			Time	
			Initials	
			Date	
			Time	
			Initials	
			Date	
			Time	
			Initials	
			Date	
			Time	
			Initials	
			Date	
			Time	
			Initials	
			Date	
			Time	
			Initials	
			Date	
			Time	
			Initials	
			Date	
			Time	
			Initials	
			Date	
			Time	
			Initials	
			Date	
			Time	
			Initials	

IM Injection Site Code
1. Rt. posterior gluteal
2. Lt. posterior gluteal
3. Rt. anterior gluteal
4. Lt. anterior gluteal
5. Rt. anterolateral thigh
6. Lt. anterolateral thigh
7. Rt. deltoid
8. Lt. deltoid

Indicate the number of the site used with each IM dose given.

Record site with time.

Signatures/Initials

ALLERGIES ____________ DIAGNOSIS ____________

ROOM NO. ______ NAME ____________ DOCTOR ____________ AGE ______

FIGURE 3-2 Example of a medication Kardex.

Box **3-2**   Common Drug Distribution Systems

FLOOR OR WARD STOCK SYSTEM

In the floor or ward stock system, all frequently used medications (except potentially dangerous or controlled substances) are stocked in large containers at the nursing station. This system is usually used in small hospitals, in nursing homes with no pharmacist, or where there are no direct charges to patients for the medications (such as in most government hospitals); it is also used in some emergency rooms. Medication is taken from each container as needed for each patient.

Advantages
- Few inpatient prescription orders
- Minimal return of medications
- Ready availability of medications

Disadvantages
- Increased potential for medication errors
- Potential for unapproved use of medication by hospital personnel
- Potential for unnoticed drug deterioration
- Potential for increased number of expired drugs that may be difficult to detect
- Storage and space problems
- Lack of review of medication order by pharmacist

INDIVIDUAL PRESCRIPTION ORDER SYSTEM

In the individual prescription order system, medication orders are sent to the pharmacy, which issues an individual box or bottle for each drug. The container may hold a 3- to 5-day supply of the drug. Medications are stored in a cabinet at the nursing station. They are arranged either alphabetically by drug name or according to the patient's room number. Medication is taken from each container by the nurse as needed and distributed to the patient.

Advantages
- Review of prescription by both pharmacist and nurse before administration
- Less chance for drug deterioration or drug misuse
- Smaller drug inventories needed
- Medication usually available for stat or prn usage
- Easy charging and billing process

Disadvantages
- Frequent need to return or discard unused medications
- Complex or expensive ordering, preparing, administering, controlling, and recording systems required

UNIT-DOSE SYSTEM

Single-unit packages of drugs are dispensed to fill each order. Each package is clearly labeled and may have a specific barcode and is often dispensed by the pharmacy into drawers assigned to individual patients in a special medication cart or an individual patient drug cabinet near the patient's room. (This is known as a "nurse service" format.) Every 24 hours, the pharmacist refills this cart or cabinet with all the medications required for the patient for 1 day. This is the safest and most economical method of drug distribution in use today.

Advantages
- Little nursing time is required for preparation of medications.
- Better use is made of pharmacists' skills and knowledge. The pharmacist has more information about the drug and can check each order for contraindications or drug interactions.
- Errors are reduced because no drug calculations by the nurse are required.
- There is little waste or misuse of medication because only small doses are dispensed.
- Credit can be given for unused drugs because medication packages have not been opened.
- Bar coding of medication builds in another level of patient safety.

Disadvantages
- Nurses must administer a medication prepared by someone else, which may occasionally lead to an error.
- Delays in starting medications may occur if no unit stock is available.
- This system requires pharmacists at the hospital, which may not be possible or may be very expensive.

COMPUTERIZED OR AUTOMATED DISPENSING SYSTEM

Medication orders are sent to the pharmacy, where medication is loaded into an automated drug dispensing system. There are a number of automated dispensing systems available such as Sure-Med™ and Pyxis® and they each work a little differently. In some systems, the stocked cart with the proper medications is delivered to the hospital unit. When the medication is to be administered, the nurse or sometimes a specially trained technician enters the patient's name and the drug needed, and that drug is dispensed and automatically entered into the computerized drug administration record. The cart then goes back to the pharmacy for refill. In other systems, the drug storage unit is located in the patient's care area and a pharmacy technician comes by and refills the system from processed orders sent to the pharmacy. The nurse or technician withdraws the medication for the patient according to the drug orders. The nurse or technician administers the medication and then charts it. In some systems, when the drug is given to the patient, both the patient's barcoded wrist band and a barcode on the medication are scanned and an automatic notation is made in the electronic patient record that the drug has been administered.

Advantages
- Reduced time required for nurses.
- Medication errors are reduced with scanning of barcodes on patient band and medicine.
- Medication is automatically recorded at the time of delivery.
- Tight control over drugs is possible.
- A technician might be used to give the medication.

Disadvantages
- Use of a pharmacist and special equipment increase cost.
- The nurse is highly dependent on pharmacist accuracy.

NOTE: All of these systems are in use today in the different places nurses may be working.

inspect the medication and return to the pharmacy a signed record stating that all the medication ordered was received and that it was in acceptable condition. As each medication is used, it must be accounted for on the inventory sheet by the nurse giving the medication.

The use of narcotics is carefully monitored on the hospital unit. Medication is stored in a special locked cabinet. The key to this cabinet is carried by the head nurse or by a medication nurse. This individual has the legal responsibility for the use and recording of all the narcotics during that shift, whether or not they personally give the medications to the patients. There are automated medication dispensing systems. They include narcotics plus also stock medicines that nurses withdraw by password or fingerprint instead of a key system.

When controlled substances are ordered for a patient, the nurse responsible for giving the medication first checks the order and verifies the dosage and the last time the medication was given before obtaining the key to the cabinet. The nurse must sign out all medications administered during the shift. The inventory report form is completed before the drug is removed from the cabinet. This report may be written or a patient barcode inserted and should state the patient's name, date, drug, dosage, and the signature of the nurse giving the medication. The medication given should be noted in the patient's chart, and there should also be a follow-up note about the patient's response to the medication. If a dose is ordered that is smaller than that provided (so that some medication must be discarded), or if the medication is accidentally dropped, contaminated, spilled, or otherwise made unusable and unreturnable, two nurses must sign the inventory report and describe the situation. Institutional policy may require additional actions.

At the end of each shift, the responsibility for all narcotic controlled substances and the key to the controlled substances cabinet is transferred to another nurse from the new shift. The contents of the locked cabinet are counted together by one nurse from each shift. The numbers of each ampule, tablet, and prefilled syringe in the cabinet must match the numbers listed on the inventory report form. Sealed packages are kept sealed. Opened packages of medications must each be inspected and counted. Prefilled syringes must be examined to make sure they all have the same color, the same fluid levels, and the same amounts of air within them. Both nurses must sign the inventory report, officially stating that the records and inventory are accurate at that time.

Occasionally, the inventory and the written report do not agree. Any errors in the number of remaining doses and the number listed in the inventory report must be explained. All nurses having access to the key must be asked about medication they have given.

Steps must be retraced to see if someone forgot to record any medication. Patient charts might also be checked to see if medication was given that was not signed for on the inventory report. If errors in the report cannot be found, both the pharmacy and the nursing service office must be notified. If the error is large, the hospital administrator and security police are usually contacted.

You can see that the nurse with the key has a lot of responsibility in watching over the controlled drugs on the nursing unit. This nurse is usually a very mature person, often the head nurse or a nurse who has been with the hospital for some time and has proven he or she can be trusted. It is the duty of this nurse to give the key only to other nurses authorized to administer controlled substances. Keys are never given to physicians or any other health care worker. (Sometimes a physician will want to give the medication, but the nurse should get the medication and sign the inventory report.) The nurse in charge of narcotic controlled substances should be able to monitor all activity with the controlled drugs on a daily basis so that if a pattern develops, changes are easily seen. On a hospital unit that has many patients coming from surgery, use of narcotics for these patients will be high soon after surgery but should taper off within 2 to 3 days. If a patient continues to need large or frequent doses or needs narcotics for longer than other patients with the same condition, the nurse in charge of these drugs should be suspicious. Any activity that causes concern relating to controlled substances should be noted by the head nurse.

 Memory Jogger

Controlled Substances

Always be sure to verify orders for and account for all controlled substances.

The Drug Order

Both state law and agency policy require that all medications given in hospitals must be ordered by licensed health care providers acting within their areas of professional training. This generally restricts prescriptive authority (the authority to write an order or prescription for medication) to physicians, dentists, and, in some states, nurse practitioners, nurse midwives, nurse anesthetists, and physician assistants who work for the hospital or clinic. Prescriptions for a hospitalized patient are written on the order form in the patient's chart or recorded in the electronic record, which may be seen by the pharmacy. Sometimes the order can be faxed, sent electronically, or is on a tear-off sheet sent directly to the pharmacy to get the medication. Other times the order must be transcribed, or rewritten, by the nurse or unit secretary onto a special pharmacy order form.

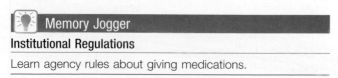

DEA #_____

ROBERT GOODFELLOW, M.D.
SARAH BOCK, R.N., A.N.P.
MARILYN EDWARDS, R.N., A.N.P.-C.
THICK FOREST PROFESSIONAL CENTER
THUNDER MILLS VILLAGE CENTER
3333 TRELLIS LANE
ST. GEORGE, MD 21043

Name _____

ADDRESS _____ DATE _____

]

☐ Label

Refill _____ times PRN NR

_____ M.D.

To ensure brand name dispensing, prescriber must write 'Dispense As Written' on the prescription.

FIGURE 3-3 Example of a prescription pad order form.

Prescriptions for patients leaving the hospital are written on regular prescription pads and taken to a pharmacy or drugstore to get the medication (Figure 3-3). Clinics or offices may work with pharmacies that will fill prescriptions for their patients. Every time a patient has a prescription filled, they should receive information about the product and how they should take it.

Whether the prescription is for hospitalized or non-hospitalized patients, the order contains the same information: the patient's full name, date, name of drug, route of administration, dose, frequency, duration, and signature of prescriber. Additional details about how to give the drug may also be written: "Take with meals," "Avoid milk products with this drug," "Do not refill," "Please label." Pharmacies require the patient's age and address on the prescription. This information may help the pharmacist ensure the right drug dosage for the patient (e.g., a child or older adult) or verify the patient's identity.

Memory Jogger

Institutional Regulations

Learn agency rules about giving medications.

In emergencies, or when the physician is not in the hospital, the physician might give the nurse either a verbal order or an order over the telephone. All agencies have policies about these types of orders. The hospital decides who may take these orders—usually the RN. The nurse taking the order is responsible for writing the order on the order form in the chart, including both the name of the nurse and the name of the doctor. Many institutions also require that a note be written to indicate that the order was read back to the physician for validation. The physician must then cosign this order, usually within 24 hours, for the order to be valid.

Medication orders may be classified into one of four types of orders:
1. The standing order
2. The emergency or "stat" order
3. The single order
4. The as-needed or "prn" order

The agency's policy clearly defines each of these types of orders and how they are carried out. Some agencies have also created a "now" order classification. A *now* order is different than a *stat* order in that the nurse has 1.5 hours to give the medication, unlike the *stat* order that must be given within minutes. The general definition of each type of order and examples of each are presented in Table 3-3. Table 3-4 lists common abbreviations used in pharmacology, which the nurse must memorize.

In an effort to cut down on medication errors, The Joint Commission (TJC), the agency that accredits or approves hospitals, has discouraged health care workers from using any abbreviations that might lead to confusion. That means that abbreviations that were used in the past (such as "hs" for nighttime, "cc" for cubic centimeter, and "QD" and "QOD" for daily and every other day) are no longer used in hospitals that wish to maintain their accreditation. Please go to the back of the text for abbreviations that must be included on each accredited organization's "Do Not Use" list.

MEDICATION ERRORS

Despite the best rules and procedures, medication errors occur in busy hospitals. Policies and procedures differ about what to do when a medication error is made. However, there are some guidelines that everyone accepts. When it is discovered that an error has been made, the nurse should immediately check the patient. Does the error pose a risk to the patient's condition (for example, giving too large a dose of insulin)? If so, the physician should be notified promptly, and any orders the physician gives must be followed. Every effort should be made to watch the patient's condition through measuring vital signs, drawing blood for tests, or any other method ordered by the physician. The nurse should also notify her nursing supervisor, record in the patient's chart exactly what happened, and fill out any other agency required reports. Whether the error is a problem for the nurse

Table **3-3**   Types of Medication Orders

DESCRIPTION	EXAMPLE
Standing Order	
Indicates that the drug is to be administered until discontinued or for a certain number of doses; hospital policy dictates that most standing orders expire after a certain number of days. A renewal order must be written by the physician before the drug may be continued.	"Amoxicillin 500 mg PO TID 10 days." "Ibuprofen 600 mg PO q6h."
Stat Order	
One-time order to be given immediately.	"Lidocaine 50 mg IV push stat."
Single Order	
One-time order to be given at specified time.	"Meperidine 100 mg IM 8 am preoperatively."
PRN Order	
Given as needed based on nurse's judgment of safety and patient need.	"Docusate 100 mg PO at bedtime prn constipation."
NOW Order	
To be given within an hour and a half.	"Lomotil II NOW for diarrhea."

Table **3-4**   Common Abbreviations Used in Pharmacology

ABBREVIATION	DEFINITION	ABBREVIATION	DEFINITION
ac	before meals	m	minim
ad lib	as desired	oz	ounce
am, AM	before noon	pc	after meals
bid	twice a day	pm, PM	after noon
$\overline{c}$	with	PO, po	by mouth
cap	capsule	PR	per rectum
comp	compound	prn	as required
D	give	Q, q	each, every
D	day	Qh, qh	every hour
dil	dilute	q2h	every 2 hours
div	divide	qid	four times daily
dos	dose	Rx	take
dr	drain	S	mark
elix	elixir	$\overline{s}$	without
ext	extract	sig	mark, write on the label
fl	fluid	ss	one half
g, gm	gram	stat	immediately
gr	grain	subcut	subcutaneous
gt (gtt)	drop(s)	tab	tablet
h	hour	tid	three times a day
IM	intramuscular	tinct, tr	tincture
IV	intravascular	ung	ointment

is often related to what happens to the patient. How and why the error was made and how it might be avoided in the future will be determined. If the nurse was careless or negligent, she may be held legally liable for any adverse consequences to the patient. Although almost every nurse has made one medication error, repeated errors will not be ignored. Research must be done in institutions to determine whether the mistakes made in that institution are most commonly due to a "system error," a unique mistake, a failure to follow the "six-rights" in giving a drug, or a deliberate wrong-doing.

In a very important Institute of Medicine (IOM) Report ("To Err is Human," IOM, 2000) about the number of errors made in medical care, estimates suggest that adverse events, which include medical errors, occur in 3% to 4% of patients. The IOM report and other studies estimate that the costs of medical errors in the United States, including lost income, disability, and need for additional health care, may be between $17 billion and $136.8 billion or more annually. These costs come from a variety of drug-related problems, including patient compliance issues and medical or medication errors. Unfortunately, estimates suggest that more than half of the adverse medical events each year are because of medical errors that could be prevented.

Because of this report, most agencies have tightened up ways to report and follow up on medication errors and some improvement has been confirmed in the most recent studies. Nurses should make every effort to know and follow the most recent agency policies to prevent errors.

LEGISLATION TO PROTECT HEALTH CARE WORKERS

Because patients have infections that may place nurses at risk, care must be taken to protect nurses and other health care workers. One of the most dangerous things nurses do is to recap the needle of a syringe that has been used in the injection of a sick patient. Recapping needles frequently leads to nurses accidentally sticking themselves. In 2001, the Needlestick Safety and Prevention Act became federal law. The object of the law is to prevent exposure in hospitals to bloodborne pathogens such as hepatitis B, hepatitis C, and human immunodeficiency virus. The law requires hospitals to follow the guidelines in the Occupational Safety and Health Administration (OSHA) Bloodborne Pathogens Standard. As part of this standard, health care institutions must have a written plan spelling out their efforts to cut the risk of needlestick injuries. In addition, employers are required to provide the safest equipment available, regardless of cost. Such equipment includes needleless products or those with engineering controls, which are built-in safety features to reduce risk. If a needlestick injury does occur, it is to be carefully recorded in a needlestick injury log. The exposure control plan, selection of safety products, and needlestick injury log must be reviewed at least every year. Many states have chosen to pass "tougher" laws, but at a minimum, every state law must meet the OSHA standard.

Get Ready for the NCLEX® Examination!

Key Points

- The nurse's authority to administer medications has grown slowly over time out of complex federal, state, and agency policies.
- These policies describe not only general procedures and rules, but also very specific responsibilities of the nurse who administers medications.
- The nurse is legally required to exercise judgment and responsibility in carrying out these tasks.
- The nurse may delegate authority to others authorized to administer medications, but keeps the responsibility for that delegation.

Additional Learning Resources

SG Go to your Study Guide for additional learning activities to help you master this chapter content.

evolve Go to your Evolve website (http://evolve.elsevier.com/Edmunds/LPN/) for additional online resources.

Review Questions for the NCLEX ® Examination

1. The patient care situation that will be most likely to cause a nurse to suspect that a colleague is engaging in substance abuse is:
   1. a patient requires scheduled doses of pain medication and verbalizes relief
   2. a patient has an order for pain medication but refuses the dosage
   3. a patient requires scheduled doses of pain medication but reports no relief
   4. a patient has an order for pain medication as needed but does not opt to take any

Get Ready for the NCLEX® Examination!—cont'd

2. Based on what you know about which groups have a high incidence of medication errors, which patient below is most likely to experience problems taking a drug?
    1. a 20-year-old woman who experiences frequent migraine headaches
    2. a 50-year-old man who underwent knee replacement surgery
    3. a 47-year-old woman who opts to use hormone replacement therapy
    4. a 9-year-old boy who experiences seizure-type activity

3. A 75-year-old female patient is experiencing difficulty taking her medication. The nurse recognizes that this is most likely the result of:
    1. inadequate amount of formalized education
    2. problems with her eyesight or coordination
    3. problems with her level of mental alertness
    4. inadequate degree of intelligence

4. The authority to administer medications is specified for nurses in:
    1. the Food and Drugs Act
    2. the nurse practice act of each state
    3. the Controlled Drugs and Substances Act
    4. Nurse Licensure Compact

5. The LVN delegates a task to a nurse's aide. The nurse should recognize that the accountability for task assignment lies with the:
    1. LVN
    2. nursing supervisor
    3. RN
    4. nurse manager

Critical Thinking Questions

1. Identify three levels of regulations the nurse must follow in giving medicines.
2. What is the major focus of each of the different forms of drug legislation?
3. Identify three categories of "scheduled" drugs, and examples of the sort of drug that fits into each schedule.
4. Review the nurse practice act in your state. Discuss at least three of your findings with the rest of the class about regulation of LPNs/LVNs.
5. Talk to nurses where you work to discover institutional policy regarding drug administration. Share your findings with the class. If you are in a hospital setting, do some agency regulations apply more to RNs than LPNs/LVNs?
6. Explain the difference between a drug order form, a prescription, and a verbal order. What does the nurse do in response to each of these items?
7. Identify the difference between *standing, stat, now, single,* and *prn* orders.
8. If it is your responsibility to take inventory of the narcotic box at the end of your shift, what should you do if you discover that an injectable narcotic is missing (i.e., the count does not match the written inventory report)?
9. What are three important things you should do if you discover you have made a medication error?
10. What should you do if you do not understand a physician's medication order?

Foundations and Principles of Pharmacology

Objectives

1. Define the key words used in pharmacology and about giving drugs.
2. Explain the differences between the chemical, generic, official, and brand names of medicines.
3. List the basic types of drug actions.
4. Describe the four basic physiologic processes that affect medications in the body.
5. Discuss the differences between side effects and adverse effects.

Key Terms

absorption (ăb-SŌRP-shŭn, p. 32)
additive effect (ĂD-ĭ-tĭv, p. 36)
adverse reactions (ăd-VŬRS, p. 35)
agonists (ĂG-ō-nĭsts, p. 32)
allergy (ĂL-ĕr-jē, p. 35)
anaphylactic reaction (ăn-ă-fĭ-LĂK-tĭk, p.35)
antagonistic effect (ăn-tăg-ŏ-NĬS-tĭk, p. 36)
antagonists (ăn-TĂG-ō-nĭsts, p. 32)
bioequivalent (BĪ-ō-ĭ-KWĬ V-ĭ-lent, p. 36)
biotransformation (BĪ-ō-trăns-fŏr-MĀ-shŭn, p. 34)
chemical name (KĔM-ĭ-kăl, p. 32)
desired action (ĂK-shŭn, p. 35)
displacement (dĭs-PLĂS-mĕnt, p. 36)
distribution (dĭs-trĭ-BŪ-shŭn, p. 33)
drug interaction (ĭn-tĕr-ĂK-shŭn, p. 36)
enteral (route) (ĔN-tĕr-ăl, p. 33)
excretion (ĕks-KRĒ-shŭn, p. 34)
first-pass (effect) (p. 34)
generic name (jĕn-ĔR-ĭk, p. 31)

half-life (p. 34)
hepatotoxic (hĕp-ă-tō-TŎK-sĭk, p. 35)
hypersensitivity (hī-pĕr-sĕn-sĭ-TĬV-ĭ-tē, p. 35)
idiosyncratic response (ĭd-ē-ō-sĭn-KRĂ-tĭk, p. 35)
incompatibility (ĭn-kŏm-păt-ĭ-BĬL-ĭ-tē, p. 36)
interference (ĭn-tŭr-FĔR-ĕns, p. 36)
nephrotoxic (nĕf-rō-TŎK-sĭk, p. 35)
official name (ō-FĬSH-ŭl, p. 32)
parenteral (route) (pĕ-RĔN-tĕr-ăl, p. 33)
partial agonists (PĂR-shăl ĂG-ō-nĭsts, p. 32)
percutaneous (route) (pĕr-kū-TĀ-nē-ŭs, p. 33)
pharmacodynamics (FĂRM-ă-kō-dĭ-NĂM-ĭks, p. 31)
pharmacokinetics (FĂRM-ă-kō-kĭNĔT-ĭks, p. 31)
pharmacotherapeutics (FĂRM-ă-kō-thĕr-ă-PŪ-tĭks, p. 31)
receptor site (rē-SĔP-tŏr, p. 32)
side effects (SĬD ĕf-FĔCTS, p. 35)
solubility (sŏl-ū-BĬL-ĭ-tē, p. 33)
synergistic effect (sĭn-ĕr-JĬS-tĭk, p. 37)
trade name (TRĀD, p. 32)

OVERVIEW

This chapter provides an overview of very basic information from chemistry, physics, anatomy, and physiology that explains the action of drugs in the body (**pharmacokinetics**, or what the body does to the drug). It also covers basic information on the effects of drugs on the functions of the body (**pharmacodynamics**, or what the drug does to the body). This information is vital in understanding **pharmacotherapeutics**, or the use of drugs in the treatment of disease (Box 4-1).

DRUG NAMES

Medications have several different names that may be confusing when you first learn to work with drugs. It is very important to know the different names of a

medication so that the wrong drug is not given to a patient. Sometimes a medication is ordered by one name for the drug and the pharmacist labels it with another name for the same drug. For example, Valium (trade name) is the same as diazepam (generic name). It is important to know whether the medication is the same or a different drug.

The most common drug name used is the **generic name**. This is the name the drug manufacturer uses for a drug, and it is the same in all countries. It is the name given to a drug before there is an official name, or when the drug has been available for many years and more than one company makes the drug. Examples would be penicillin and tetracycline. The American Pharmaceutical Association, the American Medical Association, and the U.S. Adopted Names Council

The word *drug* comes from the Dutch word *droog*, which means "dry." For centuries, most drugs used for treating health problems came from dried plants.

Medicines are those drugs used in the prevention or treatment of diseases.

Pharmacology deals with the study of drugs and the action of drugs on living organisms. It comes from the Greek words *pharmakon*, which means "drugs," and *logos*, which means "science."

Therapeutic regimen refers to all the methods to be used for treatment of disease. In addition to drug therapy, this may include plans for special diets; use of hot packs, whirlpools, or ultraviolet lights; and counseling, biofeedback, or psychotherapy.

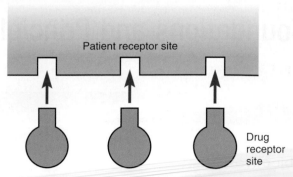

FIGURE 4-1 Drug receptor sites.

assign generic names. Generic names are not capitalized when written. An example is *warfarin*.

Another common drug name is the **trade name**, or brand name. This name is often followed by the symbol ®, which indicates that the name is registered to a specific drug maker or owner and no one else can use it. This is the drug name used in written or TV advertisements and other marketing, and it is often descriptive, easy to spell, or catchy sounding so that prescribers will remember it easily and be more likely to use it. The first letter of the trade name, and sometimes other letters, are capitalized. Examples of trade names are *Dimetapp, Lanoxin,* and *Augmentin*.

Chemical names are often the most difficult to remember, because they include the chemicals that make up the drug. These names are usually long and hyphenated, and they describe the atomic or molecular structure. An example is *ethyl 1-methyl-4-phenylisonipecotate hydrochloride,* the chemical name for meperidine (Demerol).

The final type of name is the **official name**, which is given by the Food and Drug Administration. Sometimes this name is similar to the brand or chemical name. The first letter of the official name is also capitalized. An example is *Ethacrynic acid.*

TYPES OF DRUG ACTIONS

 DRUG ATTACHMENT (DRUG-RECEPTOR BINDING)

Drugs take part in chemical reactions that change the way the body acts. They do this most commonly when the medication forms a chemical bond at a specific site in the body called a **receptor site** (Figure 4-1). The chemical reactions between a drug and a receptor site are possible only when the receptor site and the drug can fit together like pieces of a jigsaw puzzle or a key fitting into a lock. The drug attaches to the receptor site and activates the receptor; the drug has an action similar to the body's own chemicals.

Some drugs attach to the receptor site but produce only a small chemical response. These drugs are called **partial agonists**. When a drug attaches at a drug receptor site but there is no chemical drug response these are called **antagonists**. Some partial agonists and antagonists are able to compete with other chemicals or drugs already bonded to a receptor site and replace them. The Memory Jogger box summarizes the various types of receptor site activity.

 Memory Jogger

Drug Receptor Sites

Agonist: Drug attaches at receptor site and activates the receptor; the drug has an action similar to the body's own chemicals.

Antagonist: Drug attaches at drug receptor site, but no chemical drug response is produced and the drug prevents activation of the receptor.

Partial agonist: Drug attaches at drug receptor site, but only a slight chemical action is produced.

BASIC DRUG PROCESSES

Drugs must be changed chemically in the body to become usable. There are four basic processes involved in drug utilization in the body. These processes are absorption, distribution, metabolism, and excretion. Drugs have different characteristics, or pharmacokinetics, that determine to what extent these processes will be used. To understand how a drug works, the nurse must understand each of these processes for the specific drug being given.

The Process of Absorption

Absorption involves the way a drug enters the body and passes into the circulation. Absorption takes place through processes of diffusion, filtration, and osmosis. These mechanisms of absorption are more fully described in Box 4-2. How fast the drug is absorbed into the body through these processes depends on the solubility of the drug, the route of administration, and the degree of blood flow through the tissue where the medication is found.

| Box **4-2** | Mechanisms Involved in Absorption |

DIFFUSION

Diffusion is the tendency of the molecules of a substance (gas, liquid, or solid) to move from a region of high concentration to one of lower concentration.

OSMOSIS

Osmosis is the diffusion of fluid through a semipermeable membrane; the flow is primarily from the less thick or more concentrated solution to the thinner or less concentrated solution.

FILTRATION

Filtration is the passage of a substance through a filter or through a material that prevents passage of certain molecules.

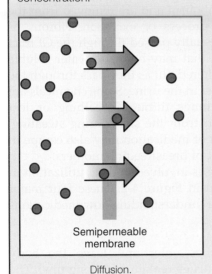

Semipermeable membrane

Diffusion.

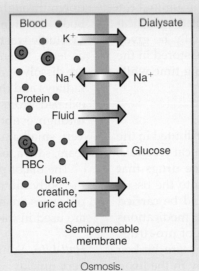

Semipermeable membrane

Osmosis.

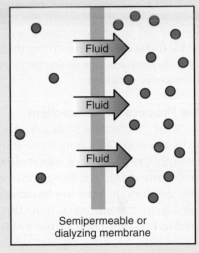

Semipermeable or dialyzing membrane

Filtration.

All medication must be dissolved in body fluid before it can enter body tissues. The ability of the medication to dissolve is called **solubility**. To achieve the best possible drug action, sometimes the medication must be dissolved quickly; at other times it should be dissolved slowly. Solubility of the drug is often controlled by the form of the medication; for example, solutions are more soluble than capsules because a liquid is absorbed faster than a tablet, which must dissolve. An injection with an oil base must be chemically changed before absorption can take place, and this holds the drug in the tissues longer, which may be the desired action. When the patient takes water with a tablet, it not only helps in swallowing but also helps dissolve the medication.

The route of administration also influences absorption. The most common medication routes are **enteral** (directly into the gastrointestinal [GI] tract through oral, nasogastric tube, or rectal administration); **parenteral** (directly into dermal, subcutaneous, or intramuscular tissue, epidurally into the cerebrospinal fluid, or into the bloodstream through intravenous [IV] injections); and **percutaneous** (through topical [skin], sublingual [under the tongue], buccal [against the cheek], or inhalation [breathing] administration).

In areas where the blood flow through tissues is very high, medication is rapidly absorbed. Examples of this include placing a nitroglycerin tablet under the tongue right next to blood vessels or spraying steroids into the nose and lungs through a nebulizer. IV medications injected into the bloodstream have the fastest

action. Oral or rectal medications usually take much longer because they must dissolve and diffuse across the barrier tissue in the GI tract (the gastric mucosa) before being carried to the body tissues where they will have their action.

The Process of Distribution

Once the medication is absorbed, it must travel throughout the body. The term **distribution** refers to the ways that drugs move by means of circulating body fluids to their sites of action in the body. The bloodstream and lymphatic system usually carry the drug throughout the whole body. The organs that have the biggest blood supply receive the medication faster, and areas of skin and fat receive the medication more slowly. Some drugs do not pass well through cell membranes with very small passages, such as those covering the placenta and the brain. These are referred to as *placental* and *blood-brain barriers*, although the *barrier* is not a complete barrier, because some drugs and some conditions make it possible for drugs to easily pass through these areas. The various types of tissues, including bone, fat, and muscle, do not absorb equal amounts of the drug. Thus the distribution is different for different drugs.

The chemical properties of a drug also affect how the drug is distributed. Some chemicals bind together with proteins such as albumin (found in the blood plasma), which serve as carriers giving a ride to drugs that are not easily dissolved. The ratio of bound chemical compared with free chemical remains the same in the blood. As more of the free chemical diffuses into the tissues, more of the bound chemical becomes unlocked and thus also available to diffuse.

Some medications are attracted to tissues other than the target receptor sites. For example, medications that dissolve easily in lipids (fats) prefer adipose, or fat tissue, and stores of the medication may build up in these areas. As the medication moving throughout the body binds at the receptor sites, more of the medication stored in adipose tissue will gradually be given up by those cells. Thus a drug that can be stored in the fat cells may remain in the body for a long time while it is slowly released.

The Process of Metabolism

Once the medication is absorbed and distributed in the body, the body's enzymes use it in chemical reactions through the process of metabolism. Some drugs that are breathed into the lungs or injected into the tissue may go directly into the bloodstream and be carried quickly to the site of action. But many medications have to be stimulated or have activation of pro-drugs before they become usable, while drugs are broken down into smaller usable parts, primarily in the liver, through a series of complex chemical reactions until they become chemically inactive. This process is called **biotransformation**. When most of a medicine goes very quickly to the liver, a lot of the medication is inactivated on its "**first-pass**" through the liver before it can be distributed to other parts of the body. That is why some medicines are given sublingually or intravenously; otherwise, patients do not get the amount of medication they require. (For example, only 1 mg of propranolol is required intravenously, but 40 mg are required when the drug is given by mouth.)

Genetic differences in the enzyme pathways in the liver also explain why people respond differently to a drug—whether they grow tolerant of the drug and seem to need larger doses, or whether they are sensitive to the drug and only need a small dose. These enzyme pathways, known as the *cytochrome P-450 system*, play

an important role in the adverse drug reactions patients may have when taking several drugs at the same time or when there are drug-food interactions.

The Process of Excretion or Elimination

All inactive chemicals, chemical by-products, and waste (often referred to as *metabolites*) finally break down through metabolism and are removed from the body through the process of **excretion**. Fibrous or insoluble waste is usually passed through the GI tract as feces. Chemicals that may be made water soluble are dissolved and filtered out as they pass through the kidneys and then lost in the urine. Some chemicals are exhaled from the lungs through breathing or lost through evaporation from the skin during sweating. Very small amounts of medication may also escape in tears, saliva, or milk of breastfeeding mothers.

The major processes involved in drug utilization in the body are shown in Figure 4-2. These four major processes are basic to understanding how medications are used in the body.

Half-Life. Some drugs enter and leave the body very quickly; other drugs remain for a long time. The standard method of describing how long it takes to metabolize and excrete a drug is the **half-life**, or the time it takes the body to remove 50% of the drug from the body. Because the rates of metabolism and excretion are usually the same for most people, the half-life helps explain the dose (how much medicine should be taken), the frequency (how often it should be taken), and the duration (how long it will last) for different drugs. If a drug has a long half-life, it may need to be taken only once a day. If a person takes too much medication with a long half-life, this may cause a serious problem because the action of the drug lasts for such a long time. If the half-life of a drug is short, such as for many antibiotics, the person must take frequent doses to keep the correct level in the blood. If a person's liver or kidneys do not function correctly, medications may not be properly metabolized or

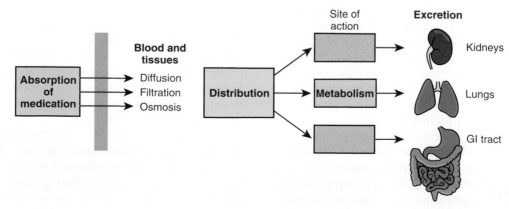

FIGURE 4-2 Processes of absorption, distribution, metabolism, and excretion. *GI*, gastrointestinal.

excreted, and this would mean that higher doses of the medication will circulate for a longer time and produce symptoms of overdosage. Drugs are often dosed based on renal and hepatic function for this reason. Therefore the function of the kidneys and liver are watched by doing repeated renal and hepatic tests.

BASICS OF DRUG ACTION

When a drug is given to a patient, it is usually possible to predict the chemical reaction that will be seen. However, because each patient is different, some unexpected chemical reactions are also seen. With each patient, giving a medication is somewhat of an experiment, so patients must be watched closely to monitor their reaction to the medication.

The expected response of the medication is called the **desired action**. This is when the medication does what is desired, and the therapeutic goal is reached (for example, meperidine [Demerol] relieves pain).

Because a medication may influence many body systems at the same time, the effect of the medication is often not restricted to the desired action. Other actions called *side effects* or *adverse reactions* may also take place. **Side effects** are usually seen as mild but annoying responses to the medication. **Adverse reactions**, or adverse effects, usually imply more severe symptoms or problems that develop because of the drug. Some adverse effects may require the patient to be hospitalized or may even be life threatening. Some side effects, such as drowsiness, may go away after the patient takes the medication for a time. Certain side effects, such as nausea, may be stopped if the dosage is reduced. Some side effects are such a problem that the medication must be changed or stopped. An example of this might be insomnia (inability to sleep) or making the patient pass out. Certainly, if severe adverse effects such as damage to the kidney (**nephrotoxic** drug) or liver (**hepatotoxic** drug) or bleeding develop, the medication must often be stopped.

Occasionally a patient may have a drug reaction that is a surprise. Strange, unique, or unpredicted responses are called **idiosyncratic responses**. These reactions may be the result of missing or defective metabolic enzymes caused by a genetic or hormonal variation. They often produce either an unexpected result, such as pain or bleeding, or an overresponse to the drug. These types of reactions are usually rare. One type of idiosyncratic response is called a *paradoxical response*. In this situation, the patient's reaction may be just the opposite of what would be expected. For example, pseudoephedrine hydrochloride, a chemical that was used until a few years ago in decongestants for children, usually produces sedation or drowsiness as a side effect. However, some children respond in the opposite way, having insomnia and tachycardia (rapid heartbeat) and are overly stimulated.

A second type of unexpected reaction is an increased reaction to a drug (**hypersensitivity**) or a sensitivity caused by antibody response to a drug (**allergy**). Some medications (sulfa products, aspirin, penicillin) and some conditions (asthma) are more likely to produce allergic reactions than others. Allergic reactions usually occur when an individual has taken the drug and the body has developed antibodies to it. When the patient takes the drug again, the antigen-antibody reaction produces hives, rash, itching, or swelling of the skin. This type of allergic reaction is very common, so ask all patients about whether they have ever had a drug reaction. Patients with an allergy to one medication may be more likely to develop an allergy to another medication, but individuals may also develop a reaction to medications they have taken before without problems.

Occasionally, the allergic reaction is so severe the patient has trouble breathing, and rarely the heart may stop. This life-threatening response is called an **anaphylactic reaction**. A patient who has a mild allergic reaction to a medication is much more likely to develop the more severe anaphylactic reaction if the medication is given again. An anaphylactic reaction is a true medical emergency because the patient may suffer paralysis of the diaphragm and swelling of the oropharynx that interfere with breathing. Patients who have anaphylactic reactions should always be warned about their allergy so they will not take the drug again, and they should wear a Medic Alert bracelet or necklace or carry identification about their allergy.

Patients often confuse an allergy with side effects—both of which may produce unpleasant symptoms. If a patient reports an "allergy" to a drug, make sure you ask the right questions to understand the exact past reaction to the drug. If the patient had nausea or stomach pain when taking aspirin, that is a side effect, but not an allergy. If the patient reported sedation when taking an antihypertensive medication, that is also not an allergy. Because patients often do not understand the difference between an allergy and a side effect, it is important to clarify the difference when patients say they have had an allergic reaction

The common responses to medications are listed in Box 4-3.

BIOEQUIVALENCE

After a new drug enters the market, a patent protects the financial interest of the drug company for some time, usually 17 years, by limiting other companies from producing that drug. After the patent ends, other companies may file an application to make the same drug under a generic name. Brand-name drugs are usually more expensive than generic drugs because the maker of the brand-name drug is attempting to recover the huge sums of money spent on research and making of the drug. Thus generic products are often less expensive.

Box 4-3 Common Responses to Medications

DESIRED EFFECT

When the desired effect takes place, the therapeutic goal is achieved. The drug does what it is supposed to do. An example is temperature reduction after taking aspirin.

SIDE EFFECT

Side effects are mild but annoying responses to medication. An example is nausea caused by an antibiotic or oral contraceptive.

ADVERSE EFFECT

Adverse effects are more severe symptoms or problems that arise because of the medication. An example is a patient who develops severe gastric bleeding from an ulcer caused by aspirin.

IDIOSYNCRATIC RESPONSE

Idiosyncratic responses are strange, unique, or unpredicted reactions. An example is blood in the urine caused by aspirin. This is rare.

PARADOXICAL REACTION

Paradoxical reactions are reactions that are the opposite of what would be expected.

ALLERGIC RESPONSE

An allergic response is an antigen-antibody reaction. The body develops hives, rashes, itching, or swelling of the skin. A rash or shortness of breath is occasionally seen in patients allergic to aspirin.

ANAPHYLACTIC RESPONSE

An anaphylactic response is a severe form of allergic reaction that is life threatening. The patient develops severe shortness of breath, may stop breathing, or may have cardiac collapse.

Box 4-4 Common Drug Interactions

ADDITIVE EFFECT

When two drugs are given together, the combined effect of the drugs is equal to either that of the single more active component of the mixture or the sum of the effects of the individual drugs.

ANTAGONISTIC EFFECT

An antagonistic effect takes place when one drug interferes with the action of another drug.

DISPLACEMENT

Displacement takes place when one drug replaces another at the drug receptor site, increasing the effect of the first drug.

INCOMPATIBILITY

Incompatibility occurs when two drugs mixed together in a syringe produce a chemical reaction, so they cannot be given.

INTERFERENCE

Interference occurs when one drug promotes the rapid excretion of another, thus reducing its activity.

SYNERGISTIC EFFECT

A synergistic effect takes place when the effect of two drugs taken at the same time is greater than the sum of the effects of each drug given alone.

Drug products seen as identical with respect to their active ingredients are known as *generic equivalents.* However, slight differences in processing or formulation may mean that the action of the generic drug in the body is slightly different from that of the brand-name product. These differences most commonly cause variations in absorption, distribution, or metabolism. Thus what product the patient actually purchases when a prescription is written for a drug may vary according to what specific brand the pharmacist dispenses. Some products are chemically the same or identical and thus **bioequivalent**. Some products are quite different, and thus the medication that is given by the pharmacist should not be changed from what the prescriber has written. This may be particularly important for some cardiac or antiseizure medications.

DRUG INTERACTIONS

When one drug changes the action of another drug, a **drug interaction** is present. These reactions often take place during the process of metabolism (or biotransformation) in the liver and are a result of the cytochrome P-450 enzyme pathways each person inherits. The actions of a number of drugs may be altered when they are taken with other drugs; these drugs include many antidepressants, theophylline, warfarin, cimetidine, ciprofloxacin, isoniazid, ketoconazole, phenytoin, zafirlukast, phenobarbital, rifampin, codeine, and morphine. Some medications are given together on purpose because the drug interactions are helpful. For example, probenecid is given with penicillin to increase the amount of penicillin that is absorbed, which is important in treating venereal disease. Other drug interactions produce adverse effects. For example, some antibiotics make birth control pills less effective, thus making it more likely a woman will get pregnant.

Several types of effects are seen with drug interactions (Box 4-4). When two drugs are given together, and the combined effect of the drugs is equal to either that of the most active drug or the sum of the effects of the individual drugs, an **additive effect** is seen. If one drug interferes with the action of another drug, it is described as an **antagonistic effect**. At times, one drug may replace another drug at a receptor site, increasing the effect of the first drug. This is called **displacement**. Sometimes **incompatibility** occurs when drugs do not mix well chemically. Attempts to mix them together in a syringe may cause a chemical reaction, so neither of the drugs can be given. **Interference** is seen when one drug promotes the rapid excretion of another drug, thus reducing its activity. Finally, if the effect of two drugs taken at the same time is greater than the sum of the effects of each drug given alone, the drugs have a **synergistic effect**. This is often seen when individuals are exposed to pollutants and toxins. *Potentiation* is one type of synergistic effect in which a drug that might produce only a small effect by itself produces a larger effect when given with another specific drug.

Food, Alcohol, and Drug Interactions

Food, alcohol, and most medications taken by mouth must travel through the liver for chemical changes before they can be used by the body. Thus the risk for drug interaction with food or alcohol is high. When taken together, food or alcohol and drugs may alter the body's ability to use a particular food or drug. Part of these interactions may be due to activation of the P-450 enzyme system or competition for receptor sites. Monoamine oxidase inhibitors are some of the drugs most noted for drug-food interactions, because they cannot be taken with aged cheese or many processed foods. Information every patient should know about possible drug interactions includes the following:

- Cigarette smoking can decrease the effect of medication or create other problems with some drugs by increasing metabolism.
- Caffeine, which is found in coffee, tea, some soft drinks, chocolate, and some medications, can also affect the action of some drugs.
- Medication should never be taken during pregnancy or by a patient trying to get pregnant without the advice of the health care provider.
- If the patient has any problem related to medication, the health care provider or a pharmacist should be contacted immediately.

Alcohol-Medication Interactions. The amount of alcohol use is very high in the U.S. population. It has been estimated that approximately 70% of adults consume alcohol at least occasionally, and up to 10% of people may drink daily. Many patients may not be aware that alcohol is one of the products that reacts most commonly with drugs. The extent to which a dose of medicine reaches its site of action is called *availability*. Alcohol can influence whether a drug is effective by changing its availability.

In an alert from the National Institute on Alcohol Abuse and Alcoholism* it was estimated that alcohol-medication interactions may be a factor in at least 25% of all emergency department admissions. An unknown number of less serious interactions go unrecognized and unrecorded. One group of individuals at high risk for alcohol-drug interactions is older adults, who take 25% to 30% of all prescription medications and also frequently drink alcohol. Older adults are more likely to suffer medication side effects compared with younger persons, and these effects tend to be more severe with advancing age.

Table 4-1 provides information about food-drug-alcohol interactions patients should know.

Drug Effects on Laboratory Tests and Blood Substances. Although medications exert a therapeutic effect in the body, they may also have effects on various natural substances in the blood, or they may alter the results of some laboratory tests. For example, the drug may increase the blood glucose level or affect the clotting time. Nurses should be aware of these changes as they look at the results of laboratory tests and try to monitor the action of a drug.

Chronotherapy. Research has shown that certain drugs are more effective at different times of the day, and drug treatment may work best when it is linked to the normal human circadian rhythm (a repetitive cycle based on a 24-hour clock). The circadian clock controls rhythms in endocrine gland secretion, metabolic processes, and behavioral activity. Certain diseases, such as asthma, angina, diabetes mellitus, and hypertension, get better or worse throughout the day according to the circadian cycle. Chronotherapy is a process that attempts to time the drug action so that it occurs when that action is most needed by the body.

PATIENT VARIABLES AFFECTING DRUG USE

Special knowledge and sometimes special medications are required for neonates, small children, adults, and older adult patients. Women who are pregnant have special risks when they take any type of medication. People of different cultures also have different attitudes about medication use. When giving medications, all these factors are important for the nurse to know and may affect the nursing care plan. (These variables are discussed in greater detail in Chapters 5 and 6.)

---

*Alcohol-medication interactions, Alcohol Alert No. 27 (PH 355), Washington DC, January 1995, National Institute on Alcohol Abuse and Alcoholism.

Table 4-1 Specific Food-Alcohol-Drug Interactions by Drug Category

MEDICATION CATEGORY	COMMON MEDICATION EXAMPLES	INTERACTIONS AND INSTRUCTIONS TO GIVE PATIENTS
Drugs for Pain		
Analgesics-antipyretics—used to relieve pain and reduce fever.	Acetaminophen (Tylenol, Tempra)	Take on an empty stomach for more rapid relief; food may slow the body's absorption of the drug. Avoid alcohol because it can increase the risk of liver damage or GI bleeding.
Analgesics-narcotics—used to suppress cough and relieve pain; often with ASA or acetaminophen.	Codeine with aspirin; codeine with acetaminophen (Tylenol #2, #3, #4); morphine (Roxanol, MS Contin); oxycodone with acetaminophen (Percocet, Roxicet); meperidine (Demerol); hydrocodone with acetaminophen (Vicodin, Lorcet)	Avoid alcohol because it increases the sedative effect of these medications. Take with meals, small snacks, or milk; these medications may cause stomach upset. Use caution when motor skills are required.
Respiratory Tract Drugs		
Antihistamines—used to relieve or prevent symptoms of colds, hay fever, and other types of allergy. They act to limit or block histamine.	Brompheniramine (Dimetapp, Bromphenex, chlorpheniramine/Chlor-Trimeton, Teldrin); diphenhydramine (Benadryl, Banophen); clemastine (Tavist); fexofenadine (Allegra); loratadine (Claritin); cetirizine (Zyrtec)	Avoid alcohol; antihistamines combined with alcohol may cause drowsiness and slowed reactions. Take prescription antihistamines on an empty stomach to increase their effectiveness.
Bronchodilators—used to treat the symptoms of bronchial asthma, chronic bronchitis, and emphysema. These medicines relieve wheezing, SOB, and dyspnea. They work by opening the air passages of the lungs.	Theophylline (Slo-bid, Uniphyl); albuterol (Ventolin, Proventil, Combivent); epinephrine (Primatene Mist)	Avoid eating or drinking large amounts of foods or beverages that contain caffeine; both bronchodilators and caffeine stimulate the central nervous system. High-fat meals may increase the amount of theophylline in the body, whereas high-carbohydrate meals may decrease it. The effect of food on theophylline products varies. Many over-the-counter cold remedies contain aspirin in combination with other active ingredients.
Antiinflammatory and Antiallergic Drugs		
Aspirin—used to reduce pain, fever, and inflammation.	Aspirin (Bayer, Ecotrin)	Aspirin can cause stomach irritation; avoid alcohol. To avoid stomach upset, take with food. Do not take with fruit juice. Buffered aspirin or enteric-coated aspirin may also reduce GI bleeding.
Corticosteroids—used to provide relief to inflamed areas. Lessen swelling, redness, itching, and allergic reactions.	Methylprednisolone (Medrol); prednisone (Deltasone); prednisolone (Pediapred, Prelone); cortisone acetate (Cortef)	Take with food or milk to decrease GI distress. Avoid alcohol; both alcohol and corticosteroids can cause stomach irritation. Also avoid foods high in sodium (salt). Check labels on food packages for sodium content. Take with food to prevent stomach upset.
NSAIDs—used to relieve pain and reduce inflammation and fever.	Ibuprofen (Advil, Motrin); naproxen (Anaprox, Aleve, Naprosyn); ketoprofen; nabumetone	Should be taken with food or milk; can irritate the stomach. Avoid taking these medications with foods or alcoholic or other beverages that tend to bother the stomach.
Drugs for Bone and Joint Disorders		
Indomethacin—used to reduce pain, swelling, stiffness, joint pain, and fever in certain types of arthritis and gout.	Indomethacin (Indocin)	Should be taken with food; can irritate the stomach. Avoid taking medication with foods or alcoholic or other beverages that tend to irritate the stomach.

Table 4-1   Specific Food-Alcohol-Drug Interactions by Drug Category—cont'd

MEDICATION CATEGORY	COMMON MEDICATION EXAMPLES	INTERACTIONS AND INSTRUCTIONS TO GIVE PATIENTS
Piroxicam—used to reduce pain, swelling, stiffness, joint pain, and fever in certain types of arthritis.	Piroxicam (Feldene)	Should be taken with a light snack; can cause stomach irritation. Avoid alcohol; can add to the possibility of stomach upset.
Diuretics		
Used to eliminate water, sodium, and chloride.	Furosemide (Lasix); hydrochlorothiazide (HydroDIURIL); triamterene (Dyrenium); bumetanide (Bumex); metolazone (Zaroxolyn); triamterene 1 hydrochlorothiazide (Dyazide, Maxzide)	Diuretics vary in their interactions with nutrients. Loss of potassium, calcium, and magnesium occurs with some diuretics. May require potassium supplement. With some diuretics, potassium loss is less significant.
Drugs for the Heart, Blood Vessels, and Blood		
Nitrates—used to relax veins and arteries to reduce work of the heart.	Nitroglycerin (Nitro-Bid, Nitro-Dur); isosorbide dinitrate (Isordil)	Use of sodium (salt) should be restricted for medication to be effective. Use with alcohol may drastically lower blood pressure. Check labels on food packages for sodium.
Antihypertensives—used to relax blood vessels, increase the supply of blood and oxygen to the heart, and lessen the heart's workload. May regulate heartbeat.	Beta blockers: atenolol (Tenormin); metoprolol (Lopressor); propranolol (Inderal); nadolol (Corgard) ACE inhibitors: captopril (Capoten); enalapril (Vasotec); lisinopril (Prinivil, Zestril); quinapril (Accupril); moexipril (Univasc)	Beta blockers: Use of sodium should be restricted for medication to be effective. Check labels on food packages for sodium content. Alcohol and propranolol in combination may dramatically lower blood pressure. ACE inhibitors: Food can decrease absorption. ACE inhibitors may increase blood levels of potassium. Avoid eating large amounts of foods high in potassium.
Anticoagulants—used to prolong clotting of the blood.	Warfarin (Coumadin)	Over 707 drugs are known to interact with this product. Check for interactions with any other drug that is ordered.
Antihyperlipidemics—HMG-CoA reductase inhibitors, or "statins," used to lower cholesterol.	Atorvastatin (Lipitor); fluvastatin (Lescol); lovastatin (Mevacor); pravastatin (Pravachol); simvastatin (Zocor)	Mevacor should be taken with the evening meal to enhance absorption. Avoid large amounts of alcohol; may increase risk of liver damage.
Antiinfectives		
Cephalosporins	Cefaclor (Ceclor, Ceclor CD); cefadroxil (Duricef); cefixime (Suprax); cefprozil (Cefzil); cephalexin (Keflex, Keftab)	Take on an empty stomach 1 hr before or 2 hr after meals. Can be taken with food if severe GI upset occurs.
Macrolides—used to treat skin, ear infections.	Erythromycin (E-Mycin, Ery-Tab, Eryc); erythromycin 1 sulfisoxazole (Pediazole); azithromycin (Zithromax); clarithromycin (Biaxin)	Macrolides vary in their reactions with food. Avoid acidic fruit juices, citrus fruits, or acidic beverages such as cola drinks; these antibiotics are acid labile (acid reduces absorption). Take on an empty stomach 1 hr before or 2 hr after meals.
Methenamine—used in treating urinary tract infections.	Mandelamine, Urex	Avoid citrus fruits and citrus juices, but cranberries, plums, prunes, and their juices help the action of this drug. Eat foods with protein, but avoid dairy products.
Metronidazole—used to treat intestinal and genital infections caused by bacteria and parasites.	Flagyl	Avoid using any form of alcohol while taking this drug; severe, prolonged vomiting and other symptoms may develop (Antabuse or disulfiram-reaction).

Continued

Table 4-1   Specific Food-Alcohol-Drug Interactions by Drug Category—cont'd

MEDICATION CATEGORY	COMMON MEDICATION EXAMPLES	INTERACTIONS AND INSTRUCTIONS TO GIVE PATIENTS
Penicillins—used to treat a wide variety of infections.	Amoxicillin (Trimox, Amoxil); ampicillin (Principen, Omnipen); penicillin V (Veetids)	Amoxicillin and bacampicillin may be taken with food, but absorption of other types of penicillins is reduced when taken with food. Avoid acidic fruit juices, citrus fruits, or acidic beverages such as cola drinks; penicillins are acid labile (acid reduces absorption). Take on an empty stomach 1 hr before or 2 hr after meals.
Quinolones	Ciprofloxacin (Cipro); levofloxacin (Levaquin); ofloxacin (Floxin);	Take on an empty stomach 1 hr before or 2 hr after meals. Can be taken with food if severe GI upset occurs. Avoid calcium-containing products, vitamins and minerals containing iron, and antacids; they significantly decrease drug concentrations. Taking with caffeine products may increase caffeine levels and produce excitability and nervousness.
Sulfonamides—used to treat stomach and urinary infections.	Sulfamethoxazole and trimethoprim (Bactrim, Septra)	Avoid alcohol; combination may cause nausea. Take on an empty stomach, if possible.
Tetracyclines—used to treat a wide variety of infections.	Tetracycline (Achromycin, Sumycin); doxycycline (Vibramycin); minocycline (Minocin)	Should not be taken within 2 hr of eating dairy products (milk, ice cream, yogurt, cheese) or taking calcium or iron supplements. Calcium forms a complex with the drug, resulting in reduced absorption of antibiotic. Take 1 hr before meals or 2 hr after.
Antifungals	Fluconazole (Diflucan); griseofulvin (Grifulvin); ketoconazole (Nizoral); itraconazole (Sporanox)	Avoid taking with dairy products or antacids. Avoid drinking alcohol or using medications or food that contain alcohol for at least 3 days after taking ketoconazole. It may produce a disulfiram-type reaction.
Drugs for Psychiatric Problems		
Antianxiety drugs	Lorazepam (Ativan); diazepam (Valium); alprazolam (Xanax)	Use with caffeine may cause excitability, nervousness, and hyperactivity and lessen the antianxiety effect. Use with alcohol may impair mental and motor functions.
Antidepressants	Paroxetine (Paxil), sertraline (Zoloft), fluoxetine (Prozac)	Avoid concurrent use with alcohol. These medications can be taken with or without food.
Lithium carbonate—regulates changes in chemical levels in the brain.	Various names	Follow the dietary and fluid intake instructions of the health care provider to avoid very serious toxic reactions.
MAO inhibitors—antidepressants	Phenelzine (Nardil); tranylcypromine (Parnate)	A very dangerous, potentially fatal interaction can occur with foods containing tyramine, a chemical in alcoholic beverages (particularly wine) and many foods (e.g., hard cheeses, chocolate, beef or chicken livers, sour cream, yogurt, raisins, bananas, avocados, soy sauce, yeast extract, meat tenderizers, sausages, anchovies). Patient may develop severe headache, nosebleed, chest pain, photosensitivity, or severe hypertension with hypertensive crisis.
Sedative-hypnotics	Various names	Do not use alcohol with any sleep medications; oversedation occurs.

Table 4-1   Specific Food-Alcohol-Drug Interactions by Drug Category—cont'd

MEDICATION CATEGORY	COMMON MEDICATION EXAMPLES	INTERACTIONS AND INSTRUCTIONS TO GIVE PATIENTS
Antacids, Antiulcer Medications, and Histamine Blockers		
Work to reduce acid in the stomach.	Cimetidine (Tagamet); famotidine (Pepcid); ranitidine (Zantac); nizatidine (Axid)	Follow specific diets given by health care provider. Avoid large amounts of caffeine; dairy products such as milk or cream may increase acid secretion. If calcium carbonate is used as a calcium supplement, avoid bran and whole-grain breads or cereals that reduce absorption of calcium.
Laxatives		
Stimulate intestine, soften stool, add bulk or fluid to stool.	Various names	Excessive use of laxatives can cause loss of essential vitamins and minerals and may require replenishment of potassium, sodium, and other nutrients through diet. Mineral oil can cause poor absorption of vitamins A, D, E, and K, and calcium. Take 2 hr before eating food.

Modified from Food & Drug Interactions, Washington DC, 2004, National Consumers League (available at http://www.nclnet.org); McKenry LM, Tessier E, Hogan MA: *Mosby's pharmacology in nursing*, ed 22, St Louis, 2006, Mosby.
ACE, Angiotensin-converting enzyme; *ASA,* acetylsalicylic acid; *GI,* gastrointestinal; *HMG-CoA,* 3-hydroxy-3-methylglutaryl coenzyme A; *hr,* hour; *MAO,* monoamine oxidase; *NSAIDs,* nonsteroidal antiinflammatory drugs; *SOB,* shortness of breath.

Get Ready for the NCLEX® Examination!

Key Points

- As you prepare to administer medications, you must be aware of the pharmacologic actions of each drug.
- You must learn about the absorption, distribution, metabolism, and excretion actions of each drug.
- The information gained through assessment of the patient added to the nurse's knowledge about the expected patient response, side effects, adverse effects, and drug interactions become the foundation for the diagnosis, planning, implementation, and evaluation of the patient's response to the medication.

Additional Learning Resources

SG Go to your Study Guide for additional learning activities to help you master this chapter content.

evolve Go to your Evolve website (http://evolve.elsevier.com/Edmunds/LPN/) for additional online resources.

Review Questions for the NCLEX® Examination

1. The nurse is administering medication. The nurse anticipates the medication with the fastest action will be:
   1. medication administered by mouth
   2. medication administered by injection
   3. medication administered topically
   4. medication administered intravenously

2. The patient is given a medication that will help him to sleep. Instead, he stays awake all night. This response to the medication is considered a(n):
   1. idiosyncratic response
   2. adverse reaction
   3. side effects
   4. anaphylactic reaction

3. The patient is prescribed a medication that leads to extremely difficulty breathing. This response to the medication is most likely to be considered a(n):
   1. adverse reaction
   2. anaphylactic reaction
   3. side effects
   4. idiosyncratic response

4. The nurse is administering two drugs and finds that one drug promotes the rapid excretion of the other drug. This type of response is most likely the result of:
   1. displacement
   2. additive effect
   3. antagonistic effect
   4. interference

5. The nurse is administering two drugs and finds that the effect of the two drugs taken together is greater than the sum of the effects of each drug were it given alone. This response is most likely to be the result of:
   1. interference
   2. synergy
   3. displacement
   4. incompatibility

Get Ready for the NCLEX® Examination!—cont'd

Critical Thinking Questions

1. Using the *Physician's Desk Reference*, a comprehensive drug handbook, or drug package inserts from a pharmacy, complete the following chart, identifying the appropriate names for each drug:

Generic Name	Chemical Name	Official Name	Brand Name
Phenobarbital	_____	_____	_____
Metronidazole	_____	_____	_____
Keflex	_____	_____	_____
Albuterol	_____	_____	_____
Valium	_____	_____	_____

2. Sometimes the brand-name version of a drug is more expensive than a generic version of the same drug. Can you always substitute a generic drug for a brand-name version? Explain.

3. To get an idea of the range of chemical reactions that can be involved with a single drug, take these steps:
   a. Pick a drug from the index of this text, look it up, and describe each of the following actions or reactions as it applies to the drug you have chosen to investigate: adverse reaction, anaphylactic reaction, desired action, drug interaction, and side effect.
   b. What did you learn about the differences in these effects or reactions? For instance, what is the difference between a side effect and an adverse reaction?
   c. Now, if time permits, repeat this exercise with another drug of your choice.

4. Choose a drug. In the second column of the following table, define the physiologic processes listed in the first column. In the third column, describe how the drug you chose is absorbed, distributed, metabolized, and excreted.
   Drug:_____

Process	Definition	Action
Absorption		
Distribution		
Metabolism		
Excretion		

5. Referring to the information you gathered in Question 4, what factors may affect these processes? Why?

6. Using Unit Three as your resource, work with a partner to find examples of each of the following types of drug interactions:
   Displacement
   Incompatibility
   Interference

7. The patient states that he is "allergic to codeine." When the nurse inquires further, the patient reports that he became severely constipated when he took codeine. Is this a drug allergy?

Lifespan and Cultural Modifications

Objectives

1. Identify specific considerations in giving medications to pediatric, pregnant, breastfeeding, or older adult patients.
2. Identify special considerations in providing care to individuals from different cultures.
3. Describe specific nursing behaviors that assist in helping patients succeed with their medication plans.

Key Terms

adolescence (ăd-ō-LĔS-ĕns, p. 43)
culture (p. 53)
geriatric (jĕr-ē-T-rĭk, p. 46)
infants (p. 44)
neonates (NĔ-ō-nāts, p. 43)

noncompliance (NŌN-cŏm-PLĪ-ăns, p. 54)
pediatric (pē-dē-ĀT-rĭk, p. 45)
regimen (RĔJ-ĭ-mĕn, p. 48)
teratogenic (TĔR-ă-tō-JĔN-ĭk, p. 49)

OVERVIEW

As the nurse learns how to give medications, he or she will see there are many differences in the medications patients take. There are differences in the patients as well. For example, small infants cannot take the same medication dosages as adults. Older adult patients may have several diseases that require many drugs; their risk for drug problems increases with every new product given. What type of special information does the nurse need to know to care for patients from birth to death?

Patient variables, or differences such as age, weight, and other diseases or medications they may be taking, affect how a drug acts in the body. Many cultural and even religious beliefs may influence whether a patient is willing to even take medication. Helping the patient understand how important it is to take a medication and how to take it properly can be a challenge. Learning about patients' backgrounds and the things that are important to the nurse will assist the nurse in helping patients to get well.

PATIENT FACTORS THAT MAY AFFECT DRUG ACTION

Before a drug can be sold, a lot of research is done, and after people begin using the new drug, much additional information is gathered. Standards have been set up by the U.S. Food and Drug Administration (FDA) to require drug companies to provide certain information to people who may prescribe, administer, or take the drugs they manufacture. This information includes a description of the therapeutic response, side effects, and adverse effects of the drug, and a list of other drugs that may interact with this drug. Information must be printed by the manufacturer and put into the drug box (the "product package insert").

General factors that influence drug activity help the nurse figure out what the response to the medication should be. Some of these patient factors or variables are listed in Box 5-1.

SPECIAL CONSIDERATIONS FOR THE PEDIATRIC PATIENT

The changes that occur as a child grows from birth to adolescence (12 to 16 years of age) have a huge or profound effect on drug action and effect. Some changes are obvious, but mild or subtle changes in their responses to drugs occur as children grow and develop.

The terms *child* or *children* cover a very broad category from neonates to 16-year-old adolescents. A very small amount of drug may have a big effect on neonates (less than 1 month of age) because of their small body mass, low body-fat content, high body-water volume, and increased membrane permeability (for example, the skin or the blood-brain barrier). Immediately after birth, several factors influence drug absorption: no gastric acid is present to help break down drugs, no intestinal bacteria or enzyme function is

Box 5-1   Patient Variables Influencing Drug Action

BODY WEIGHT

An overweight individual requires a larger dosage. An underweight individual requires a smaller dosage.

AGE

Infants and children require smaller dosages. They have smaller fat and total water content, immature enzyme systems, reduced kidney function, and variation in circulating blood proteins.

Older adults may require smaller dosages because of changes in cellular composition and functioning throughout the body (especially in the liver and kidney), the presence of several disease processes, and the necessity for many medications.

ILLNESS

The type of pathologic process influences body processes. Nephrotic syndrome, dehydration, malabsorption, or malnutrition may cause changes in blood volume and protein composition. Kidney disease produces changes in blood and electrolyte concentrations. Liver disease leads to decreased metabolism of some drugs and foods. Hyperthyroidism may produce a higher metabolic rate, which increases drug metabolism. A patient in shock may have reduced circulation with delays in drug distribution in tissues.

PREGNANCY AND BREASTFEEDING

Many drugs are contraindicated during pregnancy because of the teratogenic effect on the fetus. Medications may also be passed to the child through breast milk. Therefore no pregnant or breastfeeding mother should take any medications without contacting her health care provider. The FDA (Food and Drug Administration) requires that all drug manufacturers supply published information regarding the safety of drugs when taken during pregnancy.

GENETICS

The genetic makeup of each individual influences such factors as the cytochrome P-450 enzyme system of metabolism in the liver, as well as patient intolerance to some medications. For example, atropine is contraindicated in patients with angle-closure glaucoma, anesthetic agents may precipitate sickle cell anemia crisis, and salicylates may trigger Crigler-Najjar syndrome.

CUMULATIVE DRUG EFFECTS

A drug may reach a higher level than needed because it is administered too often, the dosage is too high, or other drugs or chemicals (such as alcohol) that increase the effect of the drug are taken at the same time. The drug may accumulate in a high concentration and produce side effects.

INDIVIDUAL PSYCHOLOGY

The patient's attitude about drug acceptability and effectiveness is important. Some patients can be given a placebo, which is made of an inert or ineffective substance, which can be as effective as real medication in certain cases. Other patients develop tolerance or a need for an increased dosage over time to produce the same effects. This is often a symptom of psychologic dependence.

DEPENDENCE

An individual may develop both a physical and a psychologic need for a drug, usually a controlled substance. This may also be termed *addiction* or *habituation*.

---

present to metabolize a drug, and the gastrointestinal (GI) transit time (the time it takes for a drug to move through the stomach and intestines) is slow. The systems that deactivate drugs in the liver are immature, and even the immaturity of the kidney and renal excretion system adds to the speed with which a drug might be eliminated in the neonate.

In **infants** (1 month to 12 to 24 months of age) and young children, the decrease in total body water, increase in body mass, decrease in membrane permeability, and changes in body fat produce less obvious changes in drug response. The infant has a high metabolic rate and a rapid turnover of body water, which result in relatively higher fluid, calorie, and drug dosage requirements per kilogram of body weight than those of the adolescent. Growth and development or maturation of drug-metabolizing systems and the development of the urinary tract also results in changes in drug response.

Absorption

Drug absorption in infants and children follows the same basic principles as in adults. However, three factors tend to be especially important in children.

First, the physiologic status of the infant or child determines the blood flow at the site of intramuscular (IM) or subcutaneous drug administration. Factors that may reduce blood flow to muscular or subcutaneous tissues include cardiovascular shock, vasoconstriction caused by sympathomimetic agents, or heart failure. In these conditions, there would be reduced absorption of any drugs injected intramuscularly or into subcutaneous tissues. In premature infants with little muscle mass, the blood supply to these areas and the resulting absorption are very irregular. In older children, muscle size and circulation in the muscles affect how rapidly a medication is absorbed. There is more rapid absorption from the deltoid muscle (shoulder and upper arm) than from the vastus lateralis muscle (thigh), and the slowest absorption is from the gluteal (buttock) muscles.

Compared with older children and adults, the instability or immaturity of different body processes in premature infants is a second influence on drug absorption from IM sites. For example, toxic drug levels may occur if the blood supply to muscle or subcutaneous tissues suddenly increases, leading to greater absorption of medication and increasing the amount of the drug entering the blood. With some drugs, there is only a small difference between the level of drug that is helpful and the level of drug that is toxic and harmful. We say that these drugs have a *narrow therapeutic margin*. Examples of these drugs are anticonvulsants, cardiac glycosides, and aminoglycoside antibiotics. With these drugs, it would be easy for an infant to get too much medicine when absorption is variable.

A final factor in drug absorption is that the skin of premature and newborn infants has a greater ability to absorb some chemicals because of its greater hydration. That is, the outside stratum corneum of the epidermal barrier in the skin may allow more fluid to enter because the system is not well developed. The transdermal route may be used with some infants to reduce the unpredictability of some medications that are usually given orally or intramuscularly (for example, theophylline). However, transdermal dosage patches available for sale are not intended for pediatric patients and would deliver doses much higher than what is needed for infants and children. Instead, rubbing the drug into the skin, putting the drug in an oil base, or using an occlusive dressing (covering the skin on which the drug is placed by wrapping the area in plastic wrap) are all different ways that may increase the absorption of topical or skin products.

Distribution

Drug distribution is determined by two factors: (1) the chemical properties of the drug itself (for example, the molecular weight), which do not vary; and (2) the physiologic factors specific to the patient, including total body water, extracellular water, protein binding, and pathologic conditions modifying physiologic function, all of which vary widely in different patient populations.

Metabolism

The biotransformation of drugs in the body into usable substances involves chemical reactions that convert a drug to an inactive or less active compound. In general, drug metabolism in infants is much slower than that in older children and adults. Because most drug metabolism takes place in the liver, the fact that the levels of cytochrome P-450 enzymes of infants are only 50% to 70% of adult values is important in treatment of children. The amounts vary for the different enzymes, but the ability to increase production of all enzymes continues until the third or fourth year of life.

Because neonates have a decreased ability to metabolize drugs, they may be at increased risk for adverse effects as a result of slow clearance rates and prolonged half-lives, particularly when drugs must be given over long periods.

Excretion

As with metabolism, the growth and maturity of the child's organs has an important effect on the child's ability to excrete the end products of the drug reactions. Problems caused by the incomplete development of the renal excretion system, including glomerular filtration, tubular secretion, and tubular reabsorption, are slowly resolved as the child develops prior to birth. However, this system may still be very immature at birth and may only slowly develop to normal over the first year of life.

This process of normal development has implications for drug clearance, particularly of common drugs such as penicillin, aminoglycosides, and digoxin, for which clearance rates may fall to 17% to 34% of the adult clearance rate. If a child is sick enough to require these drugs, the glomerular filtration rate may not improve as predicted during the first weeks and months of life. This means that adjustments must be made in dosage and dosing schedules. The child will also require more careful monitoring, and dosages should be determined based on plasma drug levels determined at intervals throughout the course of therapy.

The growth spurt and the increase in adrenal steroid and sex hormone (estrogen in girls, androgens in both sexes) levels that occur before puberty affect drug response in children who are near puberty and in adolescents. The increase in male muscle mass, increase in female body fat, and stability of the body temperature in both sexes also affect adolescent drug response.

These facts about the drug-metabolizing system in **pediatric** (infants through adolescents) patients are important to remember in looking at a child's sensitivity to medication. For example, infants and children require a total daily digoxin dose that is approximately twice that of an adult on a basis of the ratio of weight to dose. It is thought that this increased requirement for digoxin is the result of a greater binding strength of the child's developing myocardial digoxin receptors for digitalis derivatives. Variations in the development of drug receptors may make a neonate very sensitive to anesthetics such as curare but resistant to other anesthetics such as succinylcholine.

Adverse Reactions

The risk for drug-drug interactions and adverse effects is increased in very ill children and infants. Children may be exposed to drugs in three major ways: (1) transplacentally, when the drug is given to the mother during pregnancy and delivery; (2) receiving the drug as a result of direct administration; and (3) getting the drug through breast milk if the mother has taken the drug. Fetal exposure to drugs through the placenta and neonatal exposure through breast milk share a common characteristic: These are the only stages in life in which one is exposed to and affected by drugs given to another person, the mother.

The number of adverse reactions in pediatric patients is unknown. Because young children are vulnerable, their diseases are often complex, their drug therapy is often complicated, and adverse drug reactions are unavoidable or hard to assess. However, studies have generally found that rates of adverse reactions in children are equal to those in adults. The rate may be as high as 5.8% of drugs administered to children, although the rate is higher if the child is hospitalized rather than at home. Adverse drug reactions may have a large and immediate, delayed, or long-term effect on the child's neurologic and somatic development.

With younger children, it may be difficult to tell whether the child is having an adverse reaction, is just experiencing symptoms of the underlying illness, or is having a paradoxic reaction to a drug (e.g., hyperactive behavior with antihistamines or chloral hydrate, sleepiness with stimulants such as Ritalin). Over-the-counter preparations (particularly antihistamines and adrenergic drugs found in various cough syrups, cold remedies, decongestants, and nose drops) may also provoke adverse reactions in pediatric patients, and many of these medications have now been banned for this age group. A broad spectrum of reactions may be seen, varying from minor hypersensitivity reactions to more serious problems, including alterations in growth, damage to anatomic or physiologic systems, and numerous other problems.

Children are not just small adults who require a smaller dose of medication. Although we know that children do respond differently to drugs, less research has been done to determine the safety and efficacy of many specific drugs when used in children. It has only been since 1996 that the FDA has required drug companies to label all medications with specific information related to their use in different pediatric age groups. In many cases, the information gathered during research on a drug used in an adult population may be safely extended to pediatric patients. But in some cases, the FDA has required companies to file additional information about their products when used with pediatric patients. Very frequently, nurses find that drugs are labeled with "safety for use in infants and children not determined" when they look for pediatric information about a drug. Thus all drug use in very young children should be approached with caution because of their immature metabolic and elimination systems. Toxic effects may develop more quickly and stay around longer, so special dosages are required (see Chapter 9).

SPECIAL CONSIDERATIONS FOR THE GERIATRIC PATIENT

Older adult patients also react differently to drugs. Medications are absorbed, metabolized, and excreted more slowly and less completely in older adults. In **geriatric** persons (adults older than 65), problems with medications are often due to a lack of understanding of the way drugs are processed in the aging body and the body's changed response to drugs. To further complicate matters, people age differently, and their individual body systems may also age at different rates.

Absorption

The overall importance of changes in the absorption of drugs with aging is not completely clear. There may be some delay in the absorption process. Physiologic changes that affect the GI tract include a reduction in acid output, so there is a more alkaline environment, which may affect drugs that require an acid medium for absorption. Reductions in blood flow, enzyme activity, gastric emptying, and bowel motility may increase the delay in absorption of some drugs, although they probably have little if any effect on the extent of absorption. Compounds such as iron, calcium, and certain vitamins that depend on active transport mechanisms for absorption may be affected by the decreased blood flow in the aging patient's GI tract.

Distribution

The distribution of drugs in the body may also be affected by the aging process and is linked to the chemical makeup of the agent involved. There is a decline in total body water and lean body mass with aging that may result in less movement or distribution of water-soluble drugs into some tissues. If the dose of these drugs is not decreased, the patient may develop higher serum concentrations, leading to an increased effect or toxicity. Thus the usual rule is to start drugs using a low dose and then increase the dose slowly in older adult patients. Drugs that are distributed into body water or lean body mass include digoxin, cimetidine, lithium, gentamicin, meperidine, phenytoin, and theophylline.

The distribution of fat-soluble drugs may also be changed by the aging process. With aging, there is usually a decrease in lean body mass but an increase in total body fat. Thus, lipid-soluble drugs may be stored in larger amounts in fat tissues and remain in the body for a longer time. Diazepam, chlordiazepoxide, flurazepam, thiopental, antipsychotics, and some antidepressants are lipid-soluble drugs that may require a lower dose and slow increases if used in the older adult population.

Another important concern that may exist with older adult patients is a decrease in serum proteins such as albumin. Albumin is the most common protein that binds to various acidic drugs, and a large decrease in albumin may result in a greater amount of unbound drug that may circulate freely. Highly protein-bound drugs that tend to bind quickly to albumin include phenytoin, warfarin, naproxen, theophylline, phenobarbital, and some antidepressants.

Metabolism

The effect of aging on liver function is difficult to determine because there is no good marker for measuring liver, or hepatic, function. Overall, a decrease in liver mass occurs with age, along with a reduction in hepatic blood flow. The result of lowered hepatic blood flow may be seen with drugs that are mostly broken down the first time they go through the liver (high first-pass metabolism). The extent to which these drugs are metabolized depends on how fast they go through the liver. When blood flow is reduced, as may occur with aging, less of the drug is metabolized, so increased amounts of the active form may remain the blood.

In an aging liver, there may also be changes in the specific pathways or phases of metabolism during which certain chemical and molecular changes occur to prepare the drug for metabolism. During phase I metabolism, drugs are generally made more water soluble so they may be excreted in the urine. Because of age-related changes in this process, drugs that are metabolized by phase I pathways may have decreased or unchanged clearance, so the drug may stay in the body and not be eliminated. Drugs that undergo phase I metabolism include diazepam, flurazepam, chlordiazepoxide, piroxicam, quinidine, and barbiturates. Such drugs should be used with caution and at lower doses in older adult patients, and the nurse will observe these patients carefully for adverse effects. If possible, these drugs should be avoided, and other drugs that are metabolized differently (phase II metabolism) should be used. No changes with aging have been reported with drugs that are metabolized by phase II metabolic processes, including conjugation, acetylation, sulfonation, and glucuronidation.

Drugs that are metabolized by the liver may have less or reduced metabolism because of other changes in the liver and also because of the influence of other diseases. The aging liver often gets smaller, has less blood flow, is affected by changes in nutritional status, and may become overloaded with fluid from diseases such as chronic heart failure. These factors may result in a loss of "hepatic reserve," or the liver's ability to handle all the different chemicals it must process. In this situation, the patient may have more risk of adverse effects when drugs are added to the existing treatment plan.

The important point in terms of giving medications to older adult patients is to use greater care in treating each patient individually and report patient response so that the dosage may be changed, if necessary.

Excretion

Kidney, or renal, function is the single most important factor that causes adverse drug reactions. Studies show that renal function varies with aging. Biologic changes in the aging kidney include decreases in the number of nephrons; decreases in renal blood flow, glomerular filtration, and tubular secretion rate; and an increase in the number of damaged glomeruli. In addition, damage to the arterial walls of blood vessels and lowered cardiac output reduce the amount of blood that flows to the kidneys by 40% to 50% between the ages of 25 and 65. The result of these changes may be a decrease in excretion of creatinine, which is reported to decrease 10% for each decade (10 years) after age 40 years.

Creatinine is a muscle by-product, and almost all of it is removed by the kidney, making it an excellent marker to measure kidney function (or renal clearance). A drug's creatinine clearance rate is the amount of blood from which a drug is cleared per unit of time. Although creatinine clearance is used to measure renal function, it is important to note that it is only an estimate. A number of formulas can be used to determine the creatinine clearance rate, but the results may not be very accurate. Creatinine clearance can be assessed more accurately by collecting urine for 24 hours and directly measuring the amount of creatinine in it, although this may be difficult to do. However, any method of estimating creatinine clearance may not be accurate in older adult patients, who have very little muscle mass and produce very little creatinine. In addition to the normal slowing of kidney function that may occur with aging and be made worse by disease, problems leading to dehydration can also affect renal function and make the decision about how much drug to give the older adult patient even more complex.

The important factors to remember when caring for older adult patients who are taking drugs that will be excreted from the kidneys is that each patient may respond a little differently to the drug. The dosage ordered should have been adjusted based on the best creatinine clearance estimates, and low doses or longer intervals between doses are the norm if it is believed some kidney damage might be present. Drugs that depend on the kidneys for elimination include many antibiotics, some antivirals, antineoplastics, antifungals, analgesics, and many cardiac drugs.

Other kidney changes that occur with aging include a decrease in the ability of the kidney to remove only chemicals and not fluid (renal concentrating ability) and a tendency for the kidney to hold onto sodium (sodium conservation), which may affect patients on high-dose diuretics.

Adverse Reactions

Many older adults with chronic illnesses are required to take medications daily. These drugs are helpful in controlling disease, but they also present a very real hazard to older adult patients. Approximately 90% of older adults have adverse reactions to drugs, and 20% of these reactions require hospitalization. As many as 30,000 people may die each year as a result of adverse drug reactions.

Because many older adult patients take several drugs, interactions among these different drugs may also cause problems for them. These patients may see several specialists, each of whom may prescribe different medications. If the specialists don't know about all the different drugs a patient may be taking at the same time, the patient may be at risk from combining drugs that have adverse interactions with each other.

All drugs have some risk or hazard, but the medications most dangerous to the older adult patient are tranquilizers, sedatives, and other drugs that alter the mind and change what the patient thinks he or she sees, or cause the patient to become dizzy or lose balance. Diuretics and cardiac drugs such as digitalis also pose special dangers and must be given with caution and careful observation of how the patient responds. Older adult patients may become dehydrated easily, thus allowing the amount of drug in the blood to increase. This places them at greater risk for side effects and toxicity with normal dosages. Results of research show there is also a high rate of alcohol use among many older people, both living at home and in nursing homes. Thus we are now becoming aware that drug-alcohol interactions are a serious concern in this age group.

Laboratory tests should be ordered regularly to look at kidney and liver function, and the nurse should look for side effects and signs of toxicity at every visit or encounter in the hospital or nursing home–entering the room in the hospital or long term care facility, passing the resident in the hall, greeting the resident in the dining room. If the nurse notices signs or symptoms of toxic reactions or adverse effects of drugs or observes behavior that might be a side effect, this should be reported immediately to the registered nurse. These signs and symptoms include changes in level of mental function, increased fatigue, restlessness, irritability, depression, weakness, dizziness, headache, and disorientation. These problems may interfere with appetite, balance, and energy, leading to dehydration, weight loss, falls, and immobility (not being able to move around). It is important to see that these often mild symptoms may be caused by drugs and should not simply be ignored as "typical" older adult behavior. For example, an older adult who becomes confused might have a urinary infection.

Patient Teaching Considerations

Some older persons may require special teaching about how to take their prescription medications and about the danger of taking nonprescription drugs at the same time. Failure of older adult patients to follow their medication plan, or **regimen**, may be because of many reasons: the cost of the drug, difficulty in getting it from a pharmacy, poor memory, lack of desire to take the drug regularly, depression, and feelings of being overwhelmed by the responsibility of taking care of themselves. These things all contribute to older adult patients failing to follow a medication regimen. In some cases, arthritis or another disease that causes physical disability may make it difficult to open bottle lids or use an inhaler. Poor eyesight may make it hard to draw up insulin or read the dose accurately. Many older patients also diagnose each other's health problems and share medications, which may make it very difficult for the nurse to evaluate the effects of prescribed medications in a particular patient. Patients who struggle to pay for their medicines may cut pills in half or skip doses without realizing it may prevent the drug from helping them.

WOMEN'S HEALTH ISSUES

There are some drugs taken mostly by women for women's problems. These include drugs to treat female genital tract infections and supplements used during the childbearing years. Other drugs taken by women may either prepare them for pregnancy, prevent pregnancy, or help their bodies recover from the loss of fertility-related hormones as a result of aging. Some women take these drugs faithfully, some take them only part of the time, and many women never have the chance to take the medications because of lack of information or money. But all of these medications may influence a woman's quality of life.

One of the biggest problems women have faced, particularly with the increase in diets high in refined sugars, is recurrent vaginal *Candida* infection. Newer antifungal medications have cut the treatment time for vaginal fungal infections from 7 days to 1 or 2 days. Although these products were once only used by women, now men with acquired immune deficiency syndrome are also using these medications to treat the opportunistic infections that often occur with reduced immunity.

There is now a great deal of scientific data showing that eating more foods high in folate (citrus fruits, cereals, leafy greens, and whole grains) or taking a multivitamin that has folic acid protects against neural tube birth defects such as spina bifida and anencephaly. Folic acid may also reduce the risk of heart disease and stroke.

Iron supplements have long been known to be helpful for patients who suffer from anemia resulting from blood loss. Thus women of childbearing age are often placed on iron supplements. Most menopausal women would probably also benefit from a multivitamin containing 10 mg of iron or less.

Although oral contraceptive pills (OCPs) do not reduce the patient's risk of getting a sexually transmitted disease, their use has cut both the birth rate and the abortion rate. For older women, the risks associated with taking OCPs are less than those of pregnancy. However, women who smoke and use OCPs are at an increased risk of adverse side effects such as stroke.

For many years, hormone replacement therapy (HRT) was routinely used at menopause to reduce uncomfortable symptoms, such as hot flashes, and prevent calcium loss from bones. However, research has now shown that HRT may lead to increased risk of stroke, heart attack, and breast cancer in certain women. HRT is still used, but only in some women and for short periods. Although these drugs may improve quality of life, women taking HRT are now closely monitored for cardiovascular problems.

SPECIAL CONSIDERATIONS FOR PREGNANT AND BREASTFEEDING WOMEN

Pregnant and breastfeeding women may have both chronic diseases and acute problems, either of which may require drug treatment. Giving medicine to pregnant women poses a big challenge. In pregnancy, the drug is really going to two people, so you must consider how the drug may affect the growing fetus. The benefit of any drug to a pregnant patient must be carefully weighed against the possible (or potential) risk to the fetus. All mothers want to have perfect babies, so it is important for pregnant women to avoid as many drugs as possible, especially those drugs with **teratogenic** potential, or those likely to cause malformations or damage in the embryo or fetus. In addition, you must be aware of the changing body chemistry of the mother throughout the pregnancy, as well as that of the growing fetus, and how this will affect the action of the drug itself.

Since the reports in 1961 of severe fetal malformations caused by the drug thalidomide, which was given to control nausea and vomiting in pregnant women, greater precautions have been taken to consider the effect of medications on pregnant women. Medications that have been confirmed as teratogenic in humans include antithyroid compounds; aminoglycoside antibiotics; anticancer agents; androgenic hormones; tetracycline; thalidomide; warfarin (Coumadin) and other anticoagulants; lithium; diethylstilbestrol; penicillamine; vitamin A analogues; and many anticonvulsants, such as carbamazepine, primidone, valproic acid, and phenytoin. Alcohol, methadone, and cocaine also are known teratogens. The FDA has developed categories for classifying drugs according to their known level of risk to the fetus and to breastfed infants (Table 5-1; also see end of the textbook).

Factors such as what drug the mother takes, how much is taken, and the age of the fetus when the drug is taken are related to different types of malformations. Taking a drug during the first 2 weeks after conception (before implantation) results in an "all or nothing" effect. The ovum either dies from exposure to a lethal dose of a teratogen or recovers completely with no adverse effects. The critical period for morphologic, or

Table 5-1	FDA Pregnancy Risk Categories
FDA CATEGORY	**DEFINITION**
A	Adequate, well-controlled studies in pregnant women have not shown an increased risk of fetal abnormalities.
B	Animal studies have revealed no evidence of harm to the fetus; however, there are no adequate and well-controlled studies in pregnant women. **OR** Animal studies have shown an adverse effect, but adequate and well-controlled studies in pregnant women have failed to demonstrate a risk to the fetus.
C	Animal studies have shown an adverse effect, but there are no adequate and well-controlled studies in pregnant women. **OR** No animal studies have been conducted, and there are no adequate and well-controlled studies in pregnant women.
D	Adequate, well-controlled, observational studies in pregnant women have demonstrated a risk to the fetus. However, the benefits of therapy may outweigh the potential risk.
X	Adequate, well-controlled, observational studies in animals or pregnant women have demonstrated positive evidence of fetal abnormalities. The use of the product is contraindicated in women who are or may become pregnant.

From Meadows M: Pregnancy and the drug dilemma, *FDA Consumer Magazine*, 2001. Available online at www.fda.gov/fdac/features/2001/301_preg.html categories. Accessed July 2008.
FDA, Food and Drug Administration.

structural, teratogenic effects in humans last from approximately 2 to 10 weeks after the last menstrual period (Figure 5-1). This embryonic period corresponds to the time of organ development (14 to 56 days), during which any teratogenic drug taken by the mother may produce major abnormalities in the embryo. Taking a teratogen later in the pregnancy during the fetal period (57 days to term) may result in minor structural changes, but abnormalities are more likely to involve problems with growth, mental development, and reproductive organ abnormalities. Clearly, it would be best if all women could stop taking any drugs before they got pregnant.

As the fetus grows, the placenta allows most drugs and nutritional products to cross from the mother to the baby. Thus it should be assumed that what the mother eats is also "eaten" by the fetus, with the exception of some drugs such as heparin and insulin. However, the reaction of a fetus to a medication is different from that of the mother. Because of an immature blood-brain barrier, many medications are able to pass

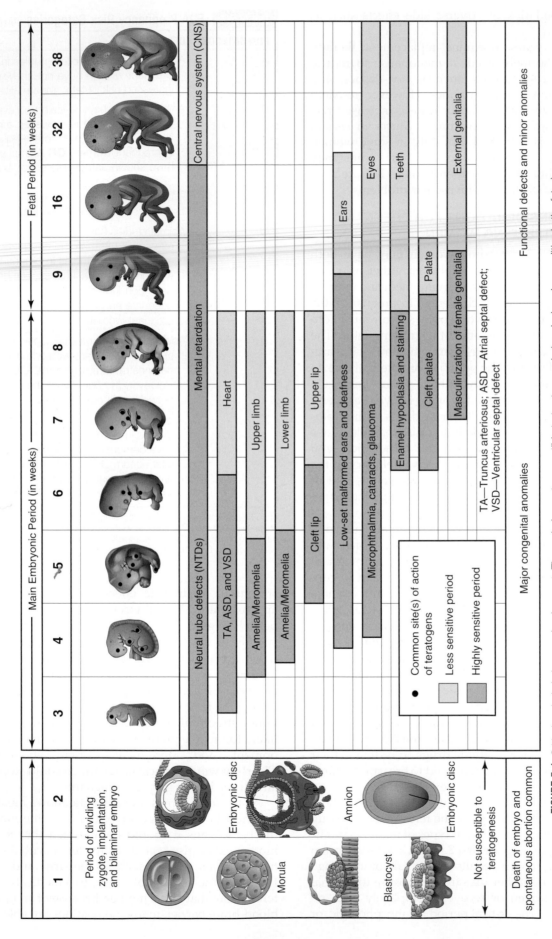

FIGURE 5-1 Critical periods in human development. The periods most susceptible to teratogenesis (producing abnormalities in the fetus) are indicated in *purple*; less sensitive stages are shown in *green*.

into the brain of the fetus, and because of the immaturity of the hepatic enzymes, the liver of the fetus is not developed enough to metabolize drugs.

Because pregnancy causes symptoms, many pregnant women require medications. The top 10 chemicals or drugs that pregnant women take are analgesics, antacids, antibiotics, antiemetics, antihistamines, diuretics, alcohol, iron supplements, sedatives, and vitamins. Anyone giving medications will wish to read the latest information to make sure that every drug given to a pregnant woman is safe.

Drugs can pass into human breast milk, and this is also a major concern for the baby. Most information about the amount of drug that goes into breast milk has come from measuring the chemical content of the drug in the milk itself. Sometimes it is possible to see the effect of the drug in the baby, but not always. Drugs that should *not* be taken by breastfeeding mothers include bromocriptine, cyclophosphamide, cyclosporine, doxorubicin, ergotamine, lithium, methotrexate, phenindione, amphetamines, nicotine, cocaine, heroin, marijuana, and phencyclidine.

If a mother is given a prescription while she is nursing, she can lessen the infant's drug exposure by taking the medication just before the infant is due to have a lengthy sleep period or right after a feeding. A bottle can then be substituted for the next scheduled feeding, and the affected breast milk can be expressed and discarded. Nevertheless, the infant should be watched for emotional changes, altered feeding habits, sleepiness, or restlessness. If short-term medication is required, the mother may need to consider stopping the breastfeeding for a short time and pumping and discarding her milk to maintain lactation until drug therapy is finished. Nursing mothers should not take sustained- or slow-release formulations or drugs with very long half-lives.

There is a growing body of knowledge about the influence of medication on breastfed babies. The FDA is currently proposing that drug manufacturers provide more information that helps identify the degree of risk to a baby from medication taken by a breastfeeding mother. The drugs are to be labeled with information about whether the drug will or will not be absorbed systemically and the degree of risk, how to minimize risk, and the data to support this information (Box 5-2).

SPECIFIC PRODUCTS USED THROUGHOUT THE LIFESPAN

Throughout the course of life, people may take many different types of medications. Some of these medications are used to help preserve health; others are given to help patients get well. Some of these common agents are discussed in this section.

| Box 5-2 | Proposed FDA Drug Labeling Guidelines for Breastfeeding Mothers |

RISK SUMMARY

For drugs that are not systemically absorbed, there is a standard statement that maternal use is not expected to result in infant exposure.

For drugs that are systemically absorbed, the risk summary must describe the following information or state that it is not available:

- State effects of drug on milk production.
- State presence of drug in human milk.
  - If drug not detected, state limits of assay.
  - If drug is detected, provide drug concentration in milk and estimated infant daily dose (actual and compared to pediatric or maternal doses).
  - State effects of the drug on the breastfed child.
- If data shows that the drug does not affect the quantity and quality of breast milk and there is reasonable certainty that either the drug is not detectable in breast milk or will not adversely affect the breastfed child, then state:
  - "The use of (name of drug) is compatible with breastfeeding."

CLINICAL CONSIDERATIONS

This section must provide, when available, information on:
- Ways to minimize exposure of the breastfed infant to the drug
- Dosing adjustments during lactation

DATA

This section must provide an overview of the data that are the basis for information in the risk summary and clinical considerations.

From the U.S. Food and Drug Administration. Center for Drug Evaluation and Research. Proposed Rule on Pregnancy and Lactation Labeling, May 28, 2008. Available at: www.fda.gov/cder/regulatory/pregnancy_labeling/default.htm

IMMUNIZATIONS

The early immunization of children against diphtheria, pertussis, tetanus, chickenpox, measles, polio, and hepatitis is a national priority. Although many children are required to have their primary immunizations before beginning elementary school, the overall quality of the nation's health would be better if these immunizations were given much earlier. Immunizations are one of the main things parents can do to protect the health of their children and one of the main things that have protected children from dying young. (See Chapter 21 for information on primary immunizations.) However, many children fail to receive these protective injections because of two factors. First, health care providers may not give immunizations because of the mistaken belief that they should be withheld if the child has a mild illness when examined. Second, parents may not have home-schooled children immunized or refuse immunizations for their children because of concern about possible adverse effects. Statistically, there is a greater chance that getting a disease will harm the child more than getting the immunization for that disease. Failure to immunize children places the whole community at risk. To encourage everyone to get immunizations, the U.S. Department of Health and Human Services created the National Vaccine Injury Compensation Program. This "no-fault" system provides payment to individuals or families of individuals who have been injured by childhood vaccines.

People who travel outside the United States, are in the military, or work in handling food are required to have immunizations against many diseases. To maintain protection against some diseases, patients must return for additional "booster" immunizations so their immunity will continue. We are learning that greater attention should be paid to immunizing more adult and geriatric patients against common diseases.

People at high risk, such as health care workers, older adults, and those who are immunocompromised, are encouraged to obtain yearly injections to help protect them against current strains of influenza. Children should also receive flu injections so that they avoid getting sick and bringing home infections to more vulnerable older adult or sick people at home.

ANTIDIABETIC AGENTS

For many years, it was not clear if it was important for patients with diabetes to maintain strict blood glucose levels. But now, tight management of blood glucose levels has been proven to reduce organ damage in the diabetic patient. When the mother's blood sugar level is controlled, there is less effect on the developing baby, who also responds to high glucose levels. These babies tend to gain more weight because their high sugar levels cause them to produce more insulin, and the blood glucose is then stored as fat.

ANTIHYPERTENSIVE AGENTS

The latest findings from research on hypertension demonstrate that lowering the blood pressure below 120/80 mm Hg reduces the patient's risk of myocardial infarction.

☀ CHOLESTEROL-LOWERING DRUGS

It has been shown that lowering cholesterol levels helps reduce atherosclerosis and decreases the risk of heart attack and stroke.

SMOKING-CESSATION PRODUCTS

Smoking has been linked to lung cancer and many other health problems. Both the smoker and those who are exposed to secondhand smoke (passive smokers) suffer. Fifty percent of cases of childhood asthma have been linked to the effects of passive smoking. It has been shown that the use of nicotine replacement products and drugs that reduce nicotine cravings, along with programs to change behavior, increase the chance that a person will be able to stop smoking. The risk of lung cancer and other adverse effects decreases in patients who are able to stop smoking.

WEIGHT-LOSS DRUGS

Although they pose some risk, weight-loss drugs, along with exercise and behavior change, may increase a person's ability to lose weight.

ANTIDEPRESSANT MEDICATIONS

Evidence exists that many people who have depression because of chemical imbalances or lack of various neurotransmitters in the brain may be helped through the use of antidepressant medications and counseling.

DRUGS FOR ERECTILE DYSFUNCTION (IMPOTENCE)

Prescriptions for drugs to treat erectile dysfunction have broken all records in terms of numbers of prescriptions written per day. These drugs are reported to increase blood circulation to the penis, thereby producing an erection. Men who have taken the drug report an amazing response that has given them potency with few side effects. It is clear that the increased physical activity associated with the return of older adults to sexual activity will place some individuals at risk for myocardial infarction. Patients with coronary heart disease should not use these drugs if they are not healthy enough to have sex. The possible long-term effects of these drugs will have to be determined through study of patients who use them repeatedly for a long time.

ASPIRIN

The benefits of aspirin in some patients who have had cardiovascular problems are clear. Research studies have shown these benefits in both men and women with a wide range of prior cardiovascular disease, ranging from a past heart attack or occlusive stroke to angina—including former coronary bypass surgery and angioplasty patients. Current guidelines for treating patients who may be having a heart attack call for them to chew and swallow a 325-mg aspirin tablet as soon as possible. This may place them at risk for bleeding, but the benefit is seen as greater than the risk.

CAFFEINE

There is growing evidence that high levels of caffeine in pregnant women may be linked to a higher rate of miscarriages. Although mothers may continue to have some caffeine, the amount should be low.

CULTURAL INFLUENCES RELATED TO MEDICATIONS

Culture guides behavior for the members of a specific group and determines what is acceptable. The **culture** of a group represents the shared values, beliefs, customs, and behavior of the members. Each new generation learns the culture of the group through both formal teaching and informal life experiences but each new generation has different experiences that make them a unique subculture. Factors such as the roles of men and women, the need for privacy or personal space, the meaning of food and nutrition, religious beliefs, the significance of transitions from one stage of life to another, and the amount of economic and personal freedom all are part of the culture of the group. Changes in the group's social and physical environment often lead to the development of different cultural practices. Subcultures may develop within the larger group based on ethnicity, when the subgroup has a common heritage, or on race, when the subgroup members share specific physical characteristics. As subcultures continue to live within the majority group, their ideas and values change, and they may grow to accept more of the practices of the dominant culture.

Over the years, cultural differences, or *diversity*, has increased among the citizens of the United States. There are many differences between the values and practices of the majority group of white, middle-class Americans and the minority subcultures that are growing in numbers. Some racial or ethnic group differences related to health care are obvious. People have different feelings, attitudes, and practices related to birth, death, and general health care. Some ethnic groups seem at risk for specific diseases. Culture often determines how they respond to suffering, pain, and loss. Culture may also direct standards of personal hygiene and need for privacy; acceptance of male and female children and tolerance of their behavior. People from different ethnic backgrounds may have differences in rate of growth and development of children; and how they adjust to life changes. The words used to talk about their feelings and attitudes, and the ideas related to health care behavior and treatments for illness, are quite different in each cultural subgroup and arise from the accepted values of the group. Good nursing care, whatever the setting, depends on the nurse having the ability to assess these differences among cultures and to adapt or change health care practices to better help the patient.

The importance of cultural diversity cannot be overemphasized. There are frequent cultures among patients in a group, between patients and care givers. Different generations have different cultural norms. Because culture often dictates behavior, recognizing that a patient's behavior may have meaning to them that is different than to you as a nurse is important.

Nurses must ask rather than making assumptions about people's beliefs.

Cultural assessment involves talking with a patient about differences and really listening to what they tell you about values, religion, dietary practices, family lines of authority, family life patterns, and beliefs and practices related to health and illness. There are usually strong cultural beliefs about important transitions in life, such as birth, marriage, and death. Patients may also have strong beliefs about such things as toilet training, common medical problems, and the use of herbs and other forms of therapy. Many of these individuals have already talked with friends, family, and religious leaders and may have incorrect notions about what is wrong with them and strong opinions about what should be done for them.

In the United States, health care workers are influenced by Western medical science and have been taught the values and beliefs of white, middle-class society. The nurses and physicians of many minority-group patients do not always share these same values and beliefs. Often today, the health care workers themselves come from a minority culture. Thus there are many challenges to talking with each other, setting priorities, and agreeing on solutions. For example, many of the health care beliefs shared by different cultural groups are based on "folk medicine" passed down through the generations of a culture. Many cultures have their own "healers" in the form of a medicine man, shaman, or curandera, whose services may be a blend of both medicine and religion. Members of the culture often seek the advice of such people before going to a Western or science-oriented health care provider. The various cures these healers suggest may be difficult to accept and include in Western health care. The fact that Western medicine has not been able to explain why some practices work does not mean they are harmful or not effective. Nurses must respect a person's cultural beliefs in all areas if they want the patient to listen to their advice and teaching.

Attempt to accept and work with the cultural practices of patients as much as possible, and do not force patients to accept care that conflicts with their personal values. Forcing a patient to accept a particular type of care may even be harmful, because feelings of guilt and being separated from the religious or cultural group are likely to threaten the patient's sense of well-being. Whether a patient is willing to take the medication provided by a nurse depends on what meaning the medication has to the patient and the individual's beliefs about its helpfulness or harm. A great deal of research is available about subcultures within the United States. If the nurse works with minority groups on a regular basis, he or she will need to learn about these subcultures to provide good care to those patients. Usually, people are proud to tell someone about their background and beliefs. Because there is growing recognition of cultural diversity, many articles and texts are being published that also provide information helpful to health care workers. However, it is important not to assume that all African Americans, American Indians, or Hispanics are the same just because they are members of a specific group. Within these larger groups are many subcultures with different histories, beliefs, languages, and values. What may be seen as acceptable behavior by one segment of the culture may be offensive to another. Take care to ask minority-group patients about what they prefer.

It is now recognized that there is also *health disparity*, or inequality in health care, for many minority-group patients. Indeed, much has been written about the "culture of poverty" and its effects on health care. Many minority-group patients are at risk for severe health problems but get less health care because of discrimination against them. Through lack of money, insurance, knowledge, or other factors, it may be difficult for them to get better care. For example, many minority-group patients do not read English well enough to understand written instructions about their health problems, get prescriptions filled, or take drugs properly. The ability to read and understand this type of information is called *health literacy*. (See Evolve for information on health literacy considerations in patient teaching.) Some individuals are afraid to seek health care because they may be in the country illegally and do not wish to draw attention to themselves.

Finally, in addition to differences in health care beliefs, values, and attitudes, drug research has also shown important differences among racial and ethnic groups in their metabolic rates, clinical responses to drugs, and side effects. In particular, cardiovascular drugs and central nervous system drugs may produce varying clinical responses in various ethnic or racial groups, particularly the Chinese and other Asian groups.

GENETICS

The mapping of the human genome and the research on genes and deoxyribonucleic acid (DNA) has shown that all individuals, no matter what race they belong to, are more similar than dissimilar. Research on individual races has concluded that African Americans are genetically the most heterogeneous (different) in their genetic profile. This may explain why this group as a whole has a greater rejection rate after organ transplantation, even with organs from living donors with similar tissue typing, and why they have particular unique responses to some types of medication. In people from some areas of the world, there are an unusually high number of cases of certain diseases, such as the thalassemia found in those of Eastern European and Mediterranean backgrounds. Research in genetics has shown that these diseases are passed down through families who carry certain genes. Hemophilia and sickle cell disease are other diseases that are the result of inherited traits in a family's DNA.

The area of genetics and the response of groups to medications is a topic of increasing interest to researchers. It has been suggested that in the future, medications might be made specifically for different races and ages as we learn more about the role that heredity plays in both disease and treatment.

SPIRITUALITY AND RELIGION

Regardless of basic ethnicity or culture, many individuals have a strong belief in a "higher power" that watches over or guides their lives, or may be asked for help in healing their illnesses. In times of sickness, people often think about religion or become more spiritual, and they try to find answers to why they have become sick or why they fail to get well. The idea of religious belief has at times been both controversial and unpopular, and many health care professionals are not comfortable talking with patients about their religious beliefs. However, it does not seem wise for a good nurse to ignore one of the most basic aspects of a person—one that affects how they view life and death. Often, all that is required is asking people about what they believe and then really listening or helping them find a religious leader to meet their spiritual needs.

Many research studies have been done about the influence of religion on health. The results suggest that people who pray have better symptom relief. People who have a strong social support network through their religion also seem to do better than those without such support. How a person of faith interprets symptoms, disease, and death, and how these beliefs influence the actions of medications, is still under study.

WHY PEOPLE DON'T TAKE THEIR MEDICINES

The goal of patient teaching for drug treatment plans is to work with patients to help them make informed decisions about taking their drugs. Many of the variables of age, culture, and belief affect a patient's willingness to take medications that are ordered. Patient difficulty with taking medications is a major unresolved problem. *Compliance* (cooperation) or *concordance* (agreement with) are the terms used to describe the patient who agrees with and follows the health care plan worked out with the health care provider. Drug **noncompliance** is when the patient does not follow the health care plan for taking medications. Patients sometimes use medications in ways that vary from the health care provider's advice because they did not agree with the plan (nonconcordance). When patients decide what medications they are and are not going to take, they may not get well and may even take drugs that are harmful.

How does drug noncompliance begin? Often patients come to a health care provider almost as a last resort after having already tried a number of remedies for their symptoms. The patient's age, sex, race, ethnic background, family, socioeconomic class, education, and past experience will have affected how the health problem is viewed and how the world in general is seen. Although today's patients are more likely to be better informed about medical care than patients were in the past, they are also more likely to be skeptical or distrusting of the medical profession. They may have read about medical mistakes and successful lawsuits, heard about bad experiences in medical care from friends, or had bad experiences themselves. They may come from a lower socioeconomic class, be less educated, or have value systems different from those of the health care provider. Patients do have underlying fears and concerns and certain expectations for their care, but they are often reluctant to express these fears and expectations because they worry others will think they are foolish.

Health care workers may often assume patients' value system is similar to their own and may not take the time to even determine the patient's beliefs about and understanding of the illness. If this has happened, the patient may not have developed trust in the health care worker. So, many times a primary reason why patients are not cooperative is because of their past bad experiences with the health care system.

Most studies of drug compliance have been done with hospital-based patients. These studies have usually found that (1) patients are unfamiliar with their medications and how to take them, and (2) patients make errors in taking medications as much as 25% to 59% of the time. The nurse must ask questions and listen to what the patient is saying. If no one learns that the patient is not taking the medication as ordered, poor outcomes may be blamed on wrong dosage, failure of the drug plan itself, or incorrect diagnosis. Drug noncompliance often increases medical costs by leading to further hospitalization, by causing nursing-home placement for older adult patients, and by increasing the use of outpatient services. It is often difficult for the nurse to learn if the patient has not taken the drugs that were ordered; patients often wish to please health care workers and may not tell them the truth.

Reasons for drug noncompliance can be classified as *errors of omission* (a prescribed medication is not taken), *errors of commission* (a medication that has not been prescribed is taken), *dosage errors* (the wrong dose is taken), and *scheduling errors* (the medication is taken on the wrong schedule, for example, once daily instead of twice daily). There are six major reasons for patient noncompliance with drugs:

1. Noncompliance rates tend to be higher for care to prevent a problem than for treatment of an existing illness. For example, patients may not remember to take calcium supplements but are more likely to take a pain pill. Also, compliance is better for "important" medications such as cardiac or anticonvulsant agents than for seemingly "less important" drugs like antacids or mild analgesics.
2. The extent of noncompliance increases with the length of therapy, as seen in chronic diseases such as diabetes, hypertension, epilepsy, and depression.
3. Noncompliance is highest for treatment regimens that require the patient to make significant changes in behavior, such as with plans to stop smoking or lose weight.
4. Poor understanding of instructions is a common cause of noncompliance.
5. People may not want to follow the treatment plan when it is very complex; for example, when many drugs are taken at different times or when drugs must be taken at frequent intervals or during the night.
6. People may not want to follow the treatment plan when there are unpleasant side effects.

Patients who have symptoms are more likely to take their medications than those who do not, especially if the symptoms are relieved by the medication. For example, patients will take pain medicine if they hurt but might not take high blood pressure medicine because they don't feel bad. The patient's age, sex, race, education, occupation, income, and marital status usually provide clues as to whether the patient will follow the instructions. People who have a stable support and family situation are more likely to follow treatment plans. For example, a husband who has a wife who will help cook special foods for the diet and remind him to take his medicine will have better success than a person who lives alone.

Although many people believe older adults are more likely not to cooperate with a treatment plan, most research indicates that aging does not affect compliance with prescribed medications. Middle-aged and younger patients are busy with careers, families, and the many activities they take part in each day and may forget about their medicines. Older adult individuals, however, typically have fewer things to do every day, and this helps them focus on taking medications as prescribed. Older adult patients have been shown to have difficulty opening some of the childproof drug bottles, and they may also experience difficulty with reading or understanding new instructions.

If the nurse establishes a good relationship with a patient, this may help the patient follow instructions. A good relationship means that the nurse and patient can share information and talk easily with each other.

Factors that have been identified as helpful in having a good relationship with the patient include the following:
- Being friendly
- Having a positive, confident approach
- Responding to patient complaints
- Encouraging patient questions
- Having a supportive, nonjudgmental method of getting information and talking to a patient who admits to noncompliance
- Encouraging patients to become actively involved in their own care
- Seeking active patient participation rather than physician- or nurse-dominated decision making
- Working together to decide the plan of care
- Identifying and resolving things that make the patient less cooperative with the plan
- Taking time to motivate and encourage the patient
- Working to help the patient be satisfied

Clearly, all these things take time, and the nurse may not always see the same patients over and over again in an office, clinic, or hospital. These positive activities can be included in the care plan as part of regular work with all patients.

Get Ready for the NCLEX Examination!

Key Points

- Efforts to make a care plan for each individual patient by taking into account the patient's culture, beliefs, and age will make it more likely that the patient will participate actively in the plan to get well.
- The problems of disease and disability belong to the patient, not the provider.
- The goal of care throughout the life cycle should be to assist patients in taking charge of their own health and learning how to get well or stay well.
- The nurse can help the patient follow the treatment plan through their own behavior.

Additional Learning Resources

SG Go to your Study Guide for additional learning activities to help you master this chapter content.

⊖volve Go to your Evolve website (http://evolve.elsevier.com/Edmunds/LPN/) for additional online resources.

Review Questions for the NCLEX Examination

1. A home health patient tells the nurse that she usually takes a particular medication only once daily instead of twice daily because of the constipation associated with that drug. The classification for this noncompliance is most likely:
   1. scheduling error
   2. dosage error
   3. error of commission
   4. error of omission

2. The nurse is working with a child who does not have the required immunizations. The nurse should recognize that this is most likely due to:
   1. parents' concerns about adverse effects
   2. parents' lack of education on the subject
   3. reasons that are unknown by the nurse and need to be determined
   4. parents' concerns about cost of injections

3. A breast feeding mother who takes a prescription drug is told the most appropriate time for her to take the medication to reduce the infant's exposure to the drug is:
   1. right before a feeding
   2. midway through a feeding
   3. right after a feeding
   4. 1 hour before a feeding

4. The nurse is selecting an intramuscular injection site for a 10-year-old child. The most appropriate site for this patient based on his age is:
   1. dorsogluteal
   2. ventrogluteal
   3. vastus lateralis
   4. deltoid

5. The nurse is administering medication to a neonate. The nurse recognizes that the patient has a decreased ability to metabolize drugs primarily as a result of:
   1. slow clearance rates and prolonged half-lives
   2. rapid clearance rates and prolonged half-lives
   3. slow clearance rates and short half-lives
   4. rapid clearance rates and short half-lives

Critical Thinking Questions

1. Look up the drug digoxin in a drug handbook. What doses are recommended for infants, children, adults, and older adult patients? What specific factors explain why these doses are different?
2. Among your classmates, discuss differences in beliefs about disease and death. What cultures produced these different beliefs? Whose beliefs are best?
3. Find resources that identify some of the different health care beliefs of various groups such as Chinese, Hispanics, and American Indians.
4. African Americans vary in their beliefs and values from other black people. Identify some of the differences in cultures of black people. If you treated everyone who is black in the same manner, what would be the likely results of your care?

Get Ready for the NCLEX® Examination!—cont'd

5. Mrs. Green is 5 months pregnant. She has severe asthma but has not been taking her asthma medication because she is afraid it would hurt her baby. What are some of the factors that should be considered when you talk to Mrs. Green about this problem?

6. Ms. Kim, an older adult Korean woman with limited English, was brought in for surgery by her grandson, who speaks English. Now it is time for her first dose of presurgery medication, but her grandson is nowhere to be found. When you approach Ms. Kim with the medication, she smiles but shakes her head no. "No," she says, shaking her head emphatically. "No pill." How can you handle this situation?

7. You and your husband plan to begin a family. What medications are safe to take if you are pregnant and have a bad cold? Diabetes? Epilepsy? What products should you definitely avoid?

8. The last time you saw a health care provider for a minor primary care problem, did you get a prescription? Did you have it filled? Why or why not? Did you take all the medication as ordered? Why or why not?

9. When you are very busy giving care to patients, what things can you do to develop a good relationship? How will this help in teaching them about taking their medications?

10. Mrs. Jones tells you that she does not want her 6-month-old child to have immunizations. What would be the most therapeutic way to communicate with her?

Objectives

1. List advantages and disadvantages of over-the-counter medications.
2. Describe some of the precautions to think about in taking herbals or other alternative or complementary therapies.

3. Identify common agents taken for health promotion.

Key Terms

alternative medicine (ăl-TĔR-nă-tĭv, p. 60)
complementary medicine (kŏm-plĕ-MĔN-tă-rē, p. 60)
health promotion (HĔLTH pră-MŌ-shun, p. 67)

herbal (ĔR-băl, p. 61)
integrative practices (ĬN-tĕ-grā-tĭv, p. 60)

OVERVIEW

When we think of patient drugs, we often forget that many of the drugs patients use are those they buy in drugstores because they learned about them from their friends, read about them in magazines or saw a television ad. More than ever before, people are learning about how to care for themselves and are more likely to purchase over-the-counter (OTC) products. Health care remedies not prescribed by health care providers also did a booming business in the United States in 2007; Americans spent $18 billion on nonprescription remedies. The majority of drugs that patients buy and use are OTC. What is safe for patients to take? What do they need to know about OTC products? What products should they take to keep them well? Can they believe the articles and stories about "wonder" drugs they can get without a prescription that promise such good results for chronic problems? How can you answer their questions?

DOCUMENTING PATIENT HEALTH CARE PRACTICES

It is important for you to be familiar with the many nonprescription products now available to patients. Many of these products contain chemicals that are useful in treating common health problems. Nurses should be familiar with these products, so that they can help patients choose the safest product for their current health concerns, problem, or illness. Some of the active chemicals in these products may make existing medical problems worse or interact with a patient's prescribed medications.

Always ask about OTC medications that patients may be taking when you ask about their drug history.

Patients often neglect to tell their providers about these products because they may regard them as harmless and not a "real drug." Many Americans consider herbal or OTC products to be safe because they are so easily available. But they may not be safe for all patients. Ask patients to bring questionable products to the attention of the patient's physician or health care provider.

It is also important to have patients bring in all herbs or drug remedies they are using so that what they are taking may be accurately recorded as patients often do not know the active ingredients or effects of natural medications they are taking. Seeing products in their original bottles or boxes gives more information that might be needed to tell if the products are safe. This action may be very helpful in preventing drug interactions or complications.

Patients who rely on complementary and alternative medicine (CAM) may be taking alternative products (herbs, supplements, or other drugs) instead of prescription drugs because of the cost, or they may use such products in addition to prescription drugs in a complementary way. When asking a patient about the use of CAM, do not make judgments about these treatments. This approach is important if you wish to have patients trust you enough to tell you the truth about what health regimens they are following or what herbal and OTC products they are taking. Understand that patients who use these different treatments do so for many reasons:

- They seek products that will keep them in good health, prevent disease, or provide treatment for health problems they now have.
- They have tried regular treatments without success.

- The regular treatments had undesirable side effects.
- There is no known therapy that will cure their problem, but they keep searching for one.
- Other people they trust in their family or community have told them about the product.
- They are seeking a cheaper or nonprescription product to replace a drug they want to use but cannot get or cannot afford.
- Regular treatment violates the patient's religious or spiritual beliefs.

OVER-THE-COUNTER MEDICATIONS

The role of OTC agents in health care today is growing, because there are now more people who are better educated and believe they should take an active role in their own health care. The Nonprescription Drug Manufacturers Association estimates that more than 100,000 products are now available over the counter. These products contain one or more of approximately 700 active chemicals and come in a variety of dosage forms, sizes, and strengths. The sales of OTC products total more than $20 billion a year.

Nonprescription medications, or *OTC products*, are defined as drugs that are thought to be safe and effective for people to use without instructions from a health care provider about how to use them. OTC products differ from prescription medications in five ways:
1. The label information is more complete than prescription-medication labels and is often written in a style easier for consumers to understand.
2. With OTCs, there is a wider margin of safety because most of these drugs have undergone a lot of testing before advertising and many have been changed by the manufacturer based on information gathered after years of OTC usage by consumers.
3. OTCs are usually advertised directly to the consumer. (Many manufacturers of prescription drugs are now following this example by advertising directly to the public and asking people to talk with their health care provider about these drugs.)
4. OTCs are widely available.
5. The dose may be lower than available with a prescription.

The most common categories of OTCs are similar to those available by prescription. These include laxatives, peptic acid disorder products (antacids, H_2 receptor antagonists), analgesics, cough and cold products (antihistamines, decongestants, expectorants, antitussives), vaginal antifungals, stop-smoking products, and topical steroids. Also, many drugs that were once available only by prescription have now been given OTC status although frequently in lower dosages.

OTCs are sold in pharmacies, grocery stores, gas stations, and many other places. Less than one half of all OTC products are sold in pharmacies. Because there are so many different names and versions of these products, it is important to learn the generic drug name instead of just the product (trade) name. Many of these products have multiple ingredients. The cost of these combination products can be more than buying all of the ingredients singly, so it is important to check out commonly used products for price comparisons.

PRODUCT LABELING

The U.S. Food and Drug Administration (FDA) requires that OTC product labels contain important information in a manner that a typical person can read and understand. Drug companies are required to use a standard labeling format for all OTCs sold in the United States. Key information, beginning with active ingredients, followed by purposes, uses, warnings, and directions, is placed in the same order on all OTC packages in an easy-to-read format. Surveys show that women are the family members most likely to buy OTC products, and they are also more likely than men to read labels before taking medications.

One of the most important things to look for on the OTC label is the presence of other chemicals in a product that might pose a risk. These "hidden" chemicals are used for different purposes: to help make the drug taste better, to help preserve the drug, to give color, and to help deliver the product or make it more stable. Consumers who have an allergy or intolerance to even small doses of any of these products may not be aware of the risk unless they read the label. Table 6-1 lists a number of common hidden chemicals in OTC products.

PATIENT TEACHING

There are some basic facts health care providers should tell patients about OTC products. Sometimes this information is printed and given out to the patient, because it is so important for patients to know about it. Whether they are given verbally or in writing, these are some of the key facts patients should learn:
- Always read the instructions on the label.
- Do not take OTC medicines in higher dosages or for a longer time than the label states.
- If you do not get well, stop treating yourself and talk with a health care professional.
- Side effects from OTCs are relatively uncommon, but it is your job to know what side effects might result from the medicines you are taking.
- Because every person is different, your response to the medicine may be different than someone else's.

Table 6-1	Common "Hidden" Ingredients in Over-the-Counter Products
HIDDEN DRUG	**OVER-THE-COUNTER CLASS THAT MAY CONTAIN THE DRUG**
Alcohol (ethanol)	Cough syrups and cold preparations, mouthwashes
Antihistamines	Analgesics, antiemetics, asthma products, cold and allergy products, dermatologic preparations, menstrual products, motion sickness products, sleep aids, topical decongestants
Antimuscarinic agents	Antidiarrheals; cold, cough, allergy preparations; hemorrhoidal products
Aspirin and other salicylates	Analgesics, antidiarrheals, cold and allergy preparations, menstrual products, sleep aids
Caffeine	Analgesics, cold and allergy products, diuretic and menstrual products, stimulants, weight control products
Estrogens	Hair creams
Local anesthetics (usually benzocaine)	Antitussives, cold sore products, dermatologic preparations, hemorrhoidal products, lozenges, teething and toothache products, weight-loss products
Sodium	Analgesics, antacids, cough syrups, laxatives
Sympathomimetics	Analgesics, asthma products, cold and allergy preparations, cough syrups, hemorrhoidal products, lozenges, menstrual products, topical decongestants, weight control products

Modified from Katzung BG: *Basic and clinical pharmacology*, ed 10, New York, 2006, McGraw Medical.

- OTC medicines often interact with other medicines, and with food or alcohol, or they might have an effect on other health problems you may have.
- If you do not understand the label, check with the pharmacist.
- Do not take medicine if the package doesn't have a label on it.
- Throw away medicines that have expired (are older than the date on the package).
- Do not use medicine that belongs to a friend.
- Buy products that treat only the symptoms you have.
- If cost is an issue, generic OTC products may be cheaper than brand name items.

Parents should know the following special information about using OTCs for children:

- Parents should never guess about the amount of medicine to give a child. Half an adult dose may be too much or not enough to be effective. This is very true of medicines such as acetaminophen (Tylenol) or ibuprofen (Advil), in which repeated overdoses may lead to poisoning of the child, liver destruction, or coma.
- If the label says to take 2 teaspoons and the dosing cup is marked with ounces only, get another measuring device. Don't try to guess how much should be given.
- Always follow the age limits listed. If the label says the product should not be given to a child younger than 2 years, DO NOT give it.
- Always use the child-resistant cap, and relock the cap after use.
- Throw away old, discolored, or expired medicine or medicine that has lost its label instructions.
- Do not give medicine containing alcohol to children.

COMPLEMENTARY AND ALTERNATIVE MEDICINE, INCLUDING HERBAL THERAPIES

Patients often believe they know more than their health care providers do about their health problems, and that their providers do not listen to them or respect their choices. These individuals often turn away from traditional Western medicine and seek other forms of alternative health care.

The practices that are known as **alternative medicine** have often been somewhat of a mystery, and the scientific basis for the action of alternative therapies has been uncertain. Because of the lack of research to explain therapeutic action, most medical and nursing schools do not teach their students about alternative medicine. Alternative therapies include herbal therapies, aromatherapy, chiropractic care, acupuncture, massage, and homeotherapy. A similar type of treatment known as **complementary medicine** includes these same basic alternative therapies and is preferred by many because it uses these therapies together with standard medical care and not as an alternative. Another term to describe this type of treatment is **integrative practices**.

Recent studies have found that 40% to 50% of Americans are using some type of alternative therapy, and even more are taking herbs and supplements. A survey estimated that in 2008 more than 48 million adults in the United States used herbal products and dietary supplements. Another survey estimated that approximately 18% of the U.S. population uses herbal therapy on a regular basis. More than half of those users said the products were important to their health and well being, and 70% may not tell their regular health care provider about what products they are taking.

The estimated number of visits to providers of alternative medicine (425 million) exceeded those to all primary care physicians (325 million). There is increasing patient interest in herbs, supplements, and homeopathic remedies, but there is little scientific information in texts and reference books about these products. Most of the books and articles about herbal therapies are written to sell products. You will want reliable information about the medicines patients are taking. Because of the widespread use of herbal products, it is crucial that you have up-to-date, balanced, and scientific material to help you understand herbal therapies and learn about strengths, weaknesses, clinical indications, proper dosages, toxicities, and interactions of different alternative drug therapies so you are able to answer patient questions accurately.

HERBAL THERAPIES AND SUPPLEMENTS

Use of **herbal** medicine (drugs made from plant sources) has long been an accepted part of health care in many cultures. China and other Asian cultures have used herbal products for centuries as an important part of medical practice. People in the United States are now using these same herbal remedies in growing numbers, because they wish to prevent disease, treat illness, and improve health. Because herbal therapies have such a long history in different cultures, this may have created the impression in the minds of some consumers that they are safe, natural, and effective. The fact that something is "natural" does not mean it is safe or effective. With the growing scientific research into use of many herbal products, there is growing belief in the health care community that if herbs are effective, then they should be used under the direction of a health care professional.

Product Labeling

Herbal preparations are not regulated anywhere in the world. Germany has done the most in terms of scientific research into the safety and efficacy of some of these herbs, but these studies have been small and do not begin to meet the scientific standard demanded by the FDA for prescription drugs. Unlike prescription and OTC drugs, the FDA does not require manufacturers to determine purity or potency of herbal products. In fact, some products have been found to contain contaminants, including prescription drugs or heavy metals, and their potency depends on many factors, such as what part of the plant is used and the climate and soil conditions where they are grown, harvested, and stored. Some herbal preparations have even resulted in toxicities.

The FDA has taken action as a result the Dietary Supplement Health and Education Act passed by Congress in 1994, which said health and disease claims are different than structure and function claims. The act says that labels cannot make claims that a product cures a disease or has a special benefit or health effect without special FDA approval. The act allows general statements about the product's function in the body. The new rules bar makers of supplements and herbal remedies from claiming to cure, prevent, or alleviate cancer, acquired immune deficiency syndrome, and other specific diseases. Companies are limited to making general claims about the product's ability to make the immune system stronger. Critics claim that most disease treatments can be described in terms of their effects on a structure or function of the body, so it will be difficult to tell the difference between structure and function claims, which are allowed, and disease claims, which are not. The herbal drug manufacturer must now use the following statement in their labeling: "This product is not intended to diagnose, treat, cure, or prevent any disease."

It might be noted that the labels on herbal products are designed to promote sales and product use and not necessarily to educate the consumer, so health professionals with a general understanding of popular herbs and supplements can talk to patients about efficacy, common side effects, risks, and interactions. When talking to the patient on admission, the nurse may ask about his or her patients' use of unconventional medicines. This might alert the physician or nurse practitioner that they need to explore these products more to avoid drug interactions with medications ordered in the hospital or clinic.

The FDA does have the authority to remove a product from the market, but this happens only after the agency can prove that the product is unsafe or ineffective. This was the case when the FDA banned products containing ephedra because of adverse cardiovascular effects and prohibited sales of kava because of concerns about liver toxicity.

Patients with medical problems should not use herbs and dietary supplements without medical supervision. When patients rely on themselves for diagnosis and treatment, they may delay the essential diagnosis of serious medical problems, and this delay may worsen their condition. Additionally, some herbal products have adverse effects and may interact with prescribed medications.

Concerns about Herbal Products and Dietary Supplements

Herbal products and dietary supplements are widely available in supermarkets and other retail outlets, as well as by mail order. Because of the wide use of alternative therapies, there has been growing interest in research on the action of various products. The scientific community has expressed concern about drugs that are not tested or regulated. Because some of these medications have "folk" acceptance, they may be cheaper than regular drugs, and there may be fewer barriers to purchasing them, so their use has increased.

As more of these products are being used over longer periods, researchers are now starting to pay attention to them. Until there are more scientific studies, health care providers should urge caution in the use of herbal products.

Pros and Cons

Safety, purity, and effectiveness are the major issues in evaluating herbal products. Important questions to consider in looking at herbal products include:

- How much of the herbal product does this product actually contain?
- What part of the plant was used to make the extract?
- What other chemicals does it contain?
- What are the active ingredients?
- What reliable information exists that this herb is useful and for what conditions?

Herbal products are made by grinding up parts of the plant and making them into pills, capsules, or liquids. One of the major criticisms of herbal products is that the plants vary so much in concentration or dosage because plants make different amounts of chemicals, depending on the soil, water, and sun where they were grown. That is, the weight of one leaf may be the same as that of another, but the amount of biologically active chemical in each leaf may vary according to the amount of sunlight, the nutrition in the soil, and the extent of watering.

Hormone replacement therapy has become a hot market for the use of "natural" products. Natural estrogens are really estrogen-like chemicals called *phytoestrogens.* Examples of plants containing natural estrogens or phytoestrogens are flaxseed, red clover sprouts, and soy flour. Herbs thought to contain chemicals that act as stimulants for hormones are licorice, ginseng, *Vitex,* and black cohosh. It generally takes 6 to 8 weeks to see an improvement in symptoms of menopause when taking these products. Again, these herbal preparations do not deliver the same amount of chemicals with each dose, and there is no way to know the purity of the product. There is also no way to know if the product will do what it claims it will do. For example, many women in China have long used an herb called *dong kwai,* claiming it reduces or eliminates hot flashes. However, research thus far has failed to find estrogen or estrogen-like chemicals in dong kwai, and its efficacy in menopause is not documented. More research is needed to determine if these are really effective.

Many nonprescription products are advertised to have the same function as prescription drugs. For example, there are herbal preparations that are supposed to act like sildenafil (Viagra). Herbal antiobesity products were sold as alternatives to fenfluramine and dexfenfluramine when these products were taken off the market. Herbal products for depression, high cholesterol, and asthma are also for sale. However, products containing St. John's wort have not been completely tested for their effectiveness as antidepressants in the United States. They may also include 6-hydroxytryptophan (closely related to another chemical linked to a rare and potentially fatal blood disorder) and ephedra, an amphetamine-like compound that may cause high blood pressure, heart irregularities, strokes, and death. The claim that garlic reduces cholesterol to an acceptable level also has not been confirmed by scientific research. Patients who take these products in place of prescription drugs should consider that they are taking an experimental drug. Because of dangers such as these, the FDA took action to remove some of these products from the market and posts information about these products on their MedWatch home page (http://www.fda.gov/medwatch/).

There is a group of industry members led by the Council for Responsible Nutrition that has developed voluntary guidelines some herbal drug makers are now using. Patients need to look for products that have been standardized by the manufacturer by measuring the amount of the key ingredient. However, the purity and potency of many products sold in the United States are unknown.

Some European countries have more extensive experience with selected herbal products than the United States. Many of the products now gaining attention in the United States have been used for years in other countries—either as OTC products or by prescription. A lot of information has been learned not only about the effects of these products, but also about how they interact with other foods and medications. For example, natural products that reduce blood glucose or blood pressure or have a sedating effect may be dangerous when taken along with prescription drugs with the same actions. Table 6-2 shows the herbs considered by non-U.S. regulatory authorities to be relatively safe and effective if used in recommended dosages and made by companies that standardize their drug making process. Table 6-3 lists herbs that are considered unsafe for use, based on reports or observations.

Table 6-4 lists a few nonherbal natural remedies that are in common use and considered both safe and effective. Sometimes the products themselves, such as calcium, may be of proven use. However, if the calcium comes from oyster shells taken from polluted waters, the shells may be filled with lead, zinc, or arsenic. A similar problem occurs with melatonin, a hormone extracted from the pineal gland of the cow. If the drug maker does not make sure that the cow is disease free, the consumer may be at risk for diseases from the cow (e.g., "mad cow" disease).

AROMATHERAPY

Essential oils extracted from the petals, leaves, bark, resins, rinds, roots, stalks, seeds, and stems of aromatic plants are used to promote health and well being. It is

Table 6-2   Herbs Considered Safe and Effective

COMMON NAME	USE FOR WHICH PROMOTED	SAFETY, EFFICACY, DOSAGE
Arnica	External remedy for healing bruises, muscle strains, and sprains; reduces inflammation	Toxic when taken orally
Black cohosh	Reduces menopausal symptoms	Clinical trials using black cohosh to relieve menopausal symptoms have yielded conflicting results. Some women experience benefits with the herb with few side effects. Appears safe, but limit use to 6 months and avoid use in those with a history of estrogen-dependent tumors.
Chamomile	Antiinflammatory, antispasmodic, antiinfective	In capsule form, FDA considers chamomile safe. Use with caution in individuals allergic to ragweed, as cross-allergenicity may occur. Allergic symptoms may include tongue thickness, tight sensation in throat, angioedema of lips and eyes, diffuse pruritus, urticaria, and pharyngeal edema. May produce sedation, so use with caution with medications that also have sedative side effects or with alcohol. Oral doses vary from 400 to 1600 mg per day (standardized to 1.2% apigenin per dose). Chamomile is often brewed as a tea; 1 heaping teaspoon of dried flowers steeped in hot water for 10 minutes may be drunk up to 3 times a day.
Chaste tree	Female hormone regulation	Safe and effective; rare indigestion
Cholesten	Serum cholesterol reduction	Safe
Echinacea	Stimulates the immune system; used in treatment or prevention of colds and flu or urinary tract infections	A wide variety of echinacea preparations and doses have been studied; results are inconsistent. *E. purpurea* seems to be modestly effective for preventing the common cold in those at risk (e.g., sick contacts). Evidence that the herb may reduce the duration of cold symptoms is mixed. Patients allergic to ragweed, with progressive autoimmune disorders, and on hepatotoxic drugs should avoid echinacea. May take 6-9 doses (1 g dried root) of echinacea juice per day for 2 weeks; very safe, no side effects.
Fennel	*Internal:* increases milk flow in lactating women; *External:* oil eases muscle and joint pain	Safe and effective
Feverfew (*Tanacetum parthenium*)	Migraine headache prevention or reduces severity and frequency; inhibits platelet aggregation	Safe and effective; take 125 mg twice daily; do not use concurrently with aspirin or warfarin (Coumadin).
Garlic (*Allium sativum*)	May lower some blood lipids; inhibits platelet aggregation; lowers blood pressure	Safe and effective; destroyed by heat; take 2.5 g/day raw or 0.4-1.2 g/day dried; do not use concurrently with aspirin, ibuprofen, or warfarin. Those taking antihypertensive medications should exercise caution and monitor BP for rare cases of orthostatic hypotension. Should be avoided by those with history of orthostasis or unexplained dizziness. A lack of standardization of garlic products and formulations makes it difficult to recommend a dose or specific product. For dyslipidemia, patients may benefit from taking 600 to 1200 mg of garlic powder daily in divided doses, or up to 4 g of raw garlic daily.
Ginger (*Zingiber officinale*)	Antiemetic, good for motion sickness; inhibits platelet aggregation	Safe and effective; take 1-2 g/day; do not use concurrently with aspirin or warfarin. Can be safely recommended in the majority of patients.
Ginkgo (*Ginkgo biloba*)	Improves blood flow to brain and extremities; improves brain tissue tolerance to hypoxia; reduces capillary fragility; alleviates vertigo and ringing in the ears; may slow dementia	Ginkgo is an option in patients with Alzheimer's disease who are also receiving medical care, but the herb has antiplatelet activity and thus may not be appropriate for patients with bleeding disorder or on antiplatelet or anticoagulation agents. Safe and effective; take 60 mg twice daily of standard extract. Only useful to elderly or debilitated persons; of no use in persons with normal brain function.

Continued

Table 6-2	Herbs Considered Safe and Effective—cont'd	
COMMON NAME	**USE FOR WHICH PROMOTED**	**SAFETY, EFFICACY, DOSAGE**
Ginseng	Taken for hot flashes but may make them worse	Safe but questionable efficacy; not an aphrodisiac; no effect on fatigue or stress. No robust clinical trials. Do not exceed labeled dosage, since adverse effects may occur. Discourage use in those anticoagulated or with cardiovascular or metabolic disease, such as hypertension and diabetes.
Goldenseal	Prevention or resolution of upper respiratory infections	Safe and effective mullein expectorant, decreases bronchial spasms; reduces colds, bronchitis
Mullein	Expectorant, decreases bronchial spasms; reduces colds, bronchitis	Safe and effective
Rose hips	Fights infections by reducing capillary fragility; contains high concentration of vitamin C	Safe and effective
St. John's wort	Antidepressant	The most commonly studied dose for depression is 300 mg taken 3 times a day, standardized to 0.3% to 0.5% hypericin per dose. Do not use in addition to other antidepressants. Depressed patients should not take without medical supervision; should be used only in the mildly depressed patient with an aversion to prescription medication. Has numerous potential drug interactions with P450 enzyme system.
Saw palmetto	Reduces benign prostatic hypertrophy	Safe and effective; take 0.5-1 g/day. Men with obstructive urinary symptoms should not self-medicate with saw palmetto. Such patients should be under medical supervision, because the symptoms of BPH can mimic other more serious disorders, such as prostate cancer and prostatitis. This herb should be reserved for men with mild BPH symptoms who have an aversion to prescription drugs and are also under medical care.
Valerian (*Valeriana officinalis*)	Mild tranquilizer and sleeping aid	Safe and effective; take 1-3 g/day; enhances the effects of other drugs that calm, sedate, or tranquilize. Chemicals may help insomnia. Mild side effects have included paradoxic stimulation (restlessness and palpitations), especially with long-term use. Valerian should not be used during pregnancy. This herb may have an additive effect with other central nervous system depressants. Patients should be cautioned regarding the operation of machinery when initiating therapy until they are accustomed to the effects. Other potential side effects include headaches, excitability, and uneasiness. Typical dosages for insomnia are 200-400 mg (standardized to 0.8%-1% valeric acids per dose) at bedtime.

Data from Edmunds MW, Mayhew MS: *Pharmacology for the primary care provider*, ed 2, St Louis, 2004, Mosby; Krinsky DL, LaValle JB, Hawkins EB, et al: *Natural therapeutics pocket guide*, ed 2, Hudson, Ohio, 2003, Lexicomp; and Hulisz DT: Top herbal products: efficacy and safety concerns (online): Available at http://www.medscape.com/viewprogram/8494. Accessed January 4, 2008.
BP, Blood pressure; *BPH*, benign prostatic hyperplasia; *FDA*, Food and Drug Administration.

also believed by some that these oils have medical properties that fight bacteria, viruses, bacterial toxins, and fungi. The scents are thought to work by triggering hormones that govern bodily functions. Massage with oils or inhaling their vapors is effective, but these oils should never be swallowed or applied near the eyes. It is believed that when these oils are applied to the skin or the vapors are inhaled, their molecules attach to oxygen molecules in the lungs and circulate through the body, helping the body to heal itself. Although the practice of aromatherapy has many followers, there is very little research presently available

to support its use. If nothing else, aromatherapy may give the patient a sense of well being and that in itself can be therapeutic.

DRUGS FOR HEALTH PROMOTION: VITAMINS AND MINERALS

Another major category of drugs used for self-care is vitamins and minerals. People in the United States are using vitamins and minerals to prevent cancer, boost immunity, cope with stress, strengthen bones, and increase their overall sense of well being. Sales of these

| Table 6-3 | Herbs Considered Unsafe | |

COMMON NAME	USE FOR WHICH PROMOTED	SAFETY, EFFICACY, DOSAGE
Blue cohosh	Labor induction; reduction of menopause symptoms	Causes birth defects in animals
Borage	Antidiarrheal, diuretic	Contains pyrrolidine alkaloids that are potentially carcinogenic and toxic to the liver
Broom (broom tops)	Miscellaneous	Toxic
Calamus	Antipyretic, digestive aid	Has produced malignancy in rats
Chaparral	Natural antioxidant, blood purity, anticancer, acne treatment	Causes severe liver damage; two cases known in which liver transplants were required
Coltsfoot	Antitussive, demulcent	Contains carcinogenic alkaloids
Comfrey	Wound healing	Obstruction of blood flow from liver; has caused cirrhosis and death
Ephedra	Anorectic, bronchodilator	Ineffective as an anorectic; effective for bronchodilation; unsafe for those with hypertension, diabetes, or thyroid disease; unsafe with caffeine; may cause serious toxic reactions when taken concurrently with MAO inhibitors
Germander	Anorectic	Causes hepatotoxicity
Jin Bu Huan	Stomachache, insomnia, antitussive	Causes hepatitis, respiratory depression with bradycardia
Licorice	Expectorant, antiulcer	Effective, but safe only in small doses for short periods; may cause sodium retention and potassium loss
Lobelia	Bronchodilator	High doses can decrease respiration, raise heart rate, and lower blood pressure
Pennyroyal	Abortion agent	Causes severe hepatotoxicity, interference with clotting
Royal jelly	Insomnia, liver ailments	Causes serious to fatal allergic reactions
Sassafras	General tonic	Contains safrole, a carcinogen
Senna (*Senna alexandrina*)	Laxative	Causes electrolyte imbalance, particularly potassium loss
Stephania magnolia	Weight loss	Causes renal toxicity
Willow bark	Antipyretic	Causes gastritis, bleeding, and Reye syndrome
Yohimbé	Aphrodisiac	Causes psychosis, loss of consciousness

Modified from Edmunds MW, Mayhew MS: *Pharmacology for the primary care provider*, ed 3, St Louis, 2009, Mosby.
MAO, Monoamine oxidase.

| Table 6-4 | Natural Remedies Other than Herbs or Vitamins | | |

NAME	SOURCE	USES	SAFETY AND EFFICACY
Chondroitin	Cow cartilage	Eases aches and pains; protects and rebuilds cartilage	Safe and effective; 400 mg/day
Dehydroepiandrosterone (DHEA)	Androgen hormone synthesized from wild yams	Alleviates cancer, heart disease, and autoimmune disease; antiaging remedy	Believed to be safe, but all side effects are not known; toxic to liver in sufficient quantities; efficacy not proven
Glucosamine	Oyster shells	Eases aches and pains; protects and rebuilds cartilage	Safe and effective if shells are not from polluted water; 500 mg/day
Melatonin	If produced from natural sources, it comes from the pineal glands of cows	Cure for jet lag; helps regulate the body's clock; sleep aid; antiaging remedy	May inhibit sex drive in men; 1-3 mg at bedtime

Modified from Edmunds MW, Mayhew MS: *Pharmacology for the primary care provider*, ed 3, St Louis, 2009, Mosby.

products are now at record highs. Patients often decide on their own that they need such products. They may or may not seek advice from a health care provider or pharmacist about what to take. Many different products are for sale, and the price varies a lot for the same product. Costs for some products are high because of the claims made about their effectiveness, but not all such claims for vitamins and minerals have been proved. Does more expensive mean better? What is fact and what is fiction about the use of vitamins and minerals?

PROS AND CONS

What is known is that vitamin and mineral supplements are useful when the patient has a deficiency, as may be the case in women in their childbearing years and in the elderly population. The American Heart Association has suggested that people should eat more fruits, vegetables, and whole grains; implement an exercise program; replace saturated fats with oils from fish and nuts; and limit salt and alcohol intake. Most official sources suggest that if a variety of healthy foods are eaten, the necessary vitamins can likely be obtained from diet alone. However, supplements may be required for some patients, mostly those who may be deficient. For supplementation, vitamins should have 50% to 150% of the recommended dietary allowance (RDA), and daily treatment should not provide more than 2 to 10 times the RDA for a specific vitamin.

There are known dangers to vitamin use, especially high-dose use. When megadoses of most vitamins are taken, the excess amount is quickly excreted in the urine with no additional benefit to the patient. Occasionally, when large doses of vitamin A are taken, the amount not used rapidly by the body may be stored in the tissues, causing the skin to turn yellow. Most vitamin products can be toxic to children, and iron can be deadly to small children. Folic acid can react with anticancer treatment medications and mask signs of vitamin B_{12} deficiency. Sometimes the body starts to rely on large doses of vitamin C when taken over a prolonged period, and the body may believe there is a deficiency when the patient returns to a normal dose. Patients with diarrhea may lose vitamin and mineral products unchanged in the stool. There is also some evidence that vitamin use may weaken the efficacy of immunizations for flu in the older adult population.

Overuse of minerals can also be dangerous. Large amounts of calcium can limit the absorption of iron and other trace elements. They can also cause constipation and reduce kidney function. Calcium is needed primarily in menopausal women and older men, particularly those who are at risk for bone loss.

Antioxidant vitamins have a prominent place in the current literature on nutritional supplements. The major antioxidant vitamins are vitamin E, or alpha-tocopherol; beta-carotene or provitamin A, which is a precursor to vitamin A; vitamin C, or ascorbic acid; and selenium. All of these vitamins are found in fruits and vegetables. Many research studies are being done to determine the mechanism of action of antioxidants. Current research suggests that when low-density lipoprotein (LDL) cholesterol is oxidized, the oxidation is often incomplete. (The analogy has been made to wood that burns incompletely in a fireplace and "pops," sending sparks against the screen.) This incomplete oxidation produces free radicals that often lead to atherosclerotic plaques. It is believed that antioxidants slow or prevent LDL cholesterol oxidation because they are oxidized better than LDL cholesterol. This slows or eliminates atherosclerosis. It is also believed that antioxidants slow the process that may cause cells to become cancerous. This has caused a large increase in the sales of antioxidants in an attempt to decrease cardiovascular disease and cancer.

Although many major research studies have looked at antioxidants and found they may have some benefits, no major clinical studies have concluded that antioxidants prevent cancer. There is evidence that those who eat fruits and vegetables regularly have less risk of cancer. However, there is no evidence that this is the result of antioxidants. Therefore, taking antioxidant vitamins may be helpful to some extent. Research has also found that vitamins C, B_6, B_{12}, and E may be helpful in preventing coronary artery disease.

Advertisers suggest that natural products are better than synthetic vitamins. However, current research concludes that vitamins are probably the same whether they are natural or synthetic, costly or cheap. In fact, natural vitamins may contain other chemicals or impurities that may make them less effective than standardized synthetic products. The most important differences are that some preparations may dissolve better than others or contain the active product in amounts that increase the absorption of other vitamins and minerals taken at the same time.

National surveys have shown that those who least need extra vitamins and minerals are the most likely to take them, including people who eat well, exercise, and do not smoke. There is no evidence that people who take vitamins live longer or suffer less illness or disease. A benefit of vitamins and minerals to the average healthy individual who consumes a variety of foods has never been proved. The United States Department of Agriculture's new MyPlate tool reminds people to balance what they are eating so they get their essential nutrition every day.

Supplements cannot make up for a poor diet or unhealthy lifestyle practices such as smoking or lack of exercise. Patients who do not eat a well-balanced diet and do eat lots of high-fat or "empty-calorie" foods may want to consider taking a multivitamin and mineral supplement. Most women in the United States 20 years of age or older eat approximately 1673 calories a day. Women who diet may eat fewer calories and may need to work harder to get the RDAs for essential vitamins and minerals. If patients cannot eat certain foods such as dairy foods, they may need to supplement their diet to make sure they are getting the nutrients they need.

An increasing amount of research suggests that taking specific nutrients may offer protection against problems such as osteoporosis, birth defects, heart disease, stroke, infectious diseases, macular degeneration, and cataracts. These products are taken to maintain or improve a person's health and well being, or for **health promotion**. Some of these products are discussed in the following sections. Chapter 24 provides a complete discussion of the types of vitamins and minerals, their actions, uses, adverse reactions, and drug interactions.

CALCIUM

In 1993, the FDA approved the use of a health claim on food and supplement labels about the role of calcium in reducing the risk of osteoporosis and the need for calcium supplements by people who do not get enough calcium from their diets. The current advice is for people older than the age of 50 to consume at least 1200 mg of calcium daily. More than three glasses of low-fat milk per day would be required to provide this much calcium. Calcium-fortified (or enriched) products such as orange juice, sardines, salmon, tofu, and other dairy products help meet the daily requirements. The calcium citrate malate found in fortified orange juice is one of the best forms of calcium because it tends to be absorbed better than other types. The calcium carbonate found in Tums and other antacids is also acceptable. Vitamin D is important for calcium absorption. It is available as a supplement in multivitamins and fortified milk and naturally from exposure of the skin to the sun. Some calcium products also come with a small amount of magnesium, which also helps calcium absorption. Calcium supplements are best absorbed when taken with food because food slows down their passage through the large intestine.

FOLIC ACID, VITAMIN B$_6$, AND VITAMIN B$_{12}$

There is now a significant amount of scientific data showing that eating foods containing folate (citrus fruits, cereals, leafy greens, and whole grains) or taking a multivitamin containing folic acid protects against fetal neural tube birth defects such as spina bifida and anencephaly and may also reduce the risk of heart disease and stroke. The neural tube of the fetus is formed within the first 28 days of pregnancy, before many women know they are pregnant. However, the evidence for folic acid in preventing neural tube defects is so strong that the U.S. Public Health Service issued an official recommendation that "all women of childbearing age in the United States who are capable of becoming pregnant should consume 0.4 mg of folic acid per day for the purpose of reducing their risk of having baby with spina bifida or other neural tube defects." This warning applies to women throughout their childbearing years. The dose of folic acid should be increased to 4 mg/day for at least 3 months before a woman plans to get pregnant.

Research has also established that modestly elevated homocysteine levels in the blood are a risk factor for heart disease. Folic acid and vitamins B$_6$ and B$_{12}$ have been shown to reduce homocysteine levels. The intake of these three B complex vitamins, found primarily in vegetables and legumes, has been shown to be low in the United States, particularly in the older adult population. Vitamin B$_{12}$ is also found in meat and fish but is not absorbed as easily by people as they age. Some experts say that those at risk for heart disease should take a supplement that contains folic acid and vitamins B$_6$ and B$_{12}$. Folic acid may be more readily absorbed from supplements and enriched foods than from other sources.

IRON

Iron has long been known to be necessary for people who suffer from anemia caused by blood loss. Thus young women of childbearing age are often given iron supplements. Most menopausal women would probably benefit from a multivitamin containing 10 milligrams of iron or less. Iron supplements for people who do not have blood loss have not been shown to be needed or desirable. High levels of iron in the blood can result in heart disease, cancer, and serious infection. However, it is hard to find a multivitamin without iron. People should take iron and calcium supplements at different times because these two minerals compete for absorption and taken together, neither one will have sufficient therapeutic action. Iron may also be very constipating, especially in some elderly patients.

SUMMARY

The scientific information about herbal products and alternative health care is still sparse. These herbal products are not benign and should be respected as important chemicals. Consumers with serious or chronic health complaints will often self-diagnose and self-treat with OTC drugs, herbs, and supplements. This is not ideal, because many of these patients need supervised medical care.

It is good practice for health professionals to advise anyone pregnant or breastfeeding to avoid use of herbal products because the effects on fetal development and breast milk excretion are unknown. Similarly, use in infants and younger children should be strongly discouraged.

If patients are taking herbal products or supplements, advise them to take the dosages that have been studied in clinical trials and not to exceed labeled amounts. Patients should avoid products with labels that fail to specify the exact amount of the herb contained per dosage unit. Generally, herbs should be taken only for a short time.

If patients tell you they are taking herbal products, take a careful history regarding any plant allergies, especially to ragweed and daisies, as many patients with allergic rhinitis (runny nose) may not know what allergens trigger their attacks. Patients who are allergic to ragweed and flowers in the daisy family (asters, chrysanthemums) may have allergic reactions to products containing echinacea and chamomile. Some herbs are photosensitizing (e.g., St. John's wort), and patients should be cautioned appropriately (especially fair-skinned individuals).

Herbal products should be discontinued at least 2 weeks prior to planned surgery, and patients should notify the anesthesiologist of herbs they have used routinely. Some herbals (e.g., garlic, ginkgo, ginseng, and ginger) may interfere with normal blood coagulation, predisposing patients to prolonged bleeding and interactions with warfarin. See other related chapters for more details on these products.

Get Ready for the NCLEX® Examination!

Key Points

- The nurse often serves, either formally or informally, as a teacher and adviser to the patient.
- It is important to be knowledgeable enough to answer questions about OTC medications, current trends in alternative therapies, and recent recommendations about vitamins and minerals.
- Keeping up on recent findings will help prepare you for this part of your nursing role.

Additional Learning Resources

SG Go to your Study Guide for additional learning activities to help you master this chapter content.

evolve Go to your Evolve website (http://evolve.elsevier.com/Edmunds/LPN/) for additional online resources.

Review Questions for the NCLEX® Examination

1. The patient is trying to decrease his daily sodium intake to help reduce his blood pressure. The over-the-counter (OTC) products that he should avoid are:
   1. diuretics
   2. cough syrups
   3. weight control products
   4. sleep aids

2. The patient has a history of fibroid tissue in her breast and wants to limit her caffeine intake. The OTC products that she should avoid are:
   1. mouthwashes
   2. cold sore products
   3. antacids
   4. analgesics

3. In talking to the patient, the nurse learns the patient is taking both the herbal medication feverfew and the prescription drug warfarin (Coumadin). The most appropriate nursing action based on this information is to:

   1. notify the physician because the practice is not safe
   2. encourage the patient to continue this practice
   3. encourage the patient to divide the dosage in half
   4. notify the physician because an allergic reaction could occur

4. The patient tells the nurse that he has been taking garlic along with his antihypertensive medication to lower his blood pressure. He also says that he feels dizzy sometimes when he stands up. The best nursing action should be:
   1. tell the patient to increase the amount of garlic and notify the physician
   2. tell the patient that he may be allergic to garlic and notify the physician
   3. tell the patient to stop taking the garlic and notify the physician
   4. tell the patient to decrease the amount of garlic and notify the physician

5. The patient tells the nurse that he has seen royal jelly advertised in an infomercial and wants to try it to treat his insomnia. The most appropriate response from the nurse should be:
   1. "This is safe to use, but you should monitor your blood pressure closely."
   2. "This is safe to use in limited amounts."
   3. "This is not a safe herbal preparation to take."
   4. "This is not safe to use unless you combine it with other herbs."

Critical Thinking Questions

1. A patient you are caring for has hypertension. He tells you that he routinely takes Sudafed for colds and sinus infections. What would you tell him?
2. Mrs. Brown is recovering from a stroke. She has been given anticoagulant therapy and is about to go home. Although she is making good progress, she is quite depressed about her appearance and her inability to walk without assistance. Her family wants her to begin taking gingko for depression. What will you tell them?

3. You develop a bad cold. When you go to the pharmacy, you see OTC medications labeled as decongestants and others labeled as antihistamines. Which will you buy and why?

4. Tylenol is a common product available in almost every home. Look at the dosages of Tylenol for infants, children, and adults. If you have a child under 2 years, a 6-year-old, and a 12-year-old, could you give them the same product? Look at the symptoms of overdosage. How easy do you think it would be to give an overdose of this medication to a child?

5. Make a list of the OTC medications in your locked medicine closet. Would any of these products be dangerous if a child were to take them? Does this information make you reconsider how you store these products?

6. Your patient says she plans to go to a health food store to buy some medication for menopausal hot flashes. What information would you give her about the products sold in these stores?

7. You discover that one of your Chinese patients makes a medicinal tea every morning. This patient has asthma and high blood pressure. What are some of the things you might want to talk about with this patient?

8. One of your very-low-income patients has been buying very expensive vitamins at a health food store. What information would you offer? What benefits exist for using these instead of less expensive vitamins available at the grocery store?

9. Which of the following individuals would you expect to need a daily multivitamin and mineral supplement: a 30-year-old woman who smokes, a thin 5-year-old boy, a 20-year-old female who is a vegetarian, a 30-year-old man who drinks lots of coffee and eats erratically, a 40-year-old woman who has had six children, a 35-year-old homeless man with cirrhosis of the liver, and a 60-year-old postal worker. Give a reason why or why not for each person.

10. Your new daughter-in-law tells you that she and your son plan to start a family. What vitamins or minerals will her health care provider most likely recommend that she take? Why?

Chapter

7

Review of Mathematical Principles

*e*volve

http://evolve.elsevier.com/Edmunds/LPN/

Objectives

1. Work basic multiplication and division problems.
2. Interpret Roman numerals correctly.

3. Apply basic rules in calculations, using fractions, decimal fractions, percentages, ratios, and proportions.

Key Terms

common denominator (dē-NŎM-ĭ-nā-tŏr, p. 73)
complex fraction (FRĂK-shŭn, p. 72)
denominator (dē-NŎM-ĭ-nā-tŏr, p. 71)
fraction (FRĂK-shŭn, p. 71)
improper fraction (ĭm-PRŎP-ĕr FRĂK-shŭn, p. 72)
mixed number (p. 72)
numerator (NŪ-mĕr-ā-tŏr, p. 71)

percent (pĕr-CĔNT, p. 76)
proper fraction (PRŎP-ĕr FRĂK-shŭn, p. 72)
proportion (prŏp-ŎR-shun, p. 75)
ratio (RĂ-shē-ō, p. 75)
Roman numeral system (RŌM- ăn NŪ-mĕr-al SĬS-tĕm, p. 71)

OVERVIEW

It is very important to give the correct dose of a medicine. This may mean that you will need to accurately calculate the dosage using basic math formulas or a calculator. Even a small error in dosage may produce a big error. (Many of you may remember that the twin babies of Actor Dennis Quaid were accidentally given a huge overdose of heparin in the neonatal intensive care unit, which made the babies' blood fail to clot.) Accuracy with dosage ensures safety.

Although most nurses feel comfortable with addition and subtraction, many can profit from a review of basic concepts in multiplication and division, as well as fractions, percentages, and proportions, to increase their speed. These number relationships form important building blocks for tasks the nurse must master. By memorizing and drilling on these basic facts, you will have confidence and speed in calculating dosages and converting from one system of measures for drugs to another. Even if one uses a calculator, it is important to know how to manually do the math problem so you can recheck calculations at the bedside when necessary to make sure you aren't making a mistake.

MULTIPLICATION AND DIVISION

Box 7-1 presents a basic grid for multiplication and division. To multiply two numbers, find one number in the top row and the other number in the left-hand column, and follow the row leading across and the column leading down from each number to where the row and the column intersect (cross each other) within the grid.

For example: What is 7 × 8? Find the number 7 on the left and follow across to the right; find the number 8 on the top and follow down from it. The two lines intersect at 56. Therefore 7 × 8 = 56. Another way to indicate that two numbers are to be multiplied is to place them in parentheses next to each other. Therefore (30)(3) means 30 × 3.

To use this grid for division, find the number on the left-hand side of the chart that is the same as the divisor (the number you are dividing by). Follow the row to the right until you come to the exact number you are dividing or the number closest to it. Follow the column up to the top to learn the number of times that larger number may be divided by the number on the left.

For example: How many times will 9 go into 81? Find 9 in the column on the left. Follow the row across until you come to 81. Follow the column up from 81 to the top, which is 9. Therefore 81 ÷ 9 = 9. If you wanted to know how many times the whole number 9 would go into 84, you would still use the column containing the number 81, because it is the closest number in that row of the grid to 84. The answer would still be 9, but there would be a remainder of 3.

Box **7-1**	Multiplication and Division Grid										
1	2	3	4	5	6	7	8	9	10	11	12
2	4	6	8	10	12	14	16	18	20	22	24
3	6	9	12	15	18	21	24	27	30	33	36
4	8	12	16	20	24	28	32	36	40	44	48
5	10	15	20	25	30	35	40	45	50	55	60
6	12	18	24	30	36	42	48	54	60	66	72
7	14	21	28	35	42	49	56	63	70	77	84
8	16	24	32	40	48	56	64	72	80	88	96
9	18	27	36	45	54	63	72	81	90	99	108
10	20	30	40	50	60	70	80	90	100	110	120
11	22	33	44	55	66	77	88	99	110	121	132
12	24	36	48	60	72	84	96	108	120	132	144

Box **7-2**	Roman Numerals and Their Values

I = 1
V = 5
X = 10
L = 50
C = 100
D = 500
M = 1000

💡 Memory Jogger

Multiplication Hint

Zero times any number is zero!

ROMAN NUMERALS

The numbers commonly used today in expressing quantity and value are called *Arabic numerals.* Examples of Arabic numerals are 1, 2, and 3. Another number system in common use is the **Roman numeral system.** Roman numerals from the values of 1 to 100 are commonly used as units of the apothecaries' system of weights and measures in writing prescriptions. They may also be used to express dates in copyrights and in formal manuscripts. Seven numerals make up the basic building blocks of the Roman numeral system (Box 7-2).

After memorizing the seven Roman numerals and their values, it is important to learn the four rules in using Roman numerals. These rules and some examples are presented in Box 7-3.

FRACTIONS

A good understanding of fractions is important to the nurse because all units of the apothecaries' system are written as common fractions for all amounts less than 1. Fractions also form the foundation in dosage calculations when medication is only available in a different dose form than the form that was ordered.

Box **7-3**	Rules in Using Roman Numerals

1. Whenever a Roman numeral is repeated, or when a smaller numeral follows a larger one, the values are added together. For example:
   II = 2 (1 + 1 = 2)
   LVII = 57 (50 + 5 + 1 + 1 = 57)
   CXIII = 113 (100 + 10 + 1 + 1 + 1 = 113)
2. Whenever a smaller Roman numeral comes before a larger Roman numeral, subtract the smaller value from the larger one. For example:
   IV = 4 (5 − 1 = 4)
   CD = 400 (500 − 100 = 400)
3. Numerals are never repeated more than three times in a sequence. For example:
   III = 3
   IV = 4
4. Whenever a smaller Roman numeral comes between two larger Roman numerals, subtract the smaller number from the numeral following it. For example:
   XIX = 19 (10 + [10 − 1] = 19)
   LIV = 54 (50 + [5 − 1] = 54)
   In expressing dosages in the apothecaries' system, lowercase rather than capital Roman numerals are used. A dot is always placed over the Roman numeral i whenever lowercase numbers are used. For example, iii or vi is the proper form rather than III or VI.

BASIC PRINCIPLES

A **fraction** is one or more equal parts of a unit. It is written as two numbers separated by a line, such as ½ or ¾. The parts of the fraction are called the *terms.* The two terms of a fraction are the **numerator** and the **denominator.** The numerator is the top number (the number above the line). The denominator is the bottom number (the number below the line). In ½, 1 is the numerator, and 2 is the denominator.

The denominator tells how many equal parts the whole has been divided into. The numerator tells how many of the parts are being used.

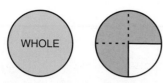

It is important not to confuse these two parts of the fraction. One way to remember which part belongs where is to think of the word *NUDE*. The *N* is on top; the *D* is on the bottom, like this:

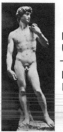

To use fractions in calculations, the numerator and the denominator must be of the same unit of measure. For example, if the numerator is in milligrams, the denominator must be in milligrams.

Fractions may be raised to higher terms by multiplying both terms of the fraction by the same number. For example, to raise ¾ to a higher term, multiply both the numerator and the denominator by 2, converting it to ⁶⁄₈. Thus ¾ and ⁶⁄₈ have the same value:

$$\frac{3}{4} \times \frac{2}{2} = \frac{6}{8}$$

Fractions are reduced to lower terms by dividing both the numerator and denominator by the same number. For example, to lower ³⁄₉ to a lower term, divide both the numerator and the denominator by 3, converting it to ⅓. Thus ³⁄₉ and ⅓ have the same value:

$$\frac{3}{9} \div \frac{3}{3} = \frac{1}{3}$$

A **proper fraction** has a numerator smaller than the denominator. The number ¾ is a proper fraction because it is less than 1; its numerator is less than its denominator.

An **improper fraction** has a numerator the same as or larger than the denominator. The number ⁶⁄₄ is an improper fraction because the numerator (6) is larger than the denominator (4).

A **mixed number** is a whole number and a proper fraction. Examples of mixed numbers are 4⅓, 3¾, and 5¹⁶⁄₃₅.

It is often necessary to change an improper fraction to a mixed number or to change a mixed number to an improper fraction when doing certain calculations. To change an improper fraction to a mixed number, divide

the denominator into the numerator. The result is the whole number (quotient) and the remainder, which is placed over the denominator of the improper fraction. For example, ¹⁷⁄₃ is an improper fraction. To convert it to a mixed number:

1. Divide the denominator (3) into the numerator (17):

$$\begin{array}{r} 5 \leftarrow \text{quotient} \\ 3\overline{)\,17} \\ \underline{-15} \\ 2 \leftarrow \text{remainder} \end{array}$$

2. Move the remainder (2) over the denominator (3).
3. Put the quotient (5) in front of the fraction:

$$5\frac{2}{3}$$

To change the mixed number 5⅔ to an improper fraction, multiply the denominator of the fraction (3) by the whole number (5), add the numerator (2), and place the sum over the denominator. For example:

$$\begin{array}{r} 3 \times 5 = 15 \\ \underline{+\ 2} \\ 17 \leftarrow \text{sum} \end{array}$$

The sum (17) goes over the denominator of the fraction: ¹⁷⁄₃ is the improper fraction.

A **complex fraction** has a fraction in either its numerator, its denominator, or both. The following are examples of complex fractions:

$$\frac{\dfrac{1}{5}}{50} \qquad \frac{\dfrac{30}{2}}{3} \qquad 3\frac{\dfrac{2}{1}}{8}$$

Complex fractions may be changed to whole numbers or to proper or improper fractions by dividing the number or fraction above the line by the number or fraction below the line. For example, to change the following complex number to a proper fraction, divide the fraction above the line by the number below the line:

$$\frac{\dfrac{1}{2}}{100} = \frac{1}{2} \div 100$$

To divide by 100, or ¹⁰⁰⁄₁, simply invert or reverse the numerator (100) and the denominator (1) and multiply by the result, or by ¹⁄₁₀₀. For example:

$$\frac{1}{2} \div 100 = \frac{1}{2} \div \frac{100}{1} = \frac{1}{2} \times \frac{1}{100}$$

$$= \frac{1}{2 \times 100} = \frac{1}{200}$$

Adding Fractions

If fractions have the same denominator, simply add the numerators and put the sum above the common denominator. For example:

$$\frac{1}{11} + \frac{3}{11} = \frac{4}{11} \quad \frac{(\text{sum of } 1+3)}{(\text{same denominator})}$$

Also:

$$\frac{2}{12} + \frac{3}{12} + \frac{6}{12} = \frac{11}{12} \quad \frac{(\text{sum of } 2+3+6)}{(\text{same denominator})}$$

If the fractions have different denominators, they must be converted to a number that each denominator has in common, or a **common denominator**. One can always find a common denominator by multiplying the two denominators by one another. Sometimes, however, both numbers will go into a smaller number. For example, in the equation $\frac{1}{12} + \frac{3}{8} + \frac{3}{4} = ?$, what is the smallest common denominator?

1. The smallest whole number all these denominators (12, 8, and 4) have in common is 24; 24, then, is the lowest common denominator.
2. Divide the lowest common denominator (24) by the denominator of each fraction (12, 8, and 4) to determine the quotient, or the answer to be used to convert each fraction to a number with the common denominator:

$$\frac{12}{24} = ?$$

$$\frac{8}{24} = ?$$

$$\frac{4}{24} = ?$$

3. Next, multiply both the numerator and the denominator of each fraction by the quotient for each. This is often easier to see if the problem is written vertically:

$$\frac{1}{12} \times \frac{2}{2} = \frac{2}{24}$$
$$+ \frac{3}{8} \times \frac{3}{3} = \frac{9}{24}$$
$$+ \frac{3}{4} \times \frac{6}{6} = \frac{18}{24}$$

4. Then add the numerators and bring down the denominator:

$$\frac{2}{24} + \frac{9}{24} + \frac{18}{24} = \frac{29}{24}$$

5. Change the improper fraction to a mixed number:

$$\frac{29}{24} = 1\frac{5}{24}$$

When adding mixed numbers, first change them to improper fractions and proceed as indicated previously.

Subtracting Fractions

If fractions have the same denominator, subtract the smaller numerator from the larger numerator. Leave the denominator the same, and then reduce to the lowest terms, if necessary. For example:

$$\frac{5}{10} - \frac{1}{10} = \frac{4}{10} = \frac{2}{5}$$

If fractions do not have the same denominator, change the fractions so they have the smallest common denominator, subtract the numerators, and leave the denominator the same. For example:

$$\frac{15}{28} - \frac{3}{14} = ?$$

Because 28 is a multiple of 14 (14 × 2 = 28), 28 is a common denominator of 28 and 14. Divide the lowest common denominator by the denominator of each fraction to determine the quotient, and multiply the numerator and denominator of the fraction by the quotient:

$$\frac{15}{28} \times \frac{1}{1} = \frac{15}{28} (\text{no change necessary})$$

$$\frac{3}{14} \times \frac{2}{2} = \frac{6}{28} (28 \div 14 = 2)$$

Subtract the numerators and leave the denominators the same:

$$\frac{15}{28} - \frac{6}{28} = \frac{9}{28}$$

When subtracting mixed numbers, first change them to improper fractions and proceed as shown in the previous examples.

Multiplying Fractions

When multiplying fractions, reduce all terms to their smallest form to simplify the calculation. For example, $\frac{12}{24}$ is the same as $\frac{1}{2}$, but $\frac{12}{24}$ is more difficult to work with. To reduce to the lowest terms, divide the same number into both the numerator and the denominator.

For example, in the fraction $\frac{2}{10}$ both 2 and 10 can be divided by 2; therefore, $\frac{2}{10} \div \frac{2}{2} = \frac{1}{5}$. Similarly, in the fraction $\frac{9}{36}$ both the numerator and the denominator can be divided by 9; therefore, $\frac{9}{36} \div \frac{9}{9} = \frac{1}{4}$.

When the fractions are in their simplest form, multiply the numerators together, and then multiply the denominators together. For example:

$$\frac{1}{20} \times \frac{5}{3} \times 3 =$$

$$\frac{1}{20} \times \frac{5}{3} \times \frac{3}{1} =$$

$$\frac{1 \times 5 \times 3}{20 \times 3 \times 1} = \frac{15}{60}$$

This can be simplified as follows:

$$\frac{15}{60} = \frac{1}{4}$$

If the number is a mixed number (a whole number and a fraction), change it to an improper fraction before solving. For example:

$$2\frac{1}{2} \times \frac{2}{3} \times 6 = \frac{5}{2} \times \frac{2}{3} \times \frac{6}{1}$$

Simplify:

$$= \frac{5}{\underset{1}{\cancel{2}}} \times \frac{\overset{1}{\cancel{2}}}{\underset{1}{\cancel{3}}} \times \frac{\overset{2}{\cancel{6}}}{1}$$

$$= \frac{10}{1} = 10$$

 Memory Jogger

Multiplying Fractions

Because 3 is a whole number, it is the same as $\frac{3}{1}$; the 1 can be added as a denominator if it makes calculations easier to understand.

Dividing Fractions

To divide a fraction by a fraction, invert (or turn upside down) the fraction that is the divisor and then multiply. For example:

$$\frac{4}{6} \div \frac{2}{6} = ?$$

Invert the divisor:

$$\frac{4}{6} \times \frac{6}{2} = ?$$

Simplify, then multiply the numerators and then the denominators:

$$\frac{\overset{2}{\cancel{4}}}{\underset{1}{\cancel{6}}} \times \frac{\overset{1}{\cancel{6}}}{\underset{1}{\cancel{2}}} = \frac{2}{1} = 2$$

If the number is a mixed number, change it to an improper fraction before solving. For example:

$$\frac{2}{3} \div 1\frac{1}{3} = ?$$

Change the mixed number to an improper fraction:

$$\frac{2}{3} \div \frac{4}{3} = ?$$

Invert the divisor:

$$\frac{2}{3} \times \frac{3}{4} = ?$$

Simplify:

$$\frac{\overset{1}{\cancel{2}}}{\underset{1}{\cancel{3}}} \times \frac{\overset{1}{\cancel{3}}}{\underset{2}{\cancel{4}}} = \frac{1}{2}$$

$$\frac{1}{1} \times \frac{1}{2} = \frac{1}{2}$$

DECIMAL FRACTIONS

A decimal fraction has a denominator of 10 or a multiple of 10. Instead of writing the denominator, a decimal point is added to the numerator. For example:

$$\frac{1}{4} = \frac{25}{100} = 0.25$$

All numbers to the left of the decimal point represent whole numbers. Numbers to the right represent fractions. Zeros may be placed to the right of the decimal without changing the value of the whole number (for example, 45 is the same as 45.0 or 45.00).

Decimals increase in value from right to left; they decrease in value from left to right. Decimals increase in value in multiples of 10. Each column in a decimal has its own value, according to where it lies in relation to the decimal point (Figure 7-1).

Adding and Subtracting Decimal Fractions

Place the numbers so that the decimal points are stacked in a straight line. Keep the columns straight. Add zeros to the right of the decimal points if necessary so that each number has an equal number of digits to the right of the decimal point. Then add or subtract as for whole numbers. The decimal point goes in the answer just below the decimal points in the problem. For example, to add 0.0678 and 1.082:

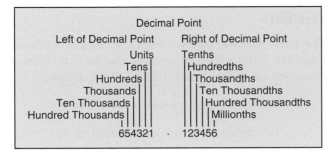

FIGURE 7-1 Values left and right of the decimal point.

$$\begin{array}{r} 0.0678 \\ 1.0820 \\ +\overline{} \\ \hline 1.1498 \end{array} \quad \text{(add one zero)}$$

Note that the decimal point in the answer is in line with the other decimal points.

To subtract 3.053 from 6.046:

$$\begin{array}{r} 6.046 \\ -3.053 \\ \hline 2.993 \end{array}$$

Multiplying and Dividing Decimal Fractions

To multiply decimal fractions, multiply the two numbers as for whole numbers. Then count the number of decimal places in the multiplicand (the number that is multiplied) and the number in the multiplier (the number you multiply by). Beginning at the right side of the product (answer), count off that total number of decimal places from right to left and insert a decimal point. For example:

44.61	Multiplicand (has two decimal places)
× 2.3	Multiplier (has one decimal place)
13383	
+89220	
102.603	Count off three places right to left and insert decimal point.

To divide by a decimal fraction, first move the decimal point in the divisor (the number you are dividing with) enough places right to make it a whole number. Then move the decimal point in the dividend (the number you are dividing) as many places as it was moved in the divisor. Place the decimal point in the quotient (answer) directly above that in the dividend. For example, to divide 32.80 by 8.2:

$$8.2\overline{)32.80} \quad \text{8.2 is the divisor; 32.80 is the dividend}$$

Move the decimal point in the divisor to the right to make it a whole number, then move it the same number of places in the dividend:

$$8.2\overline{\smash{)}\,32.80}$$

Solve the problem:

$$\begin{array}{r} 4.0 \\ 82.0\overline{)\,328.00} \\ -328.00 \\ \hline 0 \end{array}$$

A shortcut may be taken when multiplying or dividing by 10, 100, or 1000. To multiply a decimal fraction by 10, 100, or 1000, move the decimal point as many places to the right as there are zeros in the multiplier. For example:

$$0.0006 \times 1000 = ?$$

In 1000 there are three zeros, so:

$$0.0006 \times 1000 = ?$$
$$0.0006 = 0000.6 = 0.6$$

To divide a decimal fraction by 10, 100, or 1000, move the decimal place as many places to the left as there are zeros in the divisor. For example:

$$0.5 \div 100 = ?$$

The number 100 has two zeros, so:

$$0.5 \times 100 = 000.5 = 0.005$$

RATIOS

A **ratio** is a way of expressing the relationship of one number to another number, or of expressing a part of a whole number. The relationship is expressed by separating the numbers with a colon (:). The colon means division. The expression 1:2 means there is a ratio of one part to two parts. Ratios are commonly used to express concentrations of a drug in a solution.

For example, a ratio written as 1:20 means 1 part to 20 parts. The relationship may also be expressed as a fraction (e.g., 1:10 is the same as $\frac{1}{10}$).

PROPORTIONS

A **proportion** is a way of expressing a relationship of equality between two ratios. In other words, the first ratio listed is equal to the second ratio listed. The two ratios are separated by a double colon (::), which means "as." The numbers at each end of the relationship are the extremes, and the two numbers in the middle are the means. In any proportion, *the product of the extremes equals the product of the means.* This means that if one of the terms is not known, it may be calculated. The unknown term is defined by an *x*. For example:

$$5 : 500 :: 2 : x$$

(where *x* is the unknown) can be read as "5 is to 500 as 2 is to *x*" or "The relationship of 5 to 500 is the same as the relationship of 2 to *x*." Then:

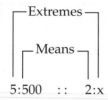

In this proportion, 5 and *x* are the extremes, and 500 and 2 are the means. Therefore:

$$5 \times x = 500 \times 2$$

To find *x*, express the proportion as a relationship of two fractions, cross multiply, and solve:

$$\frac{5}{500} = \frac{2}{x}$$

$$5x = 500 \times 2$$

$$5x = 1000$$

$$x = \frac{1000}{5}$$

$$x = 200$$

Because a proportion is a relationship of equality, both ratios in the proportion must also be written in the same system (e.g., minims are to grains as minims are to grains; milliliters are to grams as milliliters are to grams). For example:

ⓜ 15 ⓖⓡ : 60 ⓜ   ⓖⓡ :: 13 : x Correctly written

ⓜ 15 ⓜ : 60 ⓜ   ⓖⓡ :: 13 : x Incorrectly written

The calculation of ratios and proportions provides one of the major foundations in drug dosage calculations. Often you know the desired concentration of drug and need to calculate how much to give of a medication on hand. You will be able to figure how much medication to give by using the principles of proportion.

PERCENTS

The term **percent**, or the symbol %, means parts per hundred. Thus a percentage may also be expressed as a fraction or as a decimal fraction. For example:

30% means 30 parts per hundred or $^{30}/_{100}$

70% means 70 parts per hundred or $^{70}/_{100}$

Percentages should also be reduced to their lowest common denominator, when appropriate. For example:

20% is $^{20}/_{100}$ or $\frac{1}{5}$

40% is $^{40}/_{100}$ or $\frac{2}{5}$

To change a fraction to a percentage, divide the numerator by the denominator, multiply the quotient (results) by 100, and add a percent sign (%). For example, to change $^{8}/_{10}$ to a percentage:

$$8 \div 10 = 0.8$$

$$0.8 \times 100 = 80\%$$

To change $^{2}/_{5}$ to a percentage:

$$2 \div 5 = 0.4$$

$$0.4 \times 100 = 40\%$$

To change a mixed number to a percentage, first change it to an improper fraction, then proceed as noted previously. For example, to change $1\frac{1}{4}$ to a percentage:

$$\frac{5}{4} = 5 \div 4 = 1.25$$

$$1.25 \times 100 = 125\%$$

To change a ratio to a percentage, the ratio is first expressed as a fraction. The first number or term of the ratio becomes the numerator, and the second number or term becomes the denominator (e.g., 1:200 becomes $\frac{1}{200}$). The fraction is then changed to a percentage:

$$1:200 = \frac{1}{200}$$

$$1 \div 200 = 0.005$$

$$0.005 \times 100 = 0.5\%$$

To change a percentage to a ratio, the percentage becomes the numerator and is placed over the denominator of 100. For example, to change 20% and 50% to ratios:

$$20\% \text{ is } \frac{20}{100} = \frac{1}{5} \text{ or } 1:5$$

$$50\% \text{ is } \frac{50}{100} = \frac{1}{2} \text{ or } 1:2$$

$$20\% = 0.20 = \frac{20}{100} = \frac{1}{5} = 1:5$$

A percentage may easily be expressed as a decimal, a fraction, or a ratio. For example:

It is very easy to change between fractions, percentages, decimals, and ratios. The rules that summarize these changes are presented in Box 7-4.

Box 7-4   **Rules for Changing Between Percentages, Decimals, Fractions, and Ratios**

CHANGING FRACTIONS
- To change a fraction to a ratio, write the two numbers with a colon between them instead of the dividing line.
  Example: $\frac{1}{5}$ = 1:5
- To change a fraction to a decimal fraction, divide the numerator by the denominator.
  Example: $\frac{1}{5}$ = 0.20
- To change a fraction to a percentage, divide the numerator by the denominator (use as many decimal places as needed); then move the decimal point two places to the right and add the percent sign.
  Example: $\frac{1}{5}$ = 0.20 = 20%

CHANGING PERCENTAGES
- To change a percentage to a decimal fraction, move the decimal point two places to the left and omit the percent sign.
  Example: 10% = 0.10
- To change a percentage to a fraction, drop the percent sign, write the number as the numerator, write 100 as the denominator, and reduce to the lowest terms.
  Example: 10% = $\frac{10}{100}$ = $\frac{1}{10}$
- To change a percentage to a ratio, drop the percent sign, use the number as the first term and 100 as the second term, and reduce to the lowest terms; or change to a fraction and then use a colon instead of the dividing line.
  Example: 10% = 10:100 = 1:10 or 10% = $\frac{1}{10}$ = 1:10

CHANGING DECIMALS
- To change a decimal fraction to a percentage, move the decimal point two places to the right (multiply by 100) and add the percent sign.
  Example: 0.20 = 20%
- To change a decimal fraction to a common fraction, omit the decimal point and place the number over the appropriate denominator of 10, 100, or 1000, and reduce to the lowest terms.
  Example: 0.20 = $\frac{20}{100}$ = $\frac{1}{5}$
- To change a decimal fraction to a ratio, write the number as the first term; then put 10, 100, or 1000 as the second term; finally, reduce to the lowest terms.
  Example: 0.20 = 20:100 or 1:5

CHANGING RATIOS
- To change a ratio to a fraction, write the numbers with a dividing line instead of a colon.
  Example: 1:20 = $\frac{1}{20}$
- To change a ratio to a decimal fraction, divide the first term by the second term.
  Example: 1:20 = 0.05
- To change a ratio to a percentage, divide the first term by the second term, move the decimal point two places to the right in the answer, and add a percent sign.

Get Ready for the NCLEX® Examination!

Key Points

- Understand and use basic math principles to calculate correct drug dosages.
- These basic math principles include the use of multiplication, division, and Roman numerals, as well as the calculation of fractions, decimal fractions, percentages, ratios, and proportions.
- Calculations may be done manually or using a calculator.

Additional Learning Resources

SG Go to your Study Guide for additional learning activities to help you master this chapter content.

evolve Go to your Evolve website (http://evolve.elsevier.com/Edmunds/LPN/) for additional online resources.

Review Questions for the NCLEX® Examination

1. $\frac{2}{3} - \frac{1}{4} =$ ___
   1. $\frac{1}{3}$
   2. $\frac{3}{12}$
   3. $\frac{1}{4}$
   4. $\frac{5}{12}$

2. $3\frac{1}{3} \times \frac{1}{6} \times 2 =$ ___
   1. $\frac{2}{3}$
   2. $\frac{10}{9}$
   3. $\frac{4}{6}$
   4. $4\frac{5}{9}$

3. 4 : 300 :: 3: x
   Which set of numbers constitute the means?
   1. 4 and x
   2. 4 and 300
   3. 300 and 3
   4. 3 and x

Get Ready for the NCLEX® Examination!—cont'd

4. Change $\frac{2}{3}$ to a percentage.
   1. 66%
   2. 72%
   3. 45%
   4. 23%

5. Change 33 percent to a ratio.
   1. 33:10
   2. 33:1
   3. 33:1000
   4. 33:100

Critical Thinking Questions

1. Match the following mathematical expressions or components on the left with their appropriate labels on the right:
   a. $\frac{2}{3}$ _____ ratio
   b. $\frac{25}{4}$ _____ denominator
   c. $5\frac{1}{8}$ _____ improper fraction
   d. 1 _____ mixed number
   e. 3 _____ numerator
   f. 3:4 _____ percent
   g. 75% _____ proper fraction
   h. $\frac{1}{4} + \frac{2}{5} = \frac{13}{20}$ _____ common denominator

2. Review multiplication and division by doing the following problems:
   a. $7 \times 11 =$
   b. $9 \div 3 =$
   c. $8 \times 7 =$
   d. $(252)(41) =$
   e. $98 \times 7 =$
   f. $360 \div 3 =$

3. Calculate the following division problems:
   a. $516 \div 7 =$
   b. $637 \div 4 =$
   c. $7849 \div 60 =$

4. Change the following Roman numerals into Arabic numerals, and the Arabic numerals into Roman numerals:
   a. CDVIII =   e. 93 =
   b. XXXIV =   f. 562 =
   c. LXXVII =   g. 1934 =
   d. MCMXIII =   h. 2597 =

5. Find the common denominators and add or subtract (reduce, if necessary):
   a. $\frac{1}{4} + \frac{2}{5} =$
   b. $\frac{4}{25} + \frac{3}{25} =$
   c. $\frac{1}{4} + \frac{2}{3} =$
   d. $\frac{3}{4} - \frac{4}{7} =$

6. Subtract the following:
   a. $\frac{5}{6} - \frac{1}{9} =$
   b. $\frac{4}{25} - \frac{3}{20} =$

   c. $5\frac{3}{8} - 2\frac{3}{4} =$
   d. $7\frac{1}{3} - 4\frac{2}{5} =$

7. Multiply the following fractions and reduce to lowest terms:
   a. $\frac{2}{7} \times \frac{3}{5} =$
   b. $\frac{4}{11} \times \frac{3}{8} =$
   c. $\frac{5}{12} \times \frac{2}{3} \times \frac{1}{2} =$
   d. $\frac{3}{4} \times \frac{4}{5} \times \frac{2}{3} =$

8. Divide the following fractions:
   a. $\frac{5}{9} \div \frac{2}{3} =$
   b. $\frac{3}{4} \div \frac{3}{5} =$
   c. $5\frac{1}{2} \div 2\frac{3}{4} =$
   d. $7\frac{1}{5} \div 4\frac{2}{5} =$

9. Change the following decimals to fractions:
   a. 0.591 =
   b. 1.34 =
   c. 2.547 =

10. Convert to common fractions or mixed numbers in lowest terms:
    a. 1.56 =
    b. 5.27 =
    c. 3.375 =

11. Calculate the following:
    a. $11.019 + 52.70 + 7.141 =$
    b. $97.30 - 9.071 =$
    c. $1.59 \times 2.301 \times 1.977 =$
    d. $121.4 \div 8.12 =$

12. Change to a percentage:
    a. 0.65 =
    b. $5\frac{3}{8} =$
    c. $\frac{4}{9} =$

13. Change to decimal fractions:
    a. 23% =
    b. 116% =
    c. $\frac{2}{7}\% =$

14. Express as decimals:
    a. $7\frac{3}{8} =$
    b. 321% =
    c. 52% =

15. Express as percentages:
    a. 2.47 =
    b. 1.55 =
    c. $2\frac{2}{3} =$

16. Express as ratios:
    a. $\frac{1}{6}$ to $\frac{1}{5}$
    b. 2 feet to 6 inches
    c. 100 mph

17. Calculate the following:
    a. $\dfrac{3.5}{6.7} = \dfrac{x}{8.9}$
    b. $\dfrac{2}{3} = \dfrac{x}{0.49}$
    c. $0.3 : 1 :: 0.5 : x$

Mathematical Calculations Used in Pharmacology

Objectives

1. Describe the apothecaries' and household measure systems and when they might be used.
2. Use the metric system to convert from one measure to another.
3. Use common abbreviations and symbols to interpret and solve medication problems.
4. State the values of common household measures and their equivalents.
5. Compare the units used in the apothecaries', metric, and household measures systems.

Key Terms

Celsius (SĔL-sē-ĕs, p. 80)
Fahrenheit (FĂR-ĕn-HĪT, p. 80)
gram (GRĂM, p. 79)

liter (LĒ-tĕr, p. 79)
meter (MĒ-tĕr, p. 79)
metric system (MĔ-trĭk, p. 79)

OVERVIEW

Giving medicines requires the nurse to use precise weights and measures so each dose is the same. General household measures are often used when medicine is given in the home; unfortunately, it is not very accurate but patients are familiar with it. For example, 1 glass equals 8 ounces. Although one would think that this system is out of date for giving current medications, LPNs/LVNs practice in a wide variety of settings and may need to know this information. It is also important to understand household measures because this may be what patients will use in talking with you about how much medication they take. Household measures you should know are listed in Box 8-1.

Another measuring system is the apothecary system that was used primarily by pharmacists. This system is no longer recommended for use but a few medications have survived that are listed in grains (aspirin, iron, quinidine), and drops (gtts) are used in intravenous calculations. Drams and minims are no longer used. 1 grain = 60 or 64 mg of 0.06 g; 1/60 grain = 1 mg

- To convert grains to grams, divide by 15 or 16. To convert grams to milligrams, move the decimal point three places to the right. To convert grams to grains, multiple by 15 or 16.
- To convert grains to milligrams, multiple by 60 or 64. To convert milligrams to grams, move the decimal point three places to the left. To convert milligrams to grains, divided by 60 or 64.

METRIC SYSTEM

The **metric system** was developed in France and relies on a decimal system; it is built on multiples of 10 (tens, hundreds, and thousands). The metric system is the most commonly used drug measurement system. The metric system is the main system used internationally to measure weight, length, and volume.

The metric system uses **meter** (m) for the unit of length, **liter** (L) for the unit of volume, and **gram** (g) for the unit of weight. The most common measures used in the metric system are listed in Box 8-2.

 Memory Jogger

Common Metric Equivalents

Milliliters, cubic centimeters, and grams are approximately equivalent; 1 mL, or 1 cc, weighs approximately 1 g.

Relying on what you know about the decimal system, it is simple to change measures within the metric system. To change milligrams to micrograms, move the decimal point three places to the right (multiply by 1000):

$$000.00007 = 000000.07$$

To change micrograms to milligrams, move the decimal point three places to the left (divide by 1000):

$$000000.07 = 000.00007$$

Box 8-1	Common Equivalents

COMMON HOUSEHOLD EQUIVALENTS
1 teaspoon = approximately 5 mL
1 tablespoon = 3 teaspoons
1 cup = 8 ounces
1 pint = 2 cups
1 quarter = 4 cups

Box 8-2	The Metric System

MEASURES OF LENGTH (METER)
1 meter (m) = 100 centimeters (cm) = 1000 millimeters (mm)
1 centimeter (cm) = 0.01 meter (m)
1 millimeter (mm) = 0.001 meter (m)

MEASURES OF VOLUME (LITER)
1 decaliter (daL) = 10 liters (L)
1 liter (L) = 10 deciliters (dL) = 1000 milliliters (mL) or 1000 cubic centimeters (cc)

MEASURES OF WEIGHT (GRAM)
1 kilogram (kg) = 1000 grams (g)
1 gram (g) = 1000 milligrams (mg)
1 milligram (mg) = 1000 micrograms (mcg)

To change grams to milligrams, move the decimal point three places to the right (multiply by 1000):

$$1.000067 = 1000.067$$

To change milligrams to grams, move the decimal point three places to the left (divide by 1000):

$$1345.0789 = 1.3450789$$

 Memory Jogger

Metric System Prefixes

Prefixes of the metric system indicate the multiples or fractions of the unit:
- milli = one thousandth
- centi = one hundredth
- deci = one tenth
- deca = ten
- hecto = hundred
- kilo = thousand

If you have not used the metric system before, you will want to use common sense to see if the dose you calculate seems right. The number you get after doing the calculation may appear abnormally small or tremendously large. As you gain experience, common sense will help you determine whether the answer is correct. As you practice, you will soon learn shortcuts to help with mathematical calculations. You may wish to add these formulas to iPhone, personal digital assistants, or other handheld devices you use all the time. For commonly recognized measures and how they compare with the metric system, see Box 8-3.

Box 8-3	Common Equivalents for Metric Measures

METRIC EQUIVALENTS
1 meter = 39.37 inches = 3.28 feet = 1.09 yards
1 centimeter = 0.39 inch
1 millimeter = 0.04 inch
1 kilometer = 0.62 mile
1 liter = 1.06 liquid quarts
1 gram = 0.04 ounce
1 kilogram = 2.2 pounds

COMMON MEASURE EQUIVALENTS
1 inch = 25.4 millimeters
1 foot = 0.3 meter
1 yard = 0.91 meter
1 mile = 1.61 kilometers
1 ounce = 28.35 grams
1 pound = 0.45 kilogram

CONVERTING TEMPERATURE READINGS

For years, nurses have used the Fahrenheit (F) scale to take temperatures. In the last 20 years, institutions have placed increasing emphasis on the centigrade, or Celsius (C), scale for hospital use. Although electronic thermometers with digital readouts are used in some hospitals, nurses still use either Fahrenheit or Celsius mercury-based thermometers throughout other parts of the world.

Thermometers used in many hospitals come in either Fahrenheit or Celsius scale. Oral thermometers come with either a long, flat tip or oblong or stubby tips. The oblong or stubby tips may also be used for rectal or axillary temperatures.

On the **Fahrenheit** scale, 212° is the boiling point and 32° is the freezing point. Outdoor temperature thermometers generally include these points. The Fahrenheit thermometer used for medical measurement ranges from 95° to 105°, with individual divisions representing 0.2°. Because body temperature generally does not vary more than a few degrees, this smaller range is sufficient to measure the normal body temperature range of 97.6° F to 99.4° F and any common variations from normal.

The **Celsius** scale has a boiling point of 100° and a freezing point of 0°. The Celsius thermometer also has a restricted range for medical use, with each division on the scale representing 0.1°. The normal body range as measured on the Celsius scale varies from 36.5° C to 37.5° C.

Because both Fahrenheit and Celsius scales are commonly used in hospitals, the nurse must understand how to read each thermometer accurately, correctly note changes from normal, and convert from one scale to another. If you need to give a medication to help lower a high temperature, you must clearly understand the variations from normal in either scale.

The formulas for converting from one scale to another are very simple. Because the normal range of temperatures varies so little in individuals, even a little experience in changing temperatures will aid you in rapidly understanding this process.

The formula for converting Fahrenheit to Celsius is as follows:

$$(\,^\circ F - 32) \times \frac{5}{9} = \,^\circ C$$

For example:

$$102^\circ\, F \text{ is } ?\,^\circ C?$$

First, Fahrenheit temperature minus 32. Multiply that times 5, then divide by nine:

$$(102 - 32) \times \frac{5}{9} = 70 \times \frac{5}{9} = 38.9^\circ\, C$$

The formula for converting Celsius temperature to Fahrenheit temperature is as follows:

$$\left(\,^\circ C \times \frac{9}{5}\right) + 32 = \,^\circ F$$

For example:

$$40^\circ\, C \text{ is } ?\,^\circ F?$$

$$\left(40 \times \frac{9}{5}\right) + 32 = 72 + 32 = 104^\circ\, F$$

Individuals who dislike working with fractions and find decimal methods easier for temperature conversions must master two other formulas:

Changing Celsius to Fahrenheit: multiply Celsius temperature by 1.8, then add 32

Changing Fahrenheit to Celsius: subtract 32 from the Fahrenheit temperature, then divide by 1.8

Memory Jogger

Converting Temperatures

The key relationships to understand in converting temperatures are as follows:
- One degree on the Fahrenheit scale equals $\frac{9}{5}$ of one degree on the Celsius scale.
- One degree on the Celsius scale equals $\frac{5}{9}$ of one degree on the Fahrenheit scale.

Get Ready for the NCLEX® Examination!

Key Points

- The metric system is used to measure length, weight, and volume and is used internationally to describe medications.

Additional Learning Resources

SG Go to your Study Guide for additional learning activities to help you master this chapter content.

evolve Go to your Evolve website (http://evolve.elsevier.com/Edmunds/LPN/) for additional online resources.

Review Questions for the NCLEX® Examination

1. Convert 115 degrees Fahrenheit to Celsius.
   1. 43.8 degrees
   2. 44.3 degrees
   3. 45.2 degrees
   4. 46.1 degrees

2. 50 micrograms = _____ milligrams
   1. 5.0
   2. .050
   3. 500
   4. .0050

3. 15 grams = _____ milligrams
   1. .0015
   2. .015
   3. 15000
   4. 150000

4. 15 liters = _____ mL
   1. 15000
   2. 1500
   3. 150
   4. .015

5. _____ kg = 500 g
   1. 5
   2. 50
   3. 0.05
   4. 0.5

Critical Thinking Questions

Make sure that the drug ordered and the drug you have are both in the same unit of weight—for example, both grams or milligrams. To convert milligrams to grams (1000 mg = 1 g) divide the number of milligrams by 1000, or move the decimal point of the milligrams three places to the left.

Examples:
0.3 mg = 0.0003 g

Get Ready for the NCLEX® Examination!—cont'd

To convert g to mg, move the decimal point three places to the right.

Example: 0.4 g = 400 mg

1. Convert the following using the Metric system
   a. 0.2 mg = _____g
   b. 0.12 mg = _____g
   c. 4 g = _____ mg
   d. 35 mg = _____ g
   e. 0.20 g = ___mg
   f. 0.6 g = ___g

To convert weight in kilograms to pounds, multiple the kilogram weight by 2.2.

To convert weight in pounds to kilograms, divide the weight in pounds by 2.2.

To convert Celsius to **Fahrenheit,** multiply temperature by 1.8, then add 32.

To convert Fahrenheit to Celsius, subtract 32 from the temperature, then divide by 1.8.

2. Convert the following using the equivalent systems:
   a. 17 kg = ___ lb
   b. 36° C = ___ °F
   c. 137 lb = ___ kg
   d. 40° C = ___ °F
   e. 101° F = ___ °C
   f. 185 lb = _____ kg
   g. 35 kg = _____ lb

3. If 150 mL of solution contains 75 g of alcohol, how many grams of alcohol are there in 25 mL of solution?

4. It takes 7 g of a substance to make 35 mL of solution. How many milliliters of solution can be made with 42 g of the substance?

5. Phenobarbital gr 1 is prescribed. How many tablets should you give if it is available in 60 mg tablets?

Calculating Drug Dosages

Objectives

1. Use formulas to determine the dosages of tablets, capsules, or liquids.
2. Use formulas to determine the total number of tablets or capsules or the amount of liquid to be administered at a specified time.
3. Use information about the metric measurement system to accurately calculate drug dosages.
4. Calculate dosages for parenteral injections, including those for special preparations such as insulin.
5. Calculate flow rates for infusions.
6. List the rule used to calculate medication dosages for children.

Key Terms

body surface area (BSA) (p. 90)
Clark's rule (p. 89)
drop factor (DRŎP FĂC-tĕr, p. 88)

flow rate (FLŌ RĀT, p. 88)
nomogram (NŎM-Ŏ-grăm, p. 90)

OVERVIEW

How medications are ordered differs among physicians, drugs, and health care agencies. Some agencies require physicians to order generic products or only those drugs stocked by the pharmacy. Most drugs are ordered using the metric system, but occasionally another measurement system will be used; for example, heparin, a powerful blood thinner, is available in units. There are many reasons why medication orders appear in a variety of forms, and the nurse must be prepared to understand them all.

CALCULATION METHODS

Calculating dosages involves the following three steps:
1. Determine whether the drug dosage desired (what is written in the physician's order) is in the same measurement system as the drug dosage available. If they are not in the same measurement system, convert between the two systems.
2. Simplify by reducing to the lowest terms whenever possible.
3. Calculate the dosage quantity to be administered. This may be done by using fractions, ratios, or proportions. All of these calculation methods arrive at the same answer. It's simply a matter of finding which method works best for you as the nurse.
4. To avoid errors in your calculations:

- Do not use "trailing zeroes." In other words, write 2 g not 2.0 g. This is because a big error could be made if the decimal point is not seen.
- Write a zero in front of the decimal point if the answer is less than one. In other words, write 0.25 mg versus .25 mg. Again, the problem is that the dose may be wrong if the decimal is not obvious.

FRACTION METHOD

When using fractions to compute drug dosages, write an equation consisting of two fractions. First, set up a fraction showing the number of units to be given over x, the unknown number of tablets or milliliters. For example, if the physician's order states, "ibuprofen 600 mg," you would write $\frac{600 \text{ mg}}{x \text{ tablets}}$. On the other side of the equation, write a fraction showing the drug dosage as listed on the medication bottle over the number of tablets or milliliters. The ibuprofen bottle label states, "200 mg per tablet," so the second fraction is $\frac{200 \text{ mg}}{1 \text{ tablet}}$. The equation then reads:

$$\frac{600 \text{ mg}}{x \text{ tablets}} = \frac{200 \text{ mg}}{1 \text{ tablet}}$$

Note that the same units of measure are in both numerators and the same units of measure are in both denominators. Now solve for x:

$$\frac{600 \text{ mg}}{x \text{ tablets}} = \frac{200 \text{ mg}}{1 \text{ tablet}}$$

$$\frac{600}{x} = \frac{200}{1}$$

$$200x = 600$$

$$x = 3 \text{ tablets}$$

RATIO OR PROPORTION METHOD

In using the ratio method, first write the amount of the drug to be given and the quantity of the dosage (x) as a ratio. Using the previous example, this is 600 mg:x tablets. Next, complete the equation by forming a second ratio consisting of the number of units of the drug in the dosage form and the quantity of that dosage form as taken from the bottle. Again, using the previous example, the second ratio is 200 mg:1 tablet. Expressed as a proportion, this is:

$$600 \text{ mg} : x \text{ tablets} :: 200 \text{ mg} : 1 \text{ tablet}$$

Solving for x determines the dosage:

Can errors be drawn from the previous formula to show where they are in the following problem?

$$600 \times 1 = 200 \times x$$

$$600 = 200x$$

$$x = \frac{600}{200}$$

$$x = 3$$

This method, again, gives a dosage of 3 tablets.

"DESIRED OVER AVAILABLE" METHOD

A third method for drug dosage calculation combines the conversion of ordered units into available units and the computation of drug dosage into one step. The general equation for doing this is:

$$\frac{\text{Desired units} (\times \text{Converson factor}) \times}{\text{Quantity of drug form}}$$
$$\frac{\text{(caps, tabs, etc.)}}{\text{Quantity Available} (\times \text{Conversion factor})}$$
$$= x \text{ (Quantity to give)}$$

If a physician orders 10 gr of a drug and the drug is available only in 300-mg tablets, the dose may be easily calculated with this formula. Substitute 10 gr **(Desired)** for the first element of the equation. Then use a conversion factor (60 mg/1 gr) so the desired amount can be expressed in the same units as the dose available in the second portion of the formula. The second element of the equation shows the quantity of drug form (capsule or tablet) for the dose **Available** (1 tablet contains 300 mg). The completed equation then is:

$$10 \text{ gr} \times \left(\frac{60 \text{ mg}}{1 \text{ gr}} \right) \times \frac{1 \text{ tablet}}{300 \text{ mg}} = x \text{ tablets}$$

Once the conversion factor has been used, you can see the underlying relationship between dose **Desired** and dose **Available**:

$$\text{Dose } \textbf{Desired} = 10 \text{ gr} \times \frac{60 \text{ mg}}{1 \text{ gr}}$$
$$= 600 \text{ mg}$$

Thus the previous equation can be reduced to:

$$600 \text{ mg} \times \frac{1 \text{ tablet}}{300 \text{ mg}} = x; \text{ or}$$

$$\frac{(\text{Dose } \textbf{Desired}) \ 600 \text{ mg}}{(\text{Dose } \textbf{Available}) \ 300 \text{ mg}} \times 1 = x \text{ tablets}$$

$$\frac{600}{300} = 2 \text{ tablets}$$

By solving for x, you will find that the patient should receive two 300-mg tablets.

As you can see, all three methods of drug calculation (fraction, proportion, and desired over available methods) use the same information and much of the same format in solving the problems. With minor variations, they do the same thing. One or another of these methods will seem to make more sense to you or be easier to follow. Throughout the calculation sections, use the method for drug calculation that makes the most sense. Return here for review if you are having difficulty.

As a final check to yourself, ask if the answer you calculated makes sense. You will learn about the usual doses for different drugs. However, you may want to develop a plan to always recalculate the problem if your answer suggests you should give more than two tablets, ounces, and so on. Give it the "Does It Make Sense?" (DIMS) test. Always imagine looking at your answer and imagining what the dose would look like if you were to bring the dose into a patient's room. Would you bring in 45 tablespoons of a cough syrup? There is always pressure to quickly give medications. But if you always use the DIMS test, you will reduce the chance that errors will occur.

CALCULATING DOSAGES

ORAL MEDICATIONS

Although there are many forms of oral products, oral medications usually come in capsules, tablets, or liquids. Medications dispensed through the unit-dose system are packaged by the pharmacist, according to the dosage ordered. You usually do not have to calculate the medication dosage, but check the accuracy of the preparation.

When medication is ordered individually or through an open-stock system, you usually will calculate the proper drug dosage. Drug calculations are required when any of the following conditions are true:

- The drug available is in a smaller dose than that ordered.
- The drug available is in a larger dose than that ordered.
- The drug available is in a different unit of measure than that ordered.

Memory Jogger

Parentheses in Math Problems

When parentheses are used in a math problem, it all the calculations inside the parentheses should be done first, then the rest of the problem is completed.

Capsules and Tablets

Capsules cannot be broken or divided. This makes calculating the drug dosage more difficult. Additional capsules may be given to provide an accurate dosage, but a part of a capsule cannot. Manufacturers of drugs provide capsules in different dosages to help you arrive at the proper dosage. If the calculations specify that a fraction of a capsule should be given, then it is necessary to notify the prescriber for change in order for the dose. Some tablets may be easily divided if they are "scored" (Figure 9-1, *A*). Examples of unscored tablets are layered tablets (see Figure 9-1, *B*) and coated tablets (see Figure 9-1, *C*). As a general rule, if a tablet is not scored, it should *not* be broken or cut apart. Sometimes tablets may be cut to fill a smaller drug dosage order, or they may be combined to fill a larger drug dosage order.

Memory Jogger

Dosage Formula Hint

To help you remember the usual formula, remember **Desired** over **Available,** D/A, or "DA." A District Attorney (DA) often helps solve a mystery. You are helping to solve the mystery of the dosage needed.

Memory Jogger

Steps to Complete Dosage Formula

1. First change dosages to the same unit of measurement if they are different.
2. Reduce to the simplest terms.
3. Calculate the dosage, using fractions, ratios, or proportions.
4. Use common sense to check the answer.

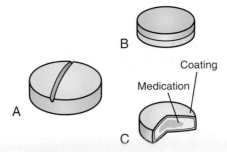

FIGURE 9-1 A, Scored tablet. **B** and **C,** Unscored tablets. The tablet in **B** is layered, and the tablet in **C** is coated.

To illustrate, here are a few examples:

The order reads, "ASA gr x stat and prn for temperature elevation." Acetylsalicylic acid (ASA) is labeled as 0.3 g/tablet:

$$\frac{\text{Dose } \textbf{Desired}}{\text{Dose } \textbf{Available}} = \frac{\text{gr } x}{0.3 \text{ g}} \times 1 = x \text{ tablets}$$

$$\left(\text{Conversation factor: } 16 \text{ gr} = 1 \text{ g, so } \frac{\text{gr } x}{16} = 0.6 \text{ g}\right)$$

$$\frac{\textbf{D}}{\textbf{A}} = \frac{0.6 \text{ g}}{0.3 \text{ g}} \times 1 = 2 \text{ tablets}$$

The order reads: "methocarbamol 1.5 g daily." The medication comes in 750-mg tablets.

$$\frac{\text{Dose } \textbf{Desired}}{\text{Dose } \textbf{Available}} = \frac{1.5 \text{ g}}{750 \text{ mg}} \times 1 = x \text{ tablets}$$

$$(\text{Conversation factor: } 1.5 \text{ g} = 1500 \text{ mg})$$

$$\frac{\textbf{D}}{\textbf{A}} = \frac{1500 \text{ mg}}{750 \text{ mg}} \times 1 = 2 \text{ tablets}$$

Liquids

The process and formulas used to calculate dosages of liquids are the same as those used to compute dosages of capsules or tablets. Only the unit of measure is different. To review:

$$\frac{\text{Dose } \textbf{Desired}}{\text{Dose } \textbf{Available}} \times \frac{\text{Drug form}}{(\text{minims; milliliters; drams})} = x \text{ (amount of liquid per dose)}$$

For example, the order reads: "phenobarbital elixir 0.2 g at bedtime." The drug is available in 20 mg/5 mL. Again, the formula is a basic proportion problem:

$$0.2 \text{ g } (= 200 \text{ mg}) : x \text{ mL} :: 20 \text{ mg} : 5 \text{ mL}$$

Written as an equation, this is:

$$200 \text{ mg} \times 5 \text{ mL} = 20 \text{ mg} \times x \text{ mL}$$

Thus:

$$\frac{(\text{Dose \textbf{Desired}})\ 200\ \text{mg}}{(\text{Dose \textbf{Available}})\ 20\ \text{mg}} \times 5\ \text{mL} = x$$

$$\frac{200\ \text{mg}}{20\ \text{mg}} \times 5\ \text{mL} = 50\ \text{mL} = \text{dose}$$

Memory Jogger

Dosage Solution Formula

$$\frac{\text{Dose \textbf{Desired}}}{\text{Dose \textbf{Available}}} \times \frac{\text{Drug form}}{(\text{Dilution or amount of solution})} = \text{Amount of solution per dose}$$

PARENTERAL MEDICATIONS

When medication is to be injected, it usually comes in one of three different forms:

1. A prefilled syringe labeled with a certain dosage in a certain volume (for example, meperidine [Demerol] 100 mg in 1 mL).
2. A single ampule or multiple-dose vial labeled with a certain dosage in a certain volume (for example, epinephrine [Adrenalin] 1:1000 in 0.1 mL).
3. A vial with a powder or crystals that must be mixed or reconstituted with sterile water or normal saline (NS) solution. This solution is the liquid dilution. The drug may be measured in grains, grams, milligrams, or units. The amount of solution to be added varies and must be calculated according to the instructions provided with the vial. Medications given intradermally or subcutaneously generally involve very small amounts of solution, whereas intravenous (IV) preparations may involve 50 mL of solution or more.

Again, proportion is the standard method for calculating this dosage:

Please change word dilution below to solution:

Dose **Available** : Dilution :: Dose **Desired** : x

Written as an equation, this becomes:

Dose Available $\times x$ = Dose Desired $\times$ Dilution

or

$$\frac{\text{Dose \textbf{Desired}}}{\text{Dose \textbf{Available}}} \times \text{Dilution} = x$$

To illustrate, here are a few examples:

The order reads: "digoxin 0.2 mg IM." The drug is available as 0.5 mg/mL.

$$\frac{(\text{Dose \textbf{Desired}})\ 0.2\ \text{mg}}{(\text{Dose \textbf{Available}})\ 0.5\ \text{mg}} \times 1\ \text{mL} = x$$

$$\frac{2}{5} \times 1\ \text{mL} = 0.4\ \text{mL}$$

Clinical Pitfall

Accurate Calculations

Again! Do not forget your common sense! If the answer tells you to inject 20 mL, you know you have made a mistake!

The order reads: "quinidine gluconate 200 mg IM (intramuscular) q6h." The medication comes in a multiple-dose vial with 80 mg/mL.

$$\frac{\textbf{D}}{\textbf{A}} = \frac{200\ \text{mg}}{80\ \text{mg}} \times 1\ \text{mL} = 2.5\ \text{mL}$$

The order reads: "Demerol 35 mg IM daily." The drug is available in 50-mg/mL ampules.

$$\frac{\textbf{D}}{\textbf{A}} = \frac{35\ \text{mg}}{50\ \text{mg}} \times 1\ \text{mL} = 0.7\ \text{mL}$$

Many chemicals are very fragile. Heat, light, and time cause the medication to change or deteriorate. To avoid these problems, some medications are manufactured as powders or crystals, making them more stable. When the medication is ordered, liquid must be added to the drug to dissolve the medication and form a solution (reconstitute the drug). The medication must then be given within a few hours or it will decay. This is often true for products that will be added to IV fluids.

Some chemicals come in a single-dose vial. When the medication is ordered, usually 1 to 2 mL of liquid is added, the solution is gently shaken to dissolve it, and the whole amount is drawn into a syringe and injected. This is very common for some antibiotics.

At other times, a vial will contain several doses of the powdered medication. The instructions for adding the liquid (diluent) must be followed carefully. Some multiple-dose vials for steroids contain the diluent in the top part of the bottle, separated from the powder in the bottom part of the container. Pushing on the top part forces the liquid down into the bottom part, dissolving the medication. The instructions are usually found on the package, on the vial label, or on the package insert in the box, and they must be followed exactly. Once powders have been dissolved in liquid or reconstituted, the bottle must be carefully labeled so that further doses may be accurately given from it. It is especially important to note the date and time the powder was dissolved, as well as the concentration of the reconstituted medication. There should be information with each vial that indicates how long the medicine can be used once it has been mixed.

To illustrate, here are a few examples:

The doctor orders an antibiotic to be given 500 mg q6h IM. The drug comes in a multiple-dose vial containing 3 g of powder. Prepare it so that 500 mg equals 1 mL. First, convert 3 g to 3000 mg. Then apply the proportion formula:

$$500 \text{ mg} : 1 \text{ mL} :: 3000 \text{ mg} : x$$
$$500 \text{ mg} \times x = 3000 \text{ mg} \times 1 \text{ mL}$$
$$\frac{3000 \text{ mg}}{500 \text{ mg}} = 6 \text{ mL}$$

Therefore 6 mL of diluent must be added to obtain a concentration of 1 mL = 500 mg/mL. Expressed more simply:

$$\frac{\text{(Drug \textbf{Available}) } 3000 \text{ mg}}{\text{(Dose \textbf{Desired}) } 500 \text{ mg}} \times 1 \text{ mL} = 6 \text{ mL to be added}$$

Thus you would add 6 mL to create the solution and then determine how much medicine to give.

The order reads: "Give 500,000 units penicillin IM." Dilute 1,000,000 units of penicillin so that 500,000 units equals 1 mL. Thus:

$$500,000 \text{ units} : 1 \text{ mL} :: 1,000,000 \text{ units} : x$$

$$\frac{1,000,000}{500,000} = 2 \text{ mL diluent}$$

or

$$\frac{\textbf{A}}{\textbf{D}} = \frac{1,000,000 \text{ units}}{500,000 \text{ units}} \times 1 \text{ mL} = 2 \text{ mL diluent to be added}$$

The order reads: "Give cephalosporin 200 mg in 1 mL IM." The drug is manufactured in 1-g units of powder. What is the amount of diluent to add?

$$\frac{\text{(Drug \textbf{Available}) } 1 \text{ g } (=1000 \text{ mg})}{\text{(Dose \textbf{Desired}) } 200 \text{ mg}} =$$
$$\frac{1000 \text{ mg}}{200 \text{ mg}} \times 1 \text{ mL} = 5 \text{ mL diluent}$$

 Memory Jogger

Dosage Formula

$$\frac{\text{Total drug \textbf{available}}}{\text{Dose \textbf{desired}}} \times 1 \text{mL} =$$

Amount of diluent that must be added to vial powder so that dose order order equals 1mL

Insulin

Insulin is a parenteral medication that replaces insulin not being made by the patient's own body. Great accuracy is important in preparing and administering insulin because the quantity given is very small, and even minor variations in dosage may produce adverse symptoms in the patient.

Calculating and preparing insulin dosages is unique in the following three ways:

1. There are many kinds of insulin, but they all come in a standardized measure called a *unit.* Insulin is available in 10-mL vials and in two strengths (concentrations): U-100 (100 units per 1 mL of solution) (Figure 9-2) and U-500 (500 units per 1 mL of solution). U-500 is five times stronger (more concentrated) than U-100. This preparation is rarely used except in patients with very large insulin needs.

2. Insulin should be drawn up in a special insulin syringe that is marked or calibrated in units (Figure 9-3).

3. The insulin order, the insulin bottle, and the insulin as drawn up should always be rechecked by another nurse for maximum accuracy. Small errors can cause big problems. It is extremely unusual to give more than 50 units of insulin.

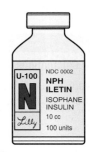

FIGURE 9-2 U-100 vial.

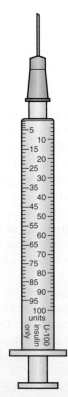

FIGURE 9-3 U-100 syringe.

When the insulin order and the syringe are both U-100, all you have to do is draw up the number of units ordered. For example, the order reads: "48 units NPH insulin] U-100 1 hour before breakfast." Using a U-100 syringe, you would draw up 48 units of NPH insulin.

When the order calls for two different types of insulin, both may be given at the same time in the same syringe. One will be short-acting (regular) insulin, and the other will be an intermediate or longer-acting type (neutral protamine Hagedorn [NPH]). Draw up the regular insulin first, then the longer-acting type. Give both in the same syringe. For example, the order reads: "20 units regular insulin U-100 and 30 units NPH U-100 before breakfast." Using a U-100 syringe, draw up 20 units of regular insulin; then draw up 30 units of NPH insulin to equal 50 units in the syringe. Be certain that you are using the correct type of insulin. The newer long-acting insulins (Lantus and Detemir) cannot be mixed with regular or rapid-acting insulins.

 Clinical Pitfall

Accurate Insulin Syringe Calculations

NOTE: You *must* be very accurate in these calculations. A small error makes a big change in insulin dosage.

Intravenous Infusions

Flow Rates. Regulating the IV infusion rate is a common nursing task. Some institutions have automatic infusion pumps that make flow-rate calculations easy. Each nurse will learn to use the equipment available. However, all nurses must learn to calculate infusion rates without relying on equipment, in case of power or equipment failures or when working in agencies where no automatic pumps are available. The completeness of physicians' orders for IV infusions varies widely. Some physicians are more specific in their instructions than others. A complete order specifies not only the type of solution and the volume to be infused (usually 500 or 1000 mL) but also the length of time the medication should be given. More commonly, the nurse is left to calculate the flow rate, or how fast the medication will be infused.

There are three mathematical procedures the nurse must be familiar with regarding IV infusions:
1. Calculating the flow rates for IV fluid administration
2. Making modifications in flow rates for infants
3. Calculating total administration time for IV fluid

To *calculate the flow rate for IV fluid administration,* two concepts must be understood: the flow rate and the drop factor. The rate at which IV fluids are given is the **flow rate**, and this is measured in drops per minute. The **drop factor** is the number of drops per milliliter of liquid and is determined by the size of the

drops. The drop factor is different for different manufacturers of IV infusion equipment, and it must be checked by reading it on the infusion set itself. Regular infusion sets generally range between 10 and 15 drops/mL. Infusion sets have different drop factors for use with blood infusion sets (usually 10 to 12 drops/mL) because the drops are larger, whereas pediatric setups use very small drops called *microdrops* (often with 50 or 60 microdrops/mL).

Once the nurse has learned the drop factor for the equipment being used, the flow rate may be calculated by using the following formula:

Drop factor × Milliliters/minute = Flow rate (drop/minute)

To illustrate, here are a few examples:

The order reads: "IV infusion to run at a slow rate to keep vein open." The rate to keep a vein open is 2 mL/min. The IV infusion set delivers 10 drops/mL. The goal is to determine the flow rate in drops/minute:

10 drops/mL (drop factor) × 2 mL/min = 20 drops/min

The order reads: "1000 mL NS to be administered in 5 hours." The drop factor is 15. To calculate the flow rate, use:

$$\frac{\text{Total of fluid to give}}{\text{Total time (minutes)}} \times \text{Drop factor (drop/milliliter)} =$$
$$\text{Flow rate (drops/minute)}$$
$$\frac{1000\ \text{mL}}{300\ \text{min}} \times 15\ \text{drops/mL} = \frac{15{,}000\ \text{drops}}{300\ \text{min}} = 50\ \text{drops/min}$$

 Memory Jogger

Intravenous Fluid Administration

- The flow rate for infusions can be calculated.
- The drop factor for infusions depends on the type of equipment and must be read from the setup label.

Flow Rates for Infants and Children. Infants and small children are very sensitive to extra amounts, or volumes, of fluids. Smaller total amounts of IV fluids are often ordered, and the infusions are given in very small drops to avoid quickly overloading the infant's circulation. This is a built-in safety mechanism to try to prevent fluid overloading as a result of accidental delivery of too much fluid.

The drop factor must be determined from the infusion setup. Usually 60 microdrops/mL is the drop factor for infants. For calculating the flow rates in infants, the same formula is used, but the microdrop drop factor must be substituted into the formula for the adult drop factor:

$$\frac{\text{Total of fluid to give}}{\text{Total time (minutes)}} \times \frac{\text{Drop factor}}{\text{(microdrops/milliliter)}} =$$
$$\text{Flow rate (drops/minute)}$$

For example, the order reads: "Give 50 mL D5W [5% dextrose in water] IV in 4 hours." The drop factor is 60 microdrops/mL. Thus:

$$\frac{50 \text{ mL}}{240 \text{ min}} \times 60 \text{ microdrops/mL} = \frac{300}{24} =$$
$$12.5 \text{ microdrops/min}$$

Total Infusion Time. Sometimes physicians' orders tell how fast they want infusions to run. To plan nursing care of the patient and to anticipate when new IV bottles may be needed, you need to calculate the total time the infusion will run.

Calculating the total administration time for IV fluid depends on calculating the total number of drops to be infused. Using this information, plus the drop factor, the total infusion time can be easily determined by using the following formula:

$$\frac{\text{Total drops to be infused}}{\text{Flow rate (drops/minute)}} \times 60 \text{ (drops/hour)} =$$
$$\text{Total infusion time (hours and minutes)}$$

To calculate the total infusion time:
1. *Determine the total number of drops ordered.* The total number of drops to be infused comes from the physician's order for the amount of fluid. This amount is multiplied by the drop factor (read from the infusion setup) to determine the total number of drops.
2. *Determine the number of minutes the IV is to flow.* The number of drops per minute (50) is multiplied by 60 to give the number of drops infused in 1 hour (3000). This figure is then divided into the total number of drops. This will give the number of hours and minutes for the total infusion.

For example, the order reads: "1000 mL D$_5$W to be given at 50 drops/min with a drop factor of 10 drops/mL." Thus:

$$1000 \text{ mL} \times 10 \text{ drops/mL} = 10,000 \text{ drops}$$

$$\frac{10,000 \text{ drops}}{3,000 \text{ drops/hr}} = 3.33 \text{ hr or 3 hr, 20 min}$$

Other Factors Influencing Flow Rates. There are many other factors that influence the flow rate of an infusion. The nurse has no control over many of them, such as the age, size, and condition of the patient; the size of the vein; the type of fluid; and the need for the fluid. Other factors may be changed or altered to assist in infusion of IV fluids: the size of the needle, the needle's position in the vein, the height of the IV pole,

the condition of the filter, the air in the air vent, and movement of the patient. If the fluid does not infuse at the calculated rate, the IV setup should be carefully checked from the IV bottle to the site of the needle's insertion.

CALCULATING DOSAGES FOR INFANTS AND CHILDREN

Drug dosages are calculated to give the highest possible blood and tissue concentration of a medication without causing overdosage or adverse effects. Because infants are very sensitive to medications, and because infants and children are so much smaller than adults, almost all dosages given to infants and children are smaller than those given to adults. Most pharmaceutical companies list the recommended dosages of their drugs for a child or infant. If this information is not listed in the instructional material provided with the medication, the nurse should question whether the medication may safely be given to a child.

Although children's dosages were once frequently calculated, there remain only a few medications that require the nurse to determine how much to give a child. In past years, there were several general rules developed to calculate these special reduced dosages for infants and children. Some were based on age, and these have fallen out of usage because children of different ages vary so much in size.

With the growing attention on having better information available for giving medications to children, there has been greater focus on accurate drug calculation for them. The Joint Commission on Accreditation of Healthcare Organizations now asks that all dosages for children be weight based, preferably in kilograms.

One of the most widely accepted methods for determining children's dosages based on body weight is known as **Clark's rule**. Again, ratios and proportions may be used to calculate the pediatric value. If we assume that an average adult weighs 150 lb and we know the adult dosage, it follows that if we know the child's weight, we can calculate the child's dosage:

Adult weight : Adult dosage :: Child's weight : *x* (Child's dosage)

For example, if the 150-lb adult dose of meperidine is 100 mg, what is the dose for a 50-lb child?

$$\frac{\text{Weight of child}}{\text{Weight of adult}} \times \text{Adult's dose} = \text{Child's dose}$$

so

$$\frac{50 \text{ lb}}{150 \text{ lb}} \times 100 \text{ mg} = \frac{100}{3} = 33 \text{ mg}$$

Other formulas substitute kilograms for pounds in calculating the correct dose. The formula remains the same. Using the problem information in the preceding column, the nurse simply divides the weight of the adult and the weight of the child by 2.2 to obtain the weights in kilograms. Clark's rule is by far the most popular method of assessing children's dosages and should be the formula used.

Medications that require very careful dosage use the **body surface area (BSA)**, or total tissue area, of the child. This is the most accurate method for determining pediatric dosages. The reason for using the BSA is that children have a greater surface area than adults in relation to their weight. For drugs that require careful dosage, charts known as *nomograms* are used to calculate the BSA in square meters. A **nomogram** is a chart that displays the relationships between two different types of data so that complex calculations are not necessary. BSA charts are constructed from height and weight data. The ratio of BSA to weight varies inversely (opposite) to length. Thus infants would have proportionally more surface area, because they weigh less and are shorter than children. These charts may be used only if the child has normal height for weight. Even with the use of standardized charts, the calculated dosages are more accurate for children than for very young infants.

An example of a nomogram used to calculate BSA is shown in Figure 9-4. A straight edge is placed from the patient's height in the left column to his weight in the right column, and the intersection on the BSA column indicates the patient's BSA. The total BSA value is determined and is put into the following formula:

Surface area of the child (m²) × Usual adult dose ÷ Surface area of an adult (1.73 m²) = Child dose

Use the nomogram to solve these two sample problems, using the BSA to calculate pediatric dosages (use 1.73 m² as the accepted adult BSA):
1. If the adult dose of kanamycin is 0.5 g, what is the pediatric dose for a 10-month-old child who weighs 22 lb and is 29 inches long?
2. If the adult dose of sulfisoxazole is 500 mg, what is the pediatric dose for an 8-year-old child who weighs 48 lb and is 47 inches tall?

Dimensional analysis is a technique used in a select few LPN/LVN programs. If your program uses dimensional analysis for drug calculations, see the Evolve website (http://evolve.elsevier.com/Edmunds/LPN/) for information on using this calculation procedure and sample problems.

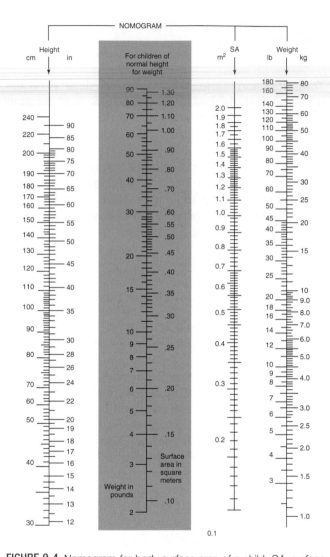

FIGURE 9-4 Nomogram for body surface area of a child. *SA*, surface area.

Get Ready for the NCLEX® Examination!

Key Points

- This chapter presented concepts and examples that illustrate common calculations you will be required to perform in administering medications.
- Mastery of this information is important for accuracy and speed.
- The foundation of multiplication facts, fractions, decimals, ratios, and proportions, added to the principles of metric, household, and apothecaries' systems, comes together in the practical application of dosage calculations.
- This chapter should be reviewed if you have difficulty with dosage calculations or need to review material you have not worked with for some time.

Get Ready for the NCLEX® Examination!—cont'd

Additional Learning Resources

SG Go to your Study Guide for additional learning activities to help you master this chapter content.

evolve Go to your Evolve website (http://evolve.elsevier.com/Edmunds/LPN/) for additional online resources.

Review Questions for the NCLEX® Examination

1. The order reads: 500 ml NS to be infused over 12 hours. The drop factor is 15. What is the total amount of time in minutes during which the infusion will occur?

   1. 67200 minutes
   2. 67.2 minutes
   3. 672 minutes
   4. 6720 minutes

2. The drop factor for infants is usually:

   1. 60 microdrops/mL
   2. 15 microdrops/mL
   3. 60 drops/mL
   4. 15 drops/mL

3. The order reads: 1000 ml NS to be given at 20 drops/minute with a drop factor of 10 drops/mL. The total infusion time is:

   1. 6 hours 14 minutes
   2. 7 hours 16 minutes
   3. 8 hours 20 minutes
   4. 9 hours 18 minutes

4. The primary reason for using the body surface area for determine pediatric dosage is that:

   1. adults have a greater surface area than children in relation to their weight
   2. children have a greater surface area than adults in relation to their weight
   3. adults have a lesser surface area than children in relation to their weight
   4. children have a lesser surface area than adults in relation to their weight

5. Which child would not be a candidate for using a nomogram?

   1. a 10-year-old with cardiac disease
   2. a 3-year-old with acute leukemia
   3. a 5-year-old with primordial dwarfism
   4. a 7-year-old with a form of autism

Drug Calculation Review

1. A patient recovering from pneumonia is being discharged from your unit. The physician orders guaifenesin (Robitussin) syrup 15 mL PO every 6 hours prn. The pharmacy sends a 500-mL bottle of guaifenesin to send home with the patient. If the patient takes one dose each night before bed, how long will a 500-mL bottle last?

2. The physician assistant orders 30 units of NPH subcutaneously. The vial contains 100 units per 1 mL. How many units of insulin must be administered?

3. The nurse practitioner orders 500 mg of the antibiotic cefazolin sulfate (Ancef) IM. The vial of powder is labeled with the following instructions: "Add 2.5 mL of sterile water for injection. This will provide an approximate volume of 330 mg/mL." How many milliliters of solution should the nurse prepare?

4. A patient is to receive 2500 mL of normal saline to infuse IV over 24 hours. The drop factor is 10 gtt = 1 mL. What is the flow rate in gtt/min of this infusion?

5. A 50-kg patient has recently experienced a myocardial infarction, and the physician orders a lidocaine infusion to suppress dysrhythmias. The order is:
   Lidocaine 500 mg in 250 mL fo D_5W at 150 microdrops (mcgtt) per minute
   What will be the rate of this IV infusion in milligrams per kilogram per minute (mg/kg/min) when the nurse uses a microdrop setup of 60 mcgtt = 1 mL?

6. The nurse practitioner has ordered 7500 units of heparin subcutaneously daily. The pharmacy has provided an ampule that contains 5000 units per 1 mL. How many milliliters will the nurse prepare for this injection?

7. As part of preoperative care, the surgeon has ordered atropine, gr $\frac{1}{300}$ IM. The multidose vial reads "1 mL = gr $\frac{1}{150}$." How many milliliters will be administered to this patient?

8. The physician orders metoprolol (Lopressor) 50 mg PO twice daily. The pharmacy has provided scored tablets of 0.1 g each. How many tablets of this antihypertensive medication should the nurse give to the patient?

9. The nurse practitioner has ordered digoxin (Lanoxin) elixir 0.25 mg PO. The nurse notes that the bottle is labeled 0.05 mg/mL. How many milliliters should be administered to the patient?

10. For an adult female patient, the physician assistant has ordered erythromycin 1 g PO at 1 pm, 2 pm, and 11 pm on the day before intestinal surgery. The nurse prepares to administer the first of the three doses and finds erythromycin 400-mg scored tablets available. How many tablets should be prepared for each dose of this intestinal antisepsis therapy?

Critical Thinking Questions

1. The drug order is for 0.6 g PO. The drug of choice is available only in 240-mg capsules. How many capsules should you give?

2. An IV infusion of tetracycline 4 mg/mL is ordered; tetracycline 500 mg/100 mL is available. The drop factor is 10 drops/mL. What is the flow rate? How much medication is received per minute?

Get Ready for the NCLEX® Examination!—cont'd

3. The drug order reads "Give 250 mL IV over 24 hours." The drop factor is 60 microdrops. What should the flow rate be? Is this IV administration rate be realistic? Why or why not?

4. The dose for a 150-lb adult of a given drug is 0.8 mg. What would be the dose for a 40-lb child? Now convert the weight to kilograms and calculate the dosage.

5. Penicillin 500,000 units q8h is ordered. The drug is available as penicillin 1,000,000 units per 5 mL. How many milliliters should be given?

6. The physician orders 0.0015 g once daily of a drug. The drug is available in tablets labeled 2.5, 1.5, and 10 mg. Which would you order, and how many would you give for each dose?

Preparing and Administering Medications

Objectives

1. Compare dosage forms for drugs given by the enteral route.
2. Outline procedures for giving medications enterally, parenterally, and percutaneously.
3. List processes to prevent human immunodeficiency virus (HIV) transmission.
4. Identify anatomy landmarks used for giving parenteral medications.

Key Terms

ampules (ĂM-pūls, p. 105)
asepsis (ā-SĔP-sĭs, p. 94)
barrel (BĂ-rŭl, p. 103)
buccal administration (BŪK-ŭl, p. 131)
capsules (CĂP-sūlz, p. 94)
elixirs (ĭ-LĬK-sĭrz, p. 94)
emulsions (ĭ-MŬL-shŭnz, p. 94)
intramuscular (IM) injections (ĭn-tră-MŬS-kū-lăr, p. 113)
intravenous (IV) route (ĭn-tră-VĒN-ĕs, p. 117)
lozenges (LŎZ-ĭn-jĕz, p. 94)
Mix-o-vial (MĬKS Ō VĪ-ăl, p. 108)
nasogastric (NG) tube (nā-zō-GĂS-trĭk, p. 97)
needle (NĒD- ăl, p. 103)
parenteral route (pĕ-RĔN-tĕr-ăl, p. 101)

percutaneous administration (pĕr-kū-TĀ-nē-ŭs, p. 126)
piggyback infusion (ĭn-FŪ-zhŭ n, p. 122)
pill (PĬL, p. 93)
plunger (PLŬN-jĭr, p. 103)
subcutaneous injections (sŭb-kū-TĀ-nē-ĕs, p. 111)
sublingual administration (sŭb-LĬNG-wăl, p. 131)
suspensions (sŭs-PĔN-shŭnz, p. 94)
syringes (sĭ-RĬN-jĕz, p. 103)
syrups (SĬR-ŭps, p. 94)
tablets (TĂB-lĕts, p. 94)
tip (TĬP, p. 103)
topical medications (TŎP-ĭ-kăl, p. 127)
vials (VĪ-ăl z, p. 105)

OVERVIEW

This chapter gives an overview of basic principles of medication administration. Section One discusses information about drugs taken by the enteral route: oral, nasogastric (NG), or rectal. Section Two describes how to give drugs parenterally. Section Three describes the methods for giving medications percutaneously.

ENTERAL MEDICATIONS

Enteral medications are given directly into the gastrointestinal (GI) tract through the oral, NG, or rectal route.

ORAL ADMINISTRATION

The most common route of administration of medications is through the mouth, or orally. The order is often written, "give PO," meaning *per os* or "by mouth." Advantages of oral preparations are as follows:

- They are easy for the nurse to give and for the patient to swallow.
- Most medications come in this form.
- It is usually not very expensive to make oral preparations.
- If a patient takes too much of an oral medication, the drug can be removed by pumping the patient's stomach (gastric lavage) or by having the patient vomit.

The major disadvantages of oral preparations are as follows:

- They cannot be given to patients with a lot of nausea, who are vomiting, or who are unconscious.
- Some chemicals are not effective if mixed with gastric secretions.
- The onset of action may vary because the drug may be slowly absorbed in the GI tract.

There are many different forms of oral medications. Each form is desired for a specific reason (for example, to increase absorption, delay absorption, or reduce gastric irritation). The term **pill** is often used by patients to describe capsules or tablets. Tablets and capsules are very common and are made up of several different chemicals. Tablets may be covered with a special coating that resists the acidic pH of the stomach but will dissolve in the alkaline pH of the intestine.

 Memory Jogger

Actions for Which the Nurse Will be Held Responsible

The nurse has responsibility to make sure patients take the medication given them. The nurse cannot know if the patient takes the medicine if the nurse doesn't see them swallow it. Even when the nurse is busy, medicine should not be left at the bedside for them to take later.

Box 10-1 summarizes the various oral dosage forms and their characteristics.

PROCEDURE FOR ADMINISTERING ORAL MEDICATIONS

The basic procedure in administration of medication is the same, regardless of type or route of administration. The equipment available and the agency policies may vary because nurses work in many different settings.

General principles that underlie all procedures include accuracy, taking responsibility, and **asepsis** (preventing of infection). The legal policies and rules, along with the nursing process and knowledge about the drug, are all part of giving medications. The steps in giving medications by the various routes are generally followed as outlined in the following sections. There are wide differences in the specific process and equipment used in administering medications and institutional procedures may require some changes in the recommended procedure. Procedure 10-1 shows the basic procedure for administering oral medications that may be used when there is no sophisticated equipment available for the process. Following these steps each time reduces the chance of medication error. This is a clean procedure and begins with cleanly washed hands.

Solid-Form Oral Medications

1. If the medicine does not come in its own unit-dose package, place all tablets or capsules together in a small paper souffle cup so the medicine is not touched.

Box **10-1**	Oral Medication Forms

Capsules are gelatin containers that hold powder or liquid medicine. Timed-release or sustained-release capsules contain granules that dissolve at different rates, providing slow and constant release of medications. Capsules are available in a variety of sizes and shapes. They provide an easy way to administer medications that have an unpleasant taste or odor. Capsules must not be opened, crushed, or chewed because irritation and excessive or lessened drug activity may be produced.

Elixirs are liquids made up of drugs dissolved in alcohol and water that may have coloring and flavoring agents added. The alcohol makes the drug more dissolvable than water alone.

Emulsions are solutions that have small droplets of water and medication dispersed in oil, or oil and medication dispersed in water. These preparations help disguise the bitter taste of a drug or increase its solubility.

Lozenges are medicine mixed with a hard sugar base to produce small, hard preparations of various sizes or shapes. Medication is released slowly when the lozenge is sucked.

Suspensions are liquids with solid, insoluble drug particles dispersed throughout. These solid particles tend to settle out in layers, so the medication must be shaken before pouring.

Syrups are liquids with a high sugar content designed to disguise the bitter taste of a drug. These are often used for pediatric patients.

Tablets are dried, powdered drugs compressed into small shapes. These shapes are small enough so that they may be swallowed whole. Tablets usually contain trademarks, designs, or words for product identification and may have a line through the middle so the tablet may be divided (this is known as a scored tablet). Tablets may also contain coatings of various types to increase solubility or absorption.

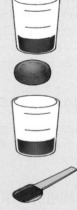

Procedure 10-1   Administering Oral Medications

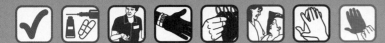

STEP ONE: GETTING READY

1. Check the accuracy of the order as written and the time to be given. Clarify any information now known about the patient or the medication, such as allergies.
2. Wash the hands well. This is essential to avoid contaminating the medication. Although it seems an obvious step, it is often neglected by busy nurses.
3. Assemble the medication equipment. Obtain the plastic medication cups, paper souffle cup, glass, water or juice, and straw if needed (*A through F*). Unlock medication cart, if necessary.

STEP TWO: PREPARING THE MEDICATION

1. Read the order on the medication form and obtain the correct medication from the cabinet or cart (*G*). Medications may come in a cardboard or plastic container, a bottle, or an individually wrapped package.
2. Compare medication order with label on container. First check for the right patient, drug, route, dosage, and time of administration.
3. Open the container and pour the correct number of tablets or capsules into the paper medication cup.
   - Do not touch the medication, but pour the medication directly into the bottle lid or the cup.
   - Return any extra medication to the container (*H*).
     ○ To avoid errors, hold the medication cup at eye level when pouring liquids (*I*).
     ○ If the unit-dose system, Pyxis dispensing machine, or nurse service is used, the medication will come in a labeled package. It is not removed from the wrapping until the nurse is at the patient's bedside (*J*).
4. Compare the information on the medication card or the medication administration record (MAR) with the label on the container. This is the second check for accuracy.
5. Close the box or replace the lid on the container, and check the information on it for the third time with the medication card or MAR. Medication lids are always replaced immediately after use.
   - Medication that requires special storage (such as refrigeration) is replaced immediately.
6. Put the medication container back on the shelf.
7. Place the cup containing the medication next to the medication card or MAR on the tray.

8. Repeat this process for each medication ordered for the patient. All of the tablets for one patient may be placed in the same medication cup.

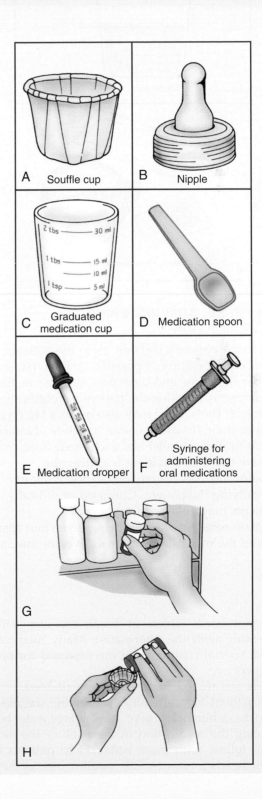

A   Souffle cup

B   Nipple

C   Graduated medication cup

D   Medication spoon

E   Medication dropper

F   Syringe for administering oral medications

G

H

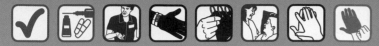

Procedure 10-1   Administering Oral Medications—cont'd

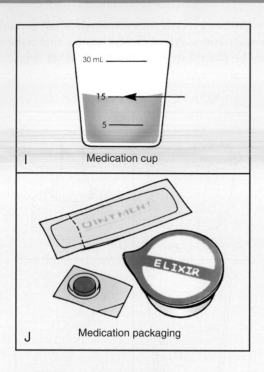

I   Medication cup

J   Medication packaging

STEP THREE: ADMINISTERING THE MEDICATION

1. Go to the patient's bedside. Help the patient into an upright position, if possible. Ask the patient his or her full name and birth date at the same time the nurse is checking the patient's identification bracelet. Their name may also be on a tag on the bed or door. If possible, scan bar code of patient's identification bracelet and each medication to help ensure the correct patient is getting the medication. Never give medication without identifying the patient. Confused or critically ill patients may answer to any name.
2. Explain what medicine is being given and answer any of the patient's questions. Give any special

instructions or teach the patient about the medication as needed. Make any special assessments required. If the patient makes any comment about the medication looking different from usual, having just taken the medication, or not having had that medication before, recheck the medication order.
3. Give the patient a glass of water or juice and have the patient place the medication in the back of his mouth, take a sip of water, and swallow. Most medication dissolves better and causes less stomach discomfort when it is taken with adequate liquid.
4. Remain at the beside until the medication is swallowed. Do not leave medication at the bedside for the patient to take later. The nurse is responsible for making certain the medication is given when ordered. The nurse cannot ensure the patient takes the medicine unless the nurse see him or her swallow it.

STEP FOUR: CONCLUDING

1. Throw away the medication cup. Wash hands.
2. Update electronic records of the MAR or note on the chart the time that the medication was given and sign their name or initials. Record accurately that the medication was given as ordered. Also record if the drug was refused or omitted and notify the charge nurse or the health care provider if the patient did not take the drug for some reason.
3. Later, check the patient again and note any responses or adverse effects that need to be recorded on the medication card or MAR and reported.

2. Do not crush tablets or break capsules without checking with the pharmacist. Many medications have special coatings that are essential for proper absorption.
3. Lozenges are to be sucked, not swallowed.
4. If a patient has difficulty swallowing the medication, have him or her take a few sips of water before placing the medication in the back of the mouth, then follow with more water. Help patients keep their heads forward while swallowing, as they do

when they eat. It is generally not helpful to tilt the head backward.
5. If the patient is unable to swallow the medication as ordered, discuss this problem with the person who ordered the medication.
6. Always give the most important tablets, such as heart medications and antibiotics, first. Other medications might even be withheld until the nurse talks with the person ordering the medications if the patient has great difficulty taking them.

Memory Jogger

General Principles that Underlie All Procedures

- Accuracy
- Acceptance of responsibility
- Asepsis

Liquid-Form Oral Medications

1. Liquids or solutions often must be shaken before they are poured. Although this is common sense, always check to make sure the lid is tightly closed before shaking the bottle.
2. Take the lid off the bottle and place the lid upside down (outer surface down) on a flat surface. This protects the inside of the lid from dirt or contamination.
3. When pouring liquids from a bottle into a plastic medication cup, hold the bottle so the label is against the hand. This prevents medicine from running down onto the label so that it cannot be read.
4. Hold the medication cup at eye level to read the proper dose. Often the medication in the cup is not level but is higher on the sides than in the middle. Read the level at the lowest point in the medication cup.
5. Wipe any extra medication from the bottle top and replace the lid quickly to avoid contamination.
6. Do not dilute a liquid medication unless ordered to do so by the physician or nurse practitioner.
7. The medication could also be drawn up from the bottle or medication cup with a syringe or a medicine dropper. These methods are useful in helping the nurse be accurate when a small dose is ordered and are often used when giving medications to infants or small children. The syringe or medicine dropper is placed halfway back in the baby's mouth, between the cheek and gums, and slowly emptied, giving the baby time to swallow it. The medication in the syringe or medicine dropper could also be emptied into a nipple on which the baby is sucking.

Lifespan Considerations

Older Adults

ADMINISTERING MEDICATIONS

Allow extra time when administering medications to older adult patients. These individuals often are slower than others in being ready to take medications, in swallowing medications and water, and in understanding the answers provided to questions about their medications. The same considerations apply to very young patients.

NASOGASTRIC ADMINISTRATION

The **nasogastric (NG) tube** is another route for enteral medication. Patients who cannot swallow or who are weak or nauseated may be able to take medications through this tube, which leads directly through the nose and into the stomach. The tubing and the clamp allow the nurse to easily give medications over a long period to patients who are unable to take food or medicine by mouth. Some patients find the NG tube so irritating to the nose that the medication must be given another way. In such cases, a percutaneous endoscopic gastrostomy (PEG) tube may be surgically placed directly through the abdomen and into the stomach.

PROCEDURE FOR ADMINISTERING NASOGASTRIC, PEG, AND JEJUNUM TUBE MEDICATIONS

The process for giving medications through a tube is similar to that given for oral medications, but with the following precautions:

- Liquid medications may be ordered for patients who have disorders of the esophagus, are in a coma, or cannot swallow. Some tablets may be crushed, mixed with 30 mL of water, and given through the NG tube.
- Because many of the patients getting medications by NG tube are seriously ill or in a coma, it is especially important to be accurate in all phases of giving the medication. The patient may not be able to help by telling the nurse if there are any problems in giving the medicine.
- Make certain that the NG tube is in the stomach. Aspirate (take out) stomach contents with a syringe, or inject (put in) 5 or 10 mL of air into the tube and listen for a gurgling sound in the abdominal area caused by the air. This may be heard by placing a stethoscope over the stomach. The nurse might also listen for breath sounds, showing that the tubing might be in the lung, by holding the tubing to the ear. Of course, medication must not be given if there is any question about where the NG tube is located. Usually the NG tube is left in place once it is put into the patient.
- The procedure for giving tubal medications is very similar to steps 1, 2, and 4 of the procedure for giving oral medications. The major difference is that the medicine must be crushed and then put into the tube rather than having the patient swallow it. Some institutions suggest all medications be crushed, mixed together in one cup and administered; other institutions wish each medication to be crushed and administered separately. If NG suction is attached to the tubing, disconnect it and clamp the suction tube shut. Clamp the NG tube and attach a bulb syringe. Next, pour the medication into the syringe, unclamp the NG tube, and let the medication run in by gravity. Add water, usually at least 50 mL or according to the institution's policy, to flush and clean out the tubing when the medicine has all passed through the tube. Reclamp the tube. The tube remains clamped for at least 30 minutes before the suction tube is reattached so that there is time for the medication to be absorbed. This procedure is shown in figure 10-1.

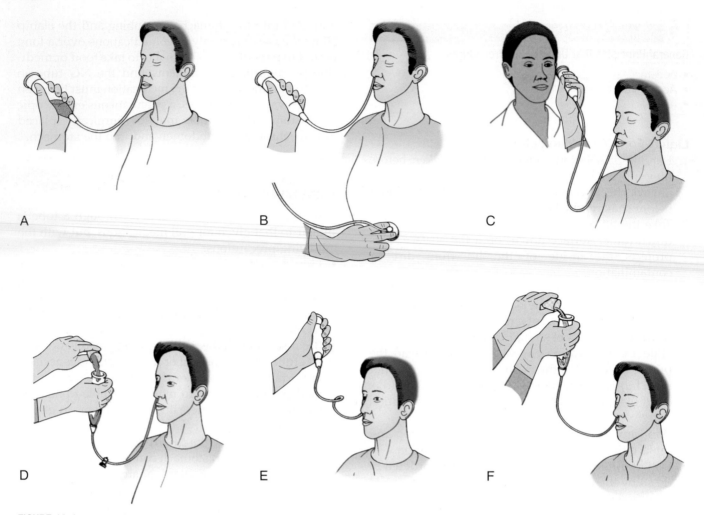

FIGURE 10-1 Administration of medication by nasogastric tube. Make certain the nasogastric tube is in place by **A,** aspirating stomach contents; **B,** listening for gurgling sound in stomach with stethoscope; or **C,** listening for breath sounds. **D,** Put the medication into tubing and **E,** let it run in by gravity. **F,** After the medication is almost out of the tubing, add water to flush the tubing.

- The process for giving medication through a PEG tube is very similar to that for the NG tube. In addition to the tubing, the PEG has a gastrostomy feeding button (a small, flexible silicone device that has a mushroom-shaped dome at one end and two small wings at the other end) that can be used to close the tube between uses. Irrigate this button with 5 to 10 mL of tap water after food and medication have been given and wiped with a cotton-tipped applicator to help keep the tube open. The PEG tube itself is to be cleaned with 25 to 50 mL of tap water after giving food to prevent it from getting clogged up. Follow institutional policy if it differs from these recommendations.

RECTAL ADMINISTRATION

When a patient has severe nausea or vomiting, medication may need to be put into the rectum, thus avoiding the mouth and stomach. Unlike an enema, when medication is given rectally, the medication is left to be absorbed and not expelled. Accurate dosage through rectal administration is somewhat more difficult and harder to predict than are the small, accurate doses used in oral medications. This is true for a variety of reasons:

- Some required medications do not come in suppository or enema form.
- Sometimes the patient has diarrhea and cannot hold the medication.
- Sometimes other rectal problems may make using this route a problem.
- If the patient has a lot of fecal material, the medication may not be well absorbed.
- Medications are not absorbed from the rectal mucosa at a standard or predictable rate.

The procedure for administering rectal medications is described in Procedure 10-2. Note that steps 1, 2, and 4 again are similar to those for administering oral medications.

Procedure 10-2   Administering Rectal Medications

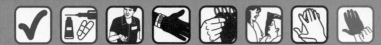

STEP ONE: GETTING READY

1. Check the medication order on the Kardex or electronic medication report sheet. Check the accuracy of the order as written and the time to be given. Clarify any information known about the patient or the medication.
2. Wash hands. This is essential to avoid contaminating the medication.
3. Assemble all the necessary equipment. In addition to the medication order or card, get the medication tray, souffle or medication cups, medication cart, lubricant, and rubber gloves.

STEP TWO: PREPARING THE MEDICATION

1. Read the medication order on the medication card or MAR and get the correct medication from the cabinet, refrigerator, or cart. Medication may come in a bottle, in a plastic container, or as a suppository wrapped in foil and kept in the refrigerator.
2. Compare the medication card or MAR with the label on the container. First check for the right patient, drug, route, dosage, and time of administration.
3. Obtain the proper amount of liquid, disposable medicated enema, or suppository. Suppositories must be firm or they cannot be properly inserted. If the suppository has melted, it may be hardened by being put in a small container of ice for a few minutes. If the unit-dose system or nurse service is used, the medication comes in a labeled package. It is not removed from the wrapping until the nurse is at the patient's bedside.
4. Compare the information on the medication card or MAR with the label on the container. This is the second check for accuracy.
5. Replace the medication container and check the information on it for the third time with the medication card or MAR. Medication such as suppositories requiring special storage (refrigeration) are to be replaced immediately.
6. Place the cup containing the medication next to the medication card or MAR on the tray. Suppositories require insertion immediately, before they melt.

STEP THREE: ADMINISTERING THE MEDICATION

1. Go to the patient's bedside. Help the patient turn over on his or her side with one leg bent over the other in a Sims' position. Protect the patient's modesty as much as possible by closing the drapes and draping the patient. Ask the patient his or her name at the same time the nurse is checking the patient's identification bracelet and bed tag. Never give medication without identifying the patient.
2. Explain what medicine is being given and answer any of the patient's questions. Give any special instructions, such as holding the medicine inside and not letting it come out, and teach the patient about the medication as needed. Make any special assessments required.
3. Put on gloves. If the nurse is giving a suppository, remove the suppository from the foil packet and place a small amount of water-soluble lubricant on the tip of the suppository and on the inserting finger. Tell the patient the procedure is ready to begin. Hold the suppository at the anal sphincter for a few seconds, and tell the patient to take a deep breath and to bear down slightly. This will relax the sphincter so the suppository may be pushed into the rectum about 1 inch (A through D). Use the fourth finger (which is smaller) for children. The patient should remain on his or her side for approximately 20 minutes. With children, it may be necessary to hold their buttocks together to prevent them from releasing the suppository.

If the medication is being given by disposable enema, the procedure is the same, except that the lubricated tip is inserted into the rectum and the 50 to 150 mL of medication is slowly squeezed from the disposable container (E through G).

STEP FOUR: CONCLUDING

1. Dispose of the foil packet or plastic containers and the gloves. Clean the medication tray or cart.
2. Leave patients with tissues to wipe themselves if needed and a way to wash their hands.
3. Wash hands.
4. Note on the medication card or MAR the time that medication was given and sign name or initials.

Procedure 10-2 Administering Rectal Medications—cont'd

Record accurately that the medication was given as ordered.

5. Check the patient again later and note any response or adverse effects that must be recorded on the medication card or MAR and reported. Medicated enemas may be given for severe asthma, to relieve constipation, or to instill steroids used to treat bowel disorders. The nurse must always look for and report any response to the medicated enema.

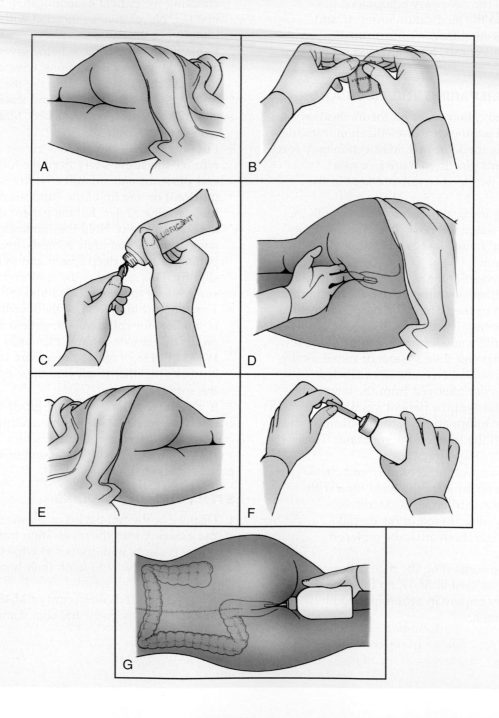

Safe Medication Administration Equation

Legal regulations
+ Nursing process
+ Knowledge about pharmacology
+ Following standard procedures =
 Safe medication administration

PARENTERAL MEDICATIONS

STANDARD PRECAUTIONS

In 1987, in an effort to protect health care workers from exposure to human immunodeficiency virus (HIV), hepatitis B virus (HBV), and other bloodborne pathogens, the Centers for Disease Control and Prevention (CDC) issued recommendations for universal precautions for all health care workers to follow. They recommend that health care workers use gloves, gowns, masks, and protective eyewear when they are likely to be exposed to patient blood or body fluids, and that they consider that all patients might be infected. In 1988, an update from the CDC clarified the specific body fluids that may be a problem (Box 10-2). Evidence has suggested that only blood, semen, vaginal fluid, and possibly breast milk could carry HIV. These precautions also apply to a variety of other body fluids and tissues (see Box 10-2), although the risk from these is unknown. In 1996, the CDC published revised guidelines, called Standard Precautions, which are considered to be the primary ways to prevent the transmission of infections.

Standard Precautions recommend the use of puncture-resistant containers for disposing of all needles and sharps. Scoop up the syringe with one hand. Do NOT put the cap back on a needle, because most needlestick injuries occur at this time. Do not break the needle off the syringe. If the syringe is supplied with a safety-cover system, be sure to slide the safety cover in place, per manufacturer instructions, prior to placing the whole syringe in the sharps container. If the syringe is supplied in a retractable needle system, simply place the whole syringe in the sharps container after use, as the needle will retract automatically after injection; in order to activate this system, be sure to administer the full volume of medication present in the syringe. With either product, if the safety feature does not activate or fails, be sure to place the whole device in the sharps container to minimize any risk of needle puncture. Place both needle and syringe in a well-marked "hazardous material" plastic canister directly after use. Research suggests that probably more needlestick injuries occur than are reported, and every effort should be made to prevent people from recapping used needles.

PARENTERAL ADMINISTRATION

The **parenteral route** (into the skin) of medication administration may be through intradermal, subcutaneous, intramuscular (IM), or intravenous (IV) injections. Drugs are administered parenterally for the following reasons:

- The patient cannot take an oral medication.
- The action of the medicine is required quickly.
- Gastric enzymes might destroy the medication.
- The medication might be removed from the body on a "first pass" through the liver before it can get to the tissues in the body where it will act.
- Medication must be given at a steady rate to provide a constant blood level.
- The medication is not available in an enteral form.

For example, vomiting or unconscious patients may receive IM or IV antibiotics; IV medication may be given in a life-threatening emergency; or a patient may receive continuous IV medication to control heart dysrhythmias.

IM and subcutaneous injections require some time for the medication to reach the bloodstream, so the onset of action may be slower than if the medication were given intravenously. If an individual is filled with fluid (edema), has large quantities of fat, or has poor circulation (for example, if in shock), the rate of absorption may be unusually long for IM or subcutaneous injections.

IV injections or infusions may be needed when medication must go directly into the bloodstream because the action of these methods is rapid. IV medications may be effective for only a short time, requiring frequent doses. Overdosage errors of IV medications can be very serious. Also, the cost is generally higher for IV medication, even though the total dose may be smaller than if the medication were given orally.

Although all medication administration should be 100% accurate, the nurse giving parenteral medication has a special responsibility for careful and accurate administration because any errors in technique or dosage may have serious consequences. Once injected, the medication cannot be withdrawn. Precise administration of drug dosage is essential. Accurately locating the site of injection is required to avoid pain and damage to tissues, nerves, or blood vessels. Aseptic (sterile) technique must be followed to lessen chances of infection. A slow and gradual rate of injection of the medication into the tissues is important for most drugs. This will reduce pain, prevent overdosage, and decrease adverse reactions such as respiratory collapse or heart dysrhythmias.

Box 10-2 Summary of Standard Precautions: Prevention of Transmission of Human Immunodeficiency Virus, Hepatitis B Virus, and Other Bloodborne Pathogens in Health Care Settings

Under Standard Precautions, blood and certain body fluids of all patients are considered to possibly contain human immunodeficiency virus (HIV), hepatitis B virus (HBV), and other bloodborne pathogens. Blood is the single most important source of transmission of HIV, HBV, and other blood-borne pathogens in health care settings. Infection control efforts for HIV, HBV, and other bloodborne pathogens must focus on preventing exposure to blood, as well as on delivery of HBV immunization.

Research has shown that only blood, semen, vaginal secretions, and possibly breast milk may transmit HIV. Although the risk is unknown, universal precautions also apply to tissues and the following fluids: cerebrospinal fluid, synovial fluid, pleural fluid, peritoneal fluid, and amniotic fluid. Standard Precautions do not apply to feces, nasal secretions, sputum, saliva (except in situations in which contamination with blood is likely, such as dental settings), sweat, tears, urine, and vomitus unless they contain visible blood. The risk of transmission of HIV and HBV from these materials is extremely low to nonexistent.

Health care workers are at risk for exposure to blood from patients and must consider all patients as possibly infected with bloodborne pathogens. Therefore health care workers must always follow infection control precautions for all patients.

PRECAUTIONS TO PREVENT TRANSMISSION OF HIV
General Precautions
- Consider all patients potentially infected.
- Wear gloves when touching blood, body fluids containing blood, and body fluids to which Standard Precautions apply; for handling items or surfaces soiled with blood or other fluids; and for doing venipuncture or other procedures involving blood. Change gloves after each contact with a patient.
- Use masks, protective eyewear or face shields, and gowns or aprons when doing procedures that may produce blood or body fluid droplets or splashes.
- Wash hands and skin surfaces immediately and thoroughly with warm soap and water if they get splashed with blood or body fluid to which universal precautions apply; wash between patients and after removal of gloves even when they are not torn or punctured.
- Take precautions to prevent injuries from needles, scalpels, and other sharp instruments during procedures, when cleaning instruments, during disposal, or when handling. To prevent needlestick injuries, needles are not to be recapped, bent or broken by hand, or removed from disposable syringes. After they are used, disposable

syringes and needles, scalpel blades, and other sharp items for disposal are to be placed in puncture-resistant containers located within the patient's room.
- Use mouthpieces, resuscitation bags, or other ventilation devices when mouth-to-mouth resuscitation is likely to be performed in emergency situations.

Special Considerations
- Health care workers who have sore, draining lesions or wet skin conditions are not to be giving direct patient care and are not to handle patient care equipment until the condition resolves.
- Pregnant health care workers are not known to be at greater risk of getting HIV infection than health care workers who are not pregnant; however, if a health care worker is infected with HIV during pregnancy, the infant is at risk of infection from perinatal transmission. Because of this risk, pregnant health care workers must be especially familiar with and strictly follow precautions to lower the risk of HIV transmission.

PRECAUTIONS FOR INVASIVE PROCEDURES
An invasive procedure is defined as any surgical entry into tissues, cavities, or organs, or repair of major traumatic injuries. General blood and body fluid precautions listed earlier, combined with the following list of precautions, are the minimal precautions for all such invasive procedures.
- All health care workers who participate in invasive procedures must use appropriate barrier procedures to prevent skin and mucous membrane contact with all patients' blood and other body fluids to which universal precautions apply.
- Gloves and surgical masks must be worn for all invasive procedures.
- Protective eyewear or face shields are to be worn for all procedures that commonly produce droplets or splashes of blood, body fluids containing blood, or other body fluids.
- Gowns or aprons made of materials providing a barrier are to be worn during an invasive procedure in which there is likely to be splashing of blood or other body fluids.
- All health care workers who perform or assist in vaginal or cesarean delivery are to wear gloves and gowns when handling the placenta or the infant until blood and amniotic fluid have been removed from the infant's skin. Gloves are worn until postdelivery care of the umbilical cord.
- If a glove is torn or a needlestick or other injury occurs, the glove is removed and a new glove put on as promptly as patient safety permits; the needle or instrument involved in the incident should also be removed from the sterile field.

Data from Centers for Disease Control: Recommendations for prevention of HIV transmission in health care settings, *Morb Mortal Wkly Rep* 36(suppl 25), 1987; Update universal precautions for prevention of transmission of human immunodeficiency virus, hepatitis B virus, and other bloodborne pathogens in health care settings, *Morb Mortal Wkly Rep* 37(24), 1988; and *Morb Mortal Wkly Rep* 38(suppl 6):9-18, 1989.

BASIC EQUIPMENT

SYRINGES

Syringes, or instruments for injecting liquids, come in 1-, 3-, 5-, 10-, 20-, and 50-mL sizes and in plastic or glass. Plastic syringes are the preferred equipment because they may be used once and thrown away. This makes them convenient in terms of packaging and disposal, but they are more expensive than glass and cannot be used with some medications; also, dosage lines or calibration may be more difficult to read. Reusable glass syringes cost far less, but they may break, may become loose with constant use, and must be cleaned, repackaged, and sterilized each time they are used. Needleless syringe systems are also now available for use, consisting of a high-pressured delivery device, a needleless syringe, and a cartridge of pressurized air deliver the medication across the dermis. Needleless systems offer a pain-free alternative, although medications available for delivery through this method are limited. Cost and medication exposure (in the form of powdered or aerosolized compounds) are risks associated with the use of a needleless system (Figure 10-2).

Syringes are made up of three main parts (Figure 10-3). The **tip** is the portion that holds the needle. The needle screws onto the tip or fits tightly so it does not fall off. The **barrel** is the container for the medication. The calibrations are printed numbers on the barrel, and they indicate the amount or volume of medication in either minims (m), milliliters (mL), units, or cubic centimeters (cc) (Figure 10-4). The **plunger** is the inner portion that fits into the barrel. The medication is forced out through the needle when the plunger is pushed into the barrel.

NEEDLES

The needle must be selected according to the needs of the medication. The **needle** is made up of the hub, or bottom part, which attaches to the syringe; the shaft, which is the hollow part through which the medication passes; and the pointed or beveled tip, which pierces the skin (Figure 10-5). The longer the pointed tip of the needle, the more easily the needle enters the skin. The

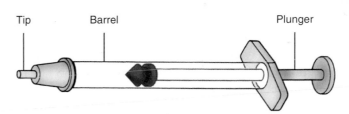

FIGURE 10-3 Parts of a syringe.

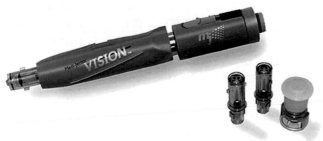

FIGURE 10-2 Sample of a Needle-Free Insulin Delivery System

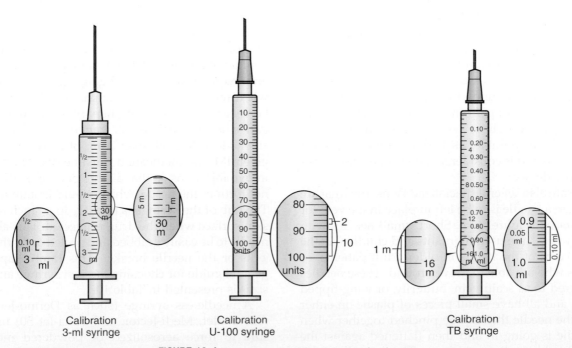

FIGURE 10-4 Comparison of different types of syringes.

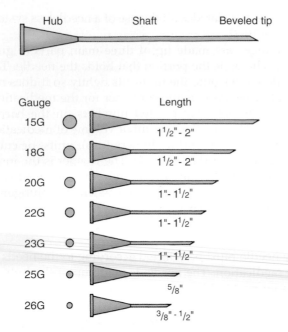

FIGURE 10-5 Parts of the needle and various needle gauges.

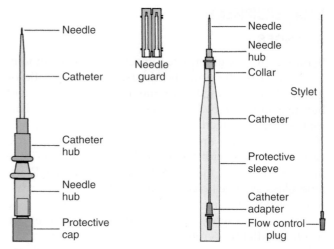

FIGURE 10-6 Over-the-needle catheters. Puncture the vein with a metal large-bore needle. Thread a 4- to 6-inch small-gauge plastic catheter inside and up into the vein before removing the metal needle. Use this type of needle when intravenous therapy must continue for several days.

Table 10-1	Suggested Guide for Selecting Syringe and Needles		
ROUTE	**GAUGE (G)**	**LENGTH (IN)**	**VOLUME TO BE INJECTED (mL)**
Intradermal	25-27	⅜-½	0.01-0.1
Subcutaneous	25-27	½-1	0.5-2
Intramuscular	20-22	1-2	0.5-2
Intravenous	15-22	½-2	Unlimited

diameter of the needle is called the *gauge*. The larger the number of the gauge, the smaller the hole. (For example, a 25-gauge needle is smaller than a 17-gauge needle.) Thick solutions require larger diameters for injection. The needle gauge is written on the needle hub and on the package. Needles also come in varying lengths, from ⅜ inch to 3 inches. Generally, the smaller the needle (larger the gauge), the shorter the needle. The smallest needles are used for intradermal or subcutaneous injections because they do not need to go very far into the skin. Filter needles are also available for use when medication is drawn from an ampule to prevent uptake of glass shards and risk of injection. Needleless systems are a recent technology that allows the administration of medication through the dermis and into the bloodstream by way of a high-pressure needleless injection. Pressurized air drives aerosolized or powdered compounds through the skin, allowing for a pain-reduced or pain-free method of rapid administration. The needleless syringe or tip used in this procedure is disposable, as it does come in contact with the skin and is considered a one-time use component of the device.

There are also several specialized IV needles that are used when a needle is to be left in place in the vein for a long period (Figure 10-6). Short, small needles with plastic "wings" are used in infants and children, in the smaller veins of the hands in older adult patients, or in adults who are able to move around. These needles are referred to as scalp vein, butterfly, or wing-tipped needles, and all have small pieces of plastic on either side of the needle that can be pinched together when the needle is going in and then flattened against the skin and held in place with tape. These needles have

a small, capped plastic tube attached to the hub that can be used when withdrawing blood specimens or injecting drugs such as heparin.

The sizes of the needle and syringe are determined by how viscous (thick) the medication is and by the amount to be injected. For example, blood is very thick and requires a 15- to 19-gauge needle. Sometimes when the volume is very small and the dosage must be very accurate (as with heparin or insulin), a small-gauge needle (such as a 27-gauge) is used so no medicine is lost. If more than 3 mL of medication is to be given IM, the medication must be divided and given in two injections so that a large pool of medicine does not form in the tissue, which would irritate the tissue. The hub of the syringe is to be ¼ to ½ inch above the skin surface when the drug is injected. This allows the needle to be easily grabbed and pulled out if the patient jerks or the needle breaks. (This rarely happens.) A general guide for choosing the best syringe and needle sizes is presented in Table 10-1.

A needleless syringe (such as Dermo-Jet, Vitajet, AdvantaJet, Medi-Jector, and Preci-Jet 50) uses pressure to force aerosolized or powdered medication across the skin into the bloodstream, or directly into

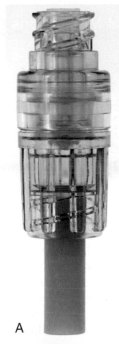

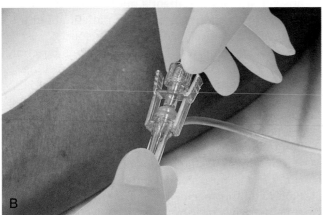

FIGURE 10-7 A, Example of a Luer Activated Valve. **B,** Needleless device using valvelike system.

site for the injection. The type of parenteral injection and the medication itself often require special equipment or injection techniques. Accurate selection of the syringe and needle and the packaging of the medication help determine the specific steps to follow in drawing up the medication.

All equipment and medication used in parenteral injections is to be clearly labeled. All packages are to be closely inspected to make certain the contents are sterile. Any equipment that appears old or has crumpled or torn packaging is to be thrown away. Check dates to make certain the sterilization date has not expired. Any medication with a questionable seal or with changes in color or appearance is to be returned promptly to the pharmacy. Any expired medications must be disposed of to ensure they are not accidentally administered.

FORMS OF PARENTERAL MEDICATIONS

Parenteral medications are supplied in a variety of different containers. Ampules, vials, Mix-o-vials, and prefilled tubes are the most common dosage forms.

Small, single- or multiple-dose glass or plastic containers of medication are called **vials**. The top of the glass container is covered first with a rubber diaphragm and then with a small aluminum lid. A tightly fitting metal band holds the rubber diaphragm in place. First the metal lid is removed, then the rubber diaphragm is cleansed with an alcohol wipe, and the needle is inserted through the rubber diaphragm into the medication. An amount of air equal to the amount of solution to be withdrawn is injected into the vial to assist the withdrawal of the medication (Figure 10-8).

The vial may contain a solution, or it may contain a powder to which a liquid must be added just before administration to make a solution. Read the label carefully to determine the type and amount of diluent that is required.

Needles are always inserted into the vial with the bevel up so the nurse may inspect the needle as it goes into the rubber stopper. The needle is always changed before administering the medication to the patient because forcing the needle through the rubber stopper may make it dull or create sharp, irregular edges called "burrs" that would produce pain when inserted into the patient.

Ampules contain one dose of medicine in a small, breakable glass container. The narrow neck of the ampule may have to be cut with a small ampule file, or may have a line (score) or ring around it, indicating a weakened area where the top can be broken off. All the medicine can be shifted to the bottom of the ampule by flicking the top lightly with a finger. Grasp the top above the scored or ringed area with an alcohol wipe or gauze pad and pull down sharply on the glass top. The top should easily fall off, allowing insertion of the needle into the ampule to draw up the medicine

tissue, and can be used for some medications and immunizations. Various needleless infusion lines are also used (Figure 10-7). This type of delivery system is growing in popularity because it removes the risks associated with reusing needles and needle disposal.

PROCEDURE FOR PREPARING AND ADMINISTERING PARENTERAL MEDICATIONS

The basic procedure for preparing and administering parenteral medications is similar to that for oral medications (Procedure 10-3). Whereas giving oral or enteral medications is a clean procedure, giving parenteral medications is a sterile procedure. So the nurse will note in the following discussion that there is greater emphasis on sterile technique in giving parenteral medications because the risk for infection is high. There is also a need to correctly determine the proper

Procedure 10-3 Preparing and Administering Parenteral Medications

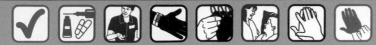

STEP ONE: GETTING READY

1. Check the medication order. Check the accuracy of the order as written and the time to be given. Clarify any information now known about the patient or the medication.
2. Wash hands. This is essential to avoid contaminating the medication and equipment. Although it seems an obvious step, it is often neglected by busy nurses.
3. Assemble all the necessary equipment. In addition to the medication order or card, obtain the medication tray, the proper size needles and syringes, alcohol swabs, tubes, and medication cart. Make certain the equipment is sterile. The expiration date on the plastic or paper wrapping should indicate when the equipment must be thrown away or sterilized again.

STEP TWO: PREPARING THE MEDICATION

1. Read the order on the medication card or MAR and obtain the correct medication from the cabinet or cart. The medication may come in an ampule, a vial, a Mix-o-vial, or an infusion set.
2. Compare the medication card or MAR with the label on the container. First check for the right patient, drug, route, dosage, and time of administration.
3. Attach the needle to the syringe, keeping the needle covered with a cap.
4. Ready the medication for withdrawal by opening the ampule, if necessary.
5. Compare the information on the medication card or MAR with the label on the container. This is the second check for accuracy.
6. Insert the needle into the medication container and fill the syringe with the proper amount of medication. (See the following discussion regarding drawing up medications from different dosage forms.) If any air bubbles are present, tap barrel of syringe so air moves into needle and can be removed. Check the information on the container for the third time with the medication card or MAR. Do not mix more than one medication in a syringe without checking to see if the medications can be mixed together.
7. Put the unused medication containers away.
8. Change the needle for a new sterile needle if medication has been withdrawn through a rubber stopper or from a multiple-dose vial.

9. Place the syringe and alcohol swabs next to the medication card or MAR on the tray.

STEP THREE: ADMINISTERING THE MEDICATION

1. Go to the patient's bedside. Help the patient get into the proper position for the injection. The patient may need to turn over, roll onto his or her side, or remove his or her gown. Ask the patient his or her name at the same time the nurse is checking the patient's identification bracelet and bed tag. Never give medication without positively identifying the patient. Confused or very ill patients may answer to any name.
2. Explain what medication is being given and answer any of the patient's questions. Give any special instructions or teach the patient about the medication as indicated. Make any special assessments required. Examine previous injection sites for signs of necrosis, infection, or swelling. Examine the site to be injected. If the patient makes any comments about the medication being different from usual, having just taken the medication, or not having had that medication before, recheck the medication order.
3. Put on gloves. Using an alcohol wipe, carefully rub the skin for several seconds to cleanse it. Following the specific procedure for intradermal, subcutaneous, or intramuscular injection (described in detail in the chapter text), insert the needle firmly, pull back slightly on the plunger to aspirate for blood, and inject the medication. (To aspirate is to look for blood, indicating that the needle has been accidentally placed in a blood vessel, artery, or vein.) If blood comes into the syringe when the plunger is pulled back, remove the needle and set the syringe aside for disposal, prepare new medication for administration, and select another site for injection.
4. Assist the patient to a comfortable position.

STEP FOUR: CONCLUDING

1. Dispose of the alcohol wipe. Return to the nursing station and dispose of the syringe and needle according to hospital procedure. Do not attempt to put the cap back on the needle, because of the risk of accidental self puncture. All hospitals have the policy that any accidental scratch or prick from a used needle must be reported because of the risk of acquired immune deficiency syndrome or

Procedure 10-3   Preparing and Administering Parenteral Medications—cont'd

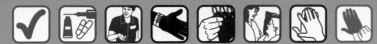

hepatitis. Clean the medication tray or cart. Wash hands.
2. Note on the medication card or MAR the time the medication was given, and sign name or initials. Record that the medication was given as ordered or was refused.

3. Check the patient again later and note any particular response or adverse effects that must be recorded and reported. Particularly note any complaints of pain, numbness, or tingling at the injection site.

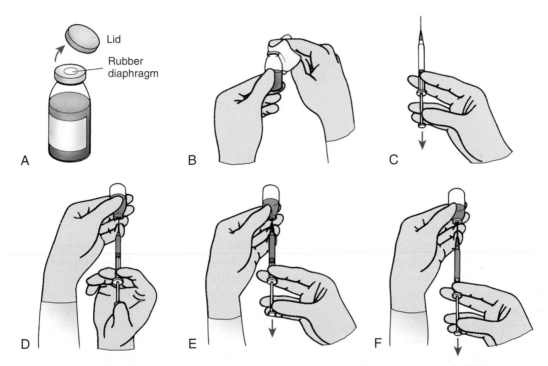

FIGURE 10-8 A, Example of a vial. **B,** Remove the metal lid and cleanse the diaphragm with an alcohol wipe. **C,** Pull into the syringe an amount of air equal to the amount of solution to be withdrawn. **D,** Insert the needle with the bevel up, and inject the air into the space above the solution. **E,** Withdraw the medication. **F,** Move the needle downward to allow needle to continue to fill.

(Figure 10-9). A filter needle is used to prevent glass shards from being drawn up into the syringe with the medication. Ampules were very common forms of medication storage in the 1960s and 1970s, after which their popularity decreased because of the availability of less expensive vials. There is interest in using ampules again as a way to reduce allergic reactions to the latex stoppers in the vials. Therefore the American Society of Health Systems Pharmacists has recommended the use of ampules whenever possible.

Occasionally two medications may be ordered that may be given in the same syringe. Two compatible medications are often ordered to be given together as a preoperative medication before surgery (for example, meperidine [Demerol] and promethazine HCl [Phenergan]). Another example is the common practice of ordering two types of insulin (for example, regular and

neutral protamine Hagedorn [NPH]) to be given together. In contrast, many antibiotics must be given in separate syringes because they chemically precipitate (harden and separate into layers) or become inactive if mixed together. It is important when mixing medications in one syringe to remember the following:

- The compatibility of the two medications must be known; check with a resource when necessary (e.g., Trissel's *Handbook on Injectable Drugs*).
- Air must be injected into both bottles before any medication is withdrawn (to avoid sucking medication already in the syringe down into another bottle).
- The medication with the shorter action or weaker dosage must be withdrawn first. (This idea can be understood if insulin is used as an example. Regular insulin acts more quickly than NPH insulin. If

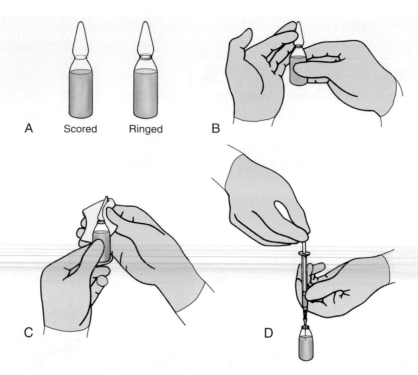

A   Scored   Ringed   B

C   D

FIGURE 10-9 A, Examples of scored and ringed ampules. **B,** Shift medication from the top to the bottom portion of the ampule by flicking the top lightly with a finger. **C,** Wrap a gauze pad around the neck of the ampule and use a snapping motion to break off top of ampule along prescored line at neck. Always break away from the body by bending the top toward you. **D,** Insert the filter needle into the ampule and draw up the medication.

regular insulin is put into the syringe first and a small amount accidentally drops into the NPH insulin bottle when this insulin is being added to the syringe, the patient usually is not affected. However, if the longer acting NPH insulin accidentally contaminates the regular insulin bottle, it could change the time at which the patient experiences the onset of the action of the insulin.)

- New guidelines for drawing up nonanimal insulin state that insulin may now be shaken before being drawn up. This reverses previous precautions.
- When regular and Lente mixtures of insulin are mixed in one syringe, they are injected within 5 minutes of drawing. If this is not possible, the effect of the regular insulin is diminished. The excess zinc from the Lente insulin binds with the regular insulin and forms a Lente-type insulin. NPH-regular insulin mixtures are stable and are absorbed as if injected separately.

Medications that come as a powder must have a solution added immediately before use. The diluent for the powder and the amount to be used are to be specified on the label. Frequently, normal saline solution or sterile water is used. The diluent may be drawn into a 1- or 2-mL syringe and added to the powder. Roll the vial carefully to make certain all the powder is dissolved in the liquid. If the powder does not completely dissolve, do not give the medication. Some of these medications come in a two-compartment vial

called a **Mix-o-vial**. The top compartment contains a sterile solution; the bottom compartment contains the medication powder. A rubber stopper separates the two areas. Pressure on the rubber plunger of the top compartment forces the rubber stopper below to fall into the bottom compartment, letting in the solution to dissolve the powder. The vial is gently rolled to help dissolve the powder, and then a needle may be inserted to withdraw the solution (Figure 10-10).

Any multiple-dose vial or newly mixed (reconstituted) powder solution must be clearly labeled when it is first opened. The date, time, and concentration are to be included, as well as the expiration time of the medication. The nurse who opened or mixed the medication also initials the label.

Many narcotics and emergency drugs (such as adrenalin) come in prefilled syringes and cartridges. These medication cartridges may be quickly slipped into a plastic holder and screwed into place; after the needle is added, the medication is administered (Figure 10-11). Prefilled syringes are particularly helpful when time is important (such as during a cardiac arrest) or when the dosage of medication rarely varies.

Medications or solutions to be given intravenously come in large plastic or glass containers that hold from 50 to 1000 mL. The opening to the glass container is plugged with a hard rubber stopper, a thin rubber diaphragm, and a metal cover. The metal cover and diaphragm are removed just before inserting the

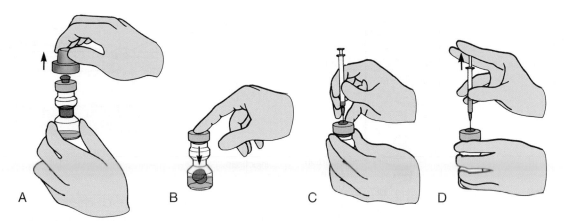

FIGURE 10-10 **A,** Remove the protective sterile cap from the Mix-o-vial. **B,** Push the rubber plunger on the top compartment; this will force the rubber stopper into the bottom compartment and let the solution dissolve the powder. The solution is mixed by gently rolling the container. **C,** The needle is inserted through the top rubber diaphragm into the solution. **D,** The required dose is withdrawn into the syringe.

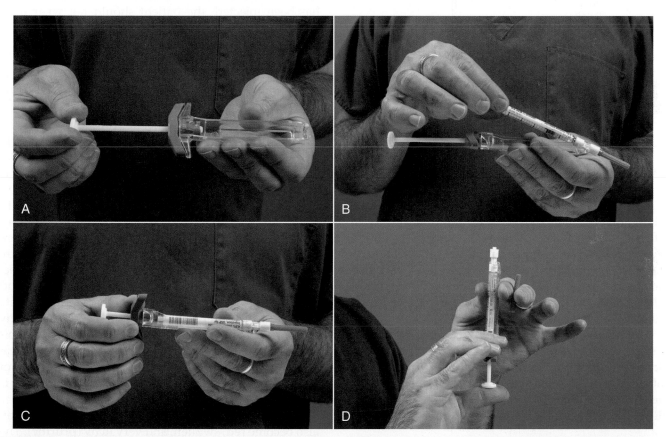

FIGURE 10-11 **A,** Example of a syringe and prefilled sterile cartridge with needle. **B,** Assembling the syringe-needle system. **C,** The cartridge slides into the syringe barrel, turns, and locks at the needle end. The plunger then screws into the cartridge end. **D,** Expel excess medication to obtain accurate dose.

infusion tube that connects the bottle to the tube through a small hole in the hard rubber stopper. In many products, there is also a second small hole in the rubber stopper that allows air to enter the container to replace the amount of medication being infused. Plastic containers come sealed in another plastic bag, which is not opened until the infusion is to begin. Air may

enter the plastic bag either at the bag opening or farther down on the infusion tubing (Figure 10-12).

Some medications, such as antibiotics, are ordered to be given every few hours. This medication comes from the pharmacy already mixed or as a solution to be injected into a smaller bottle or plastic bag, usually containing 50 to 250 mL of fluid, and hung with new

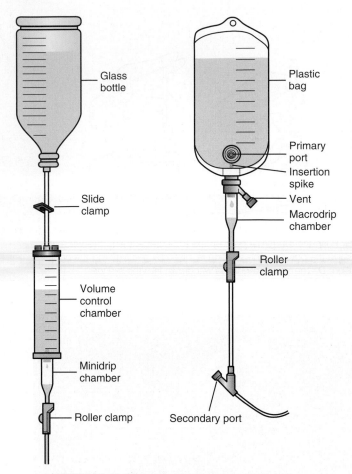

FIGURE 10-12 Intravenous bottle or bag and tubing.

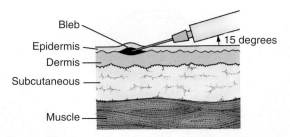

FIGURE 10-13 Anatomy of skin showing placement for intradermal injections.

of the back, and the upper chest, if these areas are reasonably hairless. Usually, just a small volume is injected, producing a small bump like a mosquito bite, called a *bleb*. The blood supply to this area of the skin is less than in other areas, so there is very slow absorption from the intradermal layer. Once the medication has been injected, the patient should not wear tight clothing over the area.

Equipment and Technique

Usually 0.01 to 0.1 mL is injected, so a needle that is both small (25 gauge) and short (⅜ inch) is used. The needle is inserted firmly at a 15-degree angle. The bevel or slanted tip of the needle is pointing upward. The medication is injected, and the needle is swiftly removed. The small bleb should be seen on the skin at the point where the medication was injected into the intradermal space.

If the injection was given for allergy or sensitivity testing, it is important to record the concentration of the medication used and the site of the injection (Figure 10-14). Many reactions to intradermal injections are not apparent for several hours or even days after injection. It is sometimes helpful to draw a circle around the injection site with a pen to help identify the site accurately at a later date when it is inspected for any reaction. The patient has an allergic reaction, or a clinically significant reaction to testing, if there is a wheal (elevated area) at the site where the diluted dose of medication was injected. The amount of swelling is measured at 5, 10, and 15 mm.

If the patient has an allergy, the injection site may also become red, swollen, and very itchy (pruritic). The patient should not scratch this area and should use cool, wet compresses to reduce the irritation. The patient should call the health care provider or go to an emergency room if he has any symptoms in any other body systems, particularly trouble breathing, shortness of breath, puffiness of the face, or hives.

Skin reactions to intradermal allergy injections or to testing for tuberculosis (purified protein derivative test) must be checked at a predetermined time after the injection. Each agency has a policy on how the patient reaction is to be evaluated and recorded. When testing is done on an outpatient basis, a reliable patient is

tubing that is "piggybacked" or "secondary" to an infusion that is already running. The existing solution is clamped off while the piggyback medication is administered, usually over 20 to 60 minutes, and then the original solution is restarted. The piggyback medication being added must be compatible with the original solution.

After studying these general procedures for administering parenteral medications, examine specific techniques necessary for administration of intradermal, subcutaneous, IM, and IV medications. The equipment, sites of injection, and technique must be completely understood.

ADMINISTERING INTRADERMAL MEDICATIONS

Intradermal injections are used to determine if someone has an allergy (allergy sensitivity testing), for tuberculosis testing, for vaccination, and for allergy desensitization shots. They are also used for injection of local anesthetics before wart removal, during suturing of the skin for minor cuts, and for minor procedures. The medication is injected into the intradermal space between the upper two layers of the skin, the epidermis, and the dermis (Figure 10-13). Injections are made into the inner aspect of the forearm, the scapular area

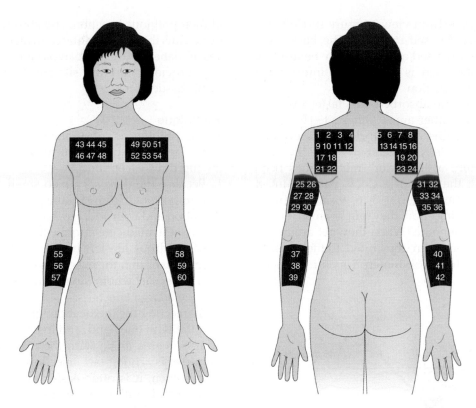

FIGURE 10-14 Sites used in intradermal skin testing for allergy.

Table 10-2	Description of Intradermal Skin Reactions	
OBSERVATION OF SKIN	**RECORDING SYMBOLS**	**REACTION**
	(0)	No reaction
	(1)	Redness or erythema of skin
	(2)	Redness and elevated lesions or papules up to 5 mm in diameter
	(3)	Redness, papules, and vesicles (fluid-filled elevated lesions) up to 5 mm
	(4)	Generalized blister larger than 5 mm

often told to look at injection site and mail in a postcard showing a picture that is most similar to the reaction. Table 10-2 shows common reactions to intradermal injections and how they are described.

ADMINISTERING SUBCUTANEOUS MEDICATIONS

Subcutaneous injections involve placing no more than 2 mL of fluid into the loose connective tissue between the dermis of the skin and the muscle layer (Figure 10-15). (This is a little deeper than the intradermal injections we have been discussing.) Because less blood is normally supplied to this area than to muscle, any medication injected here will be slowly, but completely, absorbed. This means there will be a slow onset of medication action but a long duration of drug action. Medications injected into the subcutaneous tissue are usually very strong, but concentrated into small doses. For example, insulin and heparin are the most frequently given subcutaneous injections. Because these medications are often given daily for a long time in patients with chronic illnesses, special care must be taken not to irritate the tissue with repeated injections in the same area.

Equipment and Sites for Injection
In preparing the subcutaneous injection, only a small syringe and needle are needed. Usually a 25- or 27-gauge needle is used, and one that is no longer than $\frac{5}{8}$ inch in length.

The sites used for subcutaneous injection depend on whether the nurse or the patient is giving the injection. Commonly, the nurse gives subcutaneous injections in the upper arms, upper back, or scapular region. The nurse in the hospital will often need to teach the patient how to give herself or himself the subcutaneous injection while the patient is in the hospital and can practice under the nurse's supervision. The patient is able to inject herself or himself most easily in the upper arms, anterior thighs, and abdomen. The patient should develop a rotation plan for injection sites, and this is posted with the patient's medications or by the patient's bedside. The front view in figure 10-16 shows areas usually used for self-injection. The back view shows less commonly used areas that may be used by the nurse. The site used is part of the information recorded about the injection.

Insulin injections are absorbed 50% faster from the abdomen than from other areas. Other sites for injection include arms, thighs, and buttocks. Because it may be difficult for patients to remember where they last injected the insulin, a "tape-dot" method has been developed. Using the face of a clock, patients inject themselves in the abdomen at 3, 6, 9, and then 12 o'clock. After each injection they put a small dot of tape over the injection site. When they get around to the 3 o'clock position again, they move to the extremities and then back to the abdomen, 1 inch to the side

of their previous injection, and start their new series of dots. Thus the sites are rotated in an organized manner. Teach diabetic patients to avoid injecting within 1 inch of a previous injection site for 1 month in order to avoid tissue damage.

Technique

The technique for subcutaneous injection is identical to that for other parenteral medications with the following three exceptions:

1. Because the dosages are so small and so potent, it is important to draw up the prescribed dose of medication and then add 1 to 2 minims of air. This forces all of the medicine into the tissue when it is injected so no drops are left in the needle. It is especially important that the exact dose is given, especially in children, in whom small variations in dose might have a large effect.

2. In injecting the medication, grasp the skin and hold it flat with one hand, and insert the needle firmly at a 45-degree angle with the other hand. When the nurse is giving an injection in the scapula or abdomen, it is often easier to grasp the skin with one hand, pull it up into a small roll, and insert the needle quickly at a 90-degree angle. Slowly inject the agent while watching for a small wheal or blister to appear.

3. After inserting the needle, the nurse must not aspirate or pull back on the syringe when giving heparin.

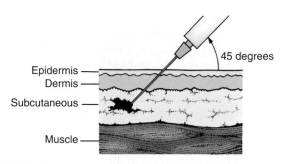

FIGURE 10-15 Anatomy of skin showing placement for subcutaneous injections.

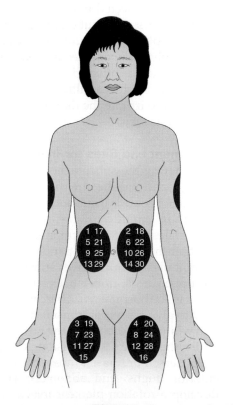
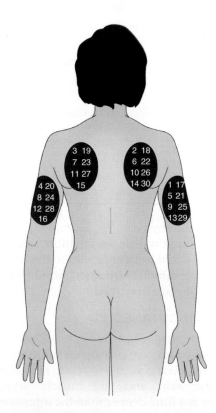

FIGURE 10-16 Body rotation sites for subcutaneous injections.

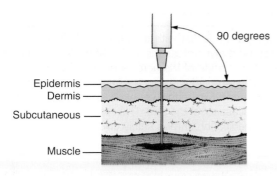

FIGURE 10-17 Anatomy of skin showing placement for intramuscular injections.

The increased vacuum on the tissues caused by aspiration would lead to damage and bruising when the heparin is injected.

ADMINISTERING INTRAMUSCULAR MEDICATIONS

The IM route is a common route for parenteral injections. Many antibiotics, preoperative sedatives, and narcotics are administered intramuscularly. In **intramuscular (IM) injections**, the medication is deposited deep into the muscle mass, past the dermis and subcutaneous tissue and into the very deepest layers of the muscle (Figure 10-17), where the rich blood supply allows for rapid and full absorption. The muscles also contain large blood vessels and nerves, so it is important to place the needle correctly to avoid damage to these structures.

Equipment

The syringe chosen has to be large enough to hold the amount of medicine to be injected. Generally, 0.5 to 2 mL is injected IM, although infants and children rarely receive more than 1 mL. On the rare occasions when more than 3 mL of medicine is ordered, give it in two doses rather than in one syringe. The needle length must be chosen to allow deeper placement of the needle. Usually 1- or ½-inch needles are used. Very obese patients may require an even longer needle; very thin or emaciated patients may require a shorter needle. The gauge of the needle is determined by the type of medication and how free-flowing it is. Usually 20- to 22-gauge needles are used.

There is substantial risk for overpenetration of the IM layer when providing injections to children. Potential dangers of needle overpenetration into the bone or periosteum may include pain and/or damage to the bone or periosteum and detachment of the needle from the syringe. New research suggests that for injections in the thigh muscle, a 1-inch needle is adequate for all children aged 6 years or younger.

For injections in the deltoid muscle of the shoulder, the recommendations include using:

- A ½-inch needle for any girl weighing 70 kg or less and for any boy weighing 75 kg or less
- A ⅝-inch needle for any girl weighing between 70 and 115 kg and for any boy weighing between 75 and 140 kg
- A ⅞- to 1-inch needle for any girl weighing 115 kg or more and for any boy weighing 140 kg or more

Sites for Injection

Five muscles are commonly used for IM injections: the deltoid, dorsogluteal, rectus femoris, vastus lateralis, and ventrogluteal muscles. Each site has advantages and disadvantages, and must be correctly identified for safe administration. These sites have been selected because they are usually away from major blood vessels and nerves, and so are safer to use. Some of these sites are not used for children. Use of the dorsogluteal site most often results in accidental injury to patients because it is close to the sciatic nerve. It is rarely used for IM injections because there have been so many lawsuits related to permanent nerve damage caused by a needle. However, if care is taken to properly identify landmarks, it is a site that may be used when other sites cannot be used. Box 10-3 summarizes the five sites for IM injections and how to identify them.

Technique

The process for giving of IM injections is the same as that for other parenteral medications, except for several additional items:

1. Carefully select the site and identify the landmarks before picking up the syringe. Have all equipment ready. This is especially true for children, who will not hold still for a prolonged time after the nurse finds the site.
2. Insert the needle firmly, usually at a 90-degree angle, and give the injection. The policy over the years when giving an IM injection is to always make sure that the needle is in the muscle and that you have not accidentally entered a vein or artery. To do this, the nurse will pull back on the plunger and check the syringe for any blood (aspirate) before injecting the medication. More recent research suggests that there is little chance of having the needle in a vein or artery and to reduce the pain of injection, the nurse does not pull back on the plunger to aspirate and, instead, injects the solution as quickly as possible. Some hospitals also suggest that the skin next to the needle be pinched to focus pain perception on the pinched area and "trick" the brain into not recognizing the pain from the injection. The nurse will need to follow the hospital policy in giving IM injections as the policy is in a state of change in many schools.
3. After withdrawing the needle, apply gentle pressure to the site with a dry cotton pad. (Use of an

Box 10-3 Sites for Intramuscular Injections

DELTOID MUSCLE

The deltoid muscle is easily reached but used infrequently because the muscle is small and can accommodate only small doses of medications. The deltoid is also near the radial nerve. No more than 2 mL may be injected here (less in children), and the medication should not be irritating and absorbed quickly. For this site, seat the patient upright or have the patient lie flat with the arms apart. Two imaginary lines can be drawn across the armpit at the level of the axilla and the lower edge of the acromion, the sharp point of the shoulder. Two more imaginary lines are then drawn down on either side, one-third and two-thirds of the way around the outer lateral aspect of the arm. This creates a small rectangle in which medication can be safely given.

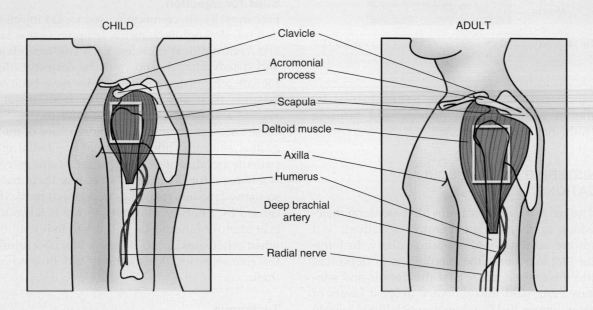

CHILD

ADULT

Clavicle
Acromonial process
Scapula
Deltoid muscle
Axilla
Humerus
Deep brachial artery
Radial nerve

DORSOGLUTEAL MUSCLE

The dorsogluteal muscle is a common injection site for adults because it is relatively free from nerves and major blood vessels. However, the muscles are not developed enough for this site to be used for children younger than 3 years of age. The patient must lie prone (on stomach) on a flat surface and point the toes inward to relax the muscles. An imaginary cross can be drawn from the anus laterally, and from the posterior superior iliac spine down the leg. The injection is given in the upper, outer quadrant of the cross. Hold the syringe perpendicular to the flat surface and inject the medication. Many nurses are afraid to use this site because the sciatic nerve may be injured when nurses fail to properly identify the landmarks.

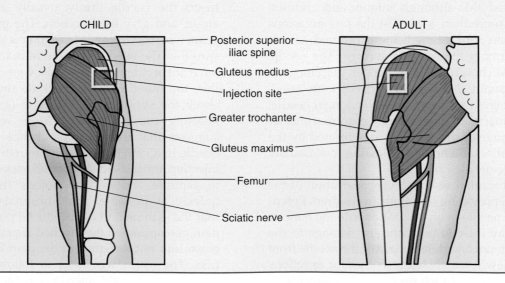

CHILD

ADULT

Posterior superior iliac spine
Gluteus medius
Injection site
Greater trochanter
Gluteus maximus
Femur
Sciatic nerve

Box 10-3   Sites for Intramuscular Injections—cont'd

RECTUS FEMORIS MUSCLE

The rectus femoris muscle lies medial to (toward the middle of the body from) the vastus lateralis muscle, but does not cross the midline of the anterior thigh. It is used in both children and adults, especially for self-injection. Injections here may be painful if the muscle is not well developed. For this site, position the patient in bed either sitting up or lying flat.

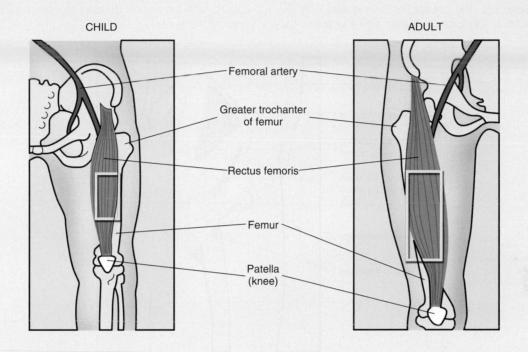

CHILD   ADULT

Femoral artery

Greater trochanter of femur

Rectus femoris

Femur

Patella (knee)

VASTUS LATERALIS MUSCLE

The vastus lateralis muscle is located on the anterior lateral thigh away from blood vessels and nerves. It can absorb a large volume of medication. This is the preferred site for intramuscular (IM) injections in infants; it is also a good site for healthy, ambulatory adults because there are few near major blood vessels and nerves. The muscle mass here tends to shrink or become smaller in elderly or very ill patients and may be inadequate. The muscle extends from one handbreadth below the greater trochanter to one handbreadth above the knee.

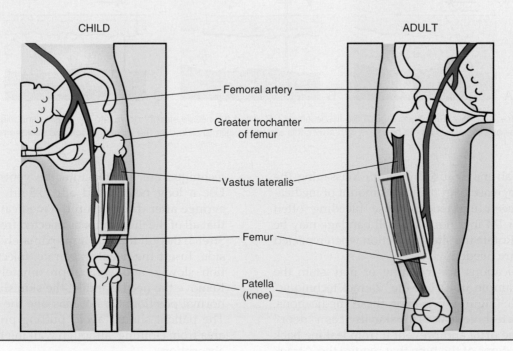

CHILD   ADULT

Femoral artery

Greater trochanter of femur

Vastus lateralis

Femur

Patella (knee)

Continued

Box 10-3	Sites for Intramuscular Injections—cont'd

VENTROGLUTEAL MUSCLE

The ventrogluteal muscle is a large muscle mass that is free of major nerves and adipose tissue, and is also remote from the rectum (minimizing the risk of contamination). Whether the site may be used for children depends on the extent of muscle development. The patient lies on the side with the upper leg flexed, or lies prone (on stomach) and points the toes inward to relax the muscles. The palm of the nurse's hand is placed on the lateral portion of the greater trochanter, the index finger on the anterior superior iliac spine, and the middle finger extended to the iliac crest. The injection is made into the center of the V formed between the index and middle fingers, with the needle directed slightly upward toward the crest of the ilium.

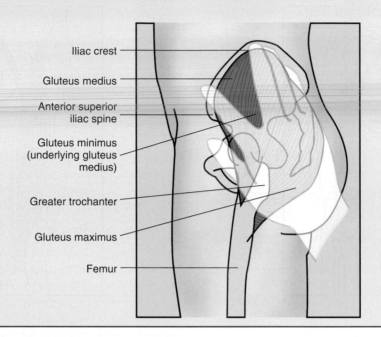

Iliac crest

Gluteus medius

Anterior superior iliac spine

Gluteus minimus (underlying gluteus medius)

Greater trochanter

Gluteus maximus

Femur

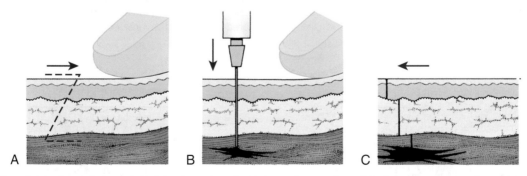

A   B   C

FIGURE 10-18 Z-track injection technique. **A,** Pull the tissue laterally. **B,** Insert the needle straight down into the muscle and inject the medication. **C,** Release the tissue as the needle is withdrawn; this allows the skin to slide over the injection track and seal the medication inside.

alcohol swab may cause burning.) Massaging the area may increase pain if a large amount of medication has been injected. Because bleeding often occurs after IM injections, a small bandage may be necessary. Rotate the site of injection when repeated injections are needed.

4. Some medications are irritating or may stain the skin (for example, iron). Use the "Z-track technique" of injection (Figure 10-18) for these medications. The Z-track technique uses the skin itself as a "door" to seal in the drug and prevent it from leaking back out. Medications of the type that require the Z-track technique are injected into the ventrogluteal site. Use a long needle and add 0.5 mL of air to the syringe after drawing up the medication to ensure that all of the medication is injected from the needle. Stretch or pull the skin approximately 1 inch to one side. Insert the needle, aspirate, inject the medication slowly, and wait approximately 5 seconds. Remove the needle and let the skin slide back to its normal position. Do not massage the injection site. The patient should avoid putting pressure on the area from clothing, although walking helps increase absorption.

ADMINISTERING INTRAVENOUS MEDICATIONS

The **intravenous (IV) route** is used when it is necessary for medication to enter the bloodstream directly. Sometimes large doses of medication must be given, either every few hours or over a long period. Because IV medication has not been exposed to other enzymes or tissues before reaching the bloodstream, the rate of absorption and the onset of action are faster. In addition, some medications cannot be given orally, and may be very painful or irritating if given IM. In emergencies, medication may be injected directly into a vein, but usually the IV medication is given on a scheduled basis or infused slowly through IV tubing or an infusion line that is already in the vein.

If a patient must have numerous medications injected daily, both the patient and the nurse generally prefer IV administration. Some patients do not like to be "tied down" by the tubing and feel general discomfort and irritation from the needle and the medication. Nurses must use greater skill to administer medication intravenously than with other routes, and must be especially careful to prevent infection at the needle site. In addition, because the effect of the medication is immediate, drug overdosages, errors in dosage calculation, or failure to control the rate of administration may produce serious problems for the patient. Thus the nurse has an increased responsibility for implementing and evaluating the medication given. Registered nurses are usually the nurses who will give these types of medicines, but LPN's/LVN's often assist in this procedure.

Equipment

IV solutions come in large-volume, plastic or glass containers, ranging from 250 to 1000 mL. Medications in vials, ampules, or prefilled syringes marked specifically "for IV use" may be added to these containers. Many hospitals receive IV solutions from the pharmacy with the medications already added.

Some hospitals have "IV teams" who can be called to insert the IV needle and start the initial medications. More frequently, the nurse has the responsibility for performing the venipuncture and starting the infusion. All hospitals have clear policies about what nurses may do in starting infusions. Most of these policies have been updated to protect the nurse from accidental exposure to HIV and HBV, which may be spread by direct contact with blood and other body fluids and may lead to the development of acquired immune deficiency syndrome and hepatitis, respectively. It is mandatory that nurses review these policies before attempting to start an IV, for their own protection and the protection of others. Policies clearly state that gloves are to be worn and state how to dispose of the equipment that is contaminated with the patient's blood.

Sites for Intravenous Needle Insertion

Needles for IV infusions are generally inserted into the smallest veins and as close to the hands as possible. Arteries are not used. As more infusion sites are needed, the needle is inserted farther and farther up the vein, closer to the patient's heart. This principle allows one vein to be used multiple times. The metacarpal, dorsal, basilic, and cephalic veins are commonly used in adults (Figure 10-19). Veins in the lower extremities; veins over sharp, bony areas or joints; and veins in areas of recent injury or surgery are to be avoided. Veins commonly used in infants and children include the scalp vein in the temporal area, veins in the dorsum of the foot, and those in the back of the hand (Figure 10-20). Elderly or emaciated patients generally have such fragile skin that needles will not stay in the veins of the hand.

Venipuncture and Intravenous Infusion

The procedures for venipuncture and starting an IV infusion are somewhat different from those with other routes of administration. Procedure 10-4 summarizes the steps involved in venipuncture and IV infusion.

Modifications in Technique for Specific Situations

Adding Medication by Syringe to an Infusion. IV medications are commonly added by syringe to an IV infusion that is already running. This is done by using the medication portal available on the IV tubing. Wear gloves while carrying out this procedure. The tubing is clamped above the self-sealing IV portal of the

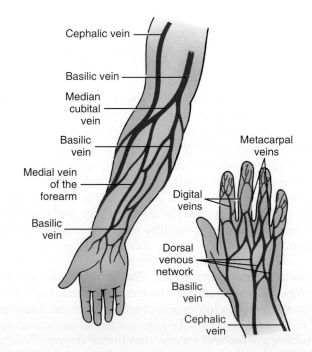

FIGURE 10-19 Intravenous sites used in the hand and forearm of adults.

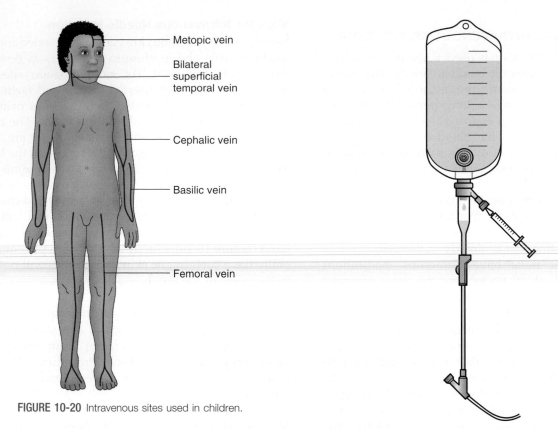

FIGURE 10-20 Intravenous sites used in children.

- Metopic vein
- Bilateral superficial temporal vein
- Cephalic vein
- Basilic vein
- Femoral vein

FIGURE 10-21 Adding medication to an intravenous (IV) plastic bag or glass bottle. Close the IV tubing with a roller clamp. Clean medication port with alcohol swab. Add the medication to the primary port of the bottle or the medication vent on the rubber stopper of the IV bag. Air must be let out of the container to equal that of the medication being injected or the medication will leak back out. Gently rotate container to mix the medication in the solution. Release the roller clamp and start the infusion.

infusion tubing. The portal is cleaned with an alcohol swab, and a syringe containing the medication is inserted through the portal. A short needle is used to avoid accidentally pushing the needle all the way through the tubing. Some institutions may use needle-less IV tubing, allowing a syringe to be attached to a luer lock site without a needle. The plunger on the syringe is drawn back until blood is seen in the tubing above the needle at the skin insertion site. This confirms that the needle is in the vein. The medication is then slowly injected into the IV line, according to the prescribed rate of infusion for that medication. Once all the medication is injected, the needle is withdrawn and the tubing is unclamped. Any blood or fluid is cleaned up, and the rate of infusion is readjusted. Then remove gloves and wash hands.

All gloves, needles, swabs, and equipment must be disposed of according to hospital policy. This may involve putting waste in the patient's waste basket and needles in a sharp's container in the room or taking them to the dirty utility room. Now wash hands again.

Adding Medication to a Plastic Bag or an IV Bottle. Make certain that the medication is compatible with the solution into which it will be injected. The top of the plastic bag or the IV glass bottle has an air portal, a tubing portal, and an injection portal (Figure 10-21). Identify the proper portal and cleanse it with an alcohol wipe. Allow the portal top to air dry. Fill the syringe

with medication and inject the medication slowly with a small needle through the medication portal into the IV container. Some plastic bags or bottles may have a needleless access port; medication may be added by locking the syringe to a luer lock site, and injecting the medication into the bag or bottle without the use of a needle. Slow administration will allow air to escape from the container while the medication is being injected. The nurse should label the bottle or bag with the date, time, dosage, and medications added and sign her initials.

Adding Medication to a Volume Control. Draw up the medication in a syringe. Fill the volume chamber with the specified amount of IV solution and clamp the tubing between the IV bottle or bag and the volume control chamber. Cleanse the medication portal on the volume control chamber with an alcohol wipe and slowly inject the medication into the chamber. Adjust the rate of flow, allowing for infusion of the fluid in the tubing and the volume control chamber within the specified time limit (Figure 10-22). Label the container

Procedure 10-4   Preparing and Administering Intravenous Medications

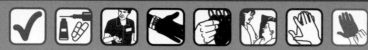

STEP ONE: GETTING READY

1. Check the medication order. Check the accuracy of the order as written and the time to be given. Clarify any information known about the patient or the medication. Complete any calculations needed for dosage, flow rate, and length of infusion.
2. Wash hands. This is essential to avoid contaminating the medication and equipment. Although it seems an obvious step, it is often neglected by busy nurses.
3. Assemble all the medication equipment. In addition to the medication order or card, obtain the medication tray, proper size needles, tubing, tape, intravenous (IV) infusion poles, alcohol swabs, and medication cart. Make certain that the equipment is sterile. The expiration date on the plastic or paper wrapping should indicate when the equipment must be thrown away or sterilized again.

STEP TWO: PREPARING THE MEDICATION

1. Read the order on the medication card or MAR, and obtain the correct medication from the cabinet or cart. Medications may come in an ampule, a vial, a Mix-o-vial, or an infusion set.
2. Compare the medication card or MAR with the label on the container. First check for the right patient, drug, route, dosage, and time of administration.
3. Attach the needle to the syringe, keeping the needle covered with a cap.
4. Ready the medication for withdrawal by opening the ampule, if necessary.
5. Compare the information on the medication card or MAR with the label on the container. This is the second check for accuracy.
6. Insert the needle into the medication container and fill the syringe with the proper amount of medication. (See the text for a discussion of drawing up medications from different dosage forms.) Check the information on the container for the third time with the medication card or MAR. Dilute the medication in the proper volume and type of solution. Always follow the manufacturer's recommendations. Do not mix medications with blood or albumin. Do not administer any solution that is hazy or cloudy or that has a precipitate or any particles in it.

- Once mixed, label the container with the medication, date, time, and initials. IV infusions are generally usable for 24 hours. Any solution not used during that time is promptly returned to the pharmacy.
- Some medications require special precautions such as shading from sunshine or infusion over a certain period.
- Make certain that the infusion is completely infused and that the tubing is cleared before other medication is added.

7. Put the unused medication containers away.
8. If using an IV bottle, remove the metal covering over the IV bottle top. Cleanse the top of the rubber diaphragm on top of the IV bottle or plastic IV bag with an alcohol wipe. Insert the needle with an unused syringe through the rubber diaphragm or medication port into the IV container and withdraw air, creating a vacuum inside the IV container. Now insert the needle with the syringe containing the medication and inject the contents into the IV container through one of the medication ports.
9. Place the syringe and alcohol preps next to the medication card or MAR on the tray. Bring other needed equipment to the bedside.

STEP THREE: INSERTING THE NEEDLE INTO THE VEIN

1. Go to the patient's bedside. Help the patient get into the proper position to receive the infusion. The patient may need to turn over, roll onto one side, or remove her or his gown. Ask the patient her or his name while at the same time checking the patient's identification bracelet and bed tag. Never give medication without positively identifying the patient.
2. Explain what medication is being given and answer any of the patient's questions. Give any special instructions or teach the patient about the medication as indicated. Make any special assessments required. Assess previous sites of injections for signs of necrosis, infection, or swelling. Examine the site to be injected. If the patient makes any comments about the medication being different from usual, having just taken the medication, or not having had that medication before, recheck the medication order.

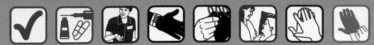

Procedure 10-4   Preparing and Administering Intravenous Medications—cont'd

3. Make sure that patient has no known allergy to adhesive tape. Before performing the venipuncture, tear strips of adhesive tape for anchoring the needle. Open up the infusion set, insert the tubing into the IV container, allow the solution to run into the tubing, and then clamp it shut. Hang the container on the IV pole.

4. Put on gloves. Use correct barrier procedures, as determined by hospital policy, to protect nurses from human immunodeficiency virus infection.

5. Apply a tourniquet 2 to 3 inches above the proposed insertion site. Use a slip knot to allow quick release of the tourniquet.

6. Identify the vein to be used and palpate it with the fingers.

7. Using an alcohol wipe, carefully rub the skin for a few seconds to cleanse. Wipe firmly in a circular pattern, moving inside to outside. Let the skin air dry.

8. Grasp the needle in the dominant hand, stretch the skin with the other hand, and stabilize the vein. With the needle bevel up at an angle less than 45 degrees, insert the needle into the skin approximately ½ inch below the point of entry into the vein. Then decrease the angle to 15 degrees and slowly push the needle into and along the vein. Blood will flow down into the tubing when the needle is in the vein.

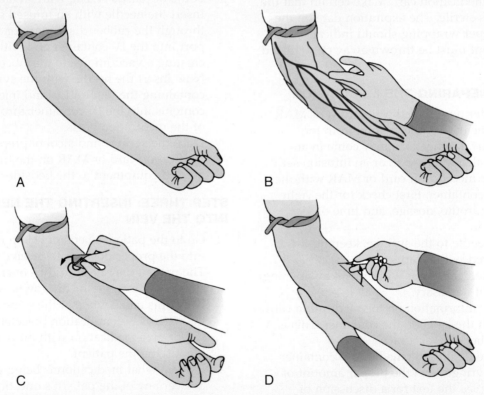

Insertion of needle for venipuncture. **A,** Select site and apply a tourniquet. **B,** Palpate vein to be used for infusion. **C,** Wipe skin with an alcohol swab, moving in a circular pattern. **D,** With the bevel up and the syringe at a 45-degree angle, the needle is inserted through the skin and into the vein. Slowly reduce the angle and thread the needle up into the vein once blood is seen in the syringe. Remove tourniquet and apply adhesive dressing.

9. Connect the tubing to the needle, release the tourniquet, and cleanse the area to remove any blood that may have gotten on the skin or tubing. Remove the gloves.

10. Anchor the tubing with adhesive tape. Mark on the tape the time that the needle was inserted and the nurses initials.

Procedure 10-4   Preparing and Administering Intravenous Medications—cont'd

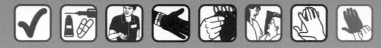

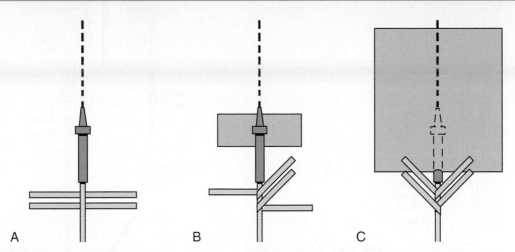

A   B   C

Taping of intravenous tubing after insertion. **A,** Place two small adhesive tape strips under the needle or the catheter with the adhesive side up. **B,** Cross adhesive tapes and fasten them securely to the skin on both sides. **C,** Place a large piece of tape over the tubing and skin to stabilize the needle. Mark the date and time of insertion and your initials or name.

11. Immobilize the arm or hand by taping it to an infusion board.
12. Adjust the rate of infusion. An infusion pump may be used to monitor the flow rate and to alert with an alarm if a problem develops. There are many types of pumps to control infusion rate. The nurse is responsible for checking the equipment's functioning and accuracy.
13. Assist the patient to a comfortable position.

STEP FOUR: CONCLUDING

1. Dispose of the alcohol wipes and gloves according to the hospital procedure. Clean the medication tray or cart and put away the equipment.
2. Note on the medication card or MAR the time the medication was given and sign name or initials.
3. Check the patient again later and note any particular responses or adverse effects that must be recorded and reported. Particularly note any complaints of pain, burning, or stinging at the needle insertion site. Note the infusion rate.

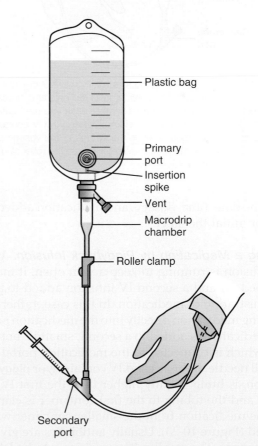

— Plastic bag

— Primary port
— Insertion spike
— Vent
— Macrodrip chamber

— Roller clamp

Secondary port

Adding intravenous (IV) push medication to an IV line. Close the IV tubing with a roller clamp. Insert the syringe with the medication into the secondary port. Inject the medication slowly. Release the IV tubing at the roller clamp and allow the infusion to resume.

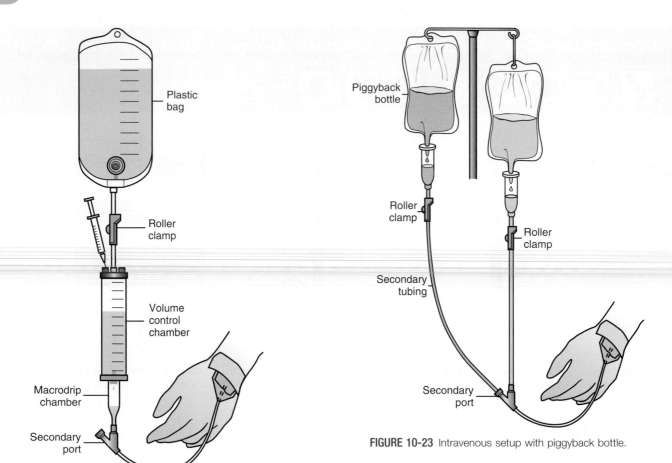

FIGURE 10-22 Adding medication to a volume control chamber. Remove the intravenous (IV) container from the pole and squeeze all the liquid from the volume control chamber back into the container. Close the IV tubing with the roller clamp. Rehang the IV container on the pole. Add the medication in the syringe to the volume control chamber through the medication portal. Reopen the roller clamp and slowly infuse the medication.

FIGURE 10-23 Intravenous setup with piggyback bottle.

with the date, time, dosage, and medication added and sign or initial the label.

Adding a Medication by Piggyback Infusion.
While an infusion is running to keep a vein open, it may be clamped off and a second IV infusion added to allow administration of medication. In this case, rather than injecting medication directly into the medication portal, the medication is added to a second, small IV bottle or bag, which is connected to the medication portal with a small needle. If this second IV container, or **piggyback infusion**, is hung slightly higher than the first IV container and the tubing to the first container is clamped off, the medication from the smaller container will be infused (Figure 10-23). Usually antibiotics are given in this manner. The smaller IV container is to be labeled with the time, date, medication, and dosage, and the nurse's initials. The order will specify the time in which the piggyback infusion should be completed. Once the smaller volume is infused, the setup is removed and the clamp on the original bottle is reopened.

Administration of Medication When There is Only an Intermittent Infusion Device.
When a butterfly or scalp vein needle is inserted and left in place, it also may become a portal for intermittent infusion. These units were formerly called *heparin locks* or *saline locks*, depending on what solution was used to flush them. They are now more often referred to as *intermittent infusion devices*. Some institutions limit LPN/LVNs from administering drugs through these systems. Follow institutional policy. If the LPN/LVN is allowed to give drugs in this manner, wear disposable gloves and use an alcohol wipe to cleanse the top of the rubber diaphragm at the end of the tubing. Pull back the plunger to aspirate blood into the tubing and then slowly inject the medication into the tubing. Follow this by inserting another syringe with 1 to 2 mL of normal saline to flush the medication out of the tubing. Some institutions also use 1 mL of heparin to help keep the tubing open. The nurse must carefully follow the hospital's policy. Clean up any spilled blood or fluid, remove the gloves, and dispose of the equipment properly. Figures 10-24 and 10-25 illustrate the taping of an intermittent infusion device and the addition of medication.

Intravenous Infusion Rates
Because so many factors influence the gravity flow, a solution may not necessarily continue to flow at the rate originally set. Therefore, IV infusions must be

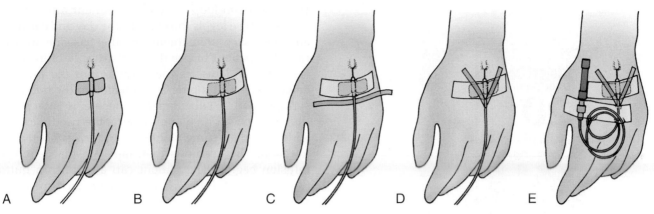

FIGURE 10-24 Taping of a butterfly needle with an intermittent infusion device. **A,** Hold the two plastic wings together and insert the butterfly needle into the vein. **B,** Flatten the plastic wings out and place a strip of adhesive tape over them. **C,** Place another strip of tape just below the wings and under the intravenous (IV) tubing, adhesive side up. **D,** Cross the tape over the wing-tips to anchor the tubing into place. **E,** Coil IV tubing and tape it into place.

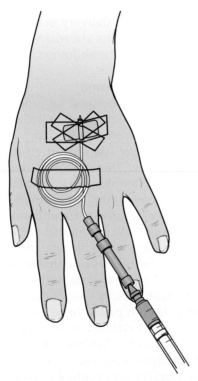

FIGURE 10-25 Adding medications through intermittent infusion device. Cleanse the main adapter plug on the end of the tubing with an alcohol wipe and allow it to air dry. Slowly inject the medication with a syringe. Withdraw the syringe and cleanse the diaphragm again with an alcohol wipe. Using another syringe containing saline, flush the reservoir with 1 to 2 mL of sterile saline. Remove syringe and cleanse diaphragm a final time with an alcohol wipe.

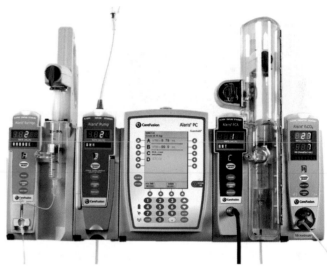

FIGURE 10-26 Example of a large Volume Infusion Pump.

monitored frequently to verify that the fluid is flowing at the intended rate. The IV flask or bag should be marked with tape to indicate the rate so that the nurse can tell at a glance whether the correct amount has been infused. The flow is calculated when the solution is originally hung, and then rechecked at least hourly. To calculate the flow rate, the number of drops delivered per milliliter must be determined. This number varies depending on the equipment used and is usually printed on the solution set packaging. A formula that can be used to calculate the drop rate is as follows:

gtt/mL of given set/60 (min in 1 hr) × total hourly volume = gtt/min

A variety of infusion pumps are available to assist in IV fluid delivery. These devices allow more accurate administration of fluids and medications than is possible with routine gravity-flow setups. Some pumps have flow rates calibrated in terms of milliliters per hour and are referred to as *volumetric pumps* (Figures 10-26 and 10-27). Others are calibrated in drops per minute and are referred to as *infusion controllers*. It is important to read the manufacturer's directions carefully before using any infusion pump or controller

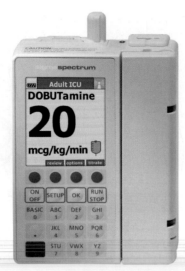

FIGURE 10-27 Example of Spectrum Infusion System.

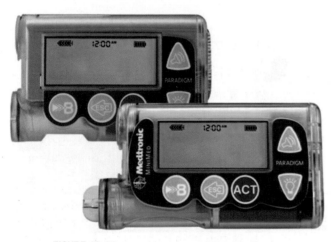

FIGURE 10-28 Example of Minimed Insulin Pump.

because there are many variations in available models. Use of these devices does not eliminate the need for frequent monitoring of the infusion and the patient.

Small pumps weighing approximately half a pound are now available as portable infusion systems for continuous drug treatment of certain patients with type 1 diabetes or cancer. The systems currently in use generally consist of a battery, a programmable electronic "brain," an electric motor and a pump, and a syringe. All of these parts can be removed as a unit from the small needle kept in place in either subcutaneous abdominal or thigh tissue in the diabetic patient or by a Silastic catheter inserted into an artery supplying the malignant tumor in a cancer patient. Some systems are designed to be worn externally over clothing, stored in a pocket, or suspended from a belt or a neck chain (Figure 10-28). Others are implanted within a subcutaneous pocket in the lower abdomen or elsewhere. The starting dosage levels and six other parameters of therapy are programmed initially by the physician.

With this open-loop system, the patient measures the blood glucose levels throughout the day and calculates any necessary adjustments in the baseline infusion rate. The patient places the day's supply of insulin in a syringe and inserts the syringe into the pump. A length of special tubing is connected to the hub of the syringe, and a subcutaneous needle is attached to the distal end. The patient inserts the needle into the abdomen in the same manner used for a subcutaneous injection. The needle is then taped in place, and the infusion begins. The patient can also push a button that releases a bolus dose to cover each meal consumed. The infusion site is changed every 2 days and kept dry to prevent bacterial contamination.

A second type of pump is a closed-loop system, sometimes called an *artificial pancreas*. This unit consists of a device that constantly measures blood glucose levels and sends information to a small computer, which calculates the needed dose of insulin and triggers the batter-powered delivery system. The insulin is then delivered through a subcutaneous needle that is usually implanted in the abdomen.

Additional Delivery Systems

Several other sites may be used for long-term administration of fluids and medication following special placement of catheters by a physician.

The *Hickman catheter* has been used for years as a venous access device. This device is commonly used for obtaining blood samples and to administer medications or hyperalimentation. This catheter and other similar venous access devices are implanted in a large vein such as the cephalic or internal jugular vein. The tip extends into the right atrium, and the end of the catheter exits the vessel through the chest wall. The end of the catheter has an intermittent infusion port attached. The flushing and special care of this tubing are required to keep it patent (open and unblocked).

Using the *epidural route*, a catheter is placed into the spinal column through a lumbar puncture. Anesthesia and narcotic analgesics are often administered by this route during surgery and postoperatively. The procedure for injecting or infusing medication through the epidural catheter follows that used for the IV route. The epidural route requires much lower doses of medication than the IV route; in addition, the effects of the medication last longer.

Percutaneous administration (PCA) and *percutaneous epidural administration (PCEA)* systems are often used in both venous and epidural sites for acute or chronic pain management (Figure 10-29). This method is also often used for short-term treatment of severe pain after surgery. The medication is delivered through an infusion pump using a microdrop infusion set. This pump allows the patient to receive a predetermined IV bolus (a preset quantity of drug injected into a vein at one time) of an analgesic (usually morphine) by using the

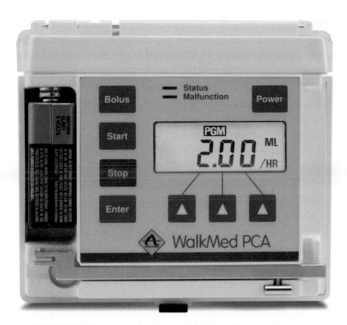

FIGURE 10-29 Example of percutaneous administration pump.

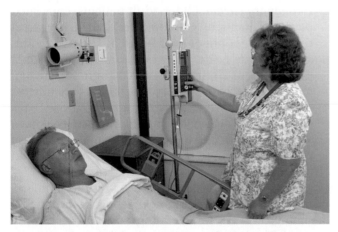

FIGURE 10-30 The nurse sets the pump to deliver an ordered dose, which the patient can administer by pushing buttons on the handheld device at his bedside.

syrige pump mechanism. Another type of device is a patient-controlled analgesia unit. Using this equipment, the patient can control when a dose of pain medication is released. The health care provider orders the dose of medication and how often the patient can receive it. The pump is then set or calibrated to deliver the ordered dose whenever the patient pushes the button (Figure 10-30). The equipment can be locked from 5 to 20 minutes after a dose is given. The lockout mechanism prevents accidental overdose or excessive dosing by the patient. The pump also records the number of times the button is pushed and the total amount of all medication given. The pump may be programmed for continuous administration, patient-activated delivery, or clinician-activated delivery. The pump also records all bolus attempts,

successful and unsuccessful, made by the patient. This helps the provider determine if the patient feels more medicine is needed than what is allowed. These systems are left in place for extended periods, and only need monitoring to ensure that the medication provided does not run out. These systems in hospitalized patients provides a method for nurses to administer medication, allow patients to self-manage their pain based on their perceived need, and avoid use of frequent IM injections.

General Nursing Actions for a Patient with an Intravenous Infusion

A patient receiving an IV infusion is to be checked hourly, and the rate of infusion closely monitored. When an infusion runs behind schedule, the infusion rate should never be increased to "catch up." Too much fluid could overwhelm infants and patients with congestive heart failure, arrhythmias, pulmonary edema, or kidney failure. Intake and output records are closely monitored. The patient should maintain an hourly output of 30 mL of urine or more. Any decrease in this level is promptly reported to the physician.

When one IV infusion has been completed and another is started, the rate is turned down very low to keep the vein open but not stopped. Using aseptic technique, the old infusion container is clamped off, the old container is exchanged for a new container, and the drip chamber is filled halfway before the tubing is unclamped and the rate is recalculated.

If the completed infusion is to be discontinued, explain to the patient what is to happen, then clamp the tubing, loosen the adhesive tape, and put on gloves. Holding a gauze pad in the nondominant hand, apply gentle pressure on the venipuncture site with the pad and carefully withdraw the needle with the dominant hand. The needle should be inspected to make sure it is intact. The area is then cleaned with an alcohol wipe and elevated, if possible, and direct pressure applied to stop any bleeding at the site. Check for bleeding after 1 to 2 minutes. Follow institutional procedure in applying an antibiotic ointment, povidone-iodine (Betadine), or just a clean pressure dressing to the area. Dispose of all contaminated equipment in the authorized way.

In evaluating the patient receiving an infusion, there are six primary areas of concern.

Failure to Infuse Properly. Occasionally, the tubing may become bent or the patient may be lying on the tubing, preventing proper infusion. At other times, the needle may become lodged against the wall of the vein; pulling back slightly on the needle and reanchoring it will start the flow again. Sometimes the rate of infusion is so slow that a small clot may form at the end of the needle, blocking the flow. The IV container might have to be elevated to keep adequate pressure for infusion, or blood pressure cuffs or tight gowns that are restricting fluid flow might have to be removed. Starting at the bottle and moving downward, check every part of the infusion setup for problems. If the IV container is placed below the needle site and the needle is in place and not obstructed, gravity causes blood to run back into the tubing. If blood fails to return to the tubing, suspect that the needle is out of place or blocked.

Infiltration. Another common complication occurs when the needle becomes dislodged from the vein, allowing infusion of medication and fluid into the tissues (infiltration). This produces pain, swelling of the area, and redness. When some kinds of medication accidentally leak into tissue, they can irritate and damage the tissue. Whenever IV infiltration is discovered, the infusion site must be carefully inspected for signs of injury. The infusion is discontinued and the physician contacted, especially if necrosis, sloughing, blistering, or unusual swelling is seen. Warm, moist compresses are then applied to the area. Sometimes other drugs are injected to counteract the medication that accidentally infused into the tissue.

Air in the Tubing. Air that is infused into a patient is potentially dangerous, producing a bubble in the bloodstream. If air is seen in the tubing, the tubing is to be immediately clamped below the air bubble and, using aseptic technique, the air is withdrawn through a syringe and a needle inserted at the piggyback portal, or at the hub of the needle. All air, fluid, and blood in the syringe is then discarded. Small amounts of air probably will not harm the patient. Should a larger amount of air actually enter the patient through the tubing, he should be placed with the head down and turned on the left side, and the physician notified. Give the patient oxygen if he complains of shortness of breath.

Signs of Infection. Redness, swelling, warmth, and burning along the course of the vein are signs of infection or inflammation of the vein (phlebitis) and are often produced or aggravated by irritating medication. They are commonly seen with medications such as potassium, antibiotics, or anticancer drugs, but may occur with any infusion. Stop the IV; the physician should be notified and warm, moist compresses applied to the area.

A contaminated infusion that causes a systemic infection is rare. If the patient suddenly develops chills, fever, nausea, vomiting, and headache, immediately stop the infusion, monitor the patient closely, and contact the health care provider. The solution is saved so that cultures may be taken.

Allergic Reactions. Some products create an allergic response in the patient. Antibiotics often cause shortness of breath, temperature elevation, or rash. Reactions to blood or blood products are also common, producing shaking chills, hematuria, and temperature elevations. Stop the medication infusion and notify the health care provider.

Circulatory Problems. Problems in the systemic circulation are produced primarily in two forms: circulating particles (which can cause pulmonary embolism) or excess fluid volume (which can cause pulmonary edema).

1. *Pulmonary embolism.* When particles of medication or pieces of a blood clot break loose and travel in the patient's bloodstream, they may become trapped in the lungs, causing shortness of breath as blood flow is blocked. Poor color, chest pain, restlessness, and coughing up blood may also be signs of pulmonary emboli. Keep infusion containers and IV lines clean, adequately dissolve medications, and use filters in the IV lines. Embolism or a traveling blood clot is an emergency. Notify the physician promptly if there is a suspicion this has happened.

2. *Pulmonary edema.* Older adult patients, emaciated patients, infants, and children are particularly sensitive to the amount of fluid infused. These individuals may have heart, lung, or kidney problems that decrease their ability to handle extra fluid. Circulatory overload may develop when fluids are infused too rapidly, or when the volume is too great. Signs of circulatory overload include dyspnea; weakness; lethargy; reduced urine output; edema; swelling of the extremities; dependent edema; weak, rapid pulse; and shallow, rapid respirations.

In some individuals, the excess fluid accumulates primarily in the lungs, producing coughing, difficulty breathing, crackles in the lung sounds, and frothy sputum. The infusion is slowed and the physician is notified if these symptoms develop.

Table 10-3 summarizes the problems that may occur with an IV infusion and the appropriate nursing actions to take.

PERCUTANEOUS MEDICATIONS

PERCUTANEOUS ADMINISTRATION

The topical application of medication for absorption through the mucous membranes or skin is called **percutaneous administration.** The medication acts locally to clean, soften, disinfect, or lubricate the skin. Many products are now given through transdermal systems to provide effects throughout the body (systemic effects).

It is difficult to predict how topical medications will be absorbed. They often have a short duration of action and require frequent applications. Some medications must be properly inhaled, spread, or shampooed to be effective. In addition, many of these medications are

Table 10-3   Common Problems with Intravenous Infusions

PROBLEM	NURSING ACTION TO TAKE
Failure to infuse properly	Check for bent tubing, needle against vein wall, or small clot at needle end; the intravenous (IV) pole may be too low, or the needle may be out of the vein. Check for damage done from tissue infusion. Stop infusion and restart it, if required.
IV infiltration	Check to see if any tissue was damaged. Notify physician of any necrosis or sloughing. Apply wet compresses to the area to reduce pain. Stop infusion and restart it, if required.
Air in tubing	Clamp tubing and remove the air with a syringe. If air was infused into the patient, put the patient in the head-down position, lying on the left side, and notify the physician.
Signs of infection	Check for local and systemic symptoms. Stop infusion, restart with a fresh setup, and notify physician. Treat symptomatically. Save the solution for testing.
Allergic reactions	Stop infusion and notify the physician or other health care provider.
Circulatory problems	Watch for symptoms of pulmonary edema: shortness of breath, poor color, weight gain, restlessness, edema. Notify the physician.
Other	Watch for symptoms of pulmonary embolus: poor color, shortness of breath, chest pain, coughing up blood. Notify the physician.

greasy or messy to apply and leave stains on clothing and bedding.

The amount of medication absorbed through the skin or mucous membranes depends on several factors:

- The size of the area covered by medication
- The concentration or strength of the drug
- The length of time the medication stays in contact with the skin

The general condition of the skin itself also makes a difference. Important factors include:

- The amount of skin irritation and breakdown
- The thickness of the skin involved
- The general hydration, nutrition, and tone of the skin

Methods of percutaneous administration include the following:

- Putting solutions onto the mucous membranes of the ear, eye, nose, mouth, or vagina
- Applying topical creams, powders, ointments, or lotions
- Inhaling aerosolized liquids or gases to carry medication to the nasal passages, sinuses, and lungs
- Application of transdermal patches or topical gel systems

PROCEDURE FOR ADMINISTERING PERCUTANEOUS MEDICATIONS

Follow the same general procedures outlined for other routes of administration when applying medications to the skin or mucous membranes. This is a clean procedure. Strictly follow the rules of safety. The general method for giving percutaneous medications is outlined in Procedure 10-5. However, the site of administration and the form of medication may require minor adjustments in the technique the nurse will use for different types of medication.

ADMINISTERING TOPICAL MEDICATIONS

Topical medications are applied directly to the area of skin requiring treatment. The most common forms of topical medications include creams, lotions, and ointments, although there are many others. Each form of topical application has specific advantages and characteristics. Several forms are discussed in Box 10-4.

Technique

1. Choose the administration site carefully. Avoid skin that has been tattooed or that has recent lesions or broken skin.
2. Always clean the skin before applying medication. This practice not only reduces the chance of infection, but also removes any remaining medication from the previous application and prevents the buildup of medication in that area. Water-based and alcohol-based products may be removed with soap and water. Oil-based products may be removed with cottonseed oil and gauze. Coal tar products may be removed with corn oil and gauze.
3. Wear gloves for protection. Many skin lesions (sores) contain infectious material that could be spread to the nurse during the treatment process. Also, many medications may be absorbed through the nurses skin as the nurse applies them unless gloves are worn.
4. Lotions are shaken until they are a uniform color and are applied by dabbing the medication onto the skin with a cotton ball or gauze. Determine through product information if the lotion is supposed to be rubbed into the area.
5. Apply ointments and creams with a tongue depressor or a cotton-tipped applicator. Medication is scooped out or squeezed onto the applicator and then applied to the patient's skin with a firm stroke. If the area is to be covered with a dressing, the

Procedure 10-5   Preparing and Administering Percutaneous Medications

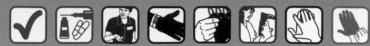

STEP ONE: GETTING READY

1. Check the medication order. Check the accuracy of the order as written and the time to be given. Clarify any information now known about the patient or the medication.
2. Wash hands. This is essential to avoid contaminating the medication. Although it seems an obvious step, it is often neglected by busy nurses.
3. Assemble all the medication equipment. In addition to the medication order or card, obtain the medication tray; medication jars, tubes, or boxes; medication cart; gloves; plastic wrap; and tongue blades.

STEP TWO: PREPARING THE MEDICATION

1. Read the order on the medication card or MAR, and obtain the correct medication from the cabinet or cart. Medications may come in bottles, disks, patches, tubes, drops, sprays, and jars. Medication containers are commonly taken to the bedside for administration.
2. Compare the medication card or MAR with the label on the container. First check for the right patient, drug, route, dosage, and time of administration.
3. Place the medication next to the medication card or MAR on the tray.

STEP THREE: ADMINISTERING THE MEDICATION

1. Go the patient's bedside. Help the patient get into a position appropriate for the medication being given. Ask the patient his or her name while at the same time checking the patient's identification bracelet and bed tag. Never give medication without positively identifying the patient. Confused or very ill patients may answer to any name.

2. Explain what medication is being given and answer any of the patient's questions. Give any special instructions or teach the patient about the medication as indicated. Make any special assessments required. If the patient makes any comments about the medication looking different from usual, having just taken the medication, or not having had that medication before, recheck the medication order.
3. Cleanse the site of previous medication if necessary. Examine for signs of irritation, infection, or swelling.
4. Compare the information on the medication card or MAR with the label on the container. This is the second check for accuracy.
5. Put on gloves.
6. Before beginning administration, check the information on the container for the third time with the medication card or MAR.
7. Follow the specific procedure for applying the solution, powder, ointment, or shampoo. Cover the area with a plastic wrap or a dressing, as ordered, to increase absorption.

STEP FOUR: CONCLUDING

1. Discard all used dressings and gloves in the dirty utility room.
2. Note on the medication card or MAR the time the medication was given and sign name or initials. Record accurately that the medication was given as ordered.
3. Check the patient again later and note any particular responses or adverse effects that must be recorded and reported.

ointment may be applied directly to the gauze with the tongue depressor and then the gauze is applied to the skin. Creams are generally rubbed into the area, whereas ointments are just spread thinly and evenly over the skin. More is not better; this is an error that both patients and nurses commonly make with ointments. Use a measurement system for dosing, when appropriate.

6. Squeeze extra medication from wet dressings so they are not dripping. Follow directions closely. Dressings may be anchored with hypoallergenic tape, or the physician may request wraps, elastic bandages, gauze pads, plastic wrap, or gloves to cover the area. These coverings increase the sticking and absorption of the medication. They may also reduce staining and grease on clothes and

Box 10-4   Common Forms of Topical Medications

ASTRINGENTS

Astringents are alcohol-based medications used for cleaning oily skin, and for cooling and soothing skin. They have a drying effect.

CREAMS

Creams are semisolid emulsions (mixture of two liquids) that contain medication and a water-soluble base. They are rubbed into the skin.

DISKS OR PATCHES

A disk or a transdermal patch is a semipermeable membrane pad containing medication that is attached to the skin by its adhesive edges. The placement of the pad and length of time it is left in place are ordered by the physician. Medications may be left in place for 24 hours, providing gradual release of medication into the skin. Some estrogen products may be left on for several days. Nitroglycerin patches are often removed during the night to reduce the amount of tolerance the patient develops to the medication. The dosage the patient gets depends on the concentration of the medication and the area of skin covered.

LOTIONS

Lotions are aqueous (watery) preparations that contain suspended materials. They cleanse or soothe the skin, or act as a drawing agent or astringent. Lotions are to be shaken thoroughly and applied sparingly by patting on the skin, not rubbing.

OINTMENTS

Ointments are semisolid preparations of medicines in an oily base, such as petrolatum or lanolin. Ointments provide good skin contact and are not easily removed. They are used sparingly, sometimes according to an application guide, and are often covered with dressings.

POWDERS

Powders are finely ground medication particles in a talc base. They are used for their drying, cooling, or protective effects.

SHAMPOOS

Shampoos are medications in an aqueous or alcohol base that are poured onto the hair, allowed to stand, and then rubbed into the hair and scalp before being rinsed off. They are designed to treat problems of the hair and scalp.

SOAPS

Medicated soaps may be used to cleanse the skin and to moisten dry skin. Some soaps also leave a residue that helps reduce bacteria and oil.

SOLUTIONS

Medicated solutions of chemicals mixed with water or normal saline are used as washes or baths, or are applied to wet dressings for wrapping the skin. Chemicals commonly used include boric acid, Burrow's solution, potassium permanganate, and silver nitrate. The mixing directions must be closely followed. Many of these solutions stain the skin and clothing.

---

bedding but may limit the patient's ability to move.

7. Many patients with skin lesions worry about their appearance. The treatment process and dressings also may draw attention to areas about which the patient feels embarrassed. These patients need to be cared for in private and given a chance to talk about their feelings about the problem and treatment. Take every chance to help the patient develop good self-esteem.

8. Many treatments for skin problems are continued after the patient leaves the hospital. Teach the patient how to apply the medication and the dressings. If possible, have the patient apply the medication and any dressings while the nurse watches.

Technique for Nitroglycerin Ointment

Medicated ointment is an increasingly common method of giving nitroglycerin to patients with chest pain from angina. When properly applied, nitroglycerin ointment (Nitrol or Nitro-Bid) can provide constant medication to help prevent anginal attacks.

To apply nitroglycerin ointment, select a site on the chest, upper arm, or flank areas. Use an area without hair. Adhesive tape applied to the skin and removed quickly will help remove small hairs. Do not shave the skin because this may cause skin irritation when medication is applied. Clean the skin gently with an alcohol wipe. The physician or health care provider will order the patient to apply a certain number of inches of nitroglycerin ointment. A measuring applicator paper that looks like a ruler is provided with the medication (Figure 10-31). The correct number of inches of medication is squeezed onto the applicator paper as a small ribbon. The applicator paper is then laid on top of the skin where the medication is to be applied. There are several ways to proceed:

1. The applicator paper is laid on the skin, ointment side down, and left in place. The area is not rubbed.

2. The applicator paper may be covered with plastic wrap that is taped in place to prevent stains on clothing. It must be changed every 3 to 6 hours, depending upon the prescriber's order.

3. The applicator paper is removed, and the area is covered with plastic wrap, spreading the nitroglycerin over a larger area.

Transdermal Delivery Systems

Disks or transdermal patches are another method of giving constant medication through the skin. Some medications using a transdermal delivery system include fentanyl, nitroglycerin, birth control pills, scopolamine, testosterone, and clonidine. Various antismoking programs also use nicotine patches. The

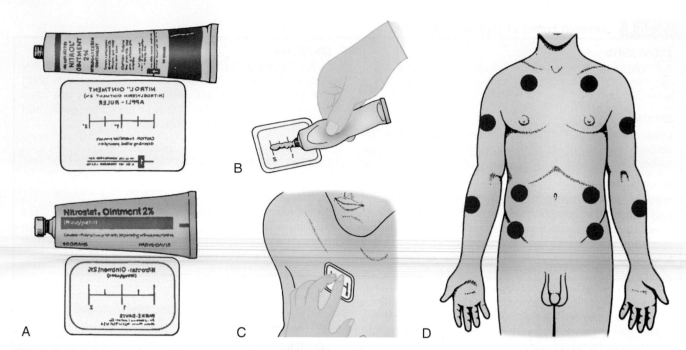

FIGURE 10-31 A, Nitroglycerin ointment and special application papers. Note that the papers are printed backward. **B,** The correct amount of ointment is squeezed onto the paper. **C,** The paper is applied to the patient's skin in one of the sites shown in **D.** Clear plastic wrap may be applied over the paper to increase absorption and protect clothing from staining.

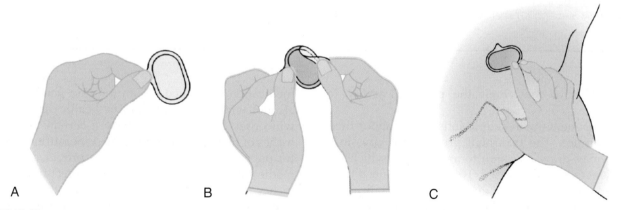

FIGURE 10-32 A, Nitroglycerin patch. **B,** Remove the plastic backing, being careful not to touch the medication inside. **C,** Place the side with medication on the patient's skin and press the adhesive edges into place.

principles for administration are similar to those for applying nitroglycerin ointment.

The medication comes packed over a semipermeable membrane and an adhesive patch. A site is chosen for application according to a standard rotation pattern. The patch is carefully picked up, and the clear plastic backing is removed from the patch, showing the medication (Figure 10-32). The medicated side is then pressed firmly onto the skin. The outer edge of the patch is adhesive and will hold the patch tightly to the skin. Patches are changed on a regular schedule, as indicated by the product, unless they become loose or come off and require replacement. Transderm-Nitro, Fentanyl patches, Nitro-Dur, and birth control patches may be worn while showering; all other medicated patches are to be applied after bathing.

ADMINISTERING MEDICATIONS TO MUCOUS MEMBRANES

The mucous membranes are the other major route of percutaneous medication administration. In general, medication is easily absorbed across mucous membranes and it is easy to reach therapeutic dosages. However, all mucous membranes do not have the same sensitivity to medication or the same ability to absorb chemicals. The blood supply under the mucous membranes also varies. These differences may be used to good advantage. For example, putting medication in an oily base will slow its absorption and might help when administering antibiotics, whereas a water-based medication would be quickly absorbed and its action would stop rapidly.

There are seven places where medications are commonly applied to mucous membranes: under the tongue (**sublingual administration**); against the cheek (**buccal administration**); in the eye, nose, or ear; or inhaled into the lung through an aerosol. Vaginal suppositories, creams, or douches also represent treatment through mucosal membranes. The medications for mucous membranes might come as tablets, drops, ointments, creams, suppositories, or metered-dose inhalers.

The procedure for applying medications to mucous membranes follows the general format already discussed. Different mucous membranes require minor changes in technique, which are listed in Procedure 10-6.

Additional Guidelines

1. All medications applied to mucous membranes must be administered aseptically or by clean technique. The nurse must wash his or her hands before preparing medications. Gloves are used to protect the nurse from infections. Standard Precautions recommended by the CDC are to be followed each time a medication is administered. Eye drops and eardrops must be instilled carefully to prevent contamination of the droppers or the spread of the infection from one eye or ear to the other. Patients must be carefully instructed if using inhalers or respiratory nebulizers so that the medication goes down into the lungs and not in the back of the nose or throat. Equipment and dressings used during medication administration must be disposed of properly.

2. Accurate recording of medication administration is made as soon as the medication is given. Medications involving site rotation are also carefully recorded. When medications are given for angina, the nurse must return within a few minutes to assess the patient's response to the medication. Additional medication may be required, or the physician may need to be called.

3. Giving medications is an excellent teaching opportunity. Take advantage of this chance to teach each time medication is given and teach the patient about the medication's actions, the important points to follow in giving the medication, and problems to report. When the medication is to be taken at home, the patient should start giving himself or herself the medicine under the nurses supervision as soon as possible. This will provide additional chances for the nurse to assess the patient's learning needs and to answer questions.

Procedure 10-6 Administering Medications to Mucous Membranes

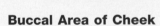
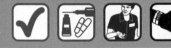

Buccal Area of Cheek

The patient holds the medication between the cheek and molar teeth (A), where it is rapidly absorbed into the bloodstream and reaches the systemic circulation without being metabolized by the liver. This site is used for nitroglycerin tablets to relieve chest pain.

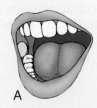

A

Ear

Localized infection or inflammation of the ear is treated by dropping a small amount of a sterile medicated solution into the ear. Very low dosages of medication are required, and the medication label must indicate that it is for otic (ear) usage. Have the medication at room temperature. The patient lies on the side with the affected ear up. Shake the medication well and draw the medication up into the dropper. In children younger than 3 years, gently pull the earlobe down and back (B); in adults, gently pull the earlobe up and out (C). This will straighten the external canal so that the medication may be dropped into the canal. Do not touch the dropper to the ear. The patient is to remain in the same position for 5 minutes to allow the medication to coat the surface of the inner canal. A cotton ball may also be inserted, if ordered. Repeat in the other ear if indicated.

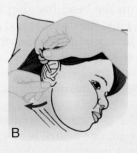
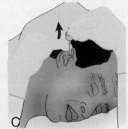

B   C

Procedure 10-6   Administering Medications to Mucous Membranes—cont'd

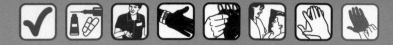

Eye

Sterile drops or ointments in very low dosage and specifically labeled for ophthalmic (eye) use may be applied to the eye. Gloves are used during the procedure. The eye may be cleaned with normal saline and cotton balls to remove exudate (discharge) or previous medication. Wipe from the nasal side out. Have the medication at room temperature. Infants may need to be restrained. Have the patient look up, and pull out the lower lid to show the conjunctival sac (D). Never touch the eye with the dropper or the ointment tip. Drop the medication or squeeze the ointment into the conjunctival sac, not onto the eye itself. Using a cotton ball, apply gentle pressure to the inner corner of the eyelid on the bone for 1 to 2 minutes to ensure adequate concentration of medication and prevent medication from draining rapidly into the nose (E). Instruct the patient to move their eyes around with eyelids closed to spread the ointment over the surface of the eye. Sterile dressings may be ordered to cover the eye at conclusion of treatment.

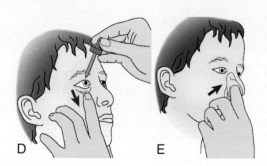

D   E

Nose

Nasal solutions act locally to treat minor congestion or infection. To instill nasal drops, draw the medication into the dropper (F). Have the patient gently blow the nose and then lie down with the head hanging back over the side of the bed (G). Hold the dropper just over one nostril, taking care not to touch the dropper to the skin, and administer the required number of nose drops. Have the patient turn the head slightly. The procedure is repeated for the other nostril. Infants may need to be restrained.

If a nasal spray or inhaler is used, the solution is shaken, the patient sits upright, one nostril is blocked, and the tip of the nasal spray is inserted into the nostril

(H). As the patient takes a deep breath, squeeze a puff of spray into the nostril (I). Wipe tip of spray bottle if medication is to be sprayed into both nostrils. Less medication is required with the spray, and the medication is rapidly absorbed into the vascular areas of the nose for prompt action.

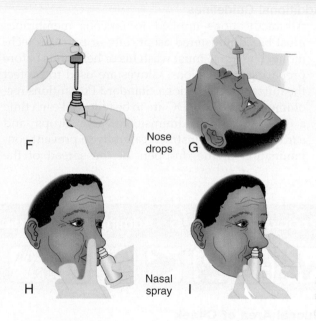

F   Nose
             drops   G

H   Nasal
             spray   I

Respiratory Mucosa

Medication may be carried through the mouth or nose and down into the respiratory tract through use of aerosol nebulizers, or metered-dose inhalers. These techniques require special equipment that must be kept very clean, and that breaks the medication up into very small particles, which can be carried with air down into the lungs where the desired action takes place.

Aerosols

Aerosols use a special nebulizer mouthpiece, and medications are diluted according to a special concentration. Oxygen is used to deliver the medication. The patient sits upright, places the nebulizer mouthpiece loosely in the mouth, and breathes in and out slowly and deeply while the oxygen is directed through the nebulizer until the medication is gone. The equipment must be cleaned after it is used.

Procedure 10-6 Administering Medications to Mucous Membranes—cont'd

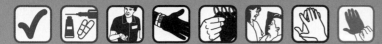

Metered-Dose Inhalers

Metered-dose inhalers are used to deliver specific amounts of corticosteroids or bronchodilators to nasal or lung tissue. These small canisters are pressurized with gas, which propels the medication out and breaks it up into small particles that can be carried deep down into the lungs as the patient takes a deep breath. The medication is carried directly to the site of action with very little systemic effect. The onset of action is rapid. Some medications are designed to be administered through the mouth, and others through the nose. It is important to read the directions completely. Shake the medication before use. If a patient can stand, he or she then leans slightly forward so his or her feet are visible. If a patient must sit upright, have the patient hold the nebulizer in the hand 1 to 2 inches in front of the mouth or at the opening of the nose *(J)*. If the patient cannot cooperate, he or she may place his lips around the mouthpiece. Have the patient exhale, then squeeze the canister in its holder as the next inspiration begins. This will carry medication down into the lungs. Have the patient hold her or his breath as long as possible before exhaling to allow the medication to settle before administering in the other nostril or taking another puff. It is important to time the squeezing of the nebulizer to ensure that medication travels in with the next breath and is not just squirted on the back of the throat or nose. The nebulizer must be cleaned with water after each use. It is important that the patient keep an adequate supply of medication on hand. Check a metered-dose canister for medication by placing it in a glass of water. *K*, Canister is full. *L*, Canister is partially filled. *M*, Canister is nearly empty.

Sublingual Mucosa

The patient places the tablet under the tongue *(N)*, where it dissolves, is rapidly absorbed through the blood vessels, and enters the systemic circulation. This site is used for nitroglycerin tablets to relieve chest pain.

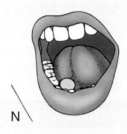

Vagina

Medication to treat local infections or irritation may be applied vaginally through creams, jellies, tablets, foams, suppositories, or irrigations (douches). Room-temperature suppositories are inserted into the vagina with a gloved hand, much like a rectal suppository is inserted. Creams, jellies, tablets, and foams are inserted with a special applicator that comes with the medication. With the patient lying down, the filled vaginal applicator is inserted as far into the vaginal canal as possible and the plunger is pushed, depositing the medication *(O)*. The patient is instructed to remain lying down for 10 to 15 minutes so all the medication can melt and coat the vaginal walls. The patient may need a perineal pad to catch any drainage or prevent staining. Gloves must be carefully discarded according to hospital regulations.

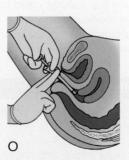

Some medicated solutions are used to wash the internal vaginal area when infection and irritation are present. These solutions are administered as douches. The patient may be on a bedpan or reclining in a bathtub. A douche bag containing a medicated solution is hung from an IV pole or shower head so that it is placed approximately 12 inches above the patient's

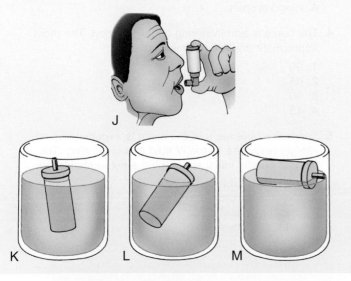

Procedure 10-6   Administering Medications to Mucous Membranes—cont'd

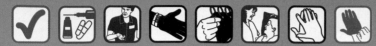

hips. The tubing is clamped shut. The vulva is gently washed by slowly unclamping the tubing, and then the douche nozzle is inserted into the vaginal canal 3 to 4 inches and pointed downward toward the patient's tail bone (coccyx). The labia are held shut while the solution is gently introduced. As much solution as possible is allowed to fill the vaginal canal

before the labia are opened and the solution flows out. Rotate the nozzle gently to allow the solution to reach and wash all areas. When all the solution has been used, the nozzle is withdrawn, all the equipment is cleaned and put away, and the gloves are discarded.

Get Ready for the NCLEX® Examination!

Key Points

- The first section of the chapter has focused on the nursing procedure in the administration of enteral medications.
- Specific steps have been outlined for giving medications orally, by NG tube, and rectally.
- Specific precautions have also been presented for administering medications by the different routes.
- The second section has stressed the procedures involved in administering parenteral medications, including the equipment, anatomic sites, and aseptic technique involved.
- The nurse should follow the standard agency procedure to ensure safe administration of parenteral medications and to protect staff from personal risk of infection.
- Percutaneous medication requires putting medication on the skin or the mucous membranes through a variety of procedures and preparations.
- The basic techniques in percutaneous administration do not usually require the accuracy and precision of parenteral or oral medications.
- The nurse's responsibility in medication administration remains significant.

Additional Learning Resources

SG Go to your Study Guide for additional learning activities to help you master this chapter content.

evolve Go to your Evolve website (http://evolve.elsevier.com/Edmunds/LPN/) for additional online resources.

Review Questions for the NCLEX ® Examination

1. The patient who would be the best candidate to receive medication by IM injection would be:

   1. the patient who has no difficulty swallowing capsules

2. the patient who is experiencing an episode of prolonged weakness
3. the patient who is in a life-threatening Code Blue situation
4. the patient who is experiencing vomiting after surgery

2. The patient has an order to receive packed red blood cells. The most appropriate needle gauge for the nurse to choose is:

   1. 25
   2. 23
   3. 21
   4. 19

3. The nurse has just administered an intradermal injection. The nurse should inspect the injection site afterward for evidence of a(n):

   1. blister
   2. bleb
   3. bruise
   4. blood droplet

4. The nurse is administering an IM injection. The most appropriate angle for administration is:

   1. 90
   2. 45
   3. 30
   4. 15

5. The nurse believes that the client is experiencing an allergic response to the IV fluid that is infusing. The highest priority initial action by the nurse should be:

   1. clamp the tubing
   2. stop the infusion
   3. monitor patient closely
   4. notify the physician

Get Ready for the NCLEX® Examination!—cont'd

Critical Thinking Questions

1. With a partner, use a jar of vitamins or aspirins or a small bottle of juice, a small paper cup, and a note card with the drug order to practice pouring and administering tablets and liquids. Prepare to demonstrate each step as your partner explains, and vice versa, to the rest of the class. As you practice, keep in mind all the steps laid out in the procedure descriptions in the text—it is not as easy as it sounds to remember everything and to do it all in the right order as well!

2. Test yourself on the administration of rectal medications by sectioning a sheet of paper off into four blocks. Label these blocks as follows: "Getting Ready," "Preparing the Medication," "Administering the Medication," and "Concluding the Process." Now fill in as many steps within each phase of administration as you can remember. Without checking your work against the book, exchange lists with a partner and fill in steps you know of that have been left out. Now answer these two questions:
   a. Did your partner's list include anything that you left out of yours? What?
   b. Did your partner add anything to your list that you had not thought of? Now check your own work against the text. How many steps in this apparently "simple" procedure did you leave out altogether?

3. Write these three headings across the top of a sheet of paper: "Dose Form," "Description," and "Indications." Now put the oral dose forms listed below in column 1, skipping at least three spaces between each.

buccal forms	elixirs	emulsions
capsules	lozenges	pills
suspensions	syrups	tablets

Now tell the difference between these forms by completing your table. How are they different not only in form, but also in indications?

4. Describe techniques and considerations unique to PEG medication administration.

5. You have just entered the medication room where Todd, another nurse, has just finished pouring capsules for Mr. Johnson, when he is called away in an emergency. As he rushes past you, he calls back, asking you to please give Mr. Johnson his medication. He points to the cup as he slips out the door. What should you do?

6. You have been responsible for Mrs. Davis's care for 2 days now, counting today. When you enter her room with her medication, she seems groggy and confused; she probably just woke up, you think. You greet her, set down the medication, but then discover that she no longer has on her identification band. However, it is time for her medication, you know her well, she answers to her name, and you do not want to delay her medication. Under these circumstances, can you administer her medication and then find out what happened to her identification band?

7. Describe Standard Precautions for preventing the transmission of HIV.

8. What is the purpose of the Z-track injection technique? Describe how it is given. Can this method be used for any IM injection?

9. Point out the differences in site, absorption, and technique between each of the following parenteral routes: intradermal, subcutaneous, IM, and IV.

10. How do you get rid of bubbles in a filled syringe? Why should you bother?

11. List as many forms of percutaneous medications as you can. Now check your work in the text; add whatever you left out. Identify unique steps in the administration of each.

12. Your patient is due to receive an oral antiemetic around the clock to control his nausea and vomiting. As you enter his room to administer his next dose, you observe him beginning to vomit. You know his medication is available as a rectal suppository. Should you administer the medication as a suppository?

Allergy and Respiratory Medications

Objectives

1. Identify major antihistamines used to treat breathing problems caused by allergies.
2. Describe the action of antitussive medications.
3. List medications used to treat and prevent asthma attacks.
4. Describe the major actions and adverse reactions of the two main categories of bronchodilators.

5. Identify at least six medications commonly used as decongestants.
6. Describe the mechanism of action for expectorants.
7. List the major contraindications to the use of nasal steroids.

Key Terms

antihistamines (ăn-tĭ-HĬS-tă-mēnz, p. 138)
antitussives (ăn-tĭ-TŬS-ĭvz, p. 142)
bronchodilators (brŏn-kō-DĪ-lă-tŏrz, p. 145)
bronchospasm (BRŎN-kō-spăzm, p. 144)
contraindications (kōn-tră-ĭn-dĭ-KĀ-shŭns, p. 139)
expectorants (ĕk-SPĔK-tŏr-ănts, p. 155)
histamine (HĬS-tă-mēn, p. 138)
leukotriene receptor inhibitors (lū-kō-TRĬ-ēn, p. 150)
ototoxic (ŏ-tō-TŎK-sĭk, p. 139)
perennial allergic rhinitis (PAR) (ă-LĔR-jĭk rī-NĪ-tĭs, p. 138)

perennial nonallergic rhinitis (PNAR) (NŎN-ă-lĕr-jĭk, p. 138)
precautions (prē-CĂW-shuns, p. 139)
prophylaxis (prŏ-fĭl-ĂK-sĭs, p. 144)
rebound effect (p. 140)
rebound vasodilation (vă-sō-dĭ-LĀ-shŭn, p. 152)
refractoriness (rē-FRĂK-tŏ-rĭ-nĕs, p. 147)
seasonal allergic rhinitis (SAR) (ă-LŪR-jĭk, p. 138)
sympathomimetics (SĬM-păth-ō-mĭ-MĔT-ĭks, p. 145)
wheezing (p. 144)
xanthines (ZĂN-thēnz, p. 145)

OVERVIEW

This chapter looks at medications that affect the respiratory system. The first section, Antihistamines, describes medications used to treat breathing problems caused by allergies. The second section discusses antitussives, or medications used to control coughing. The third section describes the several different categories of medications used for the prophylaxis (prevention) and treatment of asthma and chronic obstructive pulmonary disease (COPD). The fourth and fifth sections cover decongestants and expectorants. The final section discusses nasal steroids used to treat respiratory problems.

RESPIRATORY SYSTEM

The respiratory system is made up of the lungs and the respiratory passages (Figure 11-1). The upper respiratory system—the oral and nasal cavity, sinuses, pharynx, larynx, and trachea—provides the passages for air to move into the bronchi and lungs (the lower

respiratory system). The lungs are divided into lobes. The respiratory system acts to exchange gases (oxygen and carbon dioxide) between the blood and the air and regulates blood pH.

When you take a deep breath (inspiration), the diaphragm drops down; at the same time, the intercostal muscles contract, raising the ribs, increasing the size of the chest, and creating a negative pressure. The negative pressure causes air to rush into the lungs through the respiratory passages. When you breathe out (exhalation), the muscles relax, the pressure increases in the chest, and air is passively forced out of the lungs. Thus, the chest *works* when breathing in and *rests* when breathing out.

Any part of the respiratory passages or structures and the lungs themselves may be abnormal. Common problems requiring medication are strictures (narrowed openings) or obstructions (blockage) caused by infection or mucus, collapse of the bronchioles caused by asthma, or infectious masses or tumors. The upper airways are often the site of allergic reactions and bacterial and viral infections.

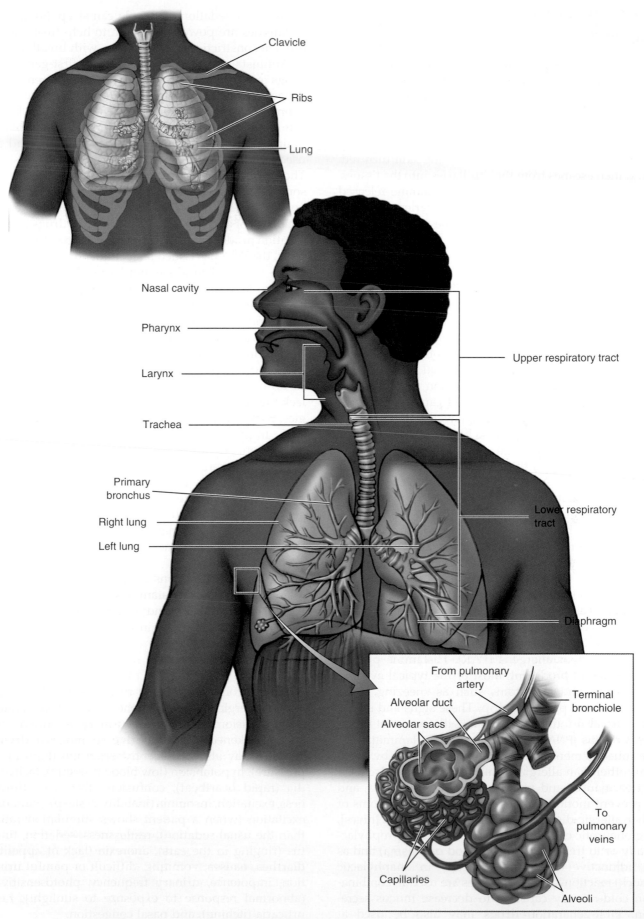

FIGURE 11-1 Organs of the respiratory system: upper respiratory tract and lower respiratory tract.

ANTIHISTAMINES

OVERVIEW

Histamine is a chemical the body produces that causes the inflammatory response. Mast cells found near capillaries and white blood cell basophils contain large amounts of histamine. When the body is injured, histamine is released, and it causes the smooth muscle and vascular system to increase blood flow by opening up the capillaries. This also makes the skin turn red. Fluid then escapes from the capillaries into the tissues, causing swelling. The amount of histamine released after an injury or an allergic reaction varies. **Antihistamines** relieve the effects of histamine on body organs and structures.

ACTION

There are two types of antihistamines. Histamine H_1-receptor antagonists do not prevent the release of histamine, but rather compete with free histamine for binding at H_1-receptor sites on the "effector structures" (e.g., vascular and nonvascular smooth muscles, salivary glands, and respiratory mucosal glands). This blocking action limits the vasodilation (opening) and bronchoconstriction, and increased capillary permeability and reduces the edema (swelling) caused by histamine. Antihistamines also limit the release of acetylcholine, producing an anticholinergic (drying) effect, particularly in the bronchioles and gastrointestinal (GI) system. Antihistamines also have a sedative effect on the central nervous system (CNS). Histamine H_2 antagonists compete with histamine at the H_2 receptor sites also, but only at the H_2 receptors located in the GI tract and so will be discussed later in the text.

USES

Antihistamine H_1 receptor antagonists are used to treat **seasonal allergic rhinitis (SAR)** and **perennial allergic rhinitis (PAR)**. Allergic rhinitis is a condition in which the patient has a reaction to either outdoor allergens (SAR) or indoor allergens (PAR). Histamine plays a central role in producing most of the typical eye and nasal signs and symptoms such as sneezing, nasal stuffiness, and postnasal drip. These signs and symptoms are also found in patients with **perennial nonallergic rhinitis (PNAR)**, which involves inflammation of the mucous membranes of the nose caused by problems other than allergies. Antihistamines are also used to treat nausea and vomiting, vertigo, insomnia, and to prevent motion sickness, and relieve symptoms of other allergic disorders (particularly urticaria [hives], angioneurotic edema, serum sickness, and prophylactically or to treat reactions to blood or plasma) and as an adjunctive (additional) therapy in anaphylactic (shock) reactions. Antihistamines are used in combination cold-remedy capsules to decrease mucus secretion. First-generation drugs may also be used at bedtime for sedation so people can sleep. Some antihistamines are powerful enough to help treat allergic bronchoconstriction that interferes with breathing.

Antihistamines are classed as either first-generation drugs or second-generation drugs. First-generation drugs are usually those products available over-the-counter (OTC) that patients use before they see a health care provider. Most of these products cross the blood-brain barrier and cause sedation (sleepiness) and are used in particular for helping older adult patients sleep. These products are very effective in helping remove some symptoms of sneezing, itching, and watery rhinorrhea when used for a short time. Because of the high incidence of overdosage of some of these drugs in combination products in children's cough and cold medications, the FDA has issued a recommendation that OTC cough and cold products not be used in infants and children less than 2 years old. Some products should not be used in children younger than 6 years.

Second-generation antihistamines are newer, more effective, and usually have a more rapid onset of relief of sneezing, pruritus (itching), and watery rhinorrhea. These drugs do not cross the blood-brain barrier and so do not cause significant sedation. These products lack the antimetic effect so their use is limited to allergies. Some are available only by prescription and some OTC. In general, they are less effective against nasal congestion. As newer drugs, they may also be more expensive. Several second generation drugs have been removed from the market because they cause lethal arrhythmias of the heart.

It is important to understand what symptoms the patient is having so that the correct medicine can be taken. This is sometimes a challenge the way OTC products are marketed.

These two generations are further divided into six main groups of antihistamines, depending on their various characteristics and actions. These groups and some specific drugs within each group are listed in Box 11-1.

ADVERSE REACTIONS

The most common adverse reactions are due to the anticholinergic activity of the drugs: constipation, blurred vision, dry mouth, urinary retention, and dried thickened secretions due to mucosal drying. Patients may also develop hypertension (high blood pressure), hypotension (low blood pressure), tachycardia (rapid heartbeat), confusion, dizziness, drowsiness, excitation, insomnia (inability to sleep), paradoxic excitation (when a patient shows stimulation rather than the usual sedation), restlessness, sedation, tinnitus (ringing in the ears), anorexia (lack of appetite), diarrhea, nausea, vomiting, difficult or painful urination, impotence, urinary frequency, photosensitivity (abnormal response to exposure to sunlight), rash, urticaria (itching), and nasal congestion.

| Box 11-1 | Major Antihistamine Groups |

FIRST GENERATION DRUGS

Alkylamines
brompheniramine
chlorpheniramine
dexchlorpheniramine

Ethanolamines
carbinoxamine
clemastine
diphenhydramine

Ethylenediamine
tripelennamine

Phenothiazine
promethazine

Piperazine
hydroxyzine

SECOND-GENERATION DRUGS

Piperidines
azatadine
cetirizine
cyproheptadine
fexofenadine
loratadine
phenindamine

Antihistamine overdosage is potentially fatal, particularly in children. Any of these products should be used with caution in children and care taken to follow recommended dosages. The symptoms of overdosage occur when the CNS is being stimulated and depressed at the same time.

DRUG DOSAGES

The dosage and delivery system for these medications should be determined based on the weight of the patient, the presence of other medical conditions, and the product. The dose will be carefully determined, based on many factors. Consult a drug handbook for common dosage recommendations.

DRUG INTERACTIONS

The sedative effect commonly seen with antihistamines is increased when other CNS depressants (such as hypnotics, sedatives, tranquilizers, depressant analgesics, and alcohol) are used along with the antihistamine. The sedative effect of antihistamines also adds to the effect of anticholinergic drugs, and they can strengthen the anticholinergic side effects of monoamine oxidase (MAO) inhibitors, as well as tricyclic antidepressants. When antihistamines are used along with ototoxic drugs (drugs that may damage hearing, such as large doses of aspirin or other salicylates, or streptomycin), the ototoxic effects on the ear may be masked. Antihistamines can decrease the effect of corticosteroids and many hormones. They may also interfere with the effects of anticholinesterase drugs.

❖NURSING IMPLICATIONS AND PATIENT TEACHING

■ Assessment

Learn as much as possible about the health history of the patient, including the presence of drug allergy, other drug use, and the presence of asthma, glaucoma, peptic ulcer, prostatic hypertrophy, bladder neck obstruction, respiratory or cardiac disease, and the possibility of pregnancy. Assess the patients work and activities to see if drowsiness might be a problem. A patient with thyroid disease or migraine headaches may be unable to take antihistamines because of the tachycardia (rapid heartbeat) produced. These conditions are either contraindications (factors that rule out the use of a drug) or precautions (factors that indicate a drug should be used with great care) for the use of antihistamines.

As you listen to the patient describe respiratory symptoms, think about whether the problem might be SAR, PAR, or PNAR. The patient may have a history of allergic reactions with allergic nasal congestion (usually seasonal in onset), runny nose, or cough related to a cold or allergy. You may observe symptoms of rhinitis: sneezing, nasal discharge, and inflamed nasal mucosa. The patient may also have edema, dermatographism (wheals, or a raised surface of the skin where it has been scratched), conjunctivitis (inflammation of the inner eyelid and eye), eczema (a chronic condition producing irritation of the skin), insect bites, or contact dermatitis. The nasal mucosa may be swollen, boggy (soft), and pale, and there may be nasal plugging or a clear, watery discharge. Increased sinus pressure may be found when pushing on or palpating the frontal or maxillary sinuses.

These drugs are so common that it is important to learn the drug effects of antihistamine use. In young children, antihistamines may cause hallucinations, convulsions, and even death. Older adult patients are also extremely sensitive to these drugs. Some products may cause teratogenic effects (deformities) in a fetus, although most first and second generation drugs are Category B drugs with a few Category C drugs. Antihistamines should be used with caution in children with a family history of sleep apnea or sudden infant death syndrome (SIDS), or in children with symptoms of Reye syndrome.

■ Diagnosis

Through reading the patient's chart, you will learn why the patient is taking this drug: they may have SAR, PAR, or PNAR, or whether the medication is being given for some other type of allergic reaction. The severity of the symptoms will help in making the nursing diagnosis and deciding what additional nursing actions need to be taken (for example, hydration of the patient [giving additional fluid]).

■ Planning

The sedative effect is common to most first generation antihistamines like diphenhydramine (Benadryl), less so with loratadine (Claritin) which is a second-generation antihistamine. The drowsiness caused by antihistamines makes it dangerous for the person taking them to operate heavy machinery or drive.

Some antihistamines may be given parenterally to treat hypersensitivity to blood products, as adjunctive therapy to analgesia, or in treating motion sickness. Most antihistamines are administered orally. Many are available in OTC preparations, although the forms with the highest dosage are available only by prescription. Most drug companies have at least one preparation available by prescription, so that people with Medicare or Medicaid benefits are able to get these drugs with their cards. Antihistamines may be administered rectally, or topically via nasal inhalation or ophthalmic solutions also.

Products that are used when a patient is hospitalized for severe respiratory difficulty are often administered by inhalation therapy by a respiratory therapist—an individual especially trained to use respiratory equipment and to assist the patient to get the most air into and out of their lungs. Watching and working with these respiratory therapists can help nurses increase their own skills to help patients breathe better.

■ Implementation

Antihistamines should be taken only when needed. The type and dosage should be chosen for the desired effect and the person being treated. For example, one of the first-generation ethanolamine derivatives makes people very sleepy, and people who do tasks that require alertness probably should not use them. Sometimes a patient is having trouble sleeping and so the doctor may want to give them a drug that will make them drowsy so they might give them a drug from the ethanolamine category. Some drugs cause less drowsiness but may not be as effective in getting rid of the symptoms.

If tolerance (increased resistance to a drug caused by repeated use) to one type of antihistamine develops, the patient might be told to switch to another type to see if it is more helpful. Medications also might be changed or rotated to keep symptoms under control.

Giving oral doses with meals or milk can limit GI side effects however, the nurse should make sure that the medication can be given with foods or milk or if they need to be taken on an empty stomach. Antihistamines given orally are usually well absorbed; parenteral administration is rarely needed. When an intramuscular (IM) preparation such as diphenhydramine is used, it should be injected deep into the muscle to prevent tissue irritation. Intravenous (IV) injection of these agents should be done slowly, with the patient lying down because of the risk of the drug causing a low blood pressure. Long-term use of topical nasal antihistamines increases the risk of sensitization, often causing a **rebound effect**, or an increase in the symptoms you are trying to stop.

Table 11-1 presents additional information on antihistamines.

■ Evaluation

The therapeutic effects of antihistamines should decrease the allergy symptoms. Watch for any adverse reactions, which are common but usually mild. Antihistamine use in children and infants is discussed in the Lifespan Considerations box.

Lifespan Considerations
Pediatric

ANTIHISTAMINES

- Infants and young children often have anticholinergic side effects or adverse effects.
- Closely watch pediatric patients with spastic paralysis or brain damage, because they often are very sensitive to these agents, and may need a lower dose.
- Anticholinergics, especially in high doses, may cause a paradoxical reaction (or the opposite reaction you would expect) of increased nervousness, confusion, or hyperexcitability.
- Where hot weather prevails or environmental temperatures are high, children receiving these agents have an increased risk of developing a rapid body temperature increase because the anticholinergic drugs suppress sweat gland activity.
- Dosage adjustments are often necessary for infants, Down syndrome patients, and blondes, because they often have an increased response to this drug category. Flushing, increased temperature, irritability, and increased pulse and respiratory rate may occur.
- Some specific products in child cough and cold remedies have now been removed from the market. Do not use adult cough or cold preparations for children because of the strong chance for overdosage.

Modified from McKenry LM, Tessier E, Hogan MA: *Mosby's pharmacology in nursing*, ed 22, St Louis, 2005, Mosby.

Older adult patients are more likely to develop side effects such as dizziness, syncope (light-headedness and fainting), confusion, dyskinesia (difficulty in movements of the body), and tremor. These are called extrapyramidal reactions. Considerations for antihistamine use in older adults are discussed in the Lifespan Considerations box.

The respiratory tract may become dry and mucus may thicken when using an antihistamine. Unless there is some reason for a fluid restriction, the patient should be encouraged to drink large amounts of water to thin secretions and keep the mucous membranes moist.

If any skin reactions occur, the patient should stop taking the drug at once and notify the health care provider. The CNS depressant effects of antihistamines may be increased if the patient takes more than the recommended dosage or drinks alcohol while using the product. This could be dangerous.

Table 11-1   Antihistamines

GENERIC NAME	TRADE NAME	COMMENTS
FIRST GENERATION DRUGS		
Alkylamines		Effective at low dosages, practical for daytime use; may cause both CNS stimulation (excitation) and depression (drowsiness); individual response varies
brompheniramine	P-Tex Dimetapp	
chlorpheniramine	Chlor-Trimeton	Low incidence of side effects; available OTC; sustained-release forms not for use in children younger than 6 yr
dexchlorpheniramine	Polaramine ♣	
Ethanolamines		Highest incidence of drowsiness, but GI side effects are infrequent
Clemastine	Tavist	
diphenhydramine	Benadryl Genahist Diphenhist Banophen	Anticholinergic, antitussive, antiemetic, and sedative properties; high incidence of CNS depressant effects; drowsiness increases with use
Phenothiazine		Strong CNS depressant effect (drowsiness); may suppress cough reflex or mask signs of intestinal obstruction, brain tumor, or overdosage from toxic drugs (see additional information on phenothiazines in third section of this chapter). Comes as oral, parental, rectal preparations.
promethazine	Phenergan	High incidence of side effects, including severe drowsiness; potent drug with prolonged action; use cautiously in ambulatory patients
Piperazine		
hydroxyzine	Vistaril	For pruritus, sedation, adjunct to analgesia, antiemetic
Miscellaneous		
azelastine	Astelin nasal spray	For SAR; avoid spraying in eyes
SECOND-GENERATION DRUGS		
Piperidines		
azatadine	Optimine	For SAR and PNAR. Comes as a spray
cetirizine	Zyrtec	For SAR and PAR; safe for patients with hypersensitivity to hydroxyzine
		May be taken with or without food
		Patients with renal or hepatic dysfunction require smaller doses
cyproheptadine	Periactin	For SAR, PAR, and hypersensitivity reactions
fexofenadine	Allegra	For SAR; analogue of terfenadine (Seldane) but not associated with cardiac dysrhythmias
	Allegra D	*Patients with renal dysfunction require special dosing*
		Watch for problems common to decongestants.
loratadine	Claritin	Place rapidly disintegrating tablets under the tongue
	Claritin D	*Patients with renal or hepatic dysfunction require special dosing* every other day. Watch for problems common to decongestants.

CNS, Central nervous system; *GI*, gastrointestinal; *OTC*, over-the-counter; *PAR*, perineal allergic rhinitis; *PNAR*, perennial nonallergic rhinitis; *SAR*, seasonal allergic rhinitis.

Lifespan Considerations
Older Adults

ANTIHISTAMINES

Older adults often have pronounced anticholinergic side or adverse effects, especially constipation, dry mouth, and urinary retention (especially in males).

- Problems with memory have been reported with continuous use of these agents, especially in older patients.
- When usual adult doses are given, some elderly people may have sedation or the opposite reaction (a paradoxical reaction) in which the patient has hyperexcitability, agitation, or confusion.
- Anticholinergic dosing in the older adult population should begin at the lowest dose with gradual increases, until maximum improvement is noted or intolerable side effects occur.
- "Start Low and Go Slow" is the common advice in giving medications to older adults.

From McKenry LM, Tessier E, Hogan MA: *Mosby's pharmacology in nursing*, ed 22, St Louis, 2005, Mosby.

■ Patient and Family Teaching

Tell the patient and family the following:

- The patient should take the medications as ordered and not take more than the recommended dosage.
- Most antihistamines cause drowsiness, so the patient must avoid tasks such as driving or activities that require alertness until they have adjusted to the drug.
- These drugs may cause dizziness, thickening of secretions, and upset stomach, which may warrant the attention of a physician, nurse, or other health care provider if they continue.
- If the medication causes stomach upset, taking it with meals or milk can decrease this problem unless there is a food-drug interaction that would prohibit this.
- The nurse might encourage a patient that although they may experience many side effects from one agent, another antihistamine may produce few side effects.
- Tolerance may develop after use of an antihistamine. If one product seems to stop working over time, the health care provider might suggest the patient try another antihistamine for better control of symptoms.
- The patient should stop using antihistamines for 48 hours before having skin tests for allergies.
- Many antihistamines can be purchased OTC; some need a prescription. Make certain the patient has a prescription if it is needed.
- The patient should not take any medications without the knowledge of the physician or other health care provider; it is especially important for the patient to not take alcohol or other sedative drugs while taking an antihistamine.
- These and all medications must be kept out of the reach of children and others for whom it is not prescribed; overdosages may be very serious.

ANTITUSSIVES

OVERVIEW

Drugs used to relieve coughing are called **antitussives**. These drugs may either: (1) act centrally on the cough center in the brain, (2) act peripherally by anesthetizing stretch receptors in the respiratory tract, or (3) act locally, primarily by soothing irritated areas in the throat. Products vary in their effectiveness. Antitussives are commonly com-bined with other drugs and are usually sold as OTC drugs. Antitussives containing controlled substances and usually require a prescription, although some states may allow codeine combination products to be sold OTC if the patient signs for them.

ACTION

The main action of an antitussive depends on whether an opioid antagonist is included. Narcotic or opioid antitussives suppress the cough reflex by acting directly on the cough center in the medulla of the brain. Nonopioid antitussives reduce the cough reflex at its source by anesthetizing stretch receptors in respiratory passages, lungs, and pleura, and by decreasing their activity.

USES

Antitussives are used for the relief of overactive or nonproductive coughs.

ADVERSE REACTIONS

Adverse reactions to antitussives include constipation, drowsiness, dry mouth, nausea, and postural hypotension (low blood pressure resulting in dizziness when a person suddenly stands up).

DRUG INTERACTIONS

Opioid antitussives have an additive effect with other CNS depressants, so the dosage should be reduced. Most antitussives increase the analgesic effect of aspirin, which may be helpful.

❖ NURSING IMPLICATIONS AND PATIENT TEACHING

■ Assessment

Learn as much as possible about the health history of the patient, including allergy to antitussives, presence of COPD that may influence the patient's response to an opioid, possibility of pregnancy, and the use of other drugs or alcohol that may cause drug interactions. These conditions may be contraindications or precautions to the use of antitussives.

Ask about a history of a nonproductive cough or a prolonged and productive cough, which may keep the patient awake at night or cause muscular pain.

▪ Diagnosis

Take care to learn why the patient has a productive cough. Signs of infection, allergy, or other problems might suggest the source of the cough.

▪ Planning

Patients with hypersensitivity (allergy) to these drugs or patients with COPD who have problems with breathing are not usually given opioid antitussives. Opioid antitussives may cause drug dependence. Some of the antitussives are Schedule II controlled substances.

These preparations may cause drowsiness, so the patient should be cautioned to avoid tasks requiring alertness after taking the medication.

▪ Implementation

Antitussives come only in oral forms. They should be used only for short periods. Short therapy decreases the risk of rebound symptoms from prolonged use or the possibility of addiction to opioid products.

Table 11-2 provides additional information on antitussives.

▪ Evaluation

Watch for therapeutic effects: the cough stops or there is a decrease in frequency and duration of coughing spells, and the patient is able to sleep better at night. Also watch the patient for adverse reactions and drug tolerance.

▪ Patient and Family Teaching

Tell the patient and family the following:
- The patient should take the medication as ordered and not alter the dosage or frequency.
- Opioid antitussives may cause drowsiness, and the patient must use caution when doing tasks that require alertness.
- Overuse of the codeine-containing antitussives may cause severe constipation and may also lead to addiction.
- Opioid antitussive drugs increase the effects of alcohol and other drugs that slow the nervous system; the patient should not take any other medications while taking an antitussive.
- The patient may become nauseated during the first few minutes after taking the medication; this problem goes away if the patient lies down.
- Many antitussives occasionally cause light-headedness, dizziness, or fainting when the patient gets up from a lying or sitting position; tell the patient to change positions slowly.
- The patient should take the drug with food or milk to decrease stomach upset if there is no food-drug interaction that would prevent that.

Table 11-2   Antitussives

GENERIC NAME	TRADE NAME	COMMENTS
Opioid Antitussives		
codeine ★		NOT FOR USE IN CHILDREN YOUNGER THAN 12 YEARS
codeine phosphate		
codeine sulfate		
hydrocodone	Hycodan	
Nonopioid Antitussives		
benzonatate	Tessalon Perles (capsules)	Anesthetizes stretch receptors; drug should not be chewed—local anesthesia of the mouth will develop
dextromethorphan	Benylin DM Robitussin DM Vicks Formula 44	Centrally depresses cough center
diphenhydramine ★	Tusstat	Potent antihistamine; safe and effective antitussive

★ Indicates "Must-Know Drugs," or the 35 drugs most prescribers use.

- This medication must be kept out of the reach of children and others for whom it is not prescribed.

ASTHMA MEDICATIONS

OVERVIEW

Asthma is a condition in which there is increased airway inflammation and mucus production, leading to bronchiolar constriction or narrowing. The patient has no trouble breathing air into the lungs, but the lumens (spaces inside the bronchial tubes) become smaller as the patient attempts to breathe out. This traps air inside the lungs. The patient feels a lack of oxygen and acts by breathing faster, trapping even more air inside the lungs. As some air is forced out through the small, mucus-lined passages during respiratory expiration, a musical respiratory sound called wheezing is heard.

The development of asthma involes the interplay between host factors, particularly genetics, deficiencies of some respiratory enzymes, and environmental exposures (reaction to an allergy, reflex response to cold, dry air, or hard exercise). For some individuals with a genetic tendency, asthma often starts in childhood. For some individuals, it becomes a chronic condition. For others, asthma may be seen only with acute illnesses or exercise.

The National Heart, Lung, and Blood Institute of the National Institutes of Health has published *Guidelines for the Diagnosis and Management of Asthma*. These guidelines recommend a stepwise plan for using asthma drugs that puts a heavy emphasis on the treatment based on the diagnostic classification. Asthma is grouped into classes of asthma severity. These classes are: (1) intermittent, (2) mild persistent, (3) moderate persistent, and (4) severe persistent. In each category, the severity and frequency of daytime symptoms, nighttime symptoms, and lung function are evaluated. The health care provider should work with the patient on prevention, identification of allergens, patient education regarding self-care, and effects of cultural and ethnic influences on asthma management. Because asthma is primarily a disease of inflammation, corticosteroids (both oral and inhaled) are also used in treatment. Some of the steroids used in treating respiratory problems are discussed briefly here and in greater detail in Chapter 20.

COPD is a slowly worsening, disabling disorder identified by abnormal tests of expiratory flow (air that is breathed out) that do not change very much over several months. The damage to the lungs results from gradual destruction of the alveolar walls (small airway disease), and parenchymal destruction, creating unequal areas of ventilation and perfusion. Thus circulating blood and inhaled air may not come together so that oxygen can be transferred to the blood, and waste products in the blood can be removed. COPD attacks or exacerbations are seen with increases in inflammation from pulmonary infections and in response to pollution and allergic or nonallergic triggers. Unlike patients with asthma, those with COPD are seldom symptom free, and the damage to the lungs is not totally reversible with COPD. Medications that dilate or open the bronchioles and help thin secretions are helpful in reducing symptoms of dyspnea (shortness of breath, difficulty or distress in breathing).

ASTHMA PROPHYLAXIS (PREVENTION) MEDICATION

ACTION

Many drugs treat the symptoms of asthma but few of them prevent the development of it. Cromolyn sodium is an asthma prophylaxis drug that works at the surface of the mst cell as a mast cell stabilizer to prevent the release of histamine, leukotrienes, and slow-reacting substances of anaphylaxis.

USES

Cromolyn is used to manage bronchial asthma in some patients. How this drug should be used is clearly described in the national guidelines. This drug has no independent, antiinflammatory, or bronchodilator activity, so they are effective primarily for prophylaxis (prevention of or protection against disease) and should not be used in an acute attack of asthma. They are also used in some patients with food allergies to prevent GI and systemic reactions; in patients with allergic rhinitis, eczema, and other forms of dermatitis; for patients with chronic urticaria; and for those with exercise-induced bronchospasm (narrowing or collapse of bronchial airways). The different formulations have different uses. A nasal inhalation (NasalCrom) of the drug is used in the treatment of the nasal symptoms associated with allergic rhinitis including runny/itching nose, sneezing, and allergic nasal congestion; and for allergic rhinitis prophylaxis. As an ophthalmic product it is used for the treatment of allergic ocular disorders such as allergic conjunctivitis, allergic keratoconjunctivitis, giant papillary conjunctictivitis, vernal keratitis, and veral keratoconjunctivitis or the product Gastrocrom is used in the treatment of systemic mastocystosis, and chronic inflammatory bowel disease such as ulcerative colitis.

ADVERSE REACTIONS

Adverse reactions to cromolyn include dizziness, headache, vertigo (feeling of dizziness or spinning), rash, nausea, bad taste in the mouth, throat irritation, damage to teeth, dysuria (painful urination), urinary frequency, bronchospasm, cough, nasal congestion, wheezing, anaphylaxis, tearing of eyes, and swollen parotid glands. Because these drugs are rapidly eliminated from the body, they are nontoxic, except to those who have a hypersensitivity to the drug.

DRUG INTERACTIONS

No drug interactions with cromolyn have been reported.

❖ NURSING IMPLICATIONS AND PATIENT TEACHING

▪ Assessment

Learn as much as possible about the health history of the patient, including specific respiratory signs and symptoms, other medications, allergy, possibility of pregnancy, and presence of infection.

The patient may have a history of allergies, asthma, bronchitis, emphysema, recurrent acute or chronic attacks of wheezing, cough with or without mucoid sputum, dyspnea, fatigue, intolerance to exercise, and in severe cases, cyanosis (bluish color to the skin). Acute upper or lower respiratory tract infections may precede the onset of acute symptoms.

▪ Diagnosis

Confirm that the patient's condition is stable. These products are not effective in an acute asthma attack. The patient should have no signs or symptoms of illness.

▪ Planning

The patient should begin taking these drugs when an acute attack of asthma is over, the airways are clear, and the patient can breathe easily.

The amount of drug the lungs are able to use depends on proper use of the nebulizer or if using an inhaler with spacer, the degree of bronchospasm present, and the amount of secretions in the tracheobronchial tree. It has been estimated that approximately 5% to 10% of the inhaled drug reaches the lungs using a standard inhaler. A spacer will increase this percentage.

▪ Implementation

Cromolyn is taken by standard inhaler. Two inhalations four times daily at regular intervals is the standard regimen.

Occasionally, cough and bronchospasm may follow administration of cromolyn. Some patients may not be able to continue using this drug, even when taking bronchodilators at the same time.

Patients must be careful when decreasing the dosage or stopping the use of cromolyn or nedocromil; this decrease in dosage can cause asthmatic symptoms to recur.

Gastrocrom is an oral concentrate which should be emptied into a half glass of water. Do not mix the solution with fruit juice, milk, or food. Medicine should be taken at least 30 minutes before meals and at bedtime.

▪ Evaluation

Symptoms of asthma should improve within 4 weeks of using cromolyn or nedocromil. The therapeutic effect is shown when the frequency of asthma attacks decrease and the intensity of the episodes lessen. Because the drug should be given when a patient's condition is stable, a visit is typically scheduled 2 weeks after the first dose and at least once more within the first 4 weeks to see how effective the medication has been.

Watch the patient carefully when the dose is being reduced or stopped. The drug regimen must be checked if there is no effect within 4 weeks.

▪ Patient and Family Teaching

Cromolyn. Tell the patient and family the following:

- The airway should be cleared of as much mucus as possible before taking the drug by having the patient cough and expectorate.
- The patient should avoid using these drugs when unable to take a deep breath and hold it or if having an asthma attack.
- These drugs are usually taken every day at regular intervals.
- If the patient is using a bronchodilator at the same time, it should be used first; then after several minutes, the cromolyn or nedocromil may be taken.
- Throat irritation, dryness of the mouth, and hoarseness may be prevented by rinsing and gargling after each dose.
- To receive the appropriate dosage of cromolyn, the patient must use the aerosol solution correctly and keep the mouthpiece clean.
- Stopping the medication quickly can make the patient have an acute attack of asthma.
- The nurse, physician, or other health care provider should be called if symptoms do not improve or if they get worse.

BRONCHODILATORS

Several types of bronchodilators may be given to open the bronchi and allow air to pass out of the lungs more freely; these include the sympathomimetics and the xanthine derivatives. The sympathomimetics are beta-adrenergic agents, and they dilate the bronchi through their action on beta-adrenergic receptors. They are also known as *adrenergic stimulants*. The xanthines act directly to relax the smooth muscle cells of the bronchi, thereby dilating or opening up the bronchi.

SYMPATHOMIMETICS

ACTION

The main action of sympathomimetic bron-chodilators like albuterol (Vospire ER, Preventil HFA) in asthma and other respiratory diseases is to relax the smooth muscle cells of the bronchi by stimulating $beta_2$-adrenergic receptors. Sympathomimetic bronchodilators also stimulate $beta_1$ receptors, which results in an increased rate and force of the heart's contractions. The sympathomimetic drugs vary in their actions on beta receptors. Some act primarily on $beta_1$ receptors that are considered cardioselective; others act primarily on $beta_2$ receptors, and others have $beta_1$ and $beta_2$ effects. If the drug action is specific to $beta_2$ receptors, there are fewer side effects.

USES

Rapid-acting beta $_2$ agonists are used to prevent or treat symptoms of bronchospasm occurring in acute and chronic asthma, bronchitis, and emphysema (COPD). Longer-acting $beta_2$ agonists are given twice daily for the long-term treatment of asthma and emphysema. They are also useful in the prevention of nocturnal asthmatic attacks. Longer-acting $beta_2$ agonists are not indicated for the treatment of acute bronchospasm.

ADVERSE REACTIONS

Adverse reactions to sympathomimetic bronchodilators include symptoms related to stimulation of other beta receptors throughout the body: dysrhythmias (irregular heartbeats), hypotension, tachycardia, anorexia, anxiety, headache, insomnia, nausea, pallor, perspiration, polyuria (excretion of a large amount of urine), restlessness, vomiting, weakness, and urinary hesitancy and retention. These symptoms get worse if there is an over dose.

DRUG INTERACTIONS

Drug interactions may occur with MAO inhibitors, tricyclic antidepressants, beta blockers (beta adrenergic antagonists), other antihypertensive agents, digoxin, potassium-losing diuretics, and caffeine-containing herbs The combination of two or more of these agents may produce an additive effect.

Many general anesthetics may cause dysrhythmias when they are used with these drugs. Nonselective beta blockers and beta-adrenergic blocking agents such as propranolol (Inderol) may block the bronchodilating effects of these beta receptor–stimulating drugs. Sympathomimetics can interfere with the action of some antihypertensive medications.

❖ NURSING IMPLICATIONS AND PATIENT TEACHING

■ Assessment

Learn as much as you can about the health history of the patient, including whether the patient is pregnant or breastfeeding or has a history of hyperthyroidism, heart disease, hypertension, diabetes, glaucoma, seizures, or psychoneurotic disease. Ask whether the patient is taking other drugs that may interact with bronchodilators or has a history of allergy. Any of these conditions may present contraindications or precautions to the use of sympathomimetic bronchodilators.

The patient may have a history of allergies, asthma, bronchitis, emphysema, recurrent acute or chronic attacks of wheezing, and cough. The patient may have had an acute upper or lower respiratory tract infection before the onset of acute symptoms.

■ Diagnosis

As you work with the patient, you will confirm that the patient is having an asthma attack or has respiratory difficulty from COPD. The asthma pattern shows the severity of asthma, and national treatment guidelines suggest that the severity of asthma determines the treatment. For example, the first-line therapy for any asthma attack is a short-acting $beta_2$ agonist. In addition, you may discover the patient needs hydration, strategies to reduce anxiety, or education about the condition.

■ Planning

To relieve bronchial spasm, $beta_2$ receptors in bronchial smooth muscle cells must be stimulated. One of the drawbacks of $beta_2$ adrenergic bronchodilators is that their effects are not limited to $beta_2$ receptors. Some agents also stimulate $beta_1$ receptors, which increase the rate and force of cardiac contraction.. Thus these $beta_2$ bronchodilator drugs should be given with extreme caution to individuals who already have cardiovascular, endocrine, or convulsive disorders that may be affected by these drugs.

■ Implementation

The routes of administration of bronchodilators vary, according to how sick the patient is (the diagnostic classification) and the preparation to be used. Drugs may be given parenterally, orally, or by oral inhalation (nebulizers, or metered-dose inhalers [MDIs]). The medications selected depend on established guidelines and whether short-term treatment or long-term management is required. A patient who is using an inhaler for the first time should be shown how to use the inhaler and given written instructions to refer to later. Research shows that many patients do not use inhalers correctly, so every time the patient comes in for health care, the nurse should ask for a demonstration of how the MDI is being used.

Use of more than one sympathomimetic agent at a time is contraindicated although a rapid-acting drug might be used when a long-acting drug taken on a regular basis is not effective

With many bronchodilators, if the drug is used too frequently, **refractoriness**, or lack of response to a drug that a patient has used before with good effectiveness, may develop. Patients also may get less relief from aerosols if they are used too often. Irritation of the bronchial tree and oropharynx may occur with use of powdered drug forms or other inhaled agents. Rinsing the mouth with water after each treatment helps reduce this problem.

Table 11-3 provides a list of sympathomimetics and other medications used for the treatment of asthma and COPD.

 Clinical Goldmine

Monitoring the Dosage

The dosage of a sympathomimetic must be carefully monitored to prevent excessive tachycardia, decreased or increased blood pressure, nausea, headache, and other CNS symptoms.

■ Evaluation

Check the patient's pulse and blood pressure to see if the heart is affected by the drug. Response to therapy varies among patients. The patient should be watched carefully to see if breathing problems have improved.

Patients should be watched for the development of tolerance, which is shown by less response to the drug.

■ Patient and Family Teaching

Tell the patient and family the following:
- The patient should take the medication as directed by the health care provider; the dosage should not be changed.
- Overuse of these drugs may result in severe side effects.
- The health care provider should be contacted if the drug is not helping the patient.
- Contact the health care provider if bronchial irritation, dizziness, chest pain, insomnia, or any change in symptoms occur.
- Drinking lots of fluid, especially water, makes the mucus thinner and helps the medication work better. This is called bronchial toilet and is a major concept of respiratory therapy.
- The patient must not take any other medications without checking first with the health care provider.
- The patient should take the last dose a few hours before bedtime so that the drug does not produce insomnia.

- The drug should be protected from light; colored solutions should be thrown away.
- Give oral medications with meals to minimize gastric irritation.
- To prevent exercise-induced bronchospasm, the usual dosage for bronchodilator inhaler for adults and children 4 years of age and older is two inhalations 15 to 30 minutes before exercise.
- Tell patient to shake the inhaler well before administering.
- Prime the inhaler with four sprays before using for the first time and again if the inhaler has not been used in the past two weeks.
- Patient should rinse their mouth with water after each administration to decrease dry mouth.
- Patient should keep a count of the total number of sprays used and discard the inhaler after 200 sprays.
- Keep the plastic mouthpiece clean to prevent medication buildup and blockage. Teach the patient to clean the mouthpiece and dry it at least once a week.

XANTHINE DERIVATIVES

ACTION

The main action of xanthine-derivative bronchodilators such as aminophylline and theophylline (Theo-24) is to relax the smooth muscle cells in the bronchi and blood vessels in the lungs. These drugs also act directly on the kidneys to produce diuresis (increased production and excretion of urine). These drugs cause CNS effects. Other actions are myocardial stimulation, increased rate of breathing, effects on metabolism, and release of epinephrine from the adrenal medulla.

USES

Xanthine derivatives are used as an alternative or adjunctive therapy to treat the symptoms of bronchospasm in acute and chronic bronchial asthma, bronchitis, and emphysema and in treating neonatal apnea. The correct way to use them is carefully described in the National Institutes of Health *Guidelines for the Diagnosis and Management of Asthma* (available at http://www.nhlbi.nih.gov/guidelines/asthma/index.htm).

ADVERSE REACTIONS

Adverse reactions to xanthine derivatives include dysrhythmias, flushing, marked hypotension, tachycardia, headache, insomnia, restlessness, diarrhea, epigastric pain, nausea, vomiting, and rash.

Overdosage causes serious adverse reactions that increase in severity, including confusion, respiratory failure, shock, bizarre behavior, extreme thirst, deliriuum (extreme confusion, often with delusions or disorientation), and hyperthermia (abnormally high

Table 11-3   Medications for Asthma and Chronic Obstructive Pulmonary Disease

GENERIC NAME	TRADE NAME	COMMENTS
Sympathomimetic Bronchodilators		
albuterol	Proventil Ventolin	Selective for beta$_2$ receptors; fewer cardiac side effects than other adrenergic drugs; fast acting, long duration of bronchodilation; comes as an inhaler with about 200 doses or in tablet form
bitolterol ephedrine sulfate	Tornalate	Nebulized over 10-15 min 2-3 times daily Long duration; used to treat milder forms of COPD
epinephrine ★	Adrenalin Chloride Primatene Mist	*Primatene Mist:* allow 1-2 min between inhalations if second dose is needed
isoetharine	Arm-A-Med Isoetharine	Use with hand nebulizer: 3-7 inhalations undiluted
isoproterenol	Isuprel Medihaler-Iso	Selective for beta receptors; helpful for those no longer benefiting from use of epinephrine; may decrease blood pressure; may turn saliva pink
metaproterenol	Alupent	More selectivity for beta$_2$ receptors in bronchi and less effect on beta$_1$ receptors of heart than isoproterenol; well absorbed from GI tract
pirbuterol salmeterol	Maxair Serevent Diskus	Long-acting inhaled beta$_2$-receptor agonist used to prevent attacks, but not in acute conditions
terbutaline	Brethine Bricanyl Tubuhaler	Negligible effect on beta$_1$ receptors; affinity for beta$_2$ receptors of the bronchial tree, peripheral vascular beds, and uterus; often effective when other drugs are not
Xanthine Bronchodilators		
aminophylline		Synthetic preparation prototype for many theophylline compounds; plays significant role in management of conditions with bronchial constriction and spasm; especially useful when differentiation cannot be made between bronchospasm and pulmonary edema; commonly prescribed by its generic name; contains 78% theophylline and 12% ethylenediamine; IM injection painful. Comes as tablets, timed release tablets, IM, rectal suppositories or rectal solutions.
dyphylline	Dylix Lufyllin	Few side effects
oxtriphylline	Choledyl SA 🍁	Less irritating to gastric mucosa; readily absorbed from GI tract; more stable and soluble than aminophylline; useful for long-term therapy of bronchospasm
theophylline	Elixophyllin Quibron Slo-Phyllin	Popular and effective drug in management of bronchial constriction and spasm; timed-release capsules slowly provide medication for 8-12 hr or 12-24 hr
Leukotriene Receptor Inhibitors		
montelukast sodium	Singulair	Well-tolerated; used for chronic asthma
zafirlukast	Accolate	Nursing women should not take this medication. Store medication at 68°-77° F and protect from light and moisture
zileuton	Zyflo	May be taken with meals and at bedtime
Corticosteroids: Systemic		
methylprednisolone		Use as required several times per day to gain control. Taper off use.
prednisolone		
prednisone ★		
Corticosteroids: Inhaled		
beclomethasone dipropionate	Qvar Beclovent	Patients usually require inhalation therapy several times a day. Patients may require instruction in use of inhalation machines or inhalers at home.

Table 11-3	Medications for Asthma and Chronic Obstructive Pulmonary Disease—cont'd	
GENERIC NAME	**TRADE NAME**	**COMMENTS**
budesonide	Pulmicort Turbuhaler	
flunisolide	AeroBid	
fluticasone	Flovent	
propionate triamcinolone acetonide	Azmacort	

GI, Gastrointestinal; *IM,* intramuscular.
★ Indicates "Must-Know Drugs," or the 35 drugs most prescribers use.

body temperature). Excessive overdosage may lead to seizures and death without warning. Children are particularly at risk for this problem.

DRUG INTERACTIONS

Xanthines may increase the CNS stimulation caused by ephedrine, sympathomimetics, and amphetamines. Cytochrome P-450 interactions between xanthines and erythromycin, lincomycin, and clindamycin may increase blood levels of theophylline. Beta-blocking agents may interfere with (antagonize) the effect of xanthines. Xanthines also increase the action of some types of diuretics. Xanthines may increase the risk of toxicity when taken with digitalis glycosides. Large doses of these agents may reverse the effect of oral anticoagulants. Lithium carbonate is excreted more rapidly in the presence of xanthines. The use of furosemide with theophylline increases the serum levels of theophylline and may cause toxicity. Xanthine derivatives shorten prothrombin and clotting times.

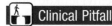

Clinical Pitfall

Factors Affecting Blood Levels

The efficacy of theophylline (Theo-Dur) is directly related to the blood levels achieved from its administration. The desired therapeutic range is considered to be 10 to 20 mcg per milliliter of serum. The factors affecting blood levels include the following:

- Differing levels of theophylline in each product
- Variance in rates of absorption
- Metabolism and elimination of each drug
- Age of the patient receiving the medication

❖ NURSING IMPLICATIONS AND PATIENT TEACHING

■ Assessment

Learn as much as possible about the health history of the patient, including whether the patient is pregnant or has a history of smoking, allergy, renal or liver dysfunction, heart disease, cardiac dysrhythmias, peptic ulcer, severe hypertension, or glaucoma. These conditions are contraindications or precautions to the use of xanthines.

■ Diagnosis

The severity of asthma or COPD is determined by history and is linked to the treatment. Look for any other problems that may require your help: need for increased hydration, insomnia, or feelings of anxiety.

■ Planning

The half-life of xanthine bronchodilators is shorter in smokers than in nonsmokers, which may make it necessary to use a higher dosage for smokers.

Some xanthine bronchodilators come in a liquid formulation with alcohol. It is not necessary to use drug formulations that contain alcohol; the addition of alcohol may be harmful to some patients.

■ Implementation

Xanthine products are available in a number of forms: capsules, sustained-release tablets and capsules, aqueous solutions and suspensions, hydroalcoholic elixirs, suppositories, rectal solutions, and IV and IM injections.

The amount of the theophylline base varies in xanthine products, and the preparations are not therapeutically equal. This inequality may cause difficulty when the patient is switched from one product to another. The health care provider will want to get blood theophylline levels to make sure that the patient is getting the right amount of medicine.

The rate of absorption of oral theophylline depends on the dosage form used. Oral liquids have the fastest absorption rate, followed by uncoated tablets. Sustained-release tablets and capsules produce inconsistent blood levels and should usually be used only at night. Food does not influence the absorption of theophylline. Absorption of rectal suppositories is slow and sometimes unpredictable. The rate of absorption for rectal solutions and IM injections is usually equivalent to that of an oral solution.

The rates of metabolism and excretion of theophylline are also variable. Xanthines are metabolized in the liver and excreted by the kidneys. The serum half-life of the drugs can range from 3 to 12 hours in adults and $1\frac{1}{4}$ to 9 hours in children. Heart failure, liver dysfunction, and pulmonary edema can slow excretion, and smoking can increase excretion. Children younger than 9 years of age actually require larger doses of theophylline than adults to maintain the same therapeutic blood levels of the drug. Thus the dosage must be prescribed on an individualized basis and be carefully monitored. It is common for an initial loading dose to be indicated.

Because of the need to increase or decrease the amount of medication based on the symptoms as well as the serum drug levels, the use of fixed-combination bronchodilator products (that is, a sympathomimetic, a xanthine, and an expectorant combined in one product) is not recommended. Fixed-combination products do not make it possible to change the doses of each individual drug, and a fixed-combination drug may lead to toxicity from some of the drugs. Use of selected sympathomimetic and xanthine bronchodilators administered at the same time, however, may have a synergistic effect. These combination products, once common, are rarely used today.

For more information about the xanthine derivatives, see Table 11-3.

▪ Evaluation

The patient's breathing status and symptoms should be watched for any change. Be alert for signs of toxicity, such as tachycardia or dysrhythmias, vomiting, dizziness, and irritability. Therapeutic blood levels of theophylline and the amount of theophylline base in each preparation will affect the patient's clinical response.

Children and older adult patients are highly sensitive to these drugs and should be carefully watched for CNS stimulation. Notify the health care provider if you suspect the drug dosage may need to be changed.

To minimize GI symptoms, administer the drug with food and water. Rectal irritation may develop from use of suppository forms.

▪ Patient and Family Teaching

Tell the patient and family the following:

- The patient should take the medications as ordered; this often means every 6 hours if taking a sustained-release medication.
- Any unusual symptoms should be reported to the health care provider—especially seizures, rapid heartbeat, irregular heartbeat, vomiting, dizziness, and irritability.
- The patient should avoid drinking large amounts of caffeine-containing drinks such as tea, coffee, cocoa, and cola drinks and not to eat charcoal-broiled foods daily.
- Some other medications interfere with the drug action if taken at the same time. The patient should avoid taking any other drugs without first checking with the nurse, physician, or other health care provider. This includes drugs the patient may buy OTC, because they may also have an effect on the respiratory system (e.g., cough syrups and hay fever and allergy medicine).
- The patient should take the medicine with a glass of water or with meals to avoid an upset stomach.
- If a dose is missed and noticed within an hour, the patient should take the prescribed dose as soon as possible. If more than an hour has passed, the dose should be skipped, and the patient should stay on the original dosing schedule.
- Some suppositories must be refrigerated, whereas others may not need refrigeration. The patient should check with the pharmacist about this.
- The health care provider should be called if use of suppositories causes burning or irritation of the rectal area.
- Encourage patients not to smoke since smoking may cause the dose to be changed.
- Teach the patient the importance of having serum blood levels drawn.

LEUKOTRIENE RECEPTOR INHIBITORS

ACTION

The **leukotriene receptor inhibitors** such as montelukast (Singulair), zafirlukast (Accolate), and ziluton (Zyflo CR) belong to the newest category of drugs used in treating asthma. These drugs are not bronchodilators but act to block receptors for the cysteinyl leukotrienes C_4, D_4, and E_4. Cysteinyl leukotrienes (leukotrienes bound to the amino acid cysteine) are potent bronchoconstrictors. By blocking receptors that control bronchoconstriction, vascular permeability, and mucus secretion, the leukotriene receptor inhibitors can reduce the symptoms of asthma.

USES

These products are substitutes for inhaled glucocorticoid therapy in patients with mild, persistent asthma who cannot take the inhaled medications. These drugs may also be added to regular therapy, because they have a different type of action. They provide medication options for patients with aspirin sensitivity. They are used for prevention and chronic asthma therapy, management of seasonal allergic rhinitis, prevention of exercise-induced bronchoconstriction in patients who are 15 years and older, and may be continued during acute attacks, although they will not reverse bronchospasm.

These drugs are rapidly absorbed orally. While it is often recommended that for pediatric dosing these products be mixed with food, food interferes with the absorption of many of these products, so they should be taken on an empty stomach. The safety of all these drugs has not been established in pregnancy. Montelukast (Singular) and zafirluklast (Accolate) are pregnancy category B(montelukast has dosing for infants from 6 months and zafirlukast has dosing for children from 5 years.) Zileuton (Zyflor CR) is category C and should not be used in breastfeeding mothers or in children younger than age of 10 .

ADVERSE REACTIONS

These drugs are generally safe and well tolerated. Headache is the most common side effect. A few individuals may have infection, nausea, and diarrhea. Singulair has quite a few minor side effects, including upper respiratory infection (URI) and otitis media for children.

DRUG INTERACTIONS

These drugs interact with warfarin, erythromycin, theophylline, MAOIs, sedative/hypnotics, barbiturates, tricyclic antidepressants, antihistamines, phenytoins, atropine/scopolamine, rifampin, and aspirin.

❖ NURSING IMPLICATIONS AND PATIENT TEACHING

■ Assessment

Learn as much as possible about the health history of the patient to determine the status of the patient's asthma and what other medications the patient might be taking. Ask about the possibility of pregnancy, breastfeeding, or liver disease.

■ Diagnosis

Carefully evaluate the patient to determine the possibility of infection, the presence of anxiety (which may cause more rapid breathing), a lack of knowledge, or anything else that may complicate the asthma treatment regimen.

■ Planning

These drugs are not started if the patient is having an acute asthma attack. They are adjunctive drugs given as part of an asthma treatment regimen. Watch to see if there might be adverse drug interactions with other medications the patient is taking. Some of these medications involve special storage requirements.

■ Implementation

Most of these medications are given once or twice daily. They are usually well tolerated, and no significant problems are associated with them.

See Table 11-3 for specific information on the drugs in this category.

■ Evaluation

Therapeutic effect is seen with a reduction in number and severity of asthma attacks. Patients should report to their health care provider if they have an increase in asthma attacks.

■ Patient and Family Teaching

Tell the patient and family the following:
- Taking food with these medications reduces the drug's absorption (except for zileuton).
- Women should not take these drugs if they are pregnant or breastfeeding, although this is a an individual decision to be made by the health care provider and patient based on risk and benefit.
- These medications should be kept out of the reach of children or others for whom they are not ordered.
- These medications are used together with other types of asthma medication. They should be continued if the patient has an acute asthma attack. The patient should not suddenly stop the medication or decrease doses.
- Zafirlukast (Accolate) must be kept protected from extremes of temperature, light, and humidity. It should be stored in the airtight container in which it is supplied.
- Teach the patient to take medications as prescribed whether they are having symptoms or not.

CORTICOSTEROIDS

ACTION

Corticosteroids are the most potent (powerful) and consistently effective medications for the long-term control of asthma. Their action on the inflammatory process may account for their effectiveness. They block the reaction to allergens and reduce airway hyperresponsiveness. They inhibit cytokine production, protein activation, and inflammatory cell migration and activation.

USES

Inhaled corticosteroids such as fluticasone (Flovent HFA) are used in the long-term control of asthma. They are often used to reduce the need for oral corticosteroids. Systemic corticosteroids are often used to get the fastest control of the disease when beginning long-term therapy although the maximum response may take up to 8 weeks. They are also used to speed recovery from moderate to severe episodes and prevent more of these episodes.

ADVERSE REACTIONS

Inhaled steroids may produce bronchospasm, cough, dysphonia (hoarseness), and oral thrush. These drugs may also produce CNS and GI side effects. In long-term or high doses, systemic effects such as slowing of growth in children and osteoporosis in adults may occur. Systemic steroids used for a short time may cause many problems, such as brief abnormalities in glucose metabolism, increased appetite, fluid retention, weight gain, mood alteration, hypertension, and peptic ulcer. Long-term use suppresses the adrenal axis and may produce serious and systemic symptoms.

DRUG INTERACTIONS

The inhaled products have a local effect and do not interact to a great extent with other drugs. However, systemic products interact with many drugs (see Chapter 20). The drugs should be used with caution with antifungals and macrolide antibiotics.

❖ NURSING IMPLICATIONS AND PATIENT TEACHING

■ Assessment

Learn everything you can about the severity of the patient's asthma. Look for symptoms of other respiratory infection, allergens, or stress that might have triggered an asthma attack. Collect information about whether the patient takes the asthma medication correctly and as prescribed. Does the patient have other conditions that could be made worse by systemic corticosteroids?

■ Diagnosis

Classify symptoms of asthma by severity, and identify asthma triggers. Diagnose needs for patient teaching. Does the patient need to take in more fluids? Does the patient need more education?

■ Planning

Develop a teaching plan to meet the educational needs that have been discovered. The health care provider will order oral products at the lowest effective dose for the shortest time possible, so plan to be watchful for adverse effects that may develop from the medication.

■ Implementation

Sometimes patients can reverse an asthma attack by controlling their breathing. Patients who learn these techniques may be fearful and unable to breathe slowly when the attack begins. Stay with the patient and offer reassurance and help with breathing exercises during an acute asthmatic attack. Also begin giving the patient extra water to reduce the thickness of secretions and help the patient cough them up and spit them out. Show the patient the proper way to hold the medication canister, take a breath, and compress the canister so that the medication is released into the lungs and not into the mouth. To insure that the medicine is at the proper angle to go into the lungs and not the

throat, if the patient can stand, they should be able to see their feet while using the inhaler. (If they cannot see their feet, they are holding the inhaler at the wrong angle). Begin teaching the patient about the disease process, the medication regimen, equipment, and procedures. Using a spacer or holder chamber device and washing out the mouth after inhalation will improve systemic absorption and decrease local side effects.

For more information about these products, see Table 11-3.

■ Evaluation

Have the patient show you how the inhaler is used. Watch for improvement in the patient's breathing. Wheezing should decrease.

■ Patient and Family Teaching

Education should focus on the disease process, triggers to asthma attacks, and appropriate therapy.

The patient and family should learn about taking the medicine and knowing when it is not effective. Make sure the patient understands when to contact the health care provider.

Explain how corticosteroid medications are used together with other products. This information should be put in writing so the patient can refer to it later.

Children need to be taught as much as possible and given the responsibility of helping to determine when they need medication, what type of medication they need, and whether it is effective.

- Teach patients who are taking inhalation corticosteroids and a bronchodilator to use the bronchodilator first and wait 5 minutes before administering the corticosteroid.
- Advise that inhalation corticosteroids should not be used to treat acute asthma attacks, but may be continued along with other inhalation agents.
- Teach patient to use the peak flow meter to monitor respiratory status.
- Teach patient correct use of inhaler and spacer for optimal effect.

DECONGESTANTS

OVERVIEW

ACTION

Decongestants directly affect the alpha receptors of blood vessels in the nasal mucosa, causing vasoconstriction. This action reduces blood flow in the edematous nasal area, resulting in decrease of the engorged turbinates and mucous membrane, which will encourage sinus drainage, improve nasal air passage, and relieve the feeling of nasal stffiness and mucosal edema. Many agents also act on beta receptors, which may cause **rebound vasodilation**, or an increase in blood flow, leading to further congestion. This problem is commonly seen with prolonged use of the medication.

USES

Decongestants are used to relieve nasal congestion that accompanies allergic rhinitis, sinusitis, and upper respiratory tract infections (URTIs). These drugs may also be used as additional therapy for middle ear infections and to decrease congestion around the eustachian tubes. Ear blockage and the pressure and pain caused by air travel may respond to nasal decongestants. Most of these products are now OTC.

ADVERSE REACTIONS

Stinging and burning as a result of mucosal dryness sometimes follow administration via nasal spray of decongestants. Rebound congestion may occur after prolonged use of topical agents. When the drugs are administered orally and absorbed from the GI tract, systemic effects such as nervousness, nausea, dizziness, tachycardia, dysrhythmia, and a transient increase in blood pressure may occur. Rarely, a severe shocklike syndrome with hypotension and coma has been reported in children. Psychologic dependence and toxic psychoses have been reported with long-term, high-dose therapy. The severity of overdosage varies, resulting in a variety of symptoms. Because of problems with inadvertent overdosage in infants and toddlers, the makers of all OTC oral cough and cold products announced in 2007 that they would remove these products from the market. This action proceeded from Food and Drug Administration regulations that these products are not to be used in infants and toddlers.

DRUG INTERACTIONS

The systemic effects of decongestants may be made stronger if they are given with other sympathomimetics, MAO inhibitors, tricyclic antidepressants, antihistamines, and thyroxine. Decongestants should be used with caution in stable hypertensive patients on guanethidine, bethanidine, or debrisoquine sulfate. Use of decongestants at the same time as high doses of digitalis or use of other drugs that may sensitize the heart to dysrhythmias should be avoided because anginal pain may result when there is coronary insufficiency.

❖ NURSING IMPLICATIONS AND PATIENT TEACHING

■ Assessment

Learn as much as possible about the patient's health history. The patient may have a history of nasal congestion, postnasal drip, nasal discharge, sneezing, sore throat, headache, itchy eyes, lacrimation (excess tear production), nasal polyps, earache, decreased hearing, URTI, or allergies.

Ask about allergy to adrenergic agents, narrow-angle glaucoma, concurrent MAO inhibitor or tricyclic antidepressant therapy, and loss of sensation in the fingers and toes. These are contraindications to the use of decongestants. Decongestants should be used cautiously by patients with hypertension, dysrhythmias, heart disease, angina, hyperthyroidism, diabetes, advanced arteriosclerotic conditions, glaucoma, prostatic hypertrophy, or chronic cough because of the possibility of systemic vasoconstriction and tachycardia. Patients with a long history of asthma and emphysema who also have degenerative heart disease should also be cautioned about the use of decongestants. Excessive use of topical decongestants may result in GI absorption that causes systemic

 Memory Jogger

Administering Decongestants

Provide the patient and family with the following instructions:
1. To administer drops:
   a. Blow the nose gently.
   b. Lie down with the head tipped back over the edge of the bed.
   c. Put 1 to 2 drops of solution on the lower nasal mucosa.
   d. Breathe through the mouth.
   e. Remain in this position for 5 minutes while turning the head from side to side; this will help the drops run back into the nose instead of down the throat.
2. The patient should always rinse the dropper after putting drops into the nose. This will help prevent growth of bacteria and fungi.
3. To administer a spray:
   a. Patients should stand so they can see their feet, or sit upright.
   b. Keep the container upright to obtain a fine mist.
   c. Gently blow the nose.
   d. Squeeze the bottle firmly in each nostril.
   e. After 3 to 5 minutes, blow the nose again.
   f. Repeat the application if congestion remains.
4. Each person in the family should use a separate bottle of nasal spray. Topical decongestants should not be shared.
5. To administer jellies:
   a. Put a small amount on the finger.
   b. Apply it to the nasal mucosa.
   c. Inhale or breathe in deeply through the nose.
6. To administer inhalers:
   a. Insert the open end of the plastic tube in each nostril.
   b. Inhale two times.
   c. Follow directions about washing and cleaning inhalers to avoid them becoming sources of infection.
7. The patient should avoid excessive use of these medications or they will cause the symptoms that the patient is trying to reduce.
8. Missed doses may be taken within an hour of the scheduled time, and then the regular schedule may be resumed. If more than 1 hour has passed, the patient should skip that dose and return to the regular schedule.

effects. The safe use of decongestants in pregnancy has not been established.

Decongestants should be used with caution in patients with hypertension, hyperthyroidism, diabetes, cardiac disease, glaucoma, or prostatic hyperplasia. Drugs containing pseudoephedrine are used in the manufacture of methamphetamines. Many states have regulations regarding the purchase of decongestants where they track and limit the number of purchases by an individual. The drugs containing decongestants are placed behind the counter at the pharmacy and individuals have to sign for them.

■ Diagnosis

To make certain the treatment is appropriate, the exact cause of the patient's problem must be found. Determine if rhinitis is related to allergy or infection.

■ Planning

Frequent and continual use of topical decongestants or use at dosages greater than recommended may result in a rebound effect. Topical decongestants should be used only in acute states, for no longer than 3 to 5 days, and should be used very carefully at low doses in older adults.

■ Implementation

Oral decongestants are considered to be more effective and longer lasting than nasal preparations because they can reach all parts of the mucous membrane in the nasal passages. The disadvantage of systemic agents is that their effects may not be limited to the nasal mucosa; they may also affect other parts of the body. This is why caution is advised for patients with certain medical conditions.

Topical forms may be supplied as drops, sprays, jellies, and oral inhalation agents. The advantage of topical administration is the rapid onset of action and direct stimulation of the nasal mucosa. Drops have a tendency to pass into the hypopharynx and then be swallowed, thus passing into the GI tract. Sprays deliver a fine mist that is easily trapped in the upper respiratory tract, so they are less likely to reach the GI tract. Topical preparations should not be used for more than 3 to 5 days because of the risk of a rebound effect. Oral preparations are more appropriate for long-term use in the rare occasions where required.

To prevent swallowing of the drug, the patient's head should be tipped back when giving nose drops. Use care not to touch the skin while administering solutions. Solutions can become contaminated with use and result in growth of bacteria and fungi.

Table 11-4 lists various nasal decongestant products.

■ Evaluation

Expect to see symptoms disappear. However, symptoms may return if there is rebound congestion following overly long use. If headache and nervousness occur, stop the treatment and contact the health care provider.

■ Patient and Family Teaching

There are many decongestants on the market that are available OTC. A lot of these OTC products contain combinations of medications to make them attractive

Table 11-4   Nasal Decongestants

GENERIC NAME	TRADE NAME	COMMENTS
Sympathomimetic Bronchodilators		
ephedrine ★	Pretz D	May produce burning, stinging, dryness of nasal mucosa, and sneezing
epinephrine	Adrenalin	Stimulates both alpha and beta receptors
Inhalers		
naphazoline	Privine	Rapid, prolonged effect; produces CNS depression when swallowed
oxymetazoline	Afrin Dristan 12 Hr Duration	Prolonged decongestant effect; often overused by patients, leading to rebound congestion when used longer than 3 days in succession
phenylephrine	Neo-Synephrine Sinex	Drug ineffective if exposed to air, strong light, or heat; very effective topical preparation but may cause marked local irritation
pseudoephedrine sulfate	Sinex Sudafed	
tetrahydrozoline	Tyzine	
xylometazoline	Otrivin	Overdose can cause extreme CNS depression in children.

CNS, Central nervous system.
★ Indicates "Must-Know Drugs," or the 35 drugs most prescribers use.

to the patient with several symptoms. These products may contain a decongestant and one or more antihistamine, analgesic, antitussive, expectorant, or anticholinergic products. Each additional medication increases the precautions for use of the product and the adverse effects that may occur. For example, drugs that contain anticholinergics cause drying of mucus secretions. They should be avoided in patients with asthma or COPD. The patient should consider whether there is a need for all of the drugs listed on the label of these combination products. Also, the types of drugs that make up even well-known products change frequently. Pharmacists are excellent sources of information about OTC medications, and patients should be encouraged to seek their professional advice before self-treating with a decongestant product.

EXPECTORANTS

OVERVIEW

ACTION

Expectorants are agents that decrease the thickness of respiratory secretions and aid in their removal. It is believed they work by increasing the amount of fluid in the respiratory tract. These thinner secretions promote ciliary action and decrease the amount of coughing while increasing the amount of sputum produced. Guaifenesin has been on the market since the 1950's but its efficacy has only recently been documented. Guaifenesin is an ingredient contained in many combination OTC cough and cold products. It is available as a single agent in both OTC medications (such as Mucinex, Robitussin, Organidin NR) and in prescription-only products (such as Humibid LA, Touro EX tablets). The drug is available in immediate-release (e.g. oral solutions), extended-release, and combination immediate/extended release formulations. Mucinex was approved in 2002 and is the only FDA-approved OTC extended-release guaifenesin product.

USES

Guaifenesin is used to treat symptoms of productive cough. These products may be useful in chronic respiratory disease when thick mucus is a complication and are indicated in patients with coughs associated with viral URIs. Table 11-5 provides a summary of expectorants. Because of cases of overdosage, the FDA has ruled that these products should not be given to children under 2 years old, and some products not to children under 6 years old. Drug companies have voluntarily removed many of these risky preparations from the market to reduce the potential for inadvertent overdose.

ADVERSE REACTIONS

GI upset is a common adverse reaction to expectorants. Dizziness, headache, and rash may also occur.

DRUG INTERACTIONS

There are no drug interactions of clinical significance with guaifenesin.

❖ NURSING IMPLICATIONS AND PATIENT TEACHING

▪ Assessment

Learn as much as possible about the health history of the patient, including the history of cough, presence of other respiratory disease, allergy, and other medications that may cause drug interactions.

▪ Diagnosis

Are there needs for hydration? Is the patient able to take water by mouth, or is he or she receiving IV fluid? Diagnose any lack of knowledge the patient may have.

Table 11-5	Expectorants	
GENERIC NAME	**TRADE NAME**	**COMMENTS**
guaifenesin	Anti-Tuss Robitussin Organidin NR Mucinex	Although there is a lack of convincing evidence to document clinical efficacy, this is a widely publicized product.
iodinated glycerol	Iophen	Codeine-guaifenesin combination drug. Patients may develop dose-related dermatitis, GI upset, or rash. Hypersensitivity, thyroid enlargement, and acute parotitis are rare. One drop is approximately equal to 3 mg.
		May be taken with juice or milk if diet allows.
iodine products	Pima SSKI	Do not use continuously, because prolonged use may lead to hypothyroidism.

GI, gastrointestinal.

Clinical Pitfall

Chronic or Persistent Cough

Chronic or persistent cough may be the result of a serious condition and should not be ignored.

▪ Planning

Expectorants are not to be used for persistent cough without the advice of a health care provider.

▪ Implementation

The patient should take an increased amount of fluid each day and breathe humidified air. This will help liquefy secretions. Medication should be taken with at least one full glass of water. (See Table 11-5.)

▪ Evaluation

Monitor to see that secretions become thinner and are decreased. If the patient uses more than the recommended dosage, adverse reactions may occur.

▪ Patient and Family Teaching

Tell the patient and family the following:
- The patient should be aware that these drugs will help make the sputum more liquid. This will make it easier to bring sputum up when the patient coughs.
- The patient should use a humidifier and drink at least 2 quarts of water daily while taking an expectorant unless there is a medication reason for fluid restriction. These actions will help get the mucus out.
- The nurse, physician, or other health care provider should be notified if the cough is present with a high fever, rash, or persistent headaches, or if the cough returns once the patient thinks it has been under control.
- The patient should use the medication only in the dosage recommended to decrease chances of side effects.
- Teach the patient to take the drug with at least one full glass of water.
- Teach the patient how to cough effectively. Patient should sit upright and take several deep breaths before trying to cough.
- Warn patient the drug may cause dizziness and to avoid driving or other activities that require alertness until response to the drug is known.

TOPICAL INTRANASAL STEROIDS

OVERVIEW

ACTION

The main action of topical intranasal steroids is an antiinflammatory effect, which decreases local congestion.

USES

Topical intranasal steroids such as flunisolide (Nasarel) are used to treat allergic, mechanical, or chemically induced local nasal inflammation or nasal polyps only when the more usual treatment has been tried and found to not work. Some patients get good allergy relief from these products and require no other medications. Although not every patient is able to take these medications, in general the medications have been found to be safe. Some patients have been able to use them for years without adverse or systemic effects.

ADVERSE REACTIONS

Adverse reactions to topical intranasal steroids include inducing an asthma attack, headache, light-headedness, loss of sense of smell, nasal irritation and dryness, nausea, nosebleeds, perforation of the nasal septum, bad taste and smell, rebound congestion, and skin rash.

DRUG INTERACTIONS

Intranasal steroids may interact with many products. Consult the earlier section on corticosteroids for more information.

❖ NURSING IMPLICATIONS AND PATIENT TEACHING

▪ Assessment

Learn as much as possible about the health history of the patient, including allergy, fungal infections, tuberculosis, ocular herpes simplex, local infections (especially of the nose, sinus, or throat), and the possibility of pregnancy. These conditions are contraindications or precautions to the use of topical nasal steroids. Ask about the patient's past experience with and response to nasal sprays.

▪ Diagnosis

Learn why the patient requires intranasal medication. Identify any other problem secondary to medication use or misuse, such as presence of adverse effects or patient education deficits.

▪ Planning

The patient receiving topical intranasal steroids should not be given smallpox vaccination or immunizations, because the immunologic response may be decreased. In the patient with latent tuberculosis or reactivated tuberculosis, close observation and possible chemoprophylaxis may be indicated. The effects of these drugs are increased in patients with hypothyroidism and cirrhosis.

▪ Implementation

The recommended dosage must not be exceeded. The dosage should be decreased when the patient begins to improve.

Table 11-6	Intranasal Steroids	
GENERIC NAME	**TRADE NAME**	**COMMENTS**
beclomethasone dipropionate	Beconase	Use after other conventional therapy has been found to be ineffective. Symptomatic relief is not immediate, so therapy should be continued even with initial minimal response. Maximal response should be seen within 3 wk or medication should be discontinued. Taper off gradually as relief is obtained.
budesonide	Rhinocort Aqua	
flunisolide	Nasarel	
	AeroBid	AeroBid comes as an inhaler
fluticasone propionate	Flonase	Comes as a MDI
mometasone-furoate	Nasonex	
Triamcinolone-acetonide	Nasacort AQ	

MDI, metered dose inhaler.

Table 11-6 provides a list of intranasal steroids.

▪ Evaluation

Watch for a reduction in nasal stuffiness, obstruction, and discharge, and for relief of sinus headaches. Also monitor how often the medication is used and what dosage is used. Watch for cracked or bleeding nasal mucosa. Be alert for adverse reactions such as signs of systemic absorption and fluid retention, increased blood pressure, weight gain, ankle edema, or evidence of local infection.

Nasal dryness and irritation are side effects and do not usually require stopping the drug. The dosage of these drugs should be gradually reduced to avoid adrenocortical insufficiency.

These drugs may decrease resistance to infection, as well as mask some common signs of infection. Elevation of blood pressure, retention of salt and fluid, and increased potassium and calcium loss may occur if the patient takes large doses. This may be treated with dietary salt restriction and potassium supplementation. Loss of the ability to smell, shortness of breath, unrelieved stuffy nose, chest tightness, or wheezing all indicate a need for intervention by a health care provider.

The patient should be watched for signs of systemic absorption, because fluid retention and temporary inhibition of pituitary-adrenal function may develop.

▪ Patient and Family Teaching

Tell the patient and family the following:
* The patient should not use these drugs if an infection is present. Patients should notify the nurse, physician, or other health care provider if an infection develops while taking this drug.
* The patient should not exceed the prescribed dosage and frequency; using the drug in the smallest effective dose for the shortest period will prevent general absorption.
* There may be temporary dryness and irritation of the nose.
* When stopping this drug, the dosage must be tapered slowly and not stopped suddenly, especially if the medicine has been used for a long period.
* The nurse, physician, or other health care provider should be notified if symptoms do not improve or if they get worse.
* Teach and have the patient return a demonstration of the correct way to administer the nasal spray or inhalers.

COMPLEMENTARY AND ALTERNATIVE THERAPIES

Allergies, asthma, and coughs and colds are some of the conditions frequently treated with alternative products. See the Complementary and Alternative Therapies box for some of the most common preparations and their use.

Complementary and Alternative Therapies

Allergy or Respiratory Problems

SYMPTOMS	HERBAL PRODUCTS OR VITAMINS/MINERALS	COMMENTS
Allergy	Grape seed, stinging nettle, coleus, vitamin C	*Grape seed:* Contraindicated in active bleeding, hemostatic disorders; potential interaction with anticoagulants, aspirin, NSAIDs, antiplatelet agents. *Coleus:* Potential interaction with anticoagulants, aspirin, NSAIDs, antiplatelet agents, methotrexate. *Vitamin C:* High doses for diabetic patients may produce falsely high blood glucose readings.
Asthma	Cordyceps, Tylophora, grape seed, coleus, vitamin C	*Cordyceps:* May interact with MAO inhibitors, anticoagulants, NSAIDs, antiplatelet agents. *Tylophora:* May interact with MAO inhibitors, anticoagulants, aspirin, NSAIDs, antiplatelet agents. *Grape seed, coleus, vitamin C:* See above.
Cold	Arabinoxylane, Echinacea, elderberry, astragalus, goldenseal, grapefruit seed extract, zinc, vitamin C	*Arabinoxylane:* High phosphorus content indicates caution in patients with renal failure. *Echinacea:* Do not use longer than 10 days; potential interaction with therapeutic immunosuppressants and corticosteroids. *Astragalus:* May interact with immunosuppressants. *Grapefruit seed extract:* Avoid taking with astemizole, cisapride, terfenadine, or other medications metabolized by cytochrome P-450 3A4 system. *Vitamin C:* See above.
Cough	Ground ivy, thyme, licorice, marshmallow	*Ground ivy:* Contraindicated in epilepsy. *Thyme:* Use with caution in patients with allergy to oregano. *Licorice:* Potential interactions with laxatives, corticosteroids, cardiac glycosides. *Marshmallow:* Potential interactions with insulin, oral hypoglycemic agents.

Modified from Krinsky DL, LaValle JB, Hawkins EB, et al: *Natural therapeutics pocket guide,* ed 2, Hudson, Ohio, 2003, Lexi-Comp, Inc.
MAO, monoamine oxidase; *NSAIDs,* nonsteroidal antiinflammatory drugs.

Get Ready for the NCLEX® Examination!

Key Points

- The following respiratory medications are used to treat allergies or respiratory system disorders: antihistamines, or allergy medications; antitussives, or medications to control cough; asthma medications (bronchodilators, leukotriene receptor inhibitors, corticosteroids); decongestants; expectorants; and nasal steroids.
- Respiratory medications are available in many forms, as both prescription and OTC medications.
- Monitoring the patient outcome, watching for development of adverse reactions, and teaching the patient about adverse reactions, administration, and dosage considerations are important responsibilities of the nurse in administering respiratory medications.

Additional Learning Resources

SG Go to your Study Guide for additional learning activities to help you master this chapter content.

evolve Go to your Evolve website (http://evolve.elsevier.com/Edmunds/LPN/) for additional online resources.

Review Questions for the NCLEX® Examination

1. A patient tells the nurse that he frequently treats his child's chronic allergies with OTC antihistamines. The most appropriate response from the nurse should be:
   1. "Antihistamines are usually not effective when given to children."
   2. "Antihistamines are excellent drugs to use to treat children."
   3. "Antihistamines can be used with children if the child is monitored closely."
   4. "Antihistamines overdosage can be fatal, especially in children."

Get Ready for the NCLEX® Examination!—cont'd

2. A nurse is doing a health history with a patient and discovers that his prescribed medications include antihistamines as well as corticosteroids. The nurse anticipates that the effect of this combination of medications will be:

   1. an increase in the effect of the corticosteroids
   2. a decrease in the effect of the corticosteroids
   3. an increase in the effect of the antihistamines
   4. a decrease in the effect of the antihistamines

3. In order to limit the GI side effects of oral antihistamines, the nurse should administer the medication with:

   1. orange juice
   2. grapefruit juice
   3. milk
   4. carbonated beverage

4. Which patient is not a candidate for treatment with antitussives?

   1. the patient with frequent headaches
   2. the patient with emphysema
   3. the patient with an overactive cough
   4. the patient with a heart murmur

5. The patient is scheduled to begin treatment with cromolyn. One of the most important pieces of information that the nurse should teach the patient about this drug is:

   1. stopping the medication quickly can make the patient have an acute attack of asthma
   2. throat irritation can be prevented by rinsing and gargling after each dose
   3. take the drug each day at regular intervals at approximately the same time
   4. prime the inhalation canister by pressing it three times before the first use

Case Study

1. Lisa Fines, 28 years old, comes to the clinic with a clear nasal discharge, red, itchy eyes, and a cough of 3 days duration.
   a. What other important information would you like to obtain from her history?
   b. What information would you like to obtain from the physical examination?
   c. What pattern of subjective and objective findings would make you believe she had seasonal allergic rhinitis? Asthma? A URI?
   d. What is the difference in treatment for seasonal allergic rhinitis, asthma, or a URTI?
   e. Would there be any modifications in the recommended treatment if Lisa were pregnant? A child younger than 2 years of age? An older adult patient with congestive heart failure?

2. Mrs. Plains is a 43-year-old African American woman who reports wheezing and tightness in her chest since early this morning. She went shopping today and has been outside during an unseasonable cold spell, which she believes is the cause of the wheezing. She has had one other episode of wheezing that occurred 3 days ago while she was outside in the cold. She has a slight cough that is productive of a small amount of clear sputum. For the last 3 or 4 days, she has awakened at night, particularly early in the morning, with dyspnea and a cough. She has no other symptoms.

Physical examination: Afebrile and in no acute distress.
Cardiovascular: Heart rate 84 beats/min, blood pressure 114/84 mm Hg.
Respiratory: Breath sounds equal throughout both sides; scattered monophonic expiratory wheezes throughout lung fields.

   a. The physician decides that Mrs. Plains has a mild persistent, reversible airway obstruction that is responsive to bronchodilators and corticosteroids. She is started on an oral inhaler. What might the doctor order? Give the name, dosage, frequency, and patient instructions for each medication you select.

NAME DOSAGE FREQUENCY PATIENT INSTRUCTIONS
   a. _____
   b. _____
   c. _____

   b. Mrs. Plains comes back in 1 month. Two weeks ago she had a cold with nasal congestion, sneezing, and a sore throat. Since then, the cough has worsened, and she is now producing large amounts of purulent sputum. What do you think has happened?
   c. The physician orders erythromycin ethyl succinate (EES) one tablet PO every 6 hours. Why?
   d. Mrs. Plains returns 1 month later. Her cough and sputum production have resolved. She continues to have wheezing when she goes out in the cold. What self-management plans would you discuss with her?

Drug Calculation Review

1. Order: Theophylline (Theo-24) 300 mg by mouth once a day Supply: Theophylline 100-mg tablets
   Question: How many tablets of theophylline are needed with each dose?

2. Order: Albuterol 4 mg by mouth three times daily Supply: Albuterol 2-mg tablets
   Question: How many tablets of albuterol are needed with each dose?

3. A 20-year-old woman presents to the emergency department with itching and red wheals on her extremities. The physician orders diphenhydramine (Benadryl) 25 mg IM stat. You note that the multiple-dose vial reads 50 mg/1 mL. How many milliliters should you prepare for this injection?

Get Ready for the NCLEX® Examination!—cont'd

Critical Thinking Questions

1. Ms. Allbright comes into the clinic stating that her antihistamine dosage requires adjustment. The nurse asks her to describe her symptoms, and she gives the nurse the classic symptoms indicating a need for antihistamine. What are the signs and symptoms that require an antihistamine?

2. The health care provider listens to the nurse's report of Ms. Allbright's complaints and then shakes his head. He tells the nurse that Ms. Allbright has been taking a decongestant for an extended time. The health care provider suspects that the patient has built up a possible psychologic dependence, leading to overuse and rebound reactions. What symptoms would lead the nurse to suspect that Ms. Allbright is undergoing rebound phenomenon? How might the nurse determine that the medication is not working?

3. Mr. Tracy enters the clinic with a severe cough. He demands loudly that he be given "cough drops right away!" What questions will the nurse ask Mr. Tracy about his cough? In what situations would you not want to suppress a cough?

4. The health care provider agrees that Mr. Tracy should be given something to relieve his coughing. What class of drugs is commonly used to relieve coughing? What is "symptomatic relief"? Why are these medications used in nonproductive coughs?

5. Mr. Tracy has been prescribed an antitussive. Develop a patient teaching plan that includes a discussion of possible adverse reactions and drug interactions. What will the nurse tell Mr. Tracy?

6. Ms. Henry has just been told she has asthma. She tells the nurse she has "suspected it for quite some time, but it is a surprise anyway." She asks the nurse to tell her what causes asthma. Then she asks the nurse to explain why she has to take medication right now, when she has not had an "attack" for several weeks. Explain the differences between treatment and prophylaxis and why she needs prophylactic therapy.

7. Ms. Henry has never used an inhaler before. Draw up a teaching plan for Ms. Henry, showing her how to place the cannister properly and how to inhale. Include strategies for reducing the coughing reaction and for care of the inhaler itself.

8. Ms. Rochester has had several nasal polyps removed and has been placed on intranasal steroids. She is worried about taking any kind of steroid. "I wouldn't mind as much, I guess, if I just knew what to watch out for," she says. Identify the most common adverse reactions to nasal steroids; compare them with adverse reactions to systemic steroids.

9. Why are antitussives generally not recommended for patients with COPD?

10. Why would a patient be asked to discontinue seasonal allergy antihistamines before receiving a purified protein derivative for tuberculosis screening or before skin testing for other allergies?

11. A nurse is working in a community clinic. As she is leaving after her appointment, Ms. Harris tells the nurse she is going straight to the drugstore, because the doctor says she has a bad head cold, and she needs something to drain her sinuses. When the nurse reviews her medical history, she sees that the patient is taking medication to control hypertension. What information does the patient need before choosing an OTC decongestant?

Antiinfective Medications

Objectives

1. Identify the major antiinfective drug categories and the organisms against which they are effective.
2. Outline the most important things to teach the patient who is taking antiinfective medications.
3. Define spectrum and explain what this word means in antiinfective therapy.
4. List some of the most common adverse reactions to medications used to treat infections.

Key Terms

antibiotics (ăn-tĭ-bī-ŎT-ĭks, p. 162)
antimicrobials (ăn-tĭ-mī-KRŌ-bē-ălz, p. 162)
bactericidal (băk-tēr-ĭ-SĪD-ăl, p. 162)
bacteriostatic (băk-tēr-ē-ō-STĂT-ĭk, p. 162)
broad-spectrum drugs (p. 162)
generation (JĔN-ĕr-Ā-shun, p. 162)

helminthiasis (hĕl-mĭn-THĪ-ă-sĭs, p. 181)
narrow-spectrum drugs (p. 162)
pathogen (PĂTH-ō-jĕn, p. 161)
spectrum (p. 162)
superinfection (SŪ-pĕr-ĭn-fĕk-shŭn, p. 163)

OVERVIEW

This chapter describes the main information about many types of antiinfective medications. It is divided into three sections: The first section discusses major bacterial antiinfective agents; the second section describes the drugs used in treating tuberculosis (TB). The third section discusses drugs used to treat parasitic infections: amebicides, anthelmintics, and antimalarial preparations. Antifungal medications are included in Chapter 13, along with other antiviral and antiretroviral drugs used in the treatment of acquired immune deficiency syndrome (AIDS).

Because of the many different types of infections and the numerous drugs that have been developed to treat them, antiinfective drugs are some of the most commonly given drugs. Thus nurses need to learn as much as possible about these drugs and what to teach patients who are taking them.

Organisms of many different types are always on the skin and inside the body of a healthy individual. These organisms do not make a person ill unless there is some alteration in the skin barrier or a change that makes the person at higher risk, such as being pregnant or having AIDS. Infants, young children, and older adults have the greatest risk of infection, as do people with poor circulation, poor nutritional status, or multiple diseases, and those who often come in contact with people who have infections.

An organism that causes infection is a **pathogen**. As a very basic summary of important definitions,

pathogenic organisms that cause disease because of their ability to divide rapidly and overwhelm the immune system or produce toxins come in a variety of forms. *Bacteria* are a large domain of single-celled, prokaryote microorganisms. They have a wide range of shapes and characteristics. This is a generic term that is now often replaced by more specific names. A *fungus* is a member of a large group of eukaryotic organisms that include microorganisms, such as yeasts and molds; grow in irregular masses, without roots, stems, or leaves; and live and feed on other organisms. A *virus* is a small infectious agent that can replicate (reproduce itself) only inside the living cells of organisms. With few exceptions, viruses are capable of passing through fine filters that trap most bacteria. How a virus is classified depends on the features of its virion (or complete virus particle). The two main classes are ribonucleic acid (RNA) viruses and deoxyribonucleic acid (DNA) viruses. A *parasite* is an organism, protozoa, or worm that lives on or in another organism and draws its food from the other organism.

Each infection in a patient must be carefully evaluated to identify the specific organism causing the infection and the drug that will be most effective against it. Although some parasites may be seen with the naked eye, most infectious organisms are visible only under a microscope. Bacteria must be carefully cultured and tested to see which antimicrobials are effective against them (antimicrobial sensitivity). Nurses will often be asked to collect specimens for this type of testing.

Bacteria can be identified by their shape. Learning what organism is present allows the health care provider to order the medication that will best treat that particular bacteria.

Antiinfective agents, or **antimicrobials**, are chemicals that kill or damage the pathogenic organisms. Antiinfective agents are classified by their chemical structures or by their mechanisms of action. Some of these chemicals are made from other living microorganisms (such as the penicillins), and are classified as **antibiotics**. Other chemicals are synthetics (such as sulfonamides) or combinations of synthetic and naturally occurring microorganisms. Some drugs have become more refined, purified, and sensitive as a result of long-term testing. Each new group of these drugs developed from other similar drugs is called a **generation**; the original drugs are referred to as *first-generation drugs,* and later groups are called *second-generation drugs, third-generation drugs,* and so on.

Antiinfective medications work in different ways to affect pathogenic bacteria (Figure 12-1). They may attack a bacterium's internal cell processes, which are vital to its existence, or they may destroy the external cell wall, making it weaker or unable to reproduce; in some cases, they actually kill the organism. Agents that are **bactericidal** kill the bacteria; those that are **bacteriostatic** limit or slow the growth of the bacteria, weakening or eventually leading to the death of the bacteria. (The "cidal" or "static" part of the word gives a clue about the activity, whether it refers to bacteria or to fungi [fungicidal or fungistatic].) Bacteria are often classified as *gram positive* or *gram negative,* depending on whether they are stained by Gram stain. The number of organisms the medication is effective against is described in terms of its **spectrum**. Some antiinfective medications are effective against only a few gram positive or negative bacteria. These are called **narrow-spectrum drugs**. An example is a drug effective against only one type of pneumonia. Other drugs are effective against both gram negative and gram positive bacteria. These are known as **broad-spectrum drugs**. An example is Levofloxacin. A specimen must be cultured and the antibiotic that is most effective against that particular organism is then determined through sensitivity testing. The correct antibiotics must be given to destroy the pathogen and to limit the adverse effects for the patient.

Antibiotics are not effective against viral, parasitic, or fungal infections and other antimicrobials are

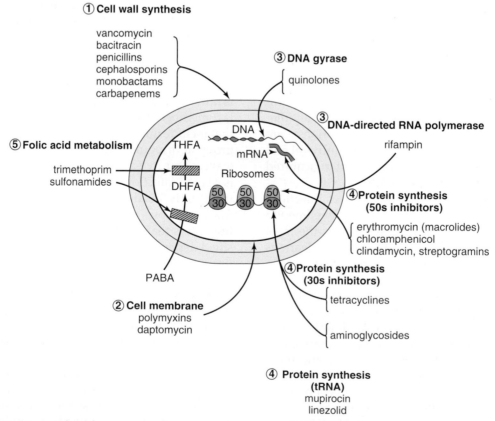

FIGURE 12-1 Sites of antimicrobial bactericidal or bacteriostatic action on bacterial pathogens. Five general actions include: (1) inhibition of synthesis or building of cell wall; (2) damage to cell membrane; (3) modificiation of nucleic acid (NA) NA synthesis; (4) modification of protein synthesis (at ribosomes); and (5) modification of energy metabolism within the cytoplasm (at the folate cycle). *PABA*, paraaminobenzoic acid; *DHFA*, dihydrofolic acid; *THFA*, tetrahydrofolic acid.

required. However, it is common for a patient with a viral or fungal infection to also develop a bacterial infection, because the body's defenses are weakened. A *secondary infection* occurs when one infection follows another. In a *mixed infection,* both infections are present at the same time.

Antibiotics may cause adverse or negative reactions. These include:

- allergy (penicillin and sulfa products cause the most allergies);
- ototoxicity, nephrotoxicity, and hepatotoxicity (damage to the ears, kidneys, and liver that may or may not be reversible if medication is stopped);
- and gastrointestinal (GI) distress so severe that it may require stopping the drug.

Antibiotics can also result in **superinfection,** when other organisms that are not sensitive to a prescribed antibiotic (for example, yeast) are able to multiply, overgrow, and get out of control because the antibiotic also killed the normal bacterias that would have kept them under control. Pseudomembranous colitis is a condition now commonly seen in hospital and nursing homes that arise from superinfections caused by *Clostridium difficile.* When an antibiotic is given when the body's natural immune system would have been effective, given for the wrong bacteria or for a virus for which it is ineffective, the pathogens are not destroyed and may become stronger. Overuse or unnecessary use of antibiotics has led to several current problems in using antibiotics: (1) patients expect and demand a prescription every time they feel ill; (2) the organisms that were weak may all have been killed over the years, leaving only the very virulent or strong pathogens; and (3) exposing organisms to antibiotics that did not kill them has led to the development of "super germs" that have built up a tolerance or resistance to common antibiotics. The result of these factors is that many common organisms infecting patients are now resistant to available drugs, and new antiinfectives have not yet been developed to fight them (Figure 12-2). Because many bacteria have developed resistance to multiple drugs, vancomycin may be a drug of last resort in many patients. Vancomycin is effective against some gram-positive bacteria that are resistant to multiple drugs and is used in cases of severe infection. Even now vancomycin has been found to be ineffective in some parts of the country for methicillin resistant streptococcus A (MRSA) infections. It is frightening to realize that there are common bacteria now for which we have no effective antibiotics. It may take several years before researchers are able to find new antiinfective drugs, and many patients may be left without effective drugs when they really do need them. One thing that can be done is to take special consideration to monitor antimicrobial use in children.

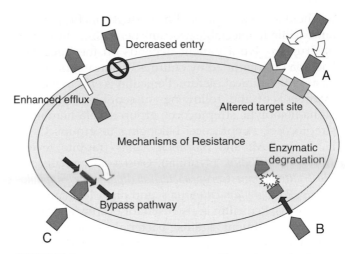

FIGURE 12-2 (Acquired bacterial resistance The major mechanisms of bacterial resistance to antibiotics are shown. These mechanisms include: (1) altered receptors or targets to which the drug cannot bind, (2) increased destruction or inactivation of the drug, (3) synthesis of resistant metabolic pathways, and (4) a decrease in the concentration of drug that reaches the receptors (by altered rates of entry or removal of drug).

Lifespan Considerations
Pediatric

ANTIMICROBIALS

- Whenever possible, blood, sputum, urine, or tissue cultures (depending on the symptoms) should be collected before beginning any antimicrobial. Once the patient has received an antibiotic, the cultures are not reliable.
- Review special dosage considerations for young children, especially those who will receive intravenous (IV) antibiotics. Safety is always important. Confirm any dosage calculations with another nurse to avoid making a dosage error; errors in children may have even more dramatic results than in adults.
- Young children who have not had previous antibiotics should be closely observed for allergic reactions.

ANTIBIOTICS

PENICILLINS

ACTION

Penicillins interfere with the creation and repair of the cell wall of the bacteria. They also bind or stick to specific enzymes that the bacteria needs so that the bacteria cannot use them. This process makes the bacterial cell weak and allows it to break down more easily (see figure 12-2).

USES

Penicillins were first used on a wide scale in the 1940's and were the main antibiotics for many years. Penicillin is the broad-spectrum drug of choice for susceptible gram-positive and gram-negative organisms. Penicillins are considered the safest antibiotics.

There are many penicillin products, including oral amoxicillin to injectable procaine penicillin. The choice of drug to give a patient depends on the infectious bacteria (as identified by cultures or smears) or on the basis of the clinical picture. Penicillin is effective in the treatment of the following susceptible organisms: alpha-hemolytic streptococci; group A beta-hemolytic streptococci; streptococci belonging to groups C, G, H, L, and M; and *Spirillum minus* (rat-bite fever), *Treponema pallidum* (syphilis), *Clostridium perfringens, Clostridium tetani, Corynebacterium diphtheriae, Staphylococcus, Pasteurella meningitidis,* and other less common organisms. Penicillin is also used for prophylactic (preventive) treatment against bacterial endocarditis in patients with rheumatic or congenital heart disease before they have dental procedures or surgery of the upper respiratory tract, genitourinary tract, or GI tract. Some penicillins may be useful against organisms used by terrorists as bioweapons.

As broad spectrum antibiotics, penicillin has been used for almost every type of infection, including those for which they were not effective. Over the years, overuse and inappropriate use of penicillin has led to the development of penicillin-resistant strains of disease. These penicillin-resistant strains of bacteria produce a chemical called *penicillinase*. β-lactamase (penicillinase) is an enzyme that disrupts the internal structure of penicillin and thus destroys the antimicrobial action of the drug. Although penicillin continues to be an important antibiotic, research on penicillin has led to the identification of many other types of antibiotics that may now be used to control infection.

ADVERSE REACTIONS

Adverse reactions to penicillin are many. Major reactions include neuropathy (nerve damage in a variety of places and seen with high parenteral dosages), fixed drug eruptions (usually a single spot that itches), nausea, vomiting, epigastric distress, anemia, and blood dyscrasias. Allergy to penicillin has also become a problem, producing rash, erythema (redness or inflammation), urticaria (hives), angioedema (swelling of the skin and mucous membranes), laryngeal edema (swelling of the larynx), and anaphylaxis (shock). These allergic reactions may occur suddenly or after the patient has been taking the medicine for some time and may be life threatening. They may occur up to 10% of the time in patients taking penicillin products.

DRUG INTERACTIONS

Other bacteriostatic antibiotics such as tetracycline and erythromycin may decrease the bactericidal effect of penicillin. Probenecid prolongs blood levels of penicillin by blocking its renal clearance. Use of ampicillin and oral contraceptives together has produced menstrual irregularities and unplanned pregnancies because penicillin reduces the level of available hormone. Indomethacin, phenylbutazone, or aspirin may increase serum penicillin levels. Antacids may decrease the absorption of penicillin. Penicillin may change the results of some laboratory tests. For example, penicillin may cause increased bleeding time when the platelet count is normal, giving a false positive urine protein test and lupus erythematosus cell test.

 Clinical Pitfall

Drug Interactions and Women

Women who are taking oral birth control pills should use another backup method of protection if they begin taking an antibiotic. Many antibiotics, including penicillin, interfere with the action of birth control pills, leaving the woman at risk of pregnancy while taking antibiotics.

❖ NURSING IMPLICATIONS AND PATIENT TEACHING

The patient in need of antibiotic therapy may vary from being asymptomatic (showing no symptoms) to being severely ill. Look for common clues to infection, such as fever, redness, swelling, or pain.

Ask whether there is a prior history of penicillin allergy, asthma, or hypersensitivity (allergy) to procaine or tartrazine, and find out if the patient is pregnant or breastfeeding. These conditions may be contraindications or precautions to the use of penicillin. Anaphylactic (shock) reactions have occurred with both oral and parenteral penicillin therapy. Penicillin should be used with caution in patients who have many other drug allergies.

 Clinical Goldmine

Antibiotic Therapy

Whenever possible, cultures should be drawn before starting antibiotic therapy. The nurse may be asked to culture sputum, urine, blood, wound, or nonhealing sites on the skin.

With intramuscular (IM) injections, follow institutional policy about whether to aspirate (pull back on the plunger of the syringe to check for blood) to prevent medicine from accidentally being injected into a blood vessel.

Patients often spread infections to family or friends. For example, the sexual partners of patients infected with syphilis or gonorrhea must be treated also.

Penicillin changes the results of many laboratory tests, so while the patient is on penicillin therapy, the results of laboratory culture and sensitivity tests, as well as many other laboratory findings, may be incorrect.

The type and dosage of penicillin ordered depends on the pathogen and severity of the infection. Over the years, several different types of penicillin have been developed: natural penicillins (Penicillins G and V), penicillinase resistant drugs; broad-spectrum amino-penicillins; and other types of broad-spectrum drugs. Table 12-1 presents a summary of penicillins.

Take the patient's blood pressure and pulse before giving IM penicillin injections to have baseline information. The patient should be advised the first time they receive this medicine to wait 30 minutes after administration by mouth (PO) or IM administration before leaving an office or clinic. This allows time to watch for signs of adverse reactions. Also watch the patient for signs of allergic reaction, although some allergic responses may not develop for days after taking the medication.

TETRACYCLINES

ACTION

The tetracyclines are bacteriostatic agents. They act by interfering with the ability of the bacterial to make protein. Without this protein, the bacteria cannot stay alive.

USES

The tetracyclines are important broad-spectrum drugs and they are effective against many gram-negative and gram-positive organisms (see Table 12-2 on p. 170). Many other drugs are more effective so that tetracyclines are the first choice drugs in only a few diseases, such as Lyme disease, stomach ulcers caused by *Helicobacter pylori, Chlamydia,* Rocky Mountain spotted fever, cholera, and typhus. Many adolescents use tetracycline-based products in the prevention or treatment of acne.

ADVERSE REACTIONS

The tetracyclines are relatively safe, with very few serious adverse effects. They commonly produce mild episodes of nausea, vomiting, and diarrhea that may require stopping the drug. These effects are often dose related, and they result from GI irritation, changes in the normal bacteria in the bowel, and overgrowth of yeast.

The use of tetracycline in pregnancy and in children younger than 8 years of age may produce permanent yellow-brown tooth discoloration or inadequate bone or tooth development.

Photosensitivity may occur with tetracycline treatment, so the patient should avoid exposure to the sun or ultraviolet rays. Pregnant women should not use tetracyclines because they are category D agents which may damage the fetus.

Tetracycline should be used with caution in patients with poor liver function, because the drug may cause hepatotoxicity.

Superinfections may develop, particularly after long-term use. These reactions, such as diarrhea, oral thrush (*Candida* infection of the mouth), or vaginal itching, are usually irritating but mild. At other times, the superinfection may become life threatening. Overgrowth of organisms is commonly seen in AIDS patients, whose immune systems may be totally overwhelmed by a mild superinfection.

Vertigo may develop with the use of any of the tetracyclines; however, vertigo is more common with the use of minocycline.

DRUG INTERACTIONS

Patients should not drink milk or take any dairy or calcium while taking these medications. Tetracyclines bind with calcium and iron and may reduce the drug's absorption up to 50%. Tetracycline is best taken with water on an empty stomach 1 hour before eating or 2 hours after eating.

❖ NURSING IMPLICATIONS AND PATIENT TEACHING

Tetracycline products that are out of date (older than the expiration date on the label) should not be used, because it may lead to damage of the proximal renal tubules.

Doxycycline (Vibramycin) is a particularly good drug, especially for the older adult population because it may be taken twice daily and is usually tolerated even by some individuals who have reduced renal function.

MACROLIDES

ACTION

Macrolides such as erythromycin are either bacteriocidal or bacteriostatic depending on the organisms and the dose used. Marcolides weaken the bacteria by limiting the production of protein, which is essential to the life of the bacteria.

USES

The macrolides are used as alternatives to penicillin for many infections for which organisms have developed penicillin resistance. They are the drugs of choice in *Streptococcus* infections, *Haemophilus influenza, Mycoplasma pneumoniae,* and *Chlamydia* infections. They are also used in legionnaires disease and in the treatment of pertussis ("whooping cough").

ADVERSE REACTIONS

Macrolides are associated with very few serious side effects. They are often considered a safe first choice for patients with uncomplicated infection. Mild abdominal pain, nausea, and diarrhea are the most common effects. Watch for signs of superinfection.

Table 12-1 Penicillins

GENERIC NAME	TRADE NAME	COMMENTS
Natural Penicillins		
penicillin G (benzathine)	Bicillin Permapen	Long-acting IM penicillin. In children, administer parenterally in midlateral aspect of thigh. In adults, give IM in gluteal muscle. Oral dosage exhibits poor absorption and is not recommended for routine use.
penicillin G (potassium)	Pfizerpen	Given primarily to infants and children IV as 15-30 min infusions.
penicillin G (procaine, aqueous) (APPG)	Wycillin Bicillin-CR	Contains procaine to decrease injection pain; determine if patient is allergic to procaine. Give deep IM injection in gluteal muscle; aspirate before injection; rotate injection sites. Drug of choice for gonorrhea.
penicillin V ★		Stable in gastric juices; however, blood levels are higher when administered on an empty stomach. 125 mg, 250 mg, and 500 mg is equivalent to 200,000, 400,000, and 800,000 units, respectively.
penicillin V potassium		Used in treatment of mild to moderately severe infections when patient can take oral medication.
Penicillinase Resistant		
cloxacillin		Effective in treatment of *pneumococci;* also effective in treatment of group A beta-hemolytic *streptococci.*
dicloxacillin		Effective in treatment of penicillinase-producing *staphylococci.*
nafcillin		
oxacillin		Rare, reversible hepatocellular dysfunction has been reported.
Aminopenicillins: Broad-Spectrum Penicillins		
amoxicillin	Amoxil Moxilin Sumox Trimox	
amoxicillin and clavulanate potassium	Augmentin	
ampicillin	Principen	
ampicillin sodium (parenteral)		Used in treatment of a variety of serious infections and often used concomitantly with a sodium aminoglycoside or a cephalosporin.
ampicillin sodium and sulbactam sodium	Unasyn	Give either IV or IM.
bacampicillin		
Extended Spectrum		
Carbenicillin	Geocillin, Geopen	Available in both IV and IM form.
Mezlocillin	Mezlin	Available in IV form.
piperacillin		Effective against a wide number of gram-positive and gram-negative aerobic and anaerobic bacteria.
piperacillin sodium and tazobactam sodium	Zosyn	Administer by IV infusion over 30 min.
ticarcillin	Ticar	Uncomplicated urinary tract infection.
ticarcillin and clavulanate sodium	Timentin	Reduced dosage required in patient with renal impairment.

IM, Intramuscular; *IV,* intravenous.
★ Indicates "Must-Know Drugs," or the 35 drugs most prescribers use.

DRUG INTERACTIONS

Macrolides increase the action of oral anticoagulants, digoxin, and many other drugs and thus may produce both drug and kidney toxicity. A drug handbook should be consulted whenever other drugs are given along with a macrolide. Anesthetic agents and anticonvulsant drugs may interact to cause high serum drug levels and toxicity.

❖ NURSING IMPLICATIONS AND PATIENT TEACHING

The major differences between erythromycin and the newer macrolides include better GI tolerability, a broader spectrum of activity, and less dosing frequency for the newer products. Giving the medication with food reduces GI irritation.

Caution should be used when this drug is given with any other medication because of the risk of drug-drug interactions and increase of adverse effects.

The strength of erythromycin varies by product. The strength of different products are reported as the erythromycin base equivalence. Because of differences in absorption, 400 mg of ethylsuccinate is required to provide the same free erythromycin serum levels as 250 mg of erythromycin base, stearate, or estolate. This accounts for the differences in doses of different erythromycin products.

Many macrolides may be administered orally or parenterally. Topical application should be avoided to prevent sensitization. The patient should be kept well hydrated (supplied with fluids). Drinking extra fluids to ensure a minimum urine output of 1500 mL decreases the chances of renal toxicity.

All chewable forms of erythromycin must be fully chewed to obtain the complete therapeutic effect.

AMINOGLYCOSIDES

ACTION

Aminoglycosides weaken the bacteria by limiting the production of protein, which is essential to the life of the bacteria.

USES

These products, such as gentamycin and amikacin, are used in the treatment of serious aerobic gram-negative infections, including those caused by *Escherichia coli*, *Serratia*, *Proteus*, *Klebsiella*, and *Pseudomonas*; aerobic gram-negative bacteria, mycobacteria, and some protozoans. Streptomycin (SM) is used in the treatment of TB. Some products are used to sterilize the bowel before intestinal surgery.

ADVERSE REACTIONS

Aminoglycosides may cause serious adverse effects including damage to the kidney (nephrotoxicity) that is usually reversible if the drug is stopped quickly.

They may also produce permanent damage to the inner ear (ototoxicity), hearing impairment, dizziness, loss of balance, ringing in the ears, and persistent headache. Aminoglycosides have a narrow therapeutic range, so the blood levels of these drugs should be closely watched to avoid toxic levels. Dosage is calculated on the basis of the patient's weight and is increased or decreased based on blood levels so an effective level is maintained. The narrow therapeutic range (when the lowest and highest acceptable drug levels are not far apart) requires that the sample for the antibiotic blood level be drawn just before the next scheduled dose is given. This sample will show the lowest blood level of the antibiotic (found at the "trough"), rather than a blood level at a higher range (at or near the "peak"). The lowest blood level will determine whether the dosage needs to be adjusted to stay within the therapeutic range and not go above the toxic level or below the effective level. Because of the nephrotoxicity of these agents, blood urea nitrogen and creatinine levels must also be monitored during the course of therapy.

DRUG INTERACTIONS

Using this drug with many products, particularly vancomycin, increases the risk of nephrotoxicity. Ototoxicity is also increased with aspirin, furosemide, ethacrynic acid, and many other drugs.

❖ NURSING IMPLICATIONS AND PATIENT TEACHING

Some of these products are available over-the-counter (OTC) or by prescription for eye, ear, or skin infections. When given for systemic bacterial infections they must be given parenterally as they are poorly absorbed from the GI tract.

Patients should have frequent hearing and urine tests to monitor for nephrotoxicity and ototoxicity.

FLUOROQUINOLONES

ACTION

Fluroquinolones are bacteriocidal and act by interfering with bacterial DNA synthesis, which makes it difficult for the pathogens to reproduce themselves and attack other cells.

USES

There are four generations of fluoroquinolones, which are all effective against gram-negative pathogens. The newer ones are significantly more effective against gram-positive microbes. These agents are used as alternatives to other antibiotics in the treatment of respiratory, GI, gynecologic, skin, and soft-tissue infections. Ciprofloxin (Cipro) is the drug of choice for anthrax exposure in a bioterrorist attack.

ADVERSE REACTIONS

Fluoroquinolones are generally viewed as safe drugs for most patients. Nausea, vomiting, and diarrhea are the most common side effects and may occur in up to 20% of patients. Patients may also have headache, dizziness, and abnormal heart rhythms.

DRUG INTERACTIONS

Fluoroquinolones should not be taken with multivitamins or mineral supplements because they reduce the absorption of the antibiotic by as much as 90%. When taken with warfarin, fluoroquinolones will increase warfarin's anticoagulant effects. Antacids and ferrous sulfate may decrease absorption of the drugs. Patients may develop excessive nervousness, anxiety, or tachycardia if taken with coffee or other caffeine-containing products.

❖ NURSING IMPLICATIONS AND PATIENT TEACHING

Fluoroquinolones are well absorbed orally and may be given only once or twice per day. Take drug with food to decrease adverse GI effects.

CEPHALOSPORINS

ACTION

Cephalosporins are bactericidal and weaken the bacteria by interfering with building of the bacteria's cell wall.

USES

There are four generations of cephalosporins, all of which have broad spectrum activity against gram-negative organisms. In general, second- and third-generation drugs are more effective and more potent than first-generation agents against a broad group of gram-negative organisms; however, they are also less effective against gram-positive organisms. Third-generation agents are also more effective against inactivation by beta-lactamase (an enzyme that some organisms make to protect them against the action of some antibiotics). However, these agents cost more and may have more side effects. Differences among drugs within categories are primarily based on the drug's activity. Later-generation drugs are more effective against some of the organisms to which earlier generation agents have been resistant.

Cephalosporins are used for serious infections, like bacteremia and septicemia (infections of the blood); and infections of the lower respiratory tract, central nervous system (CNS), genitourinary system, joints, and bones. These drugs are also used in patients who cannot take penicillin.

ADVERSE REACTIONS

Nausea, vomiting, and diarrhea are frequent. The most common adverse effect is acute hypersensitivity. Although some patients may have only a minor rash and itching, anaphylaxis is possible. There may be severe pain at the injection site. Nephrotoxicity has been reported with some cephalosporins, and the incidence is greater in older adult patients and in patients with poor renal function.

DRUG INTERACTIONS

Alcohol taken with these products may produce a severe disulfiram reaction resulting in severe flushing, vomiting, and collapse. Other products, such as probenecid, may decrease elimination of the drugs by the kidneys.

❖ NURSING IMPLICATIONS AND PATIENT TEACHING

Must be given by the IV or IM route because it is not absorbed from the GI tract.

Patients who have had a recent and severe reaction to penicillin should not be prescribed these products.

SULFONAMIDES

ACTION

Sulfonamides have a bacteriostatic effect against a wide range of gram-positive and gram-negative microorganisms by inhibiting folic acid synthesis, which is essential for cell growth and function.

USES

Sulfonamides are usually used to treat acute and chronic urinary tract infections, particularly cystitis, pyelitis, and pyelonephritis caused by *E. coli* or *Nocardia asteroides*. Other indications include toxoplasmosis, acute otitis media caused by *H. influenzae*, and preventive therapy in cases of recurrent rheumatic fever. Susceptible organisms include *Streptococcus pyogenes*, *Streptococcus pneumoniae*, some strains of *Bacillus anthracis*, *C. diphtheriae*, *Haemophilus ducreyi*, *Chlamydia trachomatis*, and other less common organisms. Several sulfonamides are useful only in the treatment of ulcerative colitis, and as preoperative and postoperative therapy for bowel surgery.

ADVERSE REACTIONS

Adverse reactions to sulfonamides include many minor but irritating problems such as headache, drowsiness, fatigue, dizziness, vertigo (feeling of dizziness or spinning), tinnitus (ringing in the ears), hearing loss, insomnia (inability to sleep), anorexia (lack of appetite), nausea, vomiting, stomatitis (inflammation of the mouth), abdominal pain, rash, fever, malaise (weakness), pruritus (itching), dermatitis, local irritation, anaphylactic shock, crystalluria (formation of crystals in the urine), hematuria (blood in the urine), and proteinuria (large amounts of protein in the urine) may develop with overdosage and indicate that the patient may have a severe hypersensitivity to sulfonamides.

 Clinical Goldmine

Superinfection

The nurse watches for signs of superinfections, or overgrowth of normal bacteria, that may show up in the oral, vaginal, or rectal areas. These might be white, odorous discharges or areas of pus or evidence of new infection.

DRUG INTERACTIONS

Sulfonamides may increase the effect of oral anticoagulants, methotrexate, sulfonylureas, thiazide diuretics, phenytoin, and uricosuric agents. Many other drugs taken at the same time will cause the effects of sulfonamides to be increased. Penicillins may be less effective when given with a sulfonamide. The sulfonamide's effect may be decreased by local anesthetics. Antacids may cause less absorption of the sulfonamide. Sulfonamides may change the results of various laboratory tests including urine glucose.

❖ NURSING IMPLICATIONS AND PATIENT TEACHING

Warn the patient to stay out of the sun, because severe photosensitivity (abnormal response to exposure to sunlight) can occur if the patient's skin is exposed to excessive amounts of sunlight or ultraviolet light.

Sulfonamide dosage depends on the severity of the infection being treated, the drug used, and the patient's response to and tolerance of the drug. Generally, the short-acting sulfonamides are given at more frequent intervals than are the intermediate- or long-acting sulfonamides. Also, short-acting sulfonamides usually require a special first dose (initial loading dose) that is larger than the dose that will be regularly taken.

Sulfonamides are more fully and quickly absorbed when they are taken on an empty stomach. They should be taken either 1 hour before or 2 hours after meals, along with a full glass of water.

To prevent formation of crystals in the urine, the patient must drink large amounts of water while taking this medication.

It is particularly important with these drugs that the patient should take all the medication prescribed and not stop just because the symptoms have disappeared, so they do not have a relapse.

The health care provider should be notified quickly if a skin rash, blood in the urine, bruises, nausea, or other adverse effects of therapy develop because these may indicate development of more severe reactions.

MISCELLANEOUS ANTIINFECTIVE DRUGS

There are many other antiinfective agents on the market, some representing drug classes that are no longer widely used, some with very narrow uses, and some new drugs, which nurses may occasionally see ordered. Two of the most important, carbapenem and vancomycin, are described here in greater detail. A selection of other drugs are presented only in Table 12-2.

MISCELLANEOUS AGENT—CARBAPENEM

ACTION

Carbapenem is a broad-spectrum antibiotics are effective against gram-positive and gram-negative bacteria. They penetrate bacterial cells and interfere with the making of vital cell wall parts, which leads to cell death, making them bactericidal.

USES

Carbapenem is used in acute infections caused by bacterial meningitis, intraabdominal infections, skin, and skin structure infections.

ADVERSE REACTIONS

Carbapenem may produce pseudomembranous colitis, hypersensitivity reactions, and impaired renal function.

Nausea, vomiting, diarrhea, headache, rash, sepsis, constipation, apnea, shock, and pruritus were all reported.

DRUG INTERACTIONS

Carbapenem competes with probenecid, so these drugs should not be given at the same time. The drug may reduce the activity of valproic acid, which is given to prevent seizures.

❖ NURSING IMPLICATIONS AND PATIENT TEACHING

Carbapenem is administered intravenously. Reduced dose is required in patients with reduced kidney function. Watch for adverse effects, as they are frequent.

MISCELLANEOUS AGENT—VANCOMYCIN

ACTION

This drug is bacteriocidal, inhibiting the building of the bacterial cell-wall.

USES

Vancomycin is an antibiotic usually reserved for severe gram-positive infections such as *Staphylococcus aureus* and *Pneumocystis pneumoniae*. It is one of the powerful antibiotics to which most organisms are still sensitive

Table 12-2 | Broad-Spectrum Antibiotics

Tetracyclines

demeclocycline	Declomycin	Frequently associated with photosensitivity and anaphylactoid reactions. Has intermediate duration of action but broad spectrum.
doxycycline	Vibramycin Periostat	Used to prevent traveler's diarrhea. It may be taken with food. Long acting. Also available in IV form.
minocycline	Minocin Dynacin	Has delayed kidney excretion, as compared with other tetracyclines. Half-life is 11-20 hr.
oxytetracycline	Terramycin	Short-acting. Available in IM and IV forms. Diarrhea common. Give deep IM injection in gluteal mass. If pain persists after injection, ice may be applied to the area. Avoid rapid IV administration.
tetracycline	Achromycin Emtet Panmycin Sumycin Tetra 250	Short-acting. IM and topical forms available.

Macrolides

azithromycin	Zithromax Zmax	Dosage may be increased with severity of infection. Available in IV form.
clarithromycin	Biaxin	
dirithromycin	Dynabac	Take with food to enhance drug activity.
erythromycin	EES E-Mycin Erythromycin Ilosone	Comes as base or as one of five other preparations.

Aminoglycosides

amikacin	Amikin	May be used to treat unidentified infections before results of sensitivity tests are known. Do not mix with other drugs.
gentamicin	Garamycin Genoptic Genoptic SOP Gentacidin Gentak G-mycin Jenamicin	Used to treat unidentified infections. Do not mix with carbenicillin or other drugs. Available in IV, topical, and ophthalmic forms.
Kanamycin	Kantrex	Most commonly used to sterilize bowel prior to colon surgery. Available in PO, inhalation, and IV forms.
neomycin	Mycifradin Neo-fradin Neo-Tabs	Used in preoperative preparation for surgery. Oral, topical, and IV forms available.
netilmicin	Netromycin	Used in intestinal amebiasis and hepatic coma. Effective against gentamicin-resistant bacteria. Available IV.
paromomycin	Humatin	Used in treatment of hepatic coma and for parasitic infections of the intestine.
Streptomycin	Streptomycin	Used primarily for treatment of TB. Also used for tularemia and plague.
tobramycin	Nebcin	May be used in combination with penicillin or cephalosporin in treatment of unidentified infections before results of sensitivity tests are known. Do not premix with other drugs. Available in IV form.

Fluoroquinolones

		Medications are excreted primarily by renal mechanism. All dosages must be adjusted in patients with impaired renal function.
		Dosage adjustment necessary for those with decreased kidney function. Keep patients well hydrated.

Table 12-2   **Broad-Spectrum Antibiotics—cont'd**

Cinoxacin	Cinobac	Used for UTI treatment.
Ciprofloxacin	Cipro, Septra Proquin XR	Used in many infections of skin, bone, joint, and lungs. Also approved for treatment and prophylaxis of anthrax.
enoxacin	Penetrex	For treatment of UTI and gonorrhea.
gatifloxacin	Tequin	For treatment UTI, gonorrhea, and respiratory infections. Available IV.
gemifloxacin	Factive	For treatment of respiratory infections.
levofloxacin	Levaquin Quixin	For treatment of respiratory and skin infections. IV forms available.
lomefloxacin	Maxaquin	For treatment of UTI and respiratory infections.
Moxifloxacin	Avelox	For respiratory and sinus infections.
norfloxacin	Noroxin	For UTI and eye infections; ophthalmic form available.
ofloxacin	Floxin Ocuflox	For treatment of respiratory infections, UTI, and gonorrhea.
sparfloxacin	Zagam	For treatment of respiratory infections.
trovafloxacin	Trovan	For treatment of sinuses, respiratory tract, gonorrhea. IV form available.
Cephalosporins		
First Generation cefadroxil	Duricef Ultracef	
Cefazolin	Ancef, Kefzol	Available IV.
cephalexin	Keflex	
Second Generation cefaclor	Ceclor Raniclor	
cefamandole	Mandol	Available IV.
cefonicid	Monocid	Available IV.
cefoxitin	Mefoxin	Recommended by CDC in treatment schedules for gonorrhea and acute pelvic inflammatory disease.
cefprozil	Cefzil	
cefuroxime	Ceftin	Available IV and IM.
	Zinacef	See CDC treatment schedules for gonorrhea and acute pelvic inflammatory disease.
Third Generation cefdinir	Omnicef	Used in community-acquired pneumonia, chronic bronchitis, acute bacterial otitis media, acute maxillary sinusitis, pharyngitis/tonsillitis, and uncomplicated skin infections.
Cefixime	Suprax	
cefotaxime	Claforan	Give IV or IM.
cefpodoxime	Vantin	
ceftazidime	Ceptaz Fortaz Tazicef Tazidime	
ceftibuten	Cedax	
ceftizoxime	Cefizox	
ceftriaxone	Rocephin	IV form available.

Continued

Table 12-2 Broad-Spectrum Antibiotics—cont'd

Fourth Generation		
cefepime	Maxipime	Used in urinary tract infection, pneumonia, skin infections. Give IV or IM according to dosing schedule in package insert.
Sulfonamides		
sulfadiazine		Requires daily urinary output of at least 1500 mL plus alkalization to prevent crystalluria; subcutaneous and IM routes contraindicated. Used in UTI, rheumatic fever prophylaxis, and intraocular infections.
sulfamethizole		Short-acting, readily soluble sulfonamide effective in treatment of UTIs.
sulfasalazine	Azulfidine Azulfidine En-Tabs	*Ulcerative colitis:* Used in treatment of ulcerative colitis.

sulfonamide
  combination
  vaginal product
	Sultrin
	Triple Sulfa
	Trysul
		Contains equal amounts of sulfathiazole, sulfabenzamide, and sulfacetamide; reduces possibility of crystalluria because solubility of each sulfonamide exists independently in solution. Foam used in vaginal infections.

Sulfonamide Mixtures		
Trimethoprim/ sulfamethoxazole	Bactrim ✦ Bactrim DS Bactrim SS Septra Septra DS Sulfatrim	Used for acute urinary tract and otitis media infections and prophylaxis; may be used in patients with impaired renal function and for those unable to tolerate sulfonamides alone.
Miscellaneous Antiinfectives		
carbapenem	Merrem	Available IV for serious infections such as bacterial meningitis, skin and abdominal infections.
bacitracin		Used primarily OTC for minor skin infections.
colistimethate	Coly-Mycin M	Do not exceed 5 mg/kg/day in patients with normal renal function. Dosage must be altered in patients with impaired renal function.
colistin	Coly-Mycin S Otic	
polymyxin B		Do not exceed 30,000 units/kg/day. IM administration not recommended because of severe pain at injection site.
spectinomycin	Trobicin	
vancomycin	Vancocin	Should be administered IV only for treating MRSA, not IM. Rapid IV administration may cause hypotension and "red man" syndrome. Dilute solution in 200 mL of glucose or saline solution and infuse over a 60- to 90-minute period. IV infusion may cause thrombophlebitis. Drug of choice in treating *Staphylococcus* bacteria.
Ketolides		
telithromycin	Ketek	Has low potential to produce macrolide-type resistance. Rapid bactericidal activity.
Chloramphenicol		
chloramphenicol	Chloromycetin	Give PO on empty stomach. Switch from IV to oral form as soon as possible.
Lincosamides		
clindamycin	Cleocin	Give deep IM injection. Single IM injections that total 600 mg or greater not recommended. For IV therapy, do not administer as bolus. For oral administration, take on empty stomach with a full glass of water.
lincomycin	Bactramycin Lincocin Lincoject	

CDC, Centers for Disease Control and Prevention; *IM*, intramuscular; *IV*, intravenous; *MRSA*, methicillin-resistant *Staphylococcus aureus*; *OTC*, over the counter; *PO*, by mouth; *TB*, tuberculosis; *UTI*, urinary tract infection.

Table 12-3   Sensitivity of Specific Organisms to Some Broad-Spectrum Antibiotics

ANTIBIOTIC	SUSCEPTIBLE ORGANISMS AND CLINICAL DISEASE
aminoglycosides	Effective in treatment of gram-negative infections when penicillin contraindicated.
bacitracin	Restricted to use in severe illness. Effective in treatment of staphylococcal pneumonia or empyema in infants.
clindamycin	Used to treat severe infections caused by streptococci, pneumococci, staphylococci, or anaerobic bacteria when penicillin and erythromycin contraindicated.
erythromycin	Alternative treatment for patients hypersensitive to penicillins.
lincomycin	Used to treat severe infections caused by susceptible strains of streptococci, pneumococci, and staphylococci when penicillin and erythromycin contraindicated.
polymyxin B	Effective against all gram-negative organisms, with exception of *Proteus.* Effective in treatment of acute infections caused by susceptible strains of *Pseudomonas aeruginosa, Haemophilus influenzae, Escherichia coli, Enterobacter aerogenes,* and *Klebsiella pneumoniae.* Reserved for multidrug-resistant infections.
spectinomycin	Drug of choice to treat gonorrhea in patients hypersensitive to penicillins and to treat penicillinase-producing gonorrhea.
telithromycin	New product for mild to moderate respiratory infections; used for *Streptococcus pneumoniae, H. influenzae,* in acute bacterial exacerbation, chronic bronchitis, acute sinusitis, community-acquired pneumonia.
tetracyclines	Used to treat granuloma inguinale, rickettsial diseases, mycoplasmal infections, spirochetal relapsing fever, and *Chlamydia trachomatis.* Indicated in patients sensitive to penicillin, especially to treat gonorrhea or syphilis.
vancomycin	Used to treat severe infections in patients hypersensitive to penicillins or cephalosporins. Effective in treatment of staphylococcal endocarditis, osteomyelitis, pneumonia, soft-tissue infections, and methicillin-resistant staphylococcal infections. Oral dosage effective in treatment of staphylococcal enterocolitis.

(Table 12-3). It is used for treating methicillin-resistant *S. aureus* (MRSA) infections.

ADVERSE REACTIONS

May be associated with minor hypersensitivity reactions or anaphylaxis. This drug causes frequent but minor side effects such as rash on the upper body (red-man syndrome), flushing, and hypotension. Higher doses may produce nephrotoxicity and ototoxicity.

DRUG INTERACTIONS

This drug adds to the toxicity of other antibiotics such as the aminoglycosides, and other products that are ototoxic or nephrotoxic. Cholestyramine and colestipol decrease the absorption of the drug.

❖ NURSING IMPLICATIONS AND PATIENT TEACHING

This drug is usually given intravenously because it is not absorbed from the GI tract (Table 12-3).

Significant reactions to antibiotics are summarized in Table 12-4.

 Clinical Goldmine

Adverse Effects from Antibiotics

All drugs have the potential to damage the tissue of certain organs. The usual organs affected are the ear (ototoxicity to the auditory nerves), the kidney (nephrotoxicity), and the liver (hepatotoxicity). Certain antibiotics are much more likely to produce tissue damage than others. It is important to carefully identify patients who may already have damage to these organs before medication is started.

Clinical Pitfall

Allergy

Many individuals have allergic reactions to antibiotics. Allergic reactions may develop within minutes of taking the drug or may appear days after stopping the medication. Hypersensitivity may also develop after repeated use of the medication. Allergy may range from a mild skin rash or fever to severe and possibly fatal anaphylaxis, characterized by shortness of breath, paralysis of the diaphragm, laryngeal edema, and shock. Patients must be closely questioned each time antibiotic therapy is ordered to determine sensitivity reactions.

Table 12-4   Significant Adverse Reactions Produced by Specific Broad-Spectrum Antibiotics

ANTIBIOTIC	ADVERSE REACTION
aminoglycosides	Significant renal toxicity, which is usually reversible; risk of toxicity increases in patients with renal impairment. Significant auditory and vestibular ototoxicity may occur in patients on prolonged therapy or those taking higher than recommended dosages.
bacitracin	Renal toxicity leading to tubular and glomerular necrosis has been reported. Also, increased serum drug levels without an increase in drug dosage and severe pain and rash with IM injection are seen.
cephalosporins	Painful IM injections; thrombophlebitis with IV therapy. May produce hemolytic anemia and other blood dyscrasias.
clindamycin	Severe and fatal colitis characterized by abdominal cramps, diarrhea, and rectal passage of blood and mucus (these symptoms may not appear until after treatment is completed).
colistin	Renal toxicity; transient neurologic disturbances have been reported with colistimethate, as well as nephrotoxicity manifested by decreased urinary output and increased serum creatinine.
erythromycin	GI distress, sensorineural hearing loss, and hepatotoxicity possible.
lincomycin	Severe and fatal colitis characterized by abdominal cramps, diarrhea, or rectal passage of blood and mucus (these symptoms may not develop until treatment is completed). Hypotension and cardiac arrest may occur after rapid IV administration.
polymyxin B	Nephrotoxicity may develop, evidenced by proteinuria, cellular urinary casts, azotemia, decreased output, or elevated BUN. Neurotoxicity may be evidenced by irritability, weakness, drowsiness, ataxia, numbness of extremities, blurring of vision, or respiratory paralysis.
tetracycline	Black, "hairy" tongue possible; oral dosage effective in treatment of staphylococcal enterocolitis.
vancomycin	Nephrotoxicity with toxic effect increased at high serum levels or with prolonged therapy; ototoxicity may also occur.

BUN, Blood urea nitrogen; *GI*, gastrointestinal; *IM*, intramuscular; *IV*, intravenous.

Clinical Pitfall

Antibiotic Cross-Sensitivity

Cross-sensitivity exists with many antibiotics. Any person who has several drug allergies should be carefully watched when taking any type of antibiotic.

❖ NURSING IMPLICATIONS AND PATIENT TEACHING FOR ANTIBIOTICS IN GENERAL

▪ Assessment

Watch for common indicators of infection, such as fever, redness, swelling, or pain.

Find out as much as possible about the patient's health history, including prior renal damage, hepatic problems, systemic lupus erythematosus, alcoholism, or drugs that may interact with an antibiotic. Ask about pregnancy or breastfeeding, age, and occupation (i.e. If they are a cook in a restaurant or working with young children or are around people who are immunocompromised). These factors may be contraindications or precautions to antibiotic drug therapy.

▪ Diagnosis

Are there other factors that may pose a problem to the patient taking this drug? For example, patients reporting any previous allergy to one drug may also be allergic to some other drugs.

▪ Planning

Many broad-spectrum antibiotics cross the placental barrier and are secreted in breast milk.

Many of the parenteral antibiotics should be used with caution because of their toxic effects. Most antibiotics should be given with extreme caution to patients with poor renal function, but the risk of toxicity is low in patients with normal renal function.

▪ Implementation

The nurse should make certain the drugs are taken at the proper time in order to maintain blood levels of the antibiotic and for the full course of the therapy. The dosage depends on the type and the severity of the infection.

▪ Evaluation

Superinfection may occur in the patient who is taking extended antibiotic therapy. Monitor for infections in the mouth and the rectal or vaginal areas.

Because of the possibility of ototoxicity in patients taking vancomycin, watch for patient complaints of tinnitus, or ringing in the ears, which may be a sign that the patient is at risk for deafness.

With some broad-spectrum antibiotics, the nurse will monitor for liver toxicity by checking for abdominal pain, jaundice, dark urine, pale-colored stools, or weakness. Blood or mucus in the stools may indicate colitis. If large doses of antibiotics are given, the patient should be monitored closely for sensorineural hearing loss. Observe the patient for therapeutic effects, allergy, and superinfection.

■ Patient and Family Teaching

Tell the patient and family the following:

- If GI upset occurs, the patient should eat a few plain crackers with the medicine.
- The patient should take the drug exactly as prescribed, even after the symptoms disappear. Prematurely stopping the drug may lead to symptom relapse, reinfection, and development of drug resistant bacteria.
- The medication should not be saved, because out-of-date medication begins to deteoriate and may produce subtherapeutic doses.
- While taking this medication, the patient should check for signs of infection in the mouth and the anal or vaginal areas while bathing and brushing the teeth. These could be related to a superinfection.
- The patient should notify the health care provider if diarrhea develops and persists for more than 24 hours or if stools have blood or mucus.
- Liquid medication should be kept in a dark colored and light-resistant container.
- For those rare individuals who still test their urine for sugar, the patient with diabetes should know that many antibiotics change the results of a urine glucose test.
- The patient should be alert to the possibility of bone marrow depression after therapy is completed and promptly report any bruising, petechiae, sore throat, or weakness.
- A rash, hives, decreased urination, diarrhea, or other unusual symptoms may develop. Allergies can develop at any time after the patient begins treatment.
- If medication is given on an outpatient basis, 911 should be called immediately or the patient taken to an emergency room quickly if shortness of breath or difficulty breathing develops.

Table 12-5 presents a summary of the broad-spectrum antibiotics.

☀ ANTITUBERCULAR DRUGS

OVERVIEW

Tuberculosis is disease seen in ancient times and still found among poor and undernourished people. It is most commonly seen in underdeveloped nations where living conditions are crowded and unsanitary. However, it is also increasingly found in the United States among immigrants, drug users, alcoholics, and AIDS patients or others with lowered immunity. The

diagnosis of TB centuries ago was a death sentence. It is once again a frightening disease because so many drugs are no longer effective against it. It is primarily a disease of the lungs but may also be seen in bones, bladder, and other parts of the body. At present, most cases of infectious TB are found in people who have not been adequately treated with antitubercular medications and in people who contract primary TB as a result of reduced immunity from human immunodeficiency virus (HIV) infection. TB may once again become a major killer.

TB is caused by the bacterium *Mycobacterium tuberculosis,* which infects animals as well as humans. Multidrug-resistant (MDR) organisms (strains that are resistant to current drugs) are now commonly found and require vigorous methods of treatment to control infection. New guidelines for treatment of TB are published by the Centers for Disease Control and Prevention (CDC) almost every year. Because there are many new cases of TB, as well as numerous untreated cases, new state laws have been passed that take aggressive action against individuals who are infected with TB and refuse to take or complete adequate drug therapy. To control the high numbers of new cases of TB, in some states, uncooperative patients may actually be sent to prison until they have completed the required drug therapy and have been rendered noninfectious.

ACTION

The main action of antitubercular drugs take place both within or outside the cell wall of the bacteria that slow down the *M. tuberculosis* bacteria. Most drugs used to treat TB do not kill the bacterium, but they control the disease and prevent its spread to various organ systems in the infected patient or to other individuals. The drugs control the bacteria by preventing them from producing new cell walls, so new bacterial cell growth is limited. Some antitubercular drugs are bactericidal, killing the organism.

USES

Chemoprophylaxis, or taking a drug to prevent disease, is recommended when the patient is at high risk of developing active TB. The current duration of prophylactic treatment is 1 year. At present, isoniazid (INH) is the only drug recommended for prophylactic therapy. INH prophylaxis is not recommended for healthy individuals older than 35 because of their increased risk of developing hepatitis. Prophylaxis is recommended, however, if the patient is at special risk for developing TB, as indicated in Box 12-1. *Chemotherapy,* or taking a drug to treat disease, is recommended for patients with active tuberculosis.

Antitubercular drugs are classified as primary or secondary agents to describe the way they are used in treating TB. Most primary agents are

Table 12-5   Common Antitubercular Drugs

GENERIC NAME	TRADE NAME	COMMENTS
Primary Treatment Agents		
ethambutol	Myambutol ♣	Give once every 24 hr. When one other bactericidal drug is used in combination with this medication, therapy generally lasts 18-24 months. It has been used in twice-weekly regimens. Ethambutol may be taken with food; watch for optic neuritis, rash.
isoniazid	Isoniazid INH Nydrazid	Well absorbed after PO or IM administration. Dosage is determined by weight, with the usual adult dose being 5 mg/kg or 300 mg/day. Children require higher doses than adults. Give with pyridoxine to reduce incidence of peripheral neuropathies. Isoniazid is the drug of choice in the prophylactic treatment of TB infections. Watch for hepatic and neurologic toxicity.
pyrazinamide	Pyrazinamide ♣	Should be administered with at least one other antitubercular drug. Watch for hepatic toxicity and hyperuricemia, arthralgia, and arthritis.
rifampin	Rifadin Rimactane	Used in combination with other antitubercular drugs. Peak plasma concentrations occur 2-4 hr after ingestion. Watch for hepatic and hematologic toxicity.
rifapentine	Priftin	
streptomycin		Used in TB and also for other serious bacterial infections. May be given IM although injection is painful.
Retreatment Agents		
para-aminosalicylate (PAS)	Paser	May produce nausea, vomiting, diarrhea, or abdominal pain. Watch for GI distress, hepatitis.
capreomycin	Capastat Sulfate	Give deep IM. Watch for renal and eighth cranial nerve toxicity.
cycloserine	Seromycin Pulvules	Watch for psychoses, seizures, rash.
ethionamide	Trecator-SC	Take with meals or antacids to reduce GI distress. High percentage of patients cannot tolerate therapeutic dose. Dosages should never exceed 1 g/day. Usual dose is 0.5-1 g/day PO. Watch for hepatitis, GI distress, hypersensitivity.
kanamycin	Kantrex	Watch for renal and eighth cranial nerve toxicity.
Prevention In HIV Patients		
rifabutin	Mycobutin	Divided dose, taken with food, may decrease GI distress.

GI, Gastrointestinal; *IM*, intramuscular; *PO*, by mouth; *TB*, tuberculosis.

bactericidal and are necessary to sterilize the TB lesions. Secondary agents are generally less effective and more toxic than primary agents. They are used with primary agents for patients infected with partially or completely drug-resistant organisms or to treat lesions found outside the lungs.

ADVERSE REACTIONS

Mycobacterium tuberculosis is able to build up a resistance to antitubercular drugs. Use of a combination of drugs helps slow the development of bacterial resistance. Most of the antitubercular medications cause only mild and infrequent symptoms such as nausea, vomiting, and diarrhea. Most of these symptoms stop when the dosage is reduced. Some of the drugs used to treat TB are toxic to various parts of the body (for

example, the ears, kidneys, and liver). The patient must be watched closely to detect development of any of these more serious problems. All drugs are associated with some adverse reactions. Those for treating TB have many adverse reactions in the body. The most common or most serious are briefly described in the following text.

Capreomycin may cause headache, ototoxicity (hearing loss, tinnitus, vertigo), nephrotoxicity, abnormal liver function tests, maculopapular rash associated with febrile reaction, urticaria, muscle weakness, pain and swelling or excessive bleeding at the injection site, and sterile abscesses.

Ethambutol (EMB) is associated with dizziness, headache, confusion, dermatitis, abdominal pain, anorexia, nausea, vomiting, joint pain and swelling, optic neuritis (loss of vision), and loss of visual acuity.

Box 12-1	High-Priority Candidates for Tuberculosis-Preventive Therapy

Patients of all ages with a positive tuberculin test, no previous therapy, and the following:
- Known or suspected human immunodeficiency virus (HIV) infection
- Close contact with individuals with infectious, clinically active tuberculosis (TB)
- Recent tuberculin skin test conversion
- Employment in a health care job or correctional facility with exposure to large numbers of individuals who may get TB
- Medical problems that increase the risk of TB (for example, diabetes, immunosuppressive therapy, IV drug use, end-stage renal disease, malignancies, hemodialysis)
- Abnormal chest x-ray studies that show old fibrotic lesions

Patients younger than 35 years old with a positive tuberculin test, no additional risk factors, and the following:
- Being born in a high-prevalence country
- Residence in long-term care facilities (for example, nursing homes) or prisons
- Belonging to a medically underserved low-income population

Ethionamide may produce severe postural hypotension (low blood pressure when a person suddenly stands or sits up), mental depression, rash, anorexia, diarrhea, epigastric distress, jaundice, nausea, and vomiting.

INH is one of the most frequently used drugs. It may produce many neurologic disturbances in sensation and vision, as well as variable changes in electrolytes. As with many drugs, nausea, constipation, epigastric distress, and vomiting are common. Severe and sometimes fatal hepatitis may develop, even after many months of treatment. The drug also changes the results of a variety of laboratory tests. Symptoms of overdosage may occur any time from 30 minutes to 3 hours after the INH is administered. Nausea, vomiting, slurred speech, dizziness, impaired vision, and visual hallucinations may be among the early symptoms. Severe overdosage results in CNS depression, respiratory distress, coma, and severe intractable seizures.

Pyrazinamide (PZA) has been associated with photosensitivity, rashes, diarrhea, hepatocellular damage, nausea, vomiting, gout, decreased blood clotting time, and anemia.

Rifampin (RIF) may cause drowsiness, headache, generalized numbness, transient low-frequency hearing loss, visual disturbances, abdominal pain or cramps, diarrhea, epigastric distress, hepatitis, nausea, sore mouth and tongue, vomiting, and changes in blood cells. Symptoms of overdosage include nausea, vomiting, increasing lethargy, unconsciousness, liver enlargement and tenderness, and jaundice. RIF also turns the urine a reddish-orange color.

SM sulfate may produce dizziness, headache, paresthesias (numbness or tingling), vertigo, anorexia, nausea, stomatitis, vomiting, changes in blood cells, arthralgia (joint pain), hypertension (high blood pressure), hypotension (low blood pressure), myocarditis, hepatotoxicity, splenomegaly (enlarged spleen), ototoxicity, and nephrotoxicity.

DRUG INTERACTIONS

The drug treatment plan for TB is often complicated. No other drugs should be taken at the same time or right after antitubercular drugs are swallowed, or put on the skin while the patient is on antituberculosis therapy. This is because other drugs may increase the significant risk for neurotoxicity and nephrotoxicity. All drugs taken by the patient should be checked closely for drug interactions, which are very common among the antitubercular drugs.

❖ NURSING IMPLICATIONS AND PATIENT TEACHING

■ Assessment

A TB infection may develop in a patient's lungs, bones, bladder, or other organs. A patient with active TB may have symptoms such as productive cough, pain, fever, night sweats, and weight loss, or the patient may be without symptoms. The diagnosis of TB is made from the patient's history, physical examination, x-ray studies, and laboratory work. A PPD skin test is not given if there is a high probability that the patient has TB. Once the diagnosis is made, the patient may be hospitalized while treatment is started. Long-term treatment is required, and much of the treatment will be carried out when the patient is at home.

■ Diagnosis

Patients with TB often have needs for financial, nutritional, and career counseling that will interfere with them being treated. These other problems must be diagnosed and included in the treatment plan if the needs of the patient are to be considered. These individuals may have other medical problems and may be taking multiple drugs, resulting in additional problems with side effects and scheduling of dosages. The nurse must be prepared to help analyze all the needs of the patient if effective treatment is to be offered. In particular, watch to see if the patient is compliant, because treatment programs in which the patient is watched while taking the medication (directly observed therapy) may be required to protect the public from this disease.

▪ Planning

Drug resistance is likely to develop if only one drug is given for active TB. Two or more drugs should always be given to provide several ways to attach the TB bacterium. Drugs that are highly ototoxic should not be given together. Two hepatotoxic drugs should not be given together when clinically active hepatitis is present.

To prevent the development of drug resistance, be aware of the following:

- Patient compliance
- Culture conversion (sputum cultures that gradually change from positive to negative)
- Selection of appropriate drugs

The CDC Advisory Council for the Elimination of Tuberculosis has issued its recommendations for initial therapy of TB. The regimen for children and adults who do not have HIV infection is as follows:

- Use daily INH, RIF, and PZA and either EMB or SM sulfate for 8 weeks.
- EMB or SM can be added to the initial regimen if needed.
- Use INH and RIF daily or two to three times per week for 16 weeks or up to 6 months.
- Continue INH for 6 months beyond culture conversion.

Directly observe the patient take the medication. The daily dose should be given in the morning before the patient eats or drinks anything else.

The therapy of choice for uncomplicated pulmonary TB is the use of two drugs, INH and RIF, which are both intracellularly and extracellularly bactericidal. The duration of therapy is usually a minimum of 9 months. Sputum that is cultured 1 to 3 months after the initiation of INH and RIF therapy will usually be negative for the bacillus. The therapy usually continues for 6 months after sputum conversion takes place. When necessary, the combination of PZA and SM sulfate may be used to substitute for either one of the bactericidal drugs described previously. However, there is some controversy over the effectiveness of this shorter, 9-month course of therapy when INH is not used.

At present, intermittent therapy with INH and RIF is being investigated. The American Thoracic Society recommends that these two drugs be given daily for 2 to 8 weeks. Then the patient is switched to twice per week for a total of 39 weeks. The minimum duration of therapy is 9 months. The daily dosage recommendations for adults are INH 300 mg and RIF 600 mg. The twice-weekly dosage plan for adults is INH 15 mg/kg of body weight and RIF 600 mg. The American Thoracic Society recommends intermittent therapy only for uncomplicated pulmonary TB. See the new CDC guidelines for treatment of patients with MDR strains whenever they are issued.

Whenever a combination of drugs does not have both an intracellular and an extracellular bactericidal effect, therapy must continue for the traditional 18 to 24 months. This usually occurs when bacteriostatic drugs are used.

For TB patients with HIV infections, use the previous treatment schedule, but continue treatment for 9 months beyond culture conversion.

Because of the long-term nature of the required treatment, drug toxicity is a special problem. Dosages for older adult patients, unusually small adults, and patients with renal impairment should be watched. All patients should be carefully asked about symptoms of adverse reactions. If toxic effects, adverse reactions, or allergic reactions occur, all drugs should be stopped, and further evaluation should be done. Restarting drugs after toxic effects or adverse reactions have ceased should be done with caution.

In the event of an unsuccessful treatment regimen, the health care provider will evaluate for patient compliance and the presence of an MDR strain. If the problem is patient compliance, the same treatment regimen can be started again. With an MDR strain, two or more new drugs are added to the regimen, never a single drug, because drug resistance may develop more easily with only one new drug. The drugs used for retreatment for an MDR strain include *para*-aminosalicylate, capreomycin, cycloserine, ethionamide, and kanamycin.

Guidelines for the treatment of TB are frequently updated by the CDC. To avoid problems with drug resistance, the latest information should always be used in treating patients.

▪ Implementation

Antitubercular drugs should be given in single daily doses unless contraindicated. All drugs, unless stated otherwise, should be taken at the same time each day, preferably in the morning. This is especially important to decrease the chance of drug resistance with the combination of INH and RIF. When poor compliance is suspected, the care provider should directly observe that the patient is indeed taking the drugs.

If parenteral administration is required, the injection sites should be rotated and each site inspected for signs of tenderness, swelling, or redness.

If a patient does not seem to be getting better, closer monitoring to make sure the patient is taking the medicine may be necessary.

Many of these drugs cause gastric irritation, which may be reduced by taking the medication with food. INH is the only antitubercular medication that is best absorbed on an empty stomach. It should be taken as a single daily dose either 1 hour before or 2 hours after a meal. It should be taken with food only if it cannot be tolerated on an empty stomach.

See Table 12-5 for a summary of common antitubercular drugs.

■ Evaluation

Drug resistance should be suspected if the patient has been treated for TB in the past. Drugs used in the regimen for the earlier infection may be used again while waiting for the results of sensitivity studies, but at least two new drugs should also be added. Drug resistance is low in infections acquired in the United States but high in TB infections acquired from Asian, South and Central American, and African sources. Drug resistance is less likely to occur when two bactericidal drugs are given together, rather than when one bactericidal drug is given together with bacteriostatic drugs.

Vital signs should be monitored for recurrence of acute infection. Patients should be weighed at each visit to monitor their general health status. Weight loss should be reported to the physician or other health care provider. Diet changes and nutritional supplements may be indicated.

Some patients taking EMB develop psychologic changes. If the patient becomes depressed, anxious, withdrawn, or stops talking—or shows any changes in personality—these findings should be reported to the physician or other health care provider.

Because of marked toxicity of these drugs, it is essential to carefully and regularly monitor both the bacteriologic studies and the toxic side effects of the drugs. Baseline sputum smears, culture and sensitivity studies, chest x-ray studies, weight, and renal, hepatic, and hematopoietic studies should be obtained.

■ Patient and Family Teaching

Because patients must take their drugs for a long time, it is important to establish a good relationship with the patient. Clear instructions should be given about the importance of continuing to take the drugs as ordered and what problems to report to the nurse practitioner, physician, or other health care provider at the scheduled visits. It is important to stress the following instructions:

- Laboratory and diagnostic tests and frequent office visits are necessary throughout the treatment of TB. The patient must continue to meet with the nurse practitioner, physician, or other health care provider so progress can be measured.
- The drug must be taken exactly as directed. The dosage must not be altered without specific instructions from the nurse practitioner, physician, or other health care provider. It is very important to take these drugs as ordered. If a dose is missed, it should be taken as soon as it is remembered, unless it is almost time for the next dose. In that case, the missed dose should not be taken and the regular dosing schedule should be followed. Forgetting to take a dose or failing to continue with one of the drugs may cause the organisms to develop a resistance to the medication. This allows the disease process to continue, with continued risk for the patient, close family members, and contacts.
- TB is a disease that must be reported to the local health department. Family members and close contacts also need to be screened for TB.
- During the initial period of illness, patients must remember that they are contagious. Patients are usually hospitalized or kept in isolation at home. Every effort must be made to cover the mouth when coughing, to dispose of sputum and soiled tissues carefully, and to act to protect those nearby.
- The patient should remember that the whole body is involved in fighting this disease. The body requires adequate rest, nourishing food, and as restful and as quiet a recovery environment as possible.
- Any adverse reactions should be reported promptly. Symptoms to report include any episodes of easy bruising, fever, sore throat, unusual bleeding, skin rashes, mental confusion, headache, tremors, severe nausea, vomiting, diarrhea, malaise, yellowish discoloration of the skin, visual changes, excessive drowsiness, severe pain in knees, feet, or wrists, or changes in personality or affect (seem not to respond to things).
- Remind patients taking RIF that their urine will become reddish-orange in color and that this is an expected finding and does not mean there is a problem.
- Patients should not take other drugs without the knowledge and permission of the nurse practitioner, physician, or other health care provider.
- With the exception of INH (which should be taken on an empty stomach), medication should be taken with food or milk. If an aftertaste occurs, a mouthwash, juice, or sugarless gum may be used after taking the medication.
- The patient should establish a regular time each day to take their medication.
- The medication is particularly toxic and should be kept in a safe place, away from animals or children.
- The patient should wear a MedicAlert bracelet or necklace or carry some other form of emergency identification indicating the medications being taken.

ANTIPARASITIC DRUGS

OVERVIEW

Parasites affecting humans are a worldwide problem. Three major categories of drugs used to treat parasites are discussed in this section: amebicides, anthelmintics, and antimalarial products. Each major category is discussed in detail.

AMEBICIDES

ACTION

There are a wide variety of parasites and thus a wide variety of drugs used to treat them. Amebiasis is often caused by the parasite *Entamoeba histolytica.* In the United States and Canada, this infection is seen primarily in people who have traveled abroad. It is also found in those who have eaten unwashed fruits or vegetables imported from other countries, so parasitic infection could be common. The main action of an amebicide is to destroy the invading amoeba, which may be located within the GI tract or some other place in the body (extraintestinal). Infections outside the intestinal tract are much more difficult to treat. The most common extraintestinal infection is a hepatic abscess.

USES

Amebicides are the primary therapy for both intestinal and extraintestinal amebiasis. The choice of drug depends on the location of the infection.

Diiodohydroxyquin and metronidazole are also used to treat *Trichomonas vaginali* and giardiasis, which is commonly found in drinking water, particularly in other countries.

ADVERSE REACTIONS

All drugs used to treat amebiasis may cause nausea, vomiting, headache, anorexia, diarrhea, or GI distress.

Chloroquine may produce dizziness, irritability, pruritus, ototoxicity, tinnitus, vertigo, visual disturbances, or abdominal cramps.

Diiodohydroxyquin has been known to cause ataxia (poor coordination), neurotoxicity, peripheral neuropathy, optic neuritis, abdominal cramps, rectal and skin itching, constipation, and hair loss.

Paromomycin may produce vertigo, rash, ototoxicity, abdominal cramps, constipation, hematuria, and nephrotoxicity.

Symptoms of overdosage are also seen with all of these drugs and are an exaggeration and increase of the adverse effects.

DRUG INTERACTIONS

With the exception of metronidazole, there are no significant drug interactions. Combining metronidazole with alcohol can produce severe headache, flushing, cramps, nausea, and vomiting. Collapse or acute psychosis may result.

❖ NURSING IMPLICATIONS AND PATIENT TEACHING

■ Assessment

Learn as much as possible about the health history of the patient, including any allergy to drugs, current use of alcohol or disulfiram, the possibility of pregnancy, or the existence of chronic renal, cardiac, thyroid, or liver disease. These conditions are contraindications or precautions to the use of amebicides.

■ Diagnosis

The nurse might consider asking the patient questions that would help uncover additional problems that might affect the diagnosis or treatment of the problem. For example, does this patient have problems with severe diarrhea that may produce dehydration? Are there knowledge deficits about handling, washing, and storage of fruits and vegetables? Are there other problems that limit the medication therapy for this patient?

■ Planning

Four major drugs are used as amebicides. The contraindications for drug use are somewhat different, depending on the drug chosen. The specific product information should be consulted.

■ Implementation

The drug to be ordered depends on the location of the infection. Some of these drugs are specific for extraintestinal infections. Because these drugs are very toxic, the decision to treat the patient should be carefully made, and only the smallest therapeutic dosage possible should be given for the shortest period. If the initial drug is ineffective and another drug is more hazardous, retreatment with the initial drug may be advised.

Teach the patient about the method of infection and review specific methods of personal hygiene to prevent reinfection and reduce the risk of spreading infection to others.

Table 12-6 provides a summary of amebicides.

■ Evaluation

After drug therapy, periodic stool tests will be required to make certain that the disease has been eliminated. These tests may be needed monthly for up to 1 year after therapy.

Be alert to signs of toxicity. If severe symptoms appear, the drug may have to be stopped.

■ Patient and Family Teaching

Tell the patient and family the following:
- The patient should take all drugs as prescribed and not skip any doses or double the medication doses. The patient should not stop taking the medication without being advised to do so by a nurse practitioner, physician, or other health care provider.
- The patient should take this drug with or after meals to decrease the chances of stomach upset.
- Some patients experience side effects from this medication. The patient should report any new or

Table 12-6   Amebicides

GENERIC NAME	TRADE NAME	COMMENTS
chloroquine HCl	Aralen HCl	Used for amebiasis, rheumatoid arthritis, and malaria.
		Watch for ototoxicity; obtain baseline audiometry tests. May be more effective if given after other systemically absorbed amebicide therapy is completed.
doxycycline	Vibramycin	Often used for traveler's diarrhea and malaria prophylaxis.
paromomycin	Humatin	This is an aminoglycoside antibiotic often used in treatment of trichomoniasis. Used as alternative drug therapy for asymptomatic intestinal amebiasis and mild to moderate infections; may cause ototoxicity, so audiometry tests should be obtained; give medication with meals.

troublesome symptoms to the nurse practitioner, physician, or other health care provider.

- The GI system (mouth) is the point of entry for these parasites. Usually, infection comes from parasite feces getting into the food or by hand-to-mouth contamination. Food should be washed carefully before eating, and hands should be washed after going to the bathroom and before preparing foods. This is important to avoid spreading infection.
- After drug therapy has been completed, it is essential that a stool examination be performed periodically to look for reinfection or for continuing infection in people who still have amebiasis but are not symptomatic.

ANTHELMINTICS

ACTION

When a patient has worms, the infestation is called **helminthiasis**. The condition is usually caused by pinworms, roundworms, hookworms, tapeworms, or whipworms. The worm gains entrance to the body through unclean food, unwashed hands, or the skin. The diagnosis is made by finding the eggs or the parasite in the stool of the infected individual. Once the type of parasite has been identified, the health care provider may order the best medication for its destruction. The way the drug works depends on the product used.

The exact action of diethylcarbamazine citrate as an anthelmintic is not known. It is thought that it sensitizes the parasite's cuticle to allow phagocytosis by the macrophages of the host. Mebendazole blocks the glucose uptake of helminths. Piperazine paralyzes the muscles of parasites by blocking the effects of acetylcholine at the neuromuscular junction, and the parasite is removed by normal peristalsis during the bowel movement. The exact action of thiabendazole is not known, but it is thought to interfere with metabolic pathways essential for a variety of helminths.

USES

Thiabendazole is the drug of choice for cutaneous larva migrans (creeping eruption), pinworms, roundworms, *Strongyloides,* and mild cases of hookworm.

Niclosamide and paromomycin are used to treat cestodiasis (tapeworm infestation).

Piperazine and pyrantel pamoate are used to treat roundworms and pinworms. Pyrantel is also effective against hookworms.

Diethylcarbamazine citrate is used mostly in tropical areas or in patients who have been in areas where these worms are endemic. It is used to treat Bancroft filariasis, Malayan filariasis, dipetalonemiasis, or infestation with loiasis (a filarial worm dwelling in tumors in subcutaneous connective tissue and often affecting the eyes).

Mebendazole is used in single or mixed infections to treat pinworm, roundworm, hookworm, and whipworm infestations.

ADVERSE REACTIONS

Each drug has different side effects. Headache, weakness, anorexia, nausea, vomiting, abdominal pain, arthralgia, lassitude (weariness), malaise, myalgia (widespread muscle pain), and skin rash are all common reactions. Allergic reactions may occur as a result of the dead microfilaria and may be seen with fever, lymphadenitis (inflammation of the lymph nodes), pruritus, and pedal edema (foot swelling). The number of side effects increases with higher dosages and longer length of treatment.

DRUG INTERACTIONS

Anthelmintic drugs work against each other (antagonistic) if they are given together. The drugs also may interfere with a number of specific drugs, such as heparin, and a variety of laboratory tests. Specific product information should be consulted for each drug.

❖ NURSING IMPLICATIONS AND PATIENT TEACHING

▪ Assessment

Learn as much as possible about the health history of the patient, including the presence of hypertension, allergy, eye disease, intestinal obstruction, inflammatory bowel disease, malaria, the possibility of pregnancy, and hepatic, renal, or cardiac disease. These conditions are contraindications or precautions to treatment with anthelmintics.

The patient may have no symptoms or may be listless, fatigued, and irritable or have abdominal pain, diarrhea, and weight loss. The patient may also have edema (collection of large amounts of fluid in tissues), especially of the lower extremities, and a discharge from the eyes. If helminthiasis is seen commonly in the area, learn the signs and symptoms of infestation by the various helminths.

▪ Diagnosis

The nurse might ask the patient questions to help determine if there are other problems that might influence the diagnosis or treatment of the problem. For example, has the patient developed skin lesions, dehydration, or other problems that require or would affect treatment? Is there lack of information that caused this problem? Are there teaching needs to prevent reinfection? Does the patient have other problems that would interfere with or limit therapy for this problem?

▪ Planning

Severe pruritus may occur in the treatment of cutaneous larva migrans, and an antiinflammatory agent may be necessary.

Patients with a recent history of malaria should be treated with an antimalarial agent before giving them anthelmintics to prevent a relapse.

Because pinworm infections are easily transferred from person to person, all family members may need to be treated.

Piperazine can be used in the last trimester of pregnancy. However, this drug has potential neurotoxicity, so long or repeated treatment in excess of the recommended dosage should be avoided, especially in children.

▪ Implementation

Thiabendazole therapy may cause an asparagus-like odor of the urine. The patient's skin may also have an unusual odor. This medication may cause drowsiness or dizziness; therefore the patient should use caution in driving or doing tasks that require alertness.

Severe hookworm infestations may produce anemia, so iron supplementation and a diet rich in iron may be required.

The patient should store piperazine syrup and tablets in tightly closed containers to avoid evaporation or decomposition. Liquids are easier for children to take. Medication is usually given in the morning before breakfast.

Patients may develop allergic reactions to the dead microfilaria and may need treatment for symptoms. Antihistamines or corticosteroids may be necessary to reduce allergic effects, particularly in the treatment of ocular onchocerciasis.

Table 12-7 provides a summary of anthelmintics.

▪ Evaluation

Determine if the patient is taking prescribed medication as ordered and doing other things that might be part of the therapy. Collect stool specimens after every treatment to make sure the worms are gone. Check to see if the patient has had an ophthalmologic (eye) examination if currently undergoing treatment for ocular onchocerciasis.

Teach the patient the hygienic measures necessary to prevent reinfestation.

If the patient develops neurologic complications with piperazine therapy, this medication should be stopped, and another drug should be used.

▪ Patient and Family Teaching

Tell the patient and family the following:

- The patient must take this medication as ordered. Therapy usually involves an initial treatment that should kill all worms, but in some cases, a second course must be taken. It is important to report any symptoms that do not disappear after treatment.
- Worms passed in bowel movements are still alive and capable of infecting others. Care must be used to avoid transmission. For the week after treatment begins, the patient should do the following:
  - Wash the toilet seat daily with soap and water.
  - Once a week for 2 weeks, boil the sheets and underwear twice in water and disinfectant.
  - Use special precautions in handling food or drink around others.
- Worm infestations are easily transmitted, and all family members may need to be tested to see if they also have worms.
- Some people have diarrhea and abdominal discomfort while taking the medication.
- If the patient develops any signs of headache, tremors, muscle weakness, or blurred vision, or if one eye does not align properly with the other eye, the nurse practitioner, physician, or other health care provider should be alerted.
- The patient may require iron supplements and an iron-rich diet during hookworm treatment.

Table 12-7 Anthelmintics

GENERIC NAME	TRADE NAME	COMMENTS
albendazole	Albenza	For treatment of lesions from pork or dog tapeworm. Give for <132 kg: 15 mg/kg/day in two divided doses for 28 days, followed by a 14-day cycle with no medications; repeat for two more cycles. For >132 kg: 400 mg PO twice daily with meals for 28 days, followed by a 14-day cycle with no medications; repeat for two more cycles.
ivermectin	Stromectol	For treatment of intestinal parasites and onchocerciasis. Give once. Usually no repeat dose needed.
mebendazole	Vermox ✦	No special diets, fasting, or purgation before administration is necessary. Medication is taken orally by chewing, crushing, or mixing with food. Given for pinworms, roundworms, hookworms, and whipworms.
praziquantel	Biltricide	Tablet very bitter if not swallowed promptly.
pyrantel	Reese's pinworm Pin-X	Medication can be administered as single dose for treating roundworms and pinworms; hookworms require longer therapy. No special fasting or diet necessary before taking medication. Purging not necessary. Taking drug with fruit juice or milk may make it more palatable Give for roundworm, pinworm, and hookworm therapy.
thiabendazole	Mintezol	Chew tablets well before swallowing. Take drug after meals. First line agent for cutaneous larva migrans and strongyloidiasis. Also given for pinworms, roundworms, and hookworms.

PO, By mouth.

ANTIMALARIALS

ACTION

Malaria is a big problem in many countries where wetlands provide a good breeding ground for mosquitoes. Patients with malaria have periods of acute sickness followed by periods during which they are symptom free. The antimalarial drugs suppress the infection but often do not cure it. Although malaria is not commonly seen in the United States or Canada, it is becoming more frequent in Florida, other areas of the southern United States, and areas adjoining Mexico. The nurse may also see cases among immigrants, migrant farm workers, and travelers returning from areas where malaria is endemic (occurs in a regular pattern). People in the military or those traveling to or living in areas where malaria is endemic can use antimalarials to prevent malaria and treat the symptoms.

Malaria is caused by four species of the protozoan *Plasmodium.* These species are *P. falciparum, P. malariae, P. vivax,* and *P. ovale.* The protozoan parasites are transmitted to humans by the *Anopheles* mosquito.

When a mosquito bites a person infected with malaria, the protozoans enter the mosquito's stomach, where they reproduce. The resulting sporozoites make their way to the salivary glands of the mosquito. They are then transmitted to other individuals whenever the mosquito bites. The sporozoites grow and divide in the human host, entering the red blood cells of the person and maturing into the adult form of the protozoan, which then produces infection and the symptoms of malaria.

Antimalarial drugs interfere with the life cycle of *Plasmodium,* usually while it is in the red blood cells (Table 12-8). These drugs reduce the ability of the DNA to reproduce or serve as a template, thereby decreasing protein synthesis in susceptible organisms. Not all drugs are effective against all four species of *Plasmodium.* In addition, many strains of *Plasmodium* have developed resistance to commonly used drugs. The drugs used in treating malaria are not without risk, and the licensed practical or vocational nurse giving these drugs will need to study the drug information carefully.

Primaquine interferes with the metabolism of parasites. Folic acid antagonists affect the differential growth requirements and the demand for nucleic acid precursors between the host and the parasite. In sulfonamide products, there is a competitive antagonism of paraaminobenzoic acid, which is a component in folic acid synthesis. Quinine, the earliest known medication for malaria, reduces the effectiveness of *Plasmodium's* DNA to act as a template in chloroquine-resistant strains of *P. falciparum.* It also decreases the parasite's oxygen use and carbohydrate metabolism. In the human body, quinine is a skeletal muscle relaxant, antipyretic, and analgesic.

A variety of other protozoals also exist, including American and African trypanosomiasis, leishmaniasis, and *Pneumocystis carinii.* A variety of other

Table 12-8   Antimalarials

GENERIC NAME	TRADE NAME	COMMENTS
Aminoquinolines		
chloroquine HCl	Aralen HCl	Parenteral drug of choice for treating acute malarial attacks when oral therapy is ineffective. Watch for ototoxicity; obtain baseline audiometry tests.
chloroquine phosphate	Aralen Phosphate	Used for malaria suppression and treatment.
hydroxychloroquine	Plaquenil	Malaria suppression and treatment. It is a synthetic antimalarial agent. Also used occasionally to treat rheumatoid arthritis and discoid lupus.
primaquine phosphate	Primaquine Phosphate	Initiate primaquine therapy following a course of chloroquine phosphate suppressive treatment or during the last 2 wk of therapy with chloroquine phosphate.
Folic Acid Agonists		
pyrimethamine	Daraprim	*Malaria suppression:* Synthetic antimalarial. Used in combination therapy for chloroquine-resistant *Plasmodium falciparum.* Therapy should begin 2 wk before entering malaria-endemic area and be continued for 10 wk after departure.
Miscellaneous Agents		
doxycycline	Doxycycline	Used for malaria prophylaxis.
mefloquine	Lariam	Prevention and treatment of malaria.
quinine sulfate	Quinamm	This was formerly used for treatment of malaria. Now used primarily for nocturnal leg cramp treatment.
Nonmalarial Antiprotosoals		
atovaquone	Mepron	Antiprotozoal agent also used for *Pneumocystis.*
metronidazole	Flagyl MetroGel	Drug of choice in mild to severe intestinal amebiasis and treatment of hepatic abscess; effective against protozoa such as *Trichomonas vaginalis, amebiasis,* and *giardiasis.* Has been used as combination therapy in treating *Helicobacter pylori* GI infection. Metronidazole may cause changes in the ECG findings, ataxia, confusion, depression, insomnia, irritability, vertigo, flushing, pruritus, blurred vision, nasal congestion, abdominal cramps, constipation, dysuria (painful urination), polyuria (excretion of a large amount of urine), pyuria (increased white blood cells in the urine), fever, and metallic taste. Alcohol must be avoided as it produces severe vomiting reactions which may be life-threatening.
nifurtimox	Lampit	The drug of choice for American trypanosomiasis
pentamidine	NebuPent, Pentam 300	For *Pneumocystis carinii* infections and prophylaxis. Available in both inhalation and IM forms.
sodium stibogluconate	Pentostam	For leishmaniasis
suramin	Germanin	Drug of choice for African trypanosomiasis.
Trimetrexate	Neutrexin	Alternative therapy for *Pneumocystis carinii* pneumonia.

ECG, Electrocardiogram; *GI,* gastrointestinal; *IM,* intramuscular; *PO,* by mouth.

antiprotozoal medications may be used in treatment of these problems.

USES

Antimalarials are used to suppress and treat acute malaria attacks caused by erythrocytic forms of *P. ovale, P. malariae, P. vivax,* and most strains of *P. falciparum.* The 4-aminoquinoline drugs are ineffective against the gametocytes of *P. falciparum* but are used with primaquine to cure malaria caused by *P. malariae* and *P. vivax.*

ADVERSE REACTIONS

Synthetic 4- and 8-aminoquinolines may produce hypotension, electrocardiogram (ECG) changes, mild and transient headaches, pruritus, abdominal cramps, anorexia, diarrhea, nausea, vomiting, blood dyscrasias, visual blurring, reduced hearing, and tinnitus.

Folic acid antagonists may produce anorexia, atrophic glossitis (loss of papillae of the tongue), vomiting, and anemias.

Quinine poisoning is called *cinchonism* and causes diarrhea, dizziness, headache, nausea, tinnitus, visual blurring, fearfulness, confusion, excitement, hypothermia (abnormally low body temperature), syncope (lightheadedness and fainting), abdominal cramps, vomiting, anemias, pruritus, rash, urticaria, and night blindness.

All of these drugs may sometimes produce blood dyscrasias, as well as visual and neurologic changes. Overdose may produce convulsions and cardiac collapse.

DRUG INTERACTIONS

Use of any antimalarials with other drugs that cause dermatologic, ototoxic, or neurologic symptoms may produce toxicity. There are isolated drugs that interact with these preparations, so read the manufacturers' information carefully.

❖ NURSING IMPLICATIONS AND PATIENT TEACHING

▪ Assessment

Learn as much as possible about the patient's health history, including whether the patient is pregnant or has a history of allergy, psoriasis, porphyria, or glucose-6-phosphate dehydrogenase deficiency. These conditions are contraindications or precautions to the use of antimalarials.

The symptoms of malaria include periodic fever and chills, profound sweating, headache, nausea, body pains, and exhaustion. The patient may report having been in an area where malaria is endemic. Objective signs of malaria include periodic diaphoresis (sweating) and periodic cycles of fever as high as 104° to 105° F.

▪ Diagnosis

Ask the patient questions to determine if there are other relevant problems that would affect the diagnosis and treatment of this problem. Is the patient dehydrated? What is the patient's state of nutrition? Are there other chronic diseases or problems that may interfere with this therapy? Is the patient taking other medications?

▪ Planning

Because certain strains of *P. falciparum* are resistant to 4-aminoquinoline compounds, individuals infected with these strains should be treated with other antimalarial drugs such as quinine.

Individuals taking high dosages or going through prolonged antimalarial therapy may develop irreversible retinal damage to the eyes. Children are highly sensitive to 4-aminoquinoline compounds, primarily chloroquine.

Quinine should be used with care in patients with cardiac dysrhythmias. Cardiotoxicity may result with quinine use. In very sensitive individuals, reversible thrombocytopenia may occur with quinine use.

Laboratory work to measure the glucose-6-phosphate dehydrogenase level in all black patients and in those of Mediterranean ancestry may be required; antimalarial drugs may precipitate hemolysis in some vulnerable patients. The drug should be stopped if the patient develops any blood dyscrasia that is not part of the disease.

 Clinical Goldmine

Active Base of Medicine

The amount of active base of a medicine varies from product to product. The health care provider will determine the dosage based on the amount of active base in the product. The product package information lists the tablet's equivalence to the base.

▪ Implementation

Chloroquine phosphate and hydroxychloroquine are administered orally. To treat malaria, an initial loading dose is usually followed by half that dose on the next 2 days. To prevent malaria, these drugs are usually started 2 weeks before the individual enters an area where malaria is endemic. The medication is taken once weekly on the same day of the week and is continued for 8 weeks after the individual has left the area.

▪ Evaluation

Watch for the malaria symptoms to go away. If the patient requires long-term therapy, periodic complete blood cell count and urinalysis should be monitored. Check for signs and symptoms of hemolysis. An ECG may be obtained before starting quinine therapy and again during treatment if the patient develops any cardiac rhythm problems. Any report of visual problems makes a full eye examination necessary.

▪ Patient and Family Teaching

Tell the patient and family the following:
- The patient should take all the medication as ordered and not stop when the symptoms disappear.
- The nurse practitioner, physician, or other health care provider should be called as soon as possible if the patient has ringing in the ears, hearing difficulties, or any problems with vision.

- Taking medication with meals can reduce GI upset. The nurse practitioner, physician, or other health care provider should be called if there is any severe nausea, vomiting, anorexia, abdominal cramps, or diarrhea.
- This medication is particularly toxic and should be kept out of the reach of children.
- Quinine products may cause the skin to appear somewhat yellow.

- Quinine may cause dizziness and blurred vision. The patient should be very careful when driving.
- Malaria may recur. The patient should watch for symptoms to develop again and call the nurse practitioner, physician, or other health care provider as soon as possible.

Get Ready for the NCLEX® Examination!

Key Points

- A wide range of drugs are available to treat infections.
- These drugs include broad-spectrum antibiotics, antitubercular drugs, antiparasitic medications, penicillins, sulfonamides, and antifungal drugs (discussed in Chapter 13).
- Because antiinfectives are so commonly used, the nurse must be familiar with significant adverse reactions and drug interactions and should know what to teach the patient and family for each type of antibiotic.
- New antibiotics are continually being developed, partly because of research in this area and also because resistant strains of many organisms have developed (especially strains resistant to penicillin, which has been in wide use for many years).

Additional Learning Resources

SG Go to your Study Guide for additional learning activities to help you master this chapter content.

Evolve Go to your Evolve website (http://evolve.elsevier.com/Edmunds/LPN/) for additional online resources.

Review Questions for the NCLEX® Examination

1. The patient is a 35-year-old woman who is receiving ampicillin for treatment of an infection. The most important information that the nurse should teach the patient is:
   1. taking ampicillin with milk can decrease the absorption of the ampicillin
   2. taking ampicillin with oral contraceptives can result in unplanned pregnancy
   3. taking ampicillin with aspirin can block renal clearance of ampicillin
   4. taking ampicillin with orange juice can result in an increase in the absorption of ampicillin

2. The patient is scheduled to receive an intramuscular injection of penicillin. The most important action for the nurse to implement prior to administration of the injection is:
   1. take a full set of vital signs on the patient
   2. monitor the patient closely for adverse reactions
   3. question the patient about any known allergies
   4. instruct the client to wait 30 minutes before leaving

3. The patient is a 9-year-old who is being treated with tetracycline. The most important adverse reaction that the nurse should monitor this patient for is:
   1. yellow-brown tooth discoloration
   2. photosensitivity
   3. anaphylactic reaction
   4. hepatotoxicity

4. The patient has been prescribed vancomycin and is already taking one of the aminoglycosides. The most important area that the nurse should monitor this patient for is:
   1. mental status
   2. visual acuity
   3. urine output
   4. energy level

5. The patient has just been prescribed vancomycin. The most important adverse reaction that the patient should be monitored for is:
   1. blindness
   2. renal failure
   3. liver failure
   4. ringing in the ears

Case Study

Bill Ethington, 64 years old, comes into the clinic with a temperature of 104° F. He is sweating profusely, feels nauseated, and says that he feels "horrible." He reports he has never felt this way before. He sits in the chair but twists and turns, rubbing his lower back as he talks. A urine specimen is positive for red blood cells and protein, and a microscopic specimen shows bacteria and urinary casts. The nurse practitioner confirms that he has a urinary tract infection.

1. What antibiotics are used primarily for urinary tract infections and why?
2. What special instructions would you give the patient if the nurse practitioner started the patient on Gantrisin?
3. What other problems does Mr. Ethington have that need nursing or medical care?
4. Would the medication ordered be any different if this patient was a pregnant woman?
5. What other types of drugs might Mr. Ethington need?

Get Ready for the NCLEX® Examination!—cont'd

Drug Calculation Review

1. A 10-year-old child has come to the family practice clinic with complaints of fever and right ear pain for 3 days. The physician diagnoses acute bacterial otitis media and orders an injection of ceftriaxone (Rocephin) 600 mg IM. The available vial of powder is marked ceftriaxone 1 g, with the following instructions: "Reconstitute with 9.6 mL diluent to equal 100 mg/mL."
   a. How many milliliters will the nurse prepare?
   b. Where should this injection be given?
   c. Should the nurse divide the dose?

2. Order: Penicillin G 1,000,000 units intramuscular stat.
   Available: Penicillin G 600,000 units/mL
   Question: How many milliliters of penicillin should be given?.

3. Order: Infuse vancomycin 1.5 g in 150 mL of D5W IVPB (IV piggyback). Medication information states that IV vancomycin should be infused using an IV infusion device at a rate of 1 g/hr.
   Question: How many milliliters per hour should the nurse set the IV infusion device for?

4. Order: Kefzol 400 mg IM every 6 hours Reconstitution directions: Add 2 mL of 0.9% normal saline to a vial of Kefzol 500 mg to yield a total volume of 2.2 mL.
   Question: How many milliliters should be administered with each dose? (Round to the nearest tenth.)

Critical Thinking Questions

1. After a complete physical, Mrs. Wilson, age 87, has just been prescribed a broad-spectrum antibiotic, much to her surprise. Her physician has asked you to administer a first dose for her before she leaves your clinic to head for the pharmacist and then home. After the doctor leaves the room, Mrs. Johnson confides to you, "I'm worried, hon. He shouldn't have given me an antibiotic, should he? I don't have a sore throat. I have a virus." Explain to Mrs. Johnson the wide variety of indications for these drugs. Also explain why an antibiotic is sometimes ordered for a viral infection.

2. Mrs. Wilson asks you which antibiotic you will be giving her and says, "That's not penicillin, is it? The last time I took penicillin, I got an awfully scratchy throat." Why is this significant?

3. What is the most important point to emphasize in a teaching plan for a patient newly diagnosed with TB?

4. While doing volunteer work overseas, Mr. Johannsen developed malaria and had to come home. His doctor has prescribed chloroquine phosphate. Write out a teaching plan to explain to Mr. Johannsen how to control infection and reinfection, the lifelong possibility of relapses, endemic reactions, how to take his medication, and the need for follow-up examinations.

5. Ms. Keaton thinks she is allergic to penicillin, although she says she has "never been tested." What are the signs and symptoms of hypersensitivity or allergy?

6. If Ms. Keaton tells you she thinks she is allergic to penicillin because it made her "stomach sick" when she was a child, what signs or symptoms is she describing?

7. Ms. Keaton comes back to the clinic, complaining that she still has the same bladder infection as when she came to you for the first time. Her doctor switches her to a sulfonamide. "What good will that do?" she asks you. Explain the actions and uses of sulfonamides. Draw up a teaching plan for this patient, stressing the importance of taking the medication properly, symptoms that should be reported immediately to the physician or other health care provider, and symptoms of hypersensitivity.

8. Ms. Keaton calls the clinic two weeks later, stating she has "another infection like the last time." "I guess those other pills didn't work, either," she says. After she makes another appointment with her doctor, Ms. Keaton asks you if she should "just start taking the pills that were left over" until she sees the doctor. What might you suspect has happened? What would be your most appropriate answer to her question?

Objectives

1. Describe how antiviral, antiretroviral, and antifungal medications work.
2. List common medications used in treating human immunodeficiency virus (HIV), acquired immune deficiency syndrome (AIDS), and fungal infections.
3. Outline Standard Precautions the nurse takes in limiting exposure to AIDS. (Review material in Chapter 10.)

Key Terms

acquired immune deficiency syndrome
   (AIDS) (ā-KWĪ-ěrd ĬM-ū-nō-dē-FĬSH-ĭn-sē, p. 189)
antifungal medications (ăn-tī-FŬN-găl, p. 196)
antiretrovirals (ăn-tī-RĚT-rō-vī-rălz, p. 191)
human immunodeficiency virus
   (HIV) (ĬM-ū-nō-dē-FĬSH-ĭn-sē, p. 190)

mycotic infections (mī-KŎT-ĭk, p. 196)
opportunistic infections (ŏp-ŏr-TŪN-ĭst-ĭk, p. 193)
retrovirus (RĚT-rō-vī-rŭs, p. 190)
virions (VĪ-rē-ŭnz, p. 190)

OVERVIEW

Antiviral and antiretroviral drugs have two basic uses: (1) They treat a variety of common conditions caused by different viruses. These include viruses that cause herpes zoster, herpes simplex, genital herpes, varicella, and some influenza infections. Some antiviral medications are helpful in treating patients with cytomegalovirus retinitis. (2) More specialized antiviral products are used in treating the immunocompromised patient with human immunodeficiency virus (HIV) infection or for adults and children at risk for developing HIV and acquired immune deficiency syndrome (AIDs). They do not cure HIV or AIDS but they do help many patients live longer by acting to stop the production of new retroviruses by interfering with the ability of the retrovirus to replicate (reproduce).

ANTIVIRALS

OVERVIEW

A *virus* is a small infectious agent that can replicate only inside the living cells of organisms. They cannot survive without finding a host in which they may metabolize or make chemicals, grow, and reproduce. Viral infections are not suppressed by antibiotics. Antivirals interfere with the ability of the virus to carry out these reproductive functions.

ACTION AND USES

Many individuals have times when their body is not as strong at fighting infection as at other times or have low immunity. Individuals who once had varicella (chickenpox) still have the virus in their bodies. When immunity is low, patients have a greater chance of developing herpes infections from these usually quiet viruses that remained behind from the chicken pox. We now have some medications that are helpful in reducing the effects of some types of viral infections, such as herpes or influenza. Most common antiviral drugs may therefore be classed as either antiherpes, antiinfluenza, or neuraminidase inhibitors.

Antiviral drugs must enter the infected cell and act at the site of infection to be effective. The drugs often act in a very specific manner—they stop the virus from growing, but cannot kill it.

Antivirals used for herpes simplex or zoster are effective for short-term treatment, long-term suppression, and treatment of recurrence. Treatment of acute infection does not eliminate the chronic infection, which lies dormant. Resistance to the action of the drug may develop quickly.

Resistance to the antiinfluenza drugs amantadine and rimantadine has made them largely ineffective for the treatment of influenza. Neuraminidase products are effective against most strains of influenza

A and B but the product may not always be available. With concerns about Avian flu, the government has stockpiled more of these products. Zanamivir is an antiviral product that must be given by inhalation.

ADVERSE REACTIONS

Many of these antiviral drugs are given topically and may have few recognized side or adverse effects. Some of the drugs are quite new, and information about adverse effects is still being collected. All health care personnel involved with giving these drugs must read the latest product information before administering these products.

DRUG INTERACTIONS

Antivirals may also have drug interactions, often with products not usually involved in drug reactions. If giving antivirals, the nurse must read carefully about each of these products to determine if it can be given safely to the patient.

❖ NURSING IMPLICATIONS AND PATIENT TEACHING

■ Assessment

Understand clearly why the product is being ordered and what the physician or other health care provider hopes to accomplish with the drug plan. Learn all about the patient's history. Know the precautions or contraindications. What conditions exist that may help or hurt the patient's ability to take antiviral medicines as prescribed?

■ Diagnosis

Identify other problems this patient has that might limit the effectiveness of treatment. Because antivirals only lessen symptoms and cannot cure disease, the same viral infection often occurs many times, and patients may need education, comfort, and basic teaching about how to reduce pain, itching, or discharge. These patients often experience weakness and muscle wasting. Ask questions such as: Do they have adequate nutrition? Can they afford the medicine? Will they be compliant?

■ Planning

More information about antiviral medications is available every day. Review the latest information from the package inserts before giving these products.

■ Implementation

Several of these products have special storage requirements or instructions for mixing. Read the latest information to administer these products correctly.

Specific information about these products is given in Table 13-1.

■ Evaluation

Watch the patient for signs of improvement in symptoms. Watch particularly for signs of toxicity or adverse effects that are specific to the medication taken.

■ Patient and Family Teaching

Tell the patient and family the following:

- This medication is usually able to reduce or suppress symptoms, but it does not cure disease.
- The patient should be careful to follow any specific storage instructions for the medication.
- The patient should learn the specific symptoms that would indicate the development of adverse effects. If these develop, the patient should contact the health care provider or return immediately to the clinic, depending on the symptoms.
- Many patients with impaired immunity drink only bottled water to protect themselves from pathogens in impure water.
- The patient should also avoid eating sushi (a form of raw fish) and raw meat. Fruits and vegetables that cannot be peeled or scrubbed vigorously should be soaked using a solution of water to which a few drops of bleach have been added.
- Patients must learn how to protect their sexual partners from disease by using condoms and safer sex practices.

The health care provider should work with pregnant patients to admit them to the national Antiretroviral Registry. This registry is the only project to evaluate first-trimester as well as late-pregnancy exposure to antiretroviral medications. Patient confidentiality is protected. Information obtained through this registry is used to learn how to weigh the risks and benefits of treatment for pregnant women and their fetuses.

ANTIRETROVIRAL AGENTS

OVERVIEW

Acquired immune deficiency syndrome (AIDS) is a disease that causes a breakdown in the immune system, leaving the patient unable to fight infection. Because many people who develop AIDS die, it is one of the most frightening diseases. More than 98% of individuals who develop the most severe form of the disease die within 5 years of diagnosis. In some cases, advances in treatment have prolonged the lives of patients who can get the needed medications for as long as 35 years.

AIDS is a viral disease that arose in central Africa in the 1950s but is now found throughout the world. In the United States, the groups at highest risk for developing AIDS include homosexual and bisexual men, although the fastest growing group to develop AIDS is heterosexual women. Intravenous drug abusers, people in prison, female sexual partners of

Table 13-1 Antiviral Medications

Antiherpes Drugs

GENERIC NAME	TRADE NAME	COMMENTS
acyclovir	Zovirax	For initial and recurrent mucosal and cutaneous HSV-1, HSV-2, and varicella-zoster infections in immunocompromised individuals. Also for severe acute and recurrent genital herpes in patients not immunocompromised. May be used for acute treatment of herpes zoster and chickenpox lesions. Initial parenteral infusion followed by oral therapy. Dosage depends on condition, acuity, and severity.
famciclovir	Famvir	For acute herpes zoster and recurrent genital herpes.
penciclovir	Denavir	Requires prescription but may move to OTC. Used in treatment of herpes labialis, herpes simplex.
valacyclovir HCl	Valtrex	For herpes zoster and recurrent genital herpes.

Antiinfluenza Drugs

amantadine HCl	Symmetrel	For prophylaxis of influenza A virus respiratory tract illnesses in patients at high risk because of underlying disease.
rimantadine	Flumadine	For prophylaxis and treatment of illnesses caused by various strains of influenza virus. In children, used as prophylaxis against influenza A virus.

Neuraminidase Inhibitors

oseltamivir phosphate	Tamiflu	For treatment of uncomplicated acute illness from influenza in patients older than 1 yr who have been symptomatic for more than 2 days or for prophylaxis for people older than 13 yr.
zanamivir	Relenza	Treatment of uncomplicated acute illness from influenza A and B in adults and children older than 7 years who have been symptomatic for more than 2 days.

Other Antivirals

cidofovir	Vistide	Used in CMV retinitis in patients with AIDS. Given as IV infusion over 1 hr. Often given with probenecid.
foscarnet Na	Foscavir	For CMV retinitis and HSV infections.
ganciclovir	Cytovene	For CMV retinitis and infection in AIDS patients. Begun with parenteral therapy and followed with oral tablets. Watch for granulocytopenia and thrombocytopenia.
ribavirin	Virazole	For severe lower respiratory tract infections in hospitalized infants and young children with severe infections from RSV. Powder for aerosol administration only.

AIDS, Acquired immune deficiency syndrome; *CMV*, cytomegalovirus; *HCl*, hydrochloride; *HSV*, herpes simplex virus; *IV*, intravenous; *OTC*, over the counter; *RSV*, respiratory syncytial virus.

people in AIDS risk groups, and children born to mothers at risk of being HIV positive make up the other groups of people most likely to get AIDS. Minorities are overrepresented among the people who get AIDS. Recipients of blood products or of semen for artificial insemination also have developed AIDS. Because AIDS is an epidemic with a high mortality rate, it is important to understand what role medications play in slowing the advance of this disease and treating the other diseases that may result from the patient's reduced immunity.

AIDS is caused by a **retrovirus** currently named **human immunodeficiency virus (HIV)**. Retroviruses are viruses that contain ribonucleic acid (RNA) rather than deoxyribonucleic acid (DNA) as their genetic material. The HIV attaches to the CD4 protein with the help of coreceptors (CXCR4 or CCR5) found on helper T lymphocytes and other cells such as macrophages and dendritic cells. The HIV then fuses its membrane with that of the host cell and inserts its genetic material into the cytoplasm. The viral genetic material is then transcribed into double-stranded DNA called *proviral DNA*. The HIV enzyme *reverse transcriptase* is responsible for creating proviral DNA from viral RNA. Once produced, this DNA often becomes integrated into the chromosomal DNA of the host cell. The HIV DNA is then able to use the host cell's genetic machinery to create new HIV RNA genetic material and messenger RNA. The messenger RNA codes for the development of HIV polyproteins, which must be cleaved, or separated, into individual proteins by the HIV enzyme *protease* for infectious **virions** (rudimentary virus particles) to be produced. Once this occurs, new virions are assembled; these bud from the host cell's membrane and are able to infect new cells. This process is demonstrated in Figure 13-1. **Antiretrovirals** are an important group of drugs that slow the growth or prevent the duplication of retroviruses; they are used to limit the advance of HIV and AIDS.

Research and clinical drug trials continue to make changes in what we know about AIDS. This will affect what drugs we use to treat AIDS patients and how we use them. Use only the most current information about these medications and their use in HIV-positive patients.

ACTION

By interfering with the ability of a retrovirus to reproduce, or replicate, antiretroviral agents act to stop more retroviruses from being made. At present, there are a wide variety of antiretrovirals in clinical use with other products in development. These types include:

- Nucleoside reverse transcriptase inhibitors (NRTIs), which act early in the life cycle of the virus. They prevent the HIV enzyme reverse transcriptase from creating HIV proviral DNA from the viral RNA. This in turn prevents more viruses from being produced.

There are two categories of reverse transcriptase inhibitors: analogue NRTIs and analogue nonnucleoside reverse transcriptase inhibitors (NNRTIs).

- Protease inhibitors act later in the life cycle of the virus. One of the final stages of the HIV life cycle is the production of HIV polyproteins, which are coded for by viral messenger RNA. These polyproteins must be cleaved, or separated, by the HIV enzyme protease into the individual proteins necessary for the production of more infectious virions. Protease inhibitors block the HIV enzyme protease and therefore prevent these polyproteins from being cleaved. This causes noninfectious HIV virions to be produced.
- Fusion inhibitors work to prevent the AIDS virus from invading the white blood cells (WBCs) of the patient.
- HIV integrase strand transfer inhibitors are designed to slow the advancement of HIV infection by blocking the HIV integrase enzyme needed for viral multiplication.
- Multiclass combination products are combinations of several antiretroviral products into one to make it easier for the patient to take their medications.

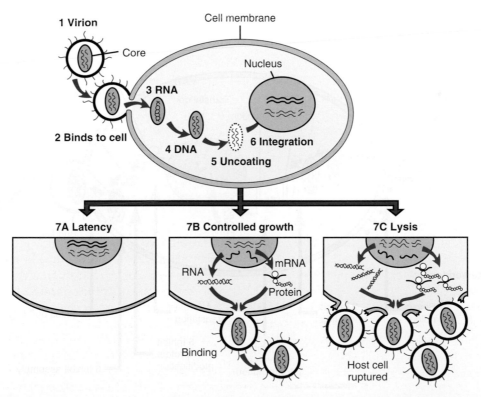

FIGURE 13-1 Infection and cellular outcomes of human immunodeficiency virus (HIV). HIV infection begins when a virion *(1)*, or virus particle, binds to the outside of a susceptible cell and fuses with it *(2)*, injecting the core proteins and two strands of viral ribonucleic acid (RNA) *(3)*. Uncoating occurs, during which the core proteins are removed, and the viral RNA is released into the infected cell's cytoplasm. The double-stranded deoxyribonucleic acid (DNA) *(4)*, or provirus, migrates to the nucleus, uncoats itself *(5)*, and is integrated into the cell's own DNA *(6)*. The provirus then can do a couple of things: remain latent *(7A)* or activate cellular mechanisms to copy its genes into RNA *(7B)*, some of which is translated into virus proteins or ribosomes. The proteins and additional RNA are then assembled into new virions that bud from the cell. The process can take place slowly, sparing the host cell *(7B)*, or so rapidly that the cell is lysed or ruptured *(7C)*.

USES

Antiretroviral agents are used to slow the advance of AIDS infection and support whatever immunity the patient still has. They may also be used to prevent HIV in infants born to HIV-infected mothers or in health care workers who have been exposed to HIV. (The effectiveness of such treatment is shown when there is no change in antibody test results from HIV-negative to HIV-positive, or seroconversion.) All of these medications are relatively new and fairly toxic, with many adverse effects and drug interactions. Pediatric antiretroviral medication usage is different than that for adults.

Figure 13-2 illustrates different stages in which drugs attack HIV. Antiretroviral medications are given only under the direction of a specialist, but the nurse may encounter patients getting these drugs when they are admitted with other health problems.

ADVERSE REACTIONS

Antiretrovirals often cause severe toxic reactions. The nurse constantly watches for symptoms of pancreatitis, peripheral neuropathy, and myopathies, as well as less serious conditions such as mouth ulcers, rash, headaches, diarrhea, and nausea. Most of these products can also cause damage to the liver or kidneys (hepatotoxic or nephrotoxic); many are associated with blood dyscrasias and peripheral neuropathies.

 Lifespan Considerations
Older Adults

ADVERSE REACTIONS

- Older immune-compromised patients may have other chronic diseases also. This may mean that they are taking 8 or 10 medications at a time. These patients often need encouragement to continue taking all their medications.
- Cost is a factor for patients who must take many of these very expensive drugs.
- Monitoring for adverse effects from some of the drugs used to treat patients with HIV is more difficult in older adult patients. Because the elderly have other health problems and take other medications, it is sometimes difficult to know which drugs are causing adverse reactions.

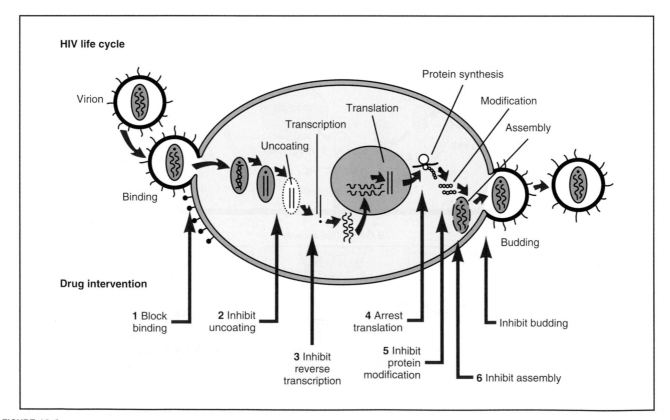

FIGURE 13-2 Human immunodeficiency virus (HIV) is subject to attack by drugs at several stages during its life cycle. Certain agents could block the binding of HIV to the CD4 receptors on the surface of helper T cells *(1)*. Other agents might keep viral ribonucleic acid (RNA) and reverse transcriptase from leaving their protein coat *(2)*. Drugs such as azidothymidine and other dideoxynucleosides prevent the reverse transcription of viral RNA into viral deoxyribonucleic acid *(3)*. Later, antisense oligonucleotides could block the translation of messenger RNA into viral proteins *(4)*. Certain compounds could interfere with viral assembly by modifying such processes *(5)*, and finally, antiviral agents such as interferon could keep the virus from assembling itself and budding out of the cell *(6)*.

DRUG INTERACTIONS

Most antiretroviral agents inhibit the cytochrome P-450 enzyme system involved in the metabolism of medications in the liver. For this reason, they should not be taken at the same time as other drugs. It is important to check with the physician or other health care provider before any medications are given to patients taking antiretroviral medications. Many of these drugs are changed when given at the same time as other drugs.

❖ NURSING IMPLICATIONS AND PATIENT TEACHING

■ Assessment

Learn all about the history and course of the disease, the medications the patient has used, and past response to the medications. Most drugs used in the treatment of AIDS are toxic to the liver. Assess for past or present history of hepatitis or hepatomegaly (enlarged liver) plus current, as well as past, alcohol use or abuse. Assess for a history of pancreatitis and symptoms of peripheral neuropathy, because these are frequently caused by medications.

Ask about AIDS-related opportunistic infections— infections that develop because the damage to the body's immune system leaves it unable to protect the patient against other infections. Opportunistic infections would not ordinarily be a problem to an individual, but because of reduced immunity, they may cause great pain and suffering in an AIDS patient. Ask the patient specifically about respiratory infections, skin lesions, and *Candida* infections.

Some of the specific questions the nurse might ask to explore related patient problems include: What are the patient's beliefs and feelings about this illness? Does the patient have a support system? Does he or she have friends and family who can help the patient when he or she is most vulnerable to infection or having problems? Does the patient have health care insurance and the means to pay for medicines? Is the patient in need of financial assistance?

■ Diagnosis

The medical diagnosis might be clear. In order to understand it, the nurse will want to understand what stage of disease the patient has (e.g., if the diagnosis is limited to exposure to HIV, or has exposure progressed to actual infection and symptoms). In addition to the medical diagnosis, the nurse will explore whether the patient has problems in the areas of hydration, nutrition, or hygiene? What are the financial needs, emotional concerns, and spiritual needs? Is there a support system in place, or is the patient going through this illness alone? Does the patient engage in unsafe sex or drug practices that put other individuals at risk? Are there knowledge deficits about HIV infection, prognosis, and treatment?

■ Planning

Compliance is a big challenge for patients with HIV infection. They must return frequently to their health care providers for tests and examinations. Because they are at risk for developing opportunistic infections as a result of their damaged immune system, patients must be taught the signs of such infections. The patients must be willing to take all the medicines that are prescribed. Antiretroviral drugs are expensive and may have complicated directions for when they need to be taken. The drugs may cause side effects. For patients who are trying to slow or halt their HIV infection, it is important to provide individual teaching, encouragement and support and help with specific problems that present obstacles to treatment goals.

Before beginning drug therapy with antiretrovirals, the helper T lymphocyte (CD4) count must be measured, and plasma HIV RNA laboratory studies must be done. These results help assess a patient's immunologic status and severity of infection. They also provide a means of measuring how well the treatment is working. A complete blood cell count (including a WBC count with differential), folate, vitamin B_{12}, ferritin, iron, and percentage of iron saturation, should also be obtained. Liver function tests and hepatitis B, C, and A serologies, as well as amylase, triglyceride, and lipase levels, will also be ordered. All of these laboratory studies are repeated during the treatment and help show treatment success or onset of adverse effects.

All of the protease inhibitors are potent inhibitors of the cytochrome P-450 enzyme system and have many contraindications to use of other drugs at the same time.

■ Implementation

In working with HIV-infected patients, be certain to follow Standard Precautions. Wear gloves when necessary to avoid exposure to lesions or bodily fluids. Patients should be taught how to take care of minor problems and when they should return for care.

Table 13-2 provides a list of important information about antiretrovirals.

■ Evaluation

Patients must see their health care provider on a frequent basis for further blood work that measures their WBC level and may indicate the presence of infection. Patients must also return to their health care provider sooner for evaluation than their regular schedule when they suspect the presence of opportunistic infections. Patients generally have fewer severe side effects with the protease inhibitors, although patients taking indinavir sulfate may develop "Crix belly." This is a syndrome characterized by elevated levels of triglycerides, cholesterol, and plasma glucose, with a weight gain of 40 lb or greater. Fat accumulates in the lower abdomen and flanks, and tissue is often lost in the arms and legs.

Table 13-2 Antiretrovirals

DRUG	CLINICAL TOXICITIES	NURSING IMPLICATIONS
Nucleoside Reverse Transcriptase Inhibitors		
Nucleoside Analogues		
didanosine (ddI) (Videx)	Pancreatitis, peripheral neuropathy, retinal depigmentation, diarrhea, headache, dry mouth, insomnia, nervousness	Medication should not be taken with food or mixed with acidic beverages; separate other drugs from ddI by 2 hr.
lamivudine (3TC) (Epivir-HBV)	Peripheral neuropathy, headache, pancreatitis (in children)	Used in combination with zidovudine.
stavudine (d4T) (Zerit, Zerit X)	Peripheral neuropathy, diarrhea, nausea, vomiting	Do not use with zidovudine.
zidovudine (ZDV, AZT) (Retrovir)	Headache, nausea, myopathy, myositis, malaise, hepatic stenosis	Nausea and headaches often resolve after 4-6 weeks of therapy; 60% CNS penetration; drug of choice for HIV CNS disease.
Nonnucleoside Reverse Transcriptase Inhibitors		
abacavir sulfate (Ziagen)	Fatal hypersensitivity reactions (discontinue immediately if any signs of hypersensitivity appear)	Question patient about any new symptoms that may suggest hypersensitivity.
delavirdine (DLV) (Rescriptor)	Rash (pruritus), headaches	When used as monotherapy, resistance can rapidly develop; antacids decrease absorption. If used with ddI, separate by 1 hr.
efavirenz (Sustiva)	Used together with other antiretroviral agents in treating HIV	Take on an empty stomach.
nevirapine (NVP) (Viramune)	Rash (Stevens-Johnson syndrome)	When used as monotherapy, resistance can rapidly develop; once-daily dosing during first 2 wk may lessen incidence of rash.
Protease Inhibitors		
amprenavir (Agenerase)	Rash, nausea, diarrhea	
atazanavir (Reyataz)	Indirect hyperbilirubinemia, prolonged PR interval, fat maldistribution, hyperglycemia	
Fosamprenavir (Lexiva)	Skin rash, diarrhea, nausea, headache, fat maldistribution	
indinavir (Crixivan)	Nephrolithiasis, nausea, abdominal pain, "Crix belly," hematuria	Should be taken 1 hr before or 2 hr after meals; increase fluids to drink >1.5 L/day to avoid renal stones; decrease rifabutin dose by half. Concurrent use with St. John's wort and other CYP3A substrates contraindicated.
nelfinavir mesylate (Viracept)	Diarrhea, nausea	Should be taken with food.
ritonavir (Norvir)	Nausea, diarrhea, taste changes, circumoral paresthesias, thrombocytopenia	Should be taken with food; used extensively with other antiviral drugs because of the numerous drug interactions. These drug-drug interactions result in greater blood levels and better efficacy.
saquinavir mesylate (Invirase)	Diarrhea, nausea, abdominal pain, ataxia, neutropenia, hemolytic anemias	Should be taken with high-fat meals.

Continued

Table 13-2 Antiretrovirals—cont'd

DRUG	CLINICAL TOXICITIES	NURSING IMPLICATIONS
Second-Generation Protease Inhibitors		
darunavir (Prezista)	Nausea, vomiting, diarrhea	
Fusion Inhibitor		
enfuvirtide (Fuzeon)	Hypersensitivity, local site reaction, diarrhea, nausea, fatigue	Must be taken by subcutaneous injection twice daily, rotating sites.
HIV Integrase Inhibitor		
raltegravir (Isentress)	Diarrhea, nausea, headache	
Combination Productions		
zidovudine/ lamivudine (Combivir)		May help compliance.
zidovudine/ lamivudine/ abacavir (Trizivir)		May help compliance.
lopinavir/ritonavir (Kaletra)		May help compliance.

CNS, Central nervous system; *HIV*, human immunodeficiency virus.

 Clinical Pitfall

Signs or Symptoms of Pancreatitis

Patients who develop any signs or symptoms of pancreatitis should have their medication stopped immediately until it is ruled out.

■ Patient and Family Teaching

Tell the patient and family the following:

- *Compliance is essential.* Patients must take their medications as ordered. With many of these drugs, taking too little medication, following the drug schedule only part of the time, or not taking the medication may result in a resistant strain of HIV that cannot be treated.
- Antiretrovirals do not cure HIV infection. Even though the patient is taking these medications they still need to prevent transmission through safe sex practices and Standard Precautions.
- Pregnant women or women who suspect they are pregnant need to seek care to minimize the risk to their fetus or neonate.

The patient should report signs and symptoms of sensorimotor peripheral neuropathy caused by several of the reverse transcriptase inhibitors. Initially, the patient feels numbness and burning, usually involving the toes. Patients may have decreased light touch, pinprick, temperature, and vibration sensation in the feet and up to the midcalf. These symptoms may be followed by sharp, shooting pains, which progress to severe, continuous burning pain that is often worse at night and requires narcotic analgesics.

 Clinical Pitfall

Prescribed Doses

Taking less than the prescribed dose can be more harmful than not taking the drug at all.

- All HIV-positive women should be warned of the high risk of HIV transmission in breast milk. The Centers for Disease Control and Prevention advises all HIV-infected women not to breastfeed.
- The patient should report all other medications being taken, including over-the-counter drugs, prescription medications, nutritional supplements obtained outside traditional medical practice, and illegal drugs.
- The patient should learn the signs and symptoms of pancreatitis.

 Clinical Pitfall

Peripheral Neuropathy

This neuropathy is usually reversible if the medication is promptly discontinued.

ANTIFUNGALS

OVERVIEW

Fungal infections are often called *opportunistic infections* because they develop when the patient's immunity is weak. Some fungal infections are kept to a localized area, whereas others may become spread throughout the patient's whole body. Fungi are more complex organisms than bacteria and thus require drugs that act in a different way than antibacterials. Antifungals often have adverse effects and their use must be closely monitored.

ACTION AND USES

A fungus is a plant that produces yeastlike or moldlike diseases called **mycotic infections** in humans. These can be either superficial infections, such as in the skin or nail, or systemic infections, such as in the lung or liver. Because fungi are found almost everywhere—in most water supplies, in the air, and in the soil—they pose a real risk for immunocompromised patients.

Antifungal medications are used orally, intravenously, topically, and vaginally to treat mycotic infections. There are a variety of antifungals; some are used primarily for vaginal yeast or fungal infections, and others are used to treat superficial or systemic infections. The actions and uses of the most common medications used to treat general fungal infections are described in Table 13-3.

Because AIDS destroys the body's immune system, patients with AIDS are prey to many opportunistic infections. Fungi the body would usually keep under control now cause some of the most problematic infections. It is important to understand how antifungal medications may be helpful in improving the general well-being of AIDS patients.

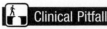

Clinical Pitfall

Adverse Reactions

Many of the adverse reactions to antifungals are similar to the symptoms of the disease they are intended to cure. It is sometimes difficult to determine if the patient needs more or less medication.

ADVERSE REACTIONS

Nausea, vomiting, and diarrhea are the most common reactions. Other products may be associated with more severe problems such as hematologic, renal, or hepatic disease.

Symptoms of overdosage include severe nausea, vomiting, and diarrhea.

Clinical Pitfall

Antifungal Drug Interactions with Alcohol

Because of severe drug interactions of some of these medications with alcohol products, assess the patient's alcohol intake patterns and make sure that the health care provider is aware of this information.

DRUG INTERACTIONS

Severe superinfection may result when antifungals are given together with prolonged corticosteroid therapy. Activity of oral anticoagulants is decreased when they

 Table **13-3**   Selected Antifungals

GENERIC NAME	TRADE NAME	COMMENTS
amphotericin B	Amphotec Fungizone IV	Reserved for use only in patients with progressive and potentially fatal fungal infections.
fluconazole	Diflucan	May require therapy for weeks.
griseofulvin microsize	Grifulvin V Grisactin	Divided doses recommended for patients unable to tolerate single doses.
griseofulvin ultramicrosize	Gris-PEG	Griseofulvin ultramicrosize has approximately 1.5 times the biologic activity of griseofulvin microsize, with no advantage in effectiveness or safety.
ketoconazole	Nizoral	Duration of treatment not specific; should be based on clinical response. Minimum treatment for candidiasis is 10 days to 2 weeks. May require therapy for up to 6 months.
nystatin	Mycostatin	Shake oral suspension well before use. Available for many routes. Use in the mouth and vaginal areas.
Terbinafine HCl	Lamisil	*Onychomycosis (infection of finger or toe nails):* Optimal clinical effect seen several months after fungus is cured and healthy nail has grown. Keep tablets cool and protect from light.
Related Drug		
Metronidazole	Flagyl	IV or PO. Dosage varies, depending on site of infection. See package insert. Not an antifungal agent but used for patients with mixed fungal and bacterial or protozoa infections.

IV, Intravenous; *PO,* by mouth.

are used at the same time as griseofulvin; it may be necessary to adjust the anticoagulant dosage. Griseofulvin activity is decreased when used at the same time as barbiturates, requiring dosage adjustments of the griseofulvin. Use of alcohol while taking antifungals potentiates, or increases, the effect of the alcohol. Because antacids, anticholinergics, and H_2 blockers (e.g., Pepcid, Zantac) change gastrointestinal (GI) pH, the patient should not take ketoconazole for at least 2 hours after taking any H_2 blockers.

Toxicity can result when flucytosine is used along with other drugs that depress bone marrow or when used during radiation therapy. Use of flucytosine with hepatotoxic or nephrotoxic drugs should be avoided. The use of flucytosine also decreases leukocyte and platelet counts and hemoglobin levels.

Metronidazole and alcohol always causes a severe reaction called a disulfiram-like reaction. With this reaction, severe nausea, vomiting, tachycardia (rapid heartbeat), flushing, and confusion develops. It is very important to warn patients not to take anything containing alcohol if they are taking metronidazole.

❖ NURSING IMPLICATIONS AND PATIENT TEACHING

▪ Assessment

Learn as much as possible about the patient's health history, including any allergy, bone marrow depression, use of alcohol or other drugs that may produce drug interactions (particularly corticosteroids), and the possibility of pregnancy. Some antifungal drugs may be teratogenic (causing deformities in the fetus).

The patient may have a history of fever and chills at the onset of infection. Itching is a common finding. A history of recent antibiotic therapy is common. The nurse may observe the classic signs of white discharge and erythema (redness or irritation) associated with thrush (Candida infection). The patient may also have a history of multiple scaly or blistered red patches on the skin, itching and soreness of infected areas, and brittle nails with yellow discoloration and separation from the nail bed.

 Memory Jogger

Antifungals

Ketoconazole: This medication has been associated with hepatic toxicity, so the patient must be monitored closely.

Flucytosine: Close monitoring of hematologic, renal, and hepatic status is essential.

Metronidazole (Flagyl) and alcohol: Counsel patients not to drink alcohol or eat alcohol-containing products while taking this medication because a severe GI and cardiovascular response may develop.

▪ Diagnosis

In addition to the medical diagnosis, what additional problems does the patient have? Are there difficulties in maintaining adequate nutrition or cleanliness or in paying for medications? Consider the need for education of the patient or family.

▪ Planning

Individuals allergic to penicillin may exhibit cross-sensitivity to antifungal agents, although this is rare. The patient may experience photosensitivity (abnormal response to exposure to sunlight) when taking these drugs.

Hepatotoxicity (usually reversible) and a few cases of hepatitis in children have been reported with ketoconazole. Liver function studies must be monitored so that any liver damage may be noted. The product should be discontinued if even a minor elevation in the liver function studies develops.

▪ Implementation

The absorption rate of griseofulvin is increased after the patient eats a fatty meal. Ketoconazole requires stomach acidity for dissolution and absorption. In patients with achlorhydria (lack of hydrochloric acid), tablets should be dissolved in several teaspoons of aqueous 0.2 NHCl solution. The patient should drink the solution with a straw to avoid staining the teeth and should follow the medication with a full glass of water. Explain to the patient how and why this is done.

Because griseofulvin is absorbed over a long period, single daily doses are often adequate. The patient must keep using the medication until the fungal infection is gone, as shown by both clinical and laboratory tests. This process may require several weeks or many months of therapy, depending on the organism responsible and the site of the infection. Use of both oral and topical antifungal agents may be required to treat some fungal infections, primarily tinea pedis (athlete's foot).

 Clinical Pitfall

Exposure to HIV

Patients who have recurrent vaginal infections that do not easily clear up and who have been exposed to HIV should be evaluated further.

▪ Evaluation

Observe the patient for therapeutic effects: chills or fever aqssociated with some infections should disappear; watch for signs of GI distress. The patient should continue to take the medication until the laboratory tests show that normal function has returned.

Nausea, vomiting, and diarrhea are symptoms of overdosage of most of the antifungal medications.

Clinical Pitfall

Liver or Renal Changes

Watch carefully for signs of liver or renal changes. These drugs are very toxic. Report all patient complaints promptly.

■ Patient and Family Teaching

Tell the patient and family the following:

- The patient should take all medication as ordered and not stop treatment when the symptoms disappear. The therapy may have to continue for many weeks before laboratory tests show that the infection is gone.
- The nurse, physician, or other health care provider should be called if the patient has any nausea, vomiting, diarrhea, or any bruising, sore throat, or fever. These drugs are very toxic, and no adverse effects should go unreported.
- The oral suspension of nystatin should be shaken thoroughly before use.

- Griseofulvin should be taken with meals that are high in fat; this causes more of the medication to be absorbed. Sometimes people taking this drug develop photosensitivity (intolerance to the sun). Alcoholic beverages should be avoided while taking griseofulvin or metronidazole.
- Cleanliness of hair, skin, and nails will help control or limit the spread of infection.
- If skin rash occurs or if nausea, vomiting, or diarrhea becomes severe in patients taking flucytosine, they should tell the nurse, physician, or other health care provider. When several capsules must be taken, they should be taken over a period of 15 minutes to avoid or reduce nausea and vomiting. If symptoms do not resolve within 2 to 3 days, the nurse, physician, or other health care provider should be called.
- Patients may be asked to use only bottled water to decrease exposure to community water supplies that may have a level of organisms that may be dangerous to immunocompromised patients.

Get Ready for the NCLEX® Examination!

Key Points

- This category of drugs is undergoing constant change as new products are added to the market. It is an area of intense research interest, and new information is being discovered every day that will help patients with immune deficiency problems.
- These are important but powerful and dangerous drugs.
- Although they are drugs ordered by specialists, these products are being used by more and more patients being seen in clinics and primary care practices. Thus the nurse will know specifics about these drugs and what to tell the patients about them.

Additional Learning Resources

SG Go to your Study Guide for additional learning activities to help you master this chapter content.

evolve Go to your Evolve website (http://evolve.elsevier.com/Edmunds/LPN/) for additional online resources.

Review Questions for the NCLEX® Examination

1. The patient has been started on an antiretroviral drug. He complains to the nurse about having mouth ulcers. The nurse recognizes this is an adverse reaction occurring because:
   1. it is indicative of an anaphylactic reaction
   2. it is an expected side effect of the medication
   3. it is unexpected toxic reaction of the medication
   4. it is indicative of liver or kidney damage

2. A major concern for patients taking antiretroviral drugs is:
   1. the number of pills required with each dosage
   2. the difficulty in swallowing the medication
   3. the cost of the prescribed medication
   4. the ineffectiveness of the medication

3. The patient has been started on metronidazole (Flagyl). One of the most important things to teach the patient is:
   1. avoid drinking orange juice while using the medication
   2. avoid drinking milk while using the medication
   3. avoid drinking grapefruit juice while using the medication
   4. avoid drinking alcohol while using the medication

4. The health care provider has ordered a nystatin suspension. The most important thing to teach the patient regarding its administration is:
   1. shake the medication thoroughly before use
   2. dilute the medication with water before use
   3. take the medication on a full stomach
   4. take the medication on an empty stomach

5. The patient has been placed on griseofulvin. In order to achieve maximum absorption of the medication, the patient should take it with a meal high in:
   1. protein
   2. carbohydrates
   3. fat
   4. cholesterol

Get Ready for the NCLEX® Examination!—cont'd

Case Study

Ms. Lucille Betts, a patient who has AIDS, comes into the clinic complaining of numbness and a burning sensation in her feet and lower legs. A physical examination shows her reflexes are good, but she has trouble feeling light touch, pinprick, temperature, and vibration in the feet and midcalf. She has been under treatment with a reverse transcriptase inhibitor.

1. What might be going on?
2. If the symptoms are ignored, what might happen?
3. What is the treatment?
4. Lucille discovers she is pregnant. What special requirements for treatment are there for pregnant women?
5. Lucille reports a thick white vaginal discharge and severe vaginal itching. What is the probable diagnosis?
6. Why are infections of this type common in immuno-compromised individuals?
7. What type of precautions should health care providers use in performing the vaginal examination on Lucille?
8. Lucille has an allergy to penicillin. Why might this be a problem for her?
9. Lucille is started on a vaginal antifungal medication. The nurse warns her that _____ is a common skin reaction associated with many antifungal medications.
10. Most vaginal infections are cured within 3 to 4 days. Is there any reason to suspect this will not be the case with Lucille?
11. Lucille is at risk for fungal infections at what other sites?

Drug Calculation Review

1. Order: Acyclovir 10 mg/kg IV over 1 hour every 8 hours
   Question: How many milligrams of acyclovir will be given for a 110-lb person?
2. Order: Amphotericin B 30 mg IV daily over 30 minutes
   Supply: Amphotericin B 30 mg in 100 mL 0.9% normal saline
   Question: How many milliliters per hour should the IV pump be set for?

Critical Thinking Questions

1. Mr. Delavan, a patient in the hospital has been given metronidazole for a systemic yeast infection; he also has AIDS and is taking several other medications as well. Why is it so important to check the ingredients of all other medications Mr. Delavan is taking? What serious problem might develop if the patient doesn't know what is in the medicines?
2. Mr. Delavan is taking a fungicide. What adverse reactions should the nurse look for in Mr. Delavan? Write up a treatment and evaluation plan for this patient.
3. A few months later, Mr. Delavan is back in the hospital. He now also has tuberculosis (TB). Mr. Delavan is a little panicky. He tells the nurse he is anxious to "get rid of it quick before it makes me sicker! How did this happen?!" Explain to Mr. Delavan why and how TB is easy for him to get now. Also explain why TB requires a long-term treatment plan and why compliance is so important. Revise the treatment and teaching plan for this patient.
4. Mr. Harris has HIV and comes to the clinic because of a severe *Candida* infection of his mouth (thrush). He is started on an antifungal medication. He returns several days later with nausea, vomiting, and severe diarrhea. What might be the source of the symptoms? What other treatment might be indicated?
5. Mr. Harris has a large, open, weeping lesion (open sore) on his leg. The doctor says this type of lesion is common in HIV-infected patients and is known as *Kaposi's sarcoma*. What precautions would should be taken in cleaning and dressing this lesion?
6. Mrs. Blake has had HIV for some time. She is 8 months pregnant. What are some of the special things the nurse would want to discuss with this prospective mother?
7. Ms. Lizz has had a bad fungal infection of her toenails. She has been taking the medication terbinafine for a couple of months. She is upset that she sees no improvement. What can the nurse tell her?
8. Ms. Sorenson comes in for her doctor's appointment complaining of a "white, itchy" vaginal discharge. She says she was seen by her doctor 10 days ago for strep throat, for which she took penicillin. Ms. Sorenson tells the nurse that she finished the antibiotics and was "fine until yesterday, when she began to get itchy". The patient asks if penicillin caused this vaginal infection or if she needs more penicillin? What would the nurse tell her?
9. Mr. Lopez arrives for his physician's appointment quite upset. He tells the nurse he is "really embarrassed by the painful lump on his lip," which appears inflamed. He states it "tingles a lot and is getting bigger every day. It feels like it is going to pop." He mentions he "just got over a bad cold." What might be Mr. Lopez's problem?

Antineoplastic Medications

Objectives

1. List the types of drugs used to treat neoplastic disease or cancer.
2. Identify the major adverse reactions associated with antineoplastic agents.

3. Develop a teaching plan for a patient taking an antineoplastic drug.

Key Terms

alkylating agents (ĂL-k-lā-tǐng, p. 201)
antibiotic preparations (ăn-tǐ-bī-ŎT-ǐk, p. 201)
antimetabolites (ăn-tǐ-mě-TĂB-ō-līts, p. 201)
Biologic Response Modifiers (BĪ-ō-LŎJ-ǐk, p. 202)
chemotherapeutic agents (kē-mō-thěr-ă-PŪ-tǐk, p. 200)

male or female hormones (HŎR-mōnz, p. 201)
malignancy (mă-LĬG-năn-sē, p. 200)
metastasis (mă-TĂS-tă-sǐs, p. 200)
mitotic inhibitors (mī-TŎT-ǐkǐn-HĪB-ǐ-tǒrs, p. 202)
neoplasms (NÊ-ō-plăz mz, p. 200)

OVERVIEW

Licensed practical and vocation nurses (LPNs/LVNs) often do not play a direct role in giving medications for cancer. There are many types of cancer and patients who have cancer are very commonly seen in areas in which LPNs/LVNs work. Every nurse should have some familiarity with the most common drugs given to fight cancer and a general awareness of why they might be ordered. Nurses are also frequently involved in administering other drugs to the cancer patient to fight the side effects of the very toxic cancer drugs.

Most cells in the body grow slowly at a rate that can be predicted. When cell growth becomes rapid and uncontrolled, **neoplasms** (abnormal growths or tumors that may be benign or malignant) may be found. These cells often have the ability to travel throughout the body, spreading this unusually rapid cell growth into other areas (**metastasis**). Cancer cells rob other tissues of the nutrients (substances that support life and growth) required for normal health. We call this out-of-control cell growth **malignancy** or cancerous growth. The causes of cancer are many—chemical, physical, hereditary, or biological. Some types of cancer are increased by patient behavior or lifestyle, such as lung cancer caused by smoking. Thus risk for developing some types of cancer may be reduced by changing eating habits, exercise, exposure to sun, or other types of behavior.

Antineoplastic agents, also called **chemotherapeutic agents**, are used to treat cancerous or malignant diseases. They slow cell growth or delay the spread of the malignant cells into other parts of the body. To achieve a cure, every malignant cell must be removed, destroyed, or crippled. Antineoplastic (anticancer) agents are most often used with other forms of treatment such as surgery and radiation. Drug therapy is rigorous, often requiring multiple drugs, intensive courses of high doses, and repeated courses of medicine if they are to be effective.

The following types of medications are used to treat neoplastic diseases: alkylating agents, antibiotic preparations, antimetabolites, hormones, natural products, and biologic response modifiers.

The types and sites of malignancies vary, and some agents are more effective than others in treating certain types of malignancies. The ideal antineoplastic agent damages the malignant cells of the patient while keeping the normal cells as healthy as possible.

Normal cells in the body do not all grow at the same rate. The cells in the gastrointestinal (GI) tract, bone marrow, hair follicles, lymph tissue, mouth, and testes or ovaries are rapidly dividing and growing. Antineoplastic drugs affect rapidly growing tumor cells, but also affect all other rapidly growing normal cells, thus producing many of the adverse reactions caused by these drugs (diarrhea, alopecia [hair loss], infertility, and the like).

There are many new, highly toxic products on the market in cancer treatment, including interferon, mitotane, and asparaginase. Antineoplastic drugs are strong and may be toxic; they are only ordered by a cancer or oncology specialist. Many drugs require intravenous (IV) administration. Even small dosage errors could have significant negative effects on the patient. Adverse reactions are common with this group of medications, and patients must be watched carefully for the development of toxicities. Hospitals may vary in whether they allow LPNs/LVNs to administer these drugs, so it is important to know institutional policy and stay within the authorized scope of practice.

Safety is a particular issue with oncology drugs. They are already toxic products and any errors in medication selected, dosage, or administration may be overwhelming to an ill patient.

Lifespan Considerations
Older Adults

ADVERSE REACTIONS
- Older adult patients are especially prone to adverse effects from these drugs and must be monitored carefully.
- Special care should be taken to give these patients plenty of water to drink (so they are hydrated). Adverse reactions such as nausea, anorexia, and diarrhea dehydrate patients.
- The older individual often does not have a lot of energy, and procedures and adverse effects make them especially tired. Monitor their strength and watch that they do not become overly exhausted.

Lifespan Considerations
Pediatric

SAFETY MEASURES
- Neoplastic drugs are particularly toxic. Particular care must be made for accurate dosing as even small errors in children could create big problems.
- Even if LPNs/LVNs are not administering these medications, they may be asked by other nurses to recheck the dosage that has been mixed, poured, or prepared as a further check for accuracy.
- Infants and small children may not be able to tell the nurse they are having problems with a drug. The nurse should watch the child carefully to watch for any changes.

ACTION AND USES

The five major types of antineoplastic agents may be used in combination or alone. There are often specific research protocols or rules that govern the use of these medications. It is important for the nurse to accurately report all reactions and adverse effects the patient might have so the action of the drug can be understood.

Alkylating agents are used to interfere with the normal process of cell division. They are some of the most widely used antineoplastic drugs. These drugs attach physically to deoxyribonucleic acid (DNA) in the tumor cell, a process called *alkylation*. As they do this, they change the structure of DNA in cancer cells and prevent it from functioning normally. There are different alkylating agents and they all attach to DNA in different ways. Working together, they are able to kill the cell or stop the production of new tumor cells. Although the alkylation occurs in the cancer cells, the killing action does not occur until the affected cell tries to divide.

This alkylating effect occurs in rapidly growing malignant cells, but it also occurs in some normal cells. Within the body, normal rapidly growing cells such as blood cells, white blood cells (WBCs) and epithelial cells lining the GI tract are also damaged. Thus as soon as the alkylating medications are given, red blood cells, WBCs, and platelets begin dying. These patients experience anemia and higher risk of infection. The death or damage to cells lining the GI tract produces nausea, vomiting, and diarrhea.

Specific **antibiotic preparations** are used, not for their antiinfective properties, but to delay or prevent cell division of the malignant cells. This action is caused by interference with DNA and ribonucleic acid synthesis. These antitumor antibiotics are obtained from bacteria and have the ability to kill cancer cells. These chemicals are more toxic than other antibiotics and their use is limited to use in treating very specific cancers.

Because the antitumor antibiotics interact with DNA in a way similar to the alkylating agents, their general actions and side effects are similar to those of the alkylating agents. However, all the antitumor antibiotics must be given intravenously or put directly into a cavity of the body using a catheter.

Antimetabolites disrupt normal cell functions by interfering with various metabolic functions of the cells and interrupt critical cell pathways in cells. Cells that are rapidly growing require large amounts of nutrients to build nucleic acids and proteins. These drugs resemble the essential building blocks of the cells but when the cancer cell attempts to use these chemicals as building blocks, the cancer cells slow their growth or die. This action is most effective in cells that are the most rapidly dividing—cancer cells, as well as normal hair and skin cells.

Some tumors may depend on **male or female hormones**, the chemicals produced by the sex glands. In patients who have these types of tumors, various hormones that counteract the effects of the hormones used by the tumors may be effective in treatment. The mechanism of action is unclear. Administering high doses of specific hormones or hormone antagonists can block the receptors in reproductive tissue tumors and slow tumor growth. An example is the use of tamoxifen to slow specific types of breast cancers that depend on estrogen for growth. Administration of the female hormone estrogen also slows the growth of prostate cancer.

In general, hormones and hormone antagonists produce few of the cytotoxic side effects seen with other antineoplastic drugs. However, as these medications may be given in high doses and for long periods, they may produce other unpleasant side effects. They rarely produce cures but may slow the growth of the cancer.

There are a variety of other primary plant extracts or alkaloids that are used as antineoplastics. These chemicals have been isolated from a number of plants, including common flowers and shrubs. Although these chemicals are structurally different, they all have the ability to stop cell division. As a group, they may be called **mitotic inhibitors**.

Taxoids and topoisomerase inhibitors are other groups of medications that have biologic properties helpful in treating cancer. They often have significant adverse effects.

Biologic response modifiers are relativity new immunologic drugs that do not kill tumor cells directly themselves, but instead stimulate the body's immune system to help it fight the cancer. They may also be helpful in minimizing the toxic effects of other antineoplastics. Specifically, some drugs work to prevent anemia, stimulate platelet production, or help prevent severe thrombocytopenia. Thus the quality of life of these patients may be better when these drugs are given.

See Figure 14-1 to see where major antineoplastic drugs act on the cells.

A mix of other drugs, most of which have been developed in the last few years, now make up the largest category of antineoplastic drugs, the miscellaneous agents. These products are used for treatment of a wide variety of conditions. Many of them have unlabeled uses, whereas, for others, clinical trials are being done to determine if they are effective and safe. Many of these drugs are being evaluated further.

 Clinical Goldmine

Use of Natural Products

Green tea has been investigated for use as a medicinal antioxidant to provide a protective effect against cancer cells. Antioxidants are viewed as helpful because of their ability to eliminate free radicals—substances that remain after normal metabolism of a chemical leaving residue that may damage the cell. (Think of the sparks that fly off from a burning log). Both green tea and, to a lesser extent, black tea have been found to have some antioxidant activity.

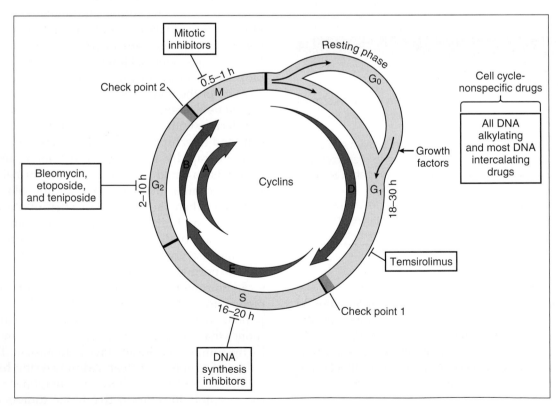

FIGURE 14-1 Cell cycle activity of antineoplastic drugs.
Cell division or replication proceeds in a cycle. In sequence, the cycle involves G1 (gap1), S (DNA synthesis), G2 (gap 2), and M (mitosis). Differentiated cells may enter a resting state called GO. Growth factors may stimulate resting cells to reenter the cell cycle. Proteins called cyclins (A,B,D,E) promote cell progress through the cycle. Two check points in the cycle which often malfunction in cancer cells are those which control entry into the critical phases of DNA synthesis and mitosis. Cell cycle-specific drugs act primarily during the designated phase of the cycle. Cell cycle-nonspecific drugs act throughout the cell cycle.

ADVERSE REACTIONS

The action of the antineoplastic agents on normal cells causes many of the adverse reactions experienced by patients on chemotherapy. Some of these reactions depend on the dose given. Nausea, vomiting, anorexia, and diarrhea are seen with almost all products. Other common reactions include alopecia (hair loss) and bone marrow depression. (Patients with bone marrow depression are more likely to get infections and may show bruising or bleeding.) Renal toxicity, hepatic toxicity, ototoxicity, ocular effects, peripheral neurotoxicity, and hypersensitivity are common among these drugs, and patients must be monitored carefully.

 Clinical Pitfall

Antineoplastic Agents

These are some of the most dangerous drugs given to patients. However, they may save the patient's life, so the benefit outweighs the risk. The nurse always watches the patient and looks for changes that might be the onset of serious adverse reactions.

Some reactions are so severe that the patient feels worse with therapy than with the malignancy. There may be no cure for the adverse effects except to stop therapy and not treat the malignancy. Knowledge about the most common adverse effects will help the nurse develop a care plan to prevent or reduce as many symptoms as possible.

DRUG INTERACTIONS

Most antineoplastic drugs interact with other medications the patient may be taking. It is very important to consult the manufacturer's guidelines before starting treatment.

NURSING IMPLICATIONS AND
❖ PATIENT TEACHING

■ Assessment

Learn everything possible about the patient's history, the type of malignancy and current status, medications taken, surgeries, allergies, and response. Many patients have numerous hospital admissions for treatment of a malignancy. Old hospital records should be read whenever possible to find accurate information and avoid the need for the patient to repeat information. The patient who comes into the hospital several times should be asked about progress since the last hospitalization. It is important to find out about the patient's emotional and physical responses to the illness, as well as cultural beliefs, spiritual and family support, and acceptance of the problem.

■ Diagnosis

What other problems does this patient have that may interfere with treatment? Are there adverse effects or disease progression that must be treated? Is the patient fearful or worried? Is money an issue?

■ Planning

Read the latest product information about the preparation, storage, and administration of antineoplastic medications. Understand and follow all warnings, precautions, and contraindications. Some preparations should be given only by a physician or other health care provider or a specially trained chemotherapy nurse. New drug information is common.

The initial dosage of antineoplastic medication is often calculated in milligrams per kilogram (mg/kg) or milligrams per square meter of body surface area (mg/m^2 BSA). These calculations are based on surface nomograms, which are provided in the drug maker's product insert. The starting dosage will be calculated by the specialist, with future adjustments based on the patient's response as measured by laboratory tests and x-ray studies.

Some medications given intravenously will damage and destroy the tissues of the skin if the IV needle becomes dislodged and medication goes into the tissue and not the veins. This is called *extravasation*. Medication must be on hand that can be immediately injected directly into the skin to counter the effect of the antitumor medicine. Failure to act quickly may result in huge areas of tissue damage, sometimes destroying the ability of the hand or arm to function.

■ Implementation

Carefully follow the dosage, frequency, and administration procedures as outlined for any drugs the nurse is authorized to give. Administration of these toxic products may pose a safety hazard to the nurse, as well as the patient, if the products are not administered properly. The syringes, bottles, and needles must be handled and disposed of carefully. There should be a special area designated for mixing these preparations.

Table 14-1 presents the product information for the major antineoplastic agents. Additional detailed information on hormones may be found in Chapter 20.

■ Evaluation

Check the patient closely for adverse effects, regularly noting subjective complaints or objective findings on the chart so the physician or other health care provider may follow the patient's progress. Teach the patient which symptoms to report to the nurse, physician, or other health care provider after discharge, when medications will be given on an outpatient basis. Table 14-1 includes a listing of common adverse effects for many of these drugs.

Table 14-1   Antineoplastic Agents

GENERIC NAME	TRADE NAME	COMMENTS
Alkylating Agents		
altretamine	Hexalen	Used for palliative treatment of patients with persistent or recurrent ovarian cancer.
busulfan	Busulfex Myleran	Used in chronic myelogenous leukemia; may produce leukopenia, anemia, thrombocytopenia, hyperpigmentation of skin, and cataracts.
carboplatin	Paraplatin	Used in ovarian carcinoma.
carmustine	BiCNU	Used in patients with brain tumors, Hodgkin disease, and multiple myeloma; may produce leukopenia, thrombocytopenia, azotemia, nausea, and vomiting; causes burning at injection site.
	Gliadel wafers	Wafer inserted into cavity after surgery. Up to 8 wafers at a time may be used. Indicated in newly diagnosed patients with high-grade malignant glioma as an adjunct to surgery and radiation; also indicated in recurrent glioblastoma multiforme patients as an adjunct to surgery; provides localized delivery of chemotherapy directly to site of tumor—the only FDA-approved brain cancer treatment capable of doing so.
chlorambucil	Leukeran ❧	Used in Hodgkin disease, chronic lymphocytic leukemia, and malignant lymphomas; may produce hyperuricemia and bone marrow depression.
cisplatin	Platinol-AQ ❧	Used in advanced bladder cancer and some metastatic testicular and ovarian tumors; may produce nausea, vomiting, leukopenia, thrombocytopenia, ototoxicity, and nephrotoxicity.
cyclophosphamide	Cytoxan Neosar	Used in Hodgkin disease, leukemia, carcinoma of ovary and breast, malignant lymphomas, multiple melanoma, and neuroblastoma; may produce anorexia, nausea, vomiting, diarrhea, cystitis, alopecia, leukopenia, thrombocytopenia, or anemia.
dacarbazine	DTIC-Dome	Used in metastatic malignant melanoma, Hodgkin disease.
estramustine	Emcyt	Used in advanced prostate cancer as palliative treatment.
ifosfamide	Ifex ❧ Ifex-Mesnex	Used in testicular cancer.
lomustine	CeeNu	Used in Hodgkin disease, some brain tumors; may produce nausea, vomiting, alopecia, anemia, leukopenia, and thrombocytopenia.
mechlorethamine	Mustargen ❧	Used in Hodgkin disease, bronchogenic carcinoma, and lymphosarcoma; may produce nausea, vomiting, jaundice, alopecia, skin rash, diarrhea, lymphocytopenia, granulocytopenia, and thrombocytopenia.
melphalan	Alkeran ❧	Used in carcinoma of ovary and for multiple myeloma; may produce nausea, vomiting, skin rash, and bone marrow depression.
oxaliplatin	Eloxatin	Used for metastatic colorectal cancer.
streptozocin	Zanosar	Used in carcinoma of the pancreas; may produce severe nausea, vomiting, and renal toxicity.
temozolomide	Temodar	Used for brain cancer.
thiotepa		Used in lymphosarcomas or carcinoma of breast, ovary, or urinary bladder; may produce nausea, vomiting, and bone marrow depression; causes pain at injection site. May be directly infiltrated into tumor.
Antitumor Antibiotics		
bleomycin	Blenoxane	Used in testicular carcinoma, lymphomas, and squamous cell carcinomas of head and neck; may cause vomiting, rash, erythema, fever, chills, pulmonary fibrosis, and pneumonitis.
dactinomycin	Cosmegen	Used in testicular or uterine carcinoma, Wilms tumor, and Ewing sarcoma; may produce anorexia, nausea, vomiting, alopecia, and bone marrow depression. Very corrosive to soft tissue.

Table 14-1   Antineoplastic Agents—cont'd

GENERIC NAME	TRADE NAME	COMMENTS
daunorubicin	Cerubidine	Used in adult leukemias; may produce nausea, vomiting, fever, chills, alopecia, and bone marrow depression. Used under strict protocols.
doxorubicin	Adriamycin Rubex	Used in acute leukemias, Wilms tumor, carcinomas of breast, ovary, and bladder, lymphomas, neuroblastomas, and soft tissue and bone sarcomas; may cause anorexia, nausea, vomiting, alopecia, fever, and bone marrow depression. Give IV.
epirubicin	Ellence	Used as a component of adjuvant therapy in patients with evidence of axillary node tumor involvement after resection of primary breast cancer. Severe local tissue necrosis develops with extravasation during administration. Watch for myocardial toxicity.
idarubicin	Idamycin PFS	Used in adult acute myeloid leukemia.
mitomycin	Mutamycin Mitozytrex	Used in adenocarcinoma of the stomach and pancreas; may cause anorexia, nausea, vomiting, headache, blurred vision, fever, and bone marrow depression.
mitoxantrone	Novantrone	Used in combination with other drugs in initial therapy for acute nonlymphatic leukemia; may cause petechiae, nausea, vomiting, diarrhea, stomatitis, sepsis, fungal infections, dyspnea, fever, and alopecia.
plicamycin	Mithramycin	For testicular cancer. Given IV daily for 8-10 days.
valrubicin	Valstar	Give as an intrabladder instillation every week for 6 weeks for bladder cancer.
Antimetabolites		
allopurinol	Aloprim Zyloprim	Used in the management of patients with leukemia, lymphoma, and solid tumor malignancies who are receiving cancer therapy that causes elevation of serum uric acid levels. May be given orally or by injection.
capecitabine	Xeloda	Prodrug of 5-fluorouracil with complex dosing schedule used in metastatic breast cancer.
clofarabine	Clolar	For childhood acute lymphoblastic leukemia. Give IV over 2 hours for 5 consecutive days.
cladribine	Leustatin	Used in treating hairy cell leukemia and unlabeled uses in a wide variety of other conditions.
cytarabine		Used in acute myelocytic or lymphocytic leukemia; may cause nausea, vomiting, anorexia, diarrhea, and bone marrow depression. Duration of treatment varies with patient response.
floxuridine	FUDR	Used in GI adenocarcinoma metastatic to liver; may produce anorexia, nausea, vomiting, diarrhea, alopecia, and bone marrow depression.
fludarabine	Fludara	Used in chronic lymphocytic leukemia. Usually given IV over 30 min for 5 consecutive days every 28 days.
fluorouracil	Adrucil	Used in carcinoma of breast, stomach, colon, and pancreas; may cause anorexia, nausea, vomiting, diarrhea, alopecia, and bone marrow depression.
gemcitabine	Gemzar	Used in adenocarcinoma of the pancreas.
mercaptopurine	Purinethol	Used in acute lymphatic leukemia and acute or chronic myelogenous leukemia; may produce hyperuricemia, hepatotoxicity, and bone marrow depression.
methotrexate	Trexall	Used in breast cancer, lymphosarcoma, and severe psoriasis; may cause nausea, vomiting, headache, rash, pruritus, stomatitis, bone marrow depression, leukopenia, and renal failure. Dosage varies depending on specific treatment requirements.
Pemetrexed	Alimta	Used for malignant mesothelioma and non-small cell lung cancer. Take on day 1 of each 21-day cycle.
pentostatin	Nipent	Used in hairy cell leukemia. Give IV every other week in well-hydrated patient.
thioguanine	Tabloid	Used in acute nonlymphocytic leukemias and chronic myelogenous leukemia; may produce nausea, vomiting, stomatitis, hyperuricemia, hepatotoxicity, and bone marrow depression. Dosage determined by individualized protocol.

Continued

Table 14-1   Antineoplastic Agents—cont'd

GENERIC NAME	TRADE NAME	COMMENTS
Hormones and Hormone Antagonists		
Hormones		
diethylstilbestrol	DES, Stilbestrol	For cancer of the prostate and breast.
estramustine	Emcyt	Used in metastatic prostatic carcinoma; may cause nausea, vomiting, diarrhea, anorexia, fluid retention, edema, leukopenia, rash, and thrombocytopenia.
ethinyl estradiol	Estinyl	Used for cancer of the prostate and breast.
fluoxymesterone	Halotestin	Used for breast cancer.
medroxyprogesterone	Depo-Provera	Used in renal or endometrial carcinoma; may cause pruritus, breast tenderness, and cerebral or pulmonary emboli.
megestrol acetate	Megace	Used in endometrial or breast carcinoma.
prednisone	Deltasone	Used for lymphomas, acute leukemia, and Hodgkin disease.
testolactone	Teslac	Used for breast cancer.
testosterone	Testred	Used for breast cancer.
triptorelin pamoate	Trelstar Depot, Trelstar LA	Used in palliative treatment of advanced prostate cancer. Given every 28 days.
Hormone Antagonists		
abarelix	Plenaxis	Palliative treatment for advanced prostate cancer.
aminoglutethimide	Cytadren	For breast, prostate, and adrenal cancer. Hydrocortisone is administered along with this drug.
anastrozole	Arimidex	First-line treatment of postmenopausal women when they have either hormone receptor–positive or hormone receptor–unknown classification of locally advanced or metastatic breast cancer.
bicalutamide	Casodex	A nonsteroidal antiandrogen used in advanced prostate cancer, along with LHRH.
exemestane	Aromasin	For the treatment of both early and advanced breast cancer in postmenopausal women whose disease has progressed after tamoxifen therapy. Also used in the prevention of prostate carcinogenesis.
flutamide	Eulexin	Used in metastatic prostatic carcinoma.
goserelin acetate	Zoladex	Used in palliative treatment of carcinoma of prostate. Give subcutaneously every 28 days in upper abdominal wall.
letrozole	Femara	Used in treatment of both early and advanced breast cancer in postmenopausal women with disease progression after antiestrogen therapy.
leuprolide	Eligard Lupron	Used in advanced prostatic carcinoma; may produce nausea, vomiting, anorexia, dizziness, headache, edema, and bone pain.
nilutamide	Nilandron	An antiandrogen used for metastatic prostate cancer, along with surgical castration. Give with or without food.
tamoxifen	Soltamox	Used in breast cancer in postmenopausal women; may produce hypercalcemia and ophthalmic changes.
toremifene citrate	Fareston	Used in treatment of metastatic breast cancer in postmenopausal women with estrogen receptor–positive or estrogen receptor–unknown tumors.
Natural Products and Mitotic Inhibitors		
docetaxel	Taxotere	Used in patients with advanced breast cancer.
etoposide	Toposar VePesid	Used in testicular tumors; may produce anorexia, nausea, vomiting, alopecia, and granulocytopenia. Duration of treatment varies with patient response.
Irinotecan	Camptosar	Used for colorectal cancer.

Table 14-1   Antineoplastic Agents—cont'd

GENERIC NAME	TRADE NAME	COMMENTS
paclitaxel	Onxol Taxol	Used in ovarian carcinoma, breast carcinoma, and AIDS-related Kaposi sarcoma.
teniposide	Vumon	Used in childhood acute lymphocytic lymphoma patients in combination with other products. Extremely corrosive to soft tissue. Give slow IV.
topotecan	Hycamtin	Used for ovarian cancer.
vinblastine	Velban	Used in Hodgkin disease, Kaposi sarcoma, lymphoma, and testicular carcinoma; may cause nausea, vomiting, malaise, headache, numbness, paresthesias, weakness, depression, and leukopenia. Usual adult dose determined by WBC counts.
vincristine	Oncovin Vincasar PFS	Used in Hodgkin disease, Wilms tumor, acute leukemia, lymphosarcoma, and neuroblastoma; may produce nausea, vomiting, diarrhea, fever, weight loss, ataxia, headache, and mouth ulcers.
vinorelbine tartrate	Navelbine	IV product used in non–small cell lung cancer. Unlabeled uses in breast cancer, ovarian carcinoma, and Hodgkin disease.
Biologic Response Modifiers and Other Miscellaneous Agents		
aldesleukin	Proleukin ✦	Used in metastatic renal cell carcinoma.
Altretamine	Hexalen	Used for ovarian cancer.
l-asparaginase	Elspar	Used with other drugs in acute lymphocytic leukemia.
bevacizumab	Avastin	Used for metastatic colorectal cancer.
cetuximab	Erbitux	Used for metastatic colorectal cancer.
erlotinib	Tarceva	Used for metastatic non–small cell lung cancer.
hydroxyurea	Droxia Hydrea ✦ Mylocel	Used in melanoma and squamous cell carcinoma. Unlabeled use for sickle cell anemia, thrombocythemia, HIV, and psoriasis. Dosage is calculated on actual weight.
imatinib	Gleevac	For chronic myeloid leukemia as palliative therapy.
interferon alfa-2a	Roferon-A	Used in hairy cell leukemia, AIDS-related Kaposi sarcoma, and chronic myelogenous leukemia.
interferon alfa-2b	Intron-A	Used in hairy cell leukemia, malignant melanoma, condyloma acuminatum, AIDS-related Kaposi sarcoma, and chronic hepatitis C and B.
levamisole	Ergamisol	Used for colon cancer.
mitotane	Lysodren	Used for inoperable adrenal cortical carcinoma.
pegaspargase	Oncaspar	Used in acute lymphocytic leukemia.
porfimer	Photofrin	A photosensitizing agent used in the treatment of esophageal cancer.
procarbazine HCl	Matulane	Used with other drugs in combination to treat Hodgkin disease. Dose is calculated on patient's actual weight.
rituximab	Rituxan	Used in treatment of Hodgkin disease.
trastuzumab	Herceptin	Used for metastatic breast cancer.

AIDS, Acquired immune deficiency syndrome; *FDA,* Food and Drug Administration; *GI,* gastrointestinal; *HIV,* human immunodeficiency virus; *LHRH,* luteinizing hormone–releasing hormone; *WBC,* white blood cell.

Nursing or pharmacologic interventions are often needed to reduce adverse effects. Some of the common problems and their treatment are included in Table 14-2.

The patient should be taught about the need to get follow-up laboratory work and x-ray studies to determine the response to medication. The nurse takes time and provides opportunities for patients to discuss their feelings and attitudes about the disease and their therapy.

■ **Patient and Family Teaching**

Tell the patient and family the following:

• Antineoplastic agents may be toxic and must be taken as ordered. The patient should learn the reason for their use, what they will do, and the possible adverse reactions. The patient may be required to sign a written consent form before many of these drugs can be administered.

• The patient should learn in detail about the possible adverse effects of these drugs. Specific plans for preventing or reducing symptoms should be developed. The patient should know which symptoms to report to the nurse, physician, or other health care provider.

• The patient's meals should be made as palatable and attractive as possible because most antineoplastic agents produce anorexia, nausea, and vomiting. The patient may be unable to eat anything at times but may find holding ice chips in the mouth to be helpful.

• The patient should learn the signs of dehydration caused by diarrhea, vomiting, and poor oral intake.

• Hair loss is usually of great concern to the patient. Provide information on wigs and toupees that might be worn until their own hair grows back. Patients with long hair may want to save lost hair and have a wig made from their own hair. There are shops that specialize in this service in many cities. The nurse may help the patient select scarves, turbans, or hats to wear. When hair begins to regrow, patients should use a very mild shampoo and conditioner.

• Patient should limit exposure to the sun by wearing long sleeves when outdoors, wearing sunscreen, sunglasses, and a hat or scarf to protect a bare scalp.

• Patients who have had surgery for cancer, such as mastectomy or amputation, should be provided with information about muscle strengthening after surgery, the postoperative recovery period, postsurgical breast reconstruction, and prosthesis use.

• There are many support groups available for specific types of cancer, and former patients may visit the hospital and talk to the patient about their colostomy or mastectomy or other needs. The patient can be referred to community resources for further information.

• Any medication taken home should be kept in a locked cabinet away from children or pets.

Table 14-2	Common Symptoms Following Chemotherapy and Their Treatment

SYMPTOMS OR PROBLEM	SUGGESTED TREATMENT
Nausea and or vomiting	Provide antiemetics. Some herbal preparations may be helpful. Drink liquids between meals and not with food.
Stomatitis	Practice good oral hygiene with soft tooth brush, water or mild salt solution; avoid alcohol-based mouthwash. Use mouth rinse such as Maalox, Xylocaine, Benadryl, BMX. Avoid hot, cold, or other products that might damage sensitive tissue. Increase fluid intake to decrease the risk of kidney damage and the formation of uric acid crystals.
Skin breakdown	Provide vitamin supplementation, practice good skin care.
Pain at surgical site	Provide analgesics or narcotics.
Dehydration	Force fluids, provide IV hydration.
Low WBC count or bone marrow suppression	Use neutropenic diet: avoid raw fish and meat, raw fruits and vegetables, or peppercorns. Watch for elevated temperatures. Stay away from other people or even use reverse isolation; provide interferon alfa-2 for severe problems.
Low platelet counts	Report any bruising, blood in urine or stools, severe fatigue, epigastric pain, difficulty clotting. Provide oprelvekin for severe problems.
Anemia	Provide epoetin alfa
Anorexia	Provide small feedings. Megestrol acetate is an appetite stimulant.
Reduced fertility	Consider sperm banking prior to chemotherapy. Chemotherapy may reduce sperm count or increase risk of genetic damage to sperm.

IV, Intravenous; *WBC*, white blood cell.

Get Ready for the NCLEX® Examination!

Key Points

- The main types of agents commonly used to treat neoplastic disease are alkylating agents, antibiotic preparations, antimetabolites, hormones, natural products, and biologic response modifiers.
- Because these drugs are highly toxic, it is especially important for the nurse to look for adverse reactions in the patient.
- Dosages must be precisely followed, and care must be taken in the preparation and disposal of syringes, bottles, and needles.

Additional Learning Resources

SG   Go to your Study Guide for additional learning activities to help you master this chapter content.

evolve   Go to your Evolve website (http://evolve.elsevier.com/Edmunds/LPN/) for additional online resources.

Review Questions for the NCLEX® Examination

1. The patient started on chemotherapy for a tumor in his lung is concerned about whether he and his wife will be able to have children after his treatments have ended. The nurse understands:
   1. sterility does not occur with chemotherapy
   2. sterility always occurs after chemotherapy
   3. that he/she should suggest the patient consider adoption, sperm banking, or rethink having children
   4. sterility might be a possibility and the nurse should suggest that the patient discuss this important concern with the health care provider

2. The patient ibeing treated with chemotherapy complains of anorexia. The most appropriate intervention to treat this is:
   1. tell the patient this is normal and not to worry about eating
   2. sympathize with the patient and report this problem to the charge nurse and put it in the nursing notes
   3. tell the patient to eat only when he is hungry
   4. tell the patient to eat small, frequent meals

3. A patient is being treated with chemotherapy and complains of experiencing nausea and vomiting. The highest priority instruction that the nurse should give the patient is:
   1. put this complaint in the nursing notes; report it to the charge nurse and ask for medicine to control nausea for the patient
   2. drink liquids between meals rather than with meals
   3. supplement his regular diet with vitamin therapy
   4. use herbal preparations to decrease nausea

4. The patient has had both surgery and chemotherapy for a fast growing cancer in his stomach. What are some of the adverse effects that might develop from chemotherapy?
   1. Anorexia, nausea, vomiting, diarrhea
   2. Sore mouth and tongue, bad odor to breath
   3. Gastric reflux, intense hunger, burping
   4. Signs of infection around the surgical incision

5. The reason that patients being treated for cancer with chemotherapy often lose their hair is because:
   1. this is a rare occurrence in some patients with some medicines. Not everyone loses hair.
   2. some patients lose hair because of an allergy to the medicine.
   3. chemotherapy targets the fastest growing cells of the tumor for destruction, but other body cells that grow fast—like hair—are also affected.
   4. chemotherapy targets the tumor cells that are very large, so the big doses of medicine required also affects the hair.

Case Study

Bonnie Taylor, 48 years old, is admitted to the hospital with a diagnosis of acute lymphoblastic leukemia (ALL). She also has a urinary tract infection when she is admitted. She has had four other admissions for chemotherapy and supportive care. She has lost weight and currently weighs 110 pounds. She is to receive platelets and a whole-blood transfusion. The medications prescribed include:

- Acetaminophen (Tylenol) 650 mg PO q4h for fever
- Gentamicin 50 mg IV q8h
- 6-Mercaptopurine (Purinethol) 200 mg PO daily

1. The usual adult daily dose of 6-mercaptopurine is 2.5 mg/kg/day. How does this compare with what is ordered?
2. The usual adult daily dose of IV gentamicin is 3 mg/kg/day in three equal doses, given every 8 hours. If the product comes in doses of 40 mg/mL, how much medication will be drawn up to be injected?
3. Why is gentamicin ordered?
4. Why is 6-mercaptopurine ordered?
5. Why might this patient have an elevated temperature? What would the nurse give her and when?
6. What other chemotherapeutic agents might be used for the treatment of leukemia?
7. Because of her condition and all of the medications she is taking, what are some of the symptoms she might also develop?

Drug Calculation Review

1. The physician orders an IV solution of cisplatin (Platinol) 10 mg in 1000 mL of dextrose 5% in 0.9% saline

Get Ready for the NCLEX® Examination!—cont'd

solution (D$_5$NS). This solution is to infuse at a rate of 1.25 mg/hr. If the drop factor is 20 gtt = 1 mL, what is the flow rate in drops per minute?

2. Order: Bleomycin 45 units IV. Supply: Bleomycin 15 units per vial
   Question: How many vials of bleomycin are needed for each dose?

3. Order: Cytoxan 10 mg/kg IV
   Question: How many mg of Cytoxan are needed for a person weighing 65 kg?

4. Order: Interferon alfa 3,000,000 International Units subcutaneously three times per week. Supply: Interferon alfa 6,000,000 International Units/mL
   Question: How many milliliters of interferon alfa are needed with each dose?

Critical Thinking Questions

1. What common action do all antineoplastic agents share? Are these antineoplastic agents generally used alone? Why or why not? Describe how treatments (chemotherapy, radiation, or surgery) might be combined.

2. What healthy, or normal, cells are also affected by antineoplastic agents? Describe several adverse reactions associated with these cells. Why does this occur?

3. Patients are closely checked before chemotherapy begins. Why is this important? What sorts of things would be important to monitor?

4. Chemotherapy is usually given by physicians. What exactly are the nurse's responsibilities when a patient is receiving chemotherapy.

5. Write out a teaching plan for explaining to a patient about the drugs they are being given and what to reasonably expect if the drug is working and detailing what adverse effects might develop.

6. Ms. Reynolds is a 30-year-old patient who is currently undergoing chemotherapy following surgery for breast cancer. She tells the nurse her 5-year-old daughter will be starting kindergarten in a few months and will need "all her shots for school soon." What things should the nurse tell the patient?

7. What things will the doctor ask the patient about in order to determine if the chemotherapy is working?

8. What laboratory tests would be helpful to determine if the patient is responding to chemotherapy?

Cardiovascular and Renal Medications

Objectives

1. Identify the approved way to give different forms of antianginal therapy.
2. Discuss the uses and general actions of cardiac drugs used to treat dysrhythmias.
3. Describe the common treatment for various types of lipoprotein disorders.
4. List the general uses and actions of cardiotonic drugs.
5. Explain the actions of different categories of drugs used to treat hypertension.
6. Identify indications for electrolyte replacement.

Key Terms

action potential duration (ĂK-shun PŌ-těn-chăl, p. 220)
congestive heart failure (CHF) (HĂRT FĀL-yŭr, p. 229)
chronotropic (KRŎ-nō-TRŌP-ĭk, p. 221)
compelling indications (p. 238)
dehydration (dē-hī-DRĀ-shŭn, p. 247)
depolarization (dē-pō-lăr-ĭ-ZĀ-shŭn, p. 221)
digitalis toxicity (dĭj-ĭ-TĂL-ĭs, p. 231)
digitalizing dose (DĬJ-ĭ-tăl-īz-ĭng, p. 231)
dromotropic (DRŎM-ō-TRŌP-ĭk, p. 221)
dysrhythmia (dĭs-RĬTH-mē-ă, p. 219)
ectopic beats (ěk-TŎP-ĭk, p. 220)
edema (ě-DĒ-mă, p. 229)
effective refractory period (rē-FRĂK-tŏr-ē, p. 220)
electrocardiogram (ECG) (ě-lěk-trō-KĂR-dē-ō-gram, p. 219)

end-organ damage (p. 238)
fluid and electrolyte mixtures (ě-LĚK-trō-līt, p. 247)
hyperlipidemia (hī-pěr-lĭp-ĭ-DĒ-mē-a, p. 224)
hyperlipoproteinemia (hī-pěr-līp-ō-PRŌT-ě-NĒ-mē-ă, p. 226)
myocardial infarction (MI) (mī-ō-KĂR-dē-ăl ĭn-FĂRK-shŭn, p. 225)
myocardium (mī-ō-KĂR-dē-ŭm, p. 219)
normal sinus rhythm (SĪ-nŭs RĬTH-ĭm, p. 219)
pacemaker (PĂS-MĀ-kěr, p. 219)
positive inotropic action (ĭ-nă-TRŌP-ĭk, p. 230)
primary hypertension (PRĪ-măr-ē hī-pěr-TĚN-shŭn, p. 233)
secondary hypertension (SĚK-ŏn-dăr-ē hī-pěr-TĚN-shŭn, p. 233)

OVERVIEW

This chapter is divided into six major sections, each with a focus on an important job of the cardiovascular, circulatory, or renal system. Some cardiovascular drugs have more than one action and are used for several reasons in the patient with cardiovascular problems. However, they are usually classified into one of the major drug categories.

The first section, Antianginals and Peripheral Vasodilators, focuses on the drugs used to treat chest pain from angina and problems with diseases causing blockage of the arteries, mostly in the legs. These drugs are widely used, and the nurse will have a major role in teaching the patient how to properly store and use them. The second section discusses the four major classes of medications used for dysrhythmias (irregular heartbeats). The antidysrhythmics are powerful drugs, and there may be many adverse reactions from some of these medications. The third section looks at lipids (fats) and the problem of lipoprotein

abnormalities. Antihyperlipidemic agents are discussed as a part of the overall therapy for lipoprotein problems. The fourth section focuses on the drugs that make the heartbeat stronger—the cardiotonics or positive inotropic agents, such as digitalis and related products. These are some of the most common drugs for patients both in and out of the hospital, and some of the "must know" drugs. Antihypertensives, diuretics, and urinary system drugs are explored in the fifth section. Because hypertension (high blood pressure) is so common, the nurse will use many of these drugs. The latest guidelines for lowering blood pressure are listed, as well as common adverse reactions to these drugs. Although most of the drugs acting on the kidney are diuretics, other agents that affect the urinary tract are also presented here. The sixth section covers fluid and electrolytes, which nurses also frequently give.

These classifications have many drugs and these sections give the most important basic information about each drug category. If the nurse reviews the anatomy and physiology of the cardiovascular and urinary systems at the same time, it will help them understand both the problems that occur in these systems and how the different drugs act to solve those problems.

CARDIOVASCULAR AND URINARY SYSTEMS

The cardiovascular system is made up of the heart, blood vessels (Figure 15-1), and blood. This system moves nutrients (substances that support life and

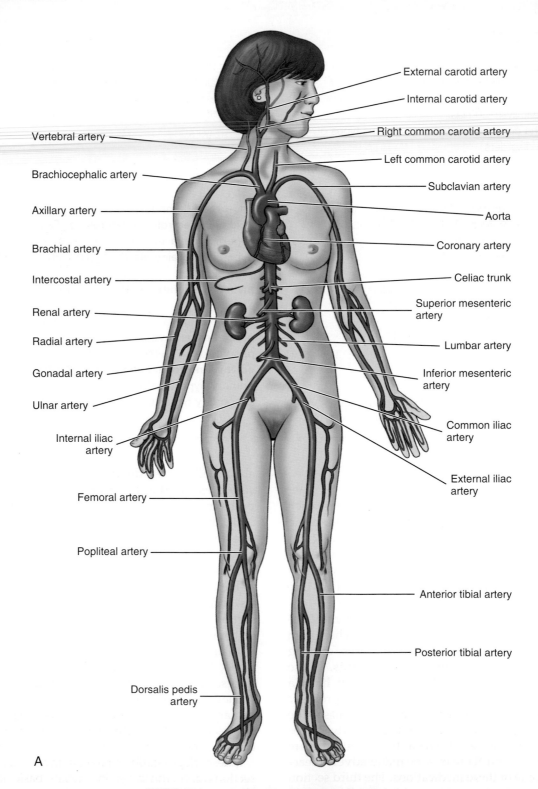

External carotid artery

Internal carotid artery

Right common carotid artery

Left common carotid artery

Subclavian artery

Aorta

Coronary artery

Celiac trunk

Superior mesenteric artery

Lumbar artery

Inferior mesenteric artery

Common iliac artery

External iliac artery

Anterior tibial artery

Posterior tibial artery

Vertebral artery

Brachiocephalic artery

Axillary artery

Brachial artery

Intercostal artery

Renal artery

Radial artery

Gonadal artery

Ulnar artery

Internal iliac artery

Femoral artery

Popliteal artery

Dorsalis pedis artery

A

FIGURE 15-1 Cardiovascular system. **A,** Major arteries.

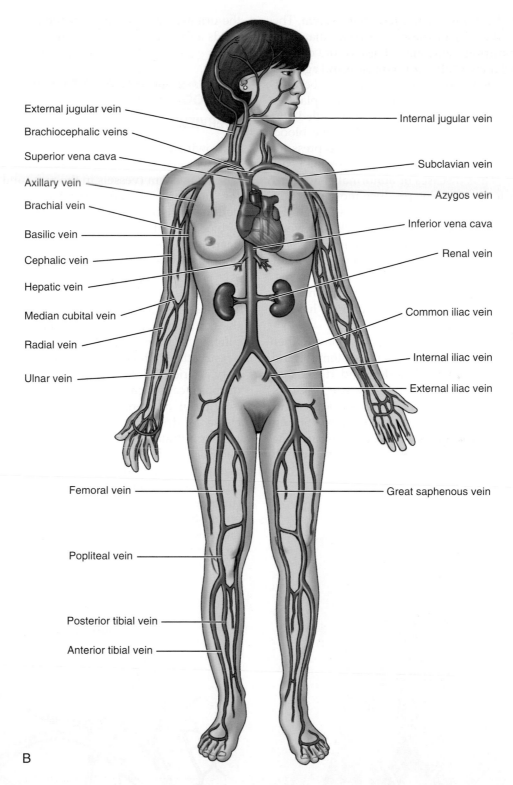

External jugular vein

Brachiocephalic veins

Superior vena cava

Axillary vein

Brachial vein

Basilic vein

Cephalic vein

Hepatic vein

Median cubital vein

Radial vein

Ulnar vein

Internal jugular vein

Subclavian vein

Azygos vein

Inferior vena cava

Renal vein

Common iliac vein

Internal iliac vein

External iliac vein

Femoral vein

Great saphenous vein

Popliteal vein

Posterior tibial vein

Anterior tibial vein

B

FIGURE 15-1, cont'd B, Major veins.

growth), waste products, gases, and hormones through the body. It also plays a role in the immune response and changes in body temperature.

Using special cardiac muscle and nerve systems, electrical impulses tell the heart muscle when to contract, forcing blood from the heart, through blood vessels, and out through the body. Arteries move blood from the heart to tissues using smaller branches called *arterioles*. Veins move blood from tissues back toward the heart, beginning with their smaller branches, called *venules*. Capillaries are very small vessels that link arterioles and venules.

The heart is the pump of the circulation system. The heart itself is fed by small coronary arteries that send nutrients to it during the resting phase of the cardiac cycle. The heart may weaken with disease and age and become less efficient. Sometimes the arteries become stiff and the walls become filled with fatty plaques from cholesterol or lipids. This condition is called *atherosclerosis.* In patients with hypertension, the blood vessels become less elastic, and the increased pressure against which the heart has to pump causes the heart to work harder. Thus diseases or abnormal conditions of the heart, arteries, or veins produce more stress on the heart itself. When blood cannot flow through the heart muscles, the muscles hurt from lack of oxygen (angina). This severe chest pain is called *angina pectoris.* In a heart attack (myocardial infarction [MI]), some of the heart muscle cells actually die and a scar forms. Medicine can often control the pain of angina and prevent heart attacks when the heart doesn't have to work so hard.

Many of the cardiovascular drugs also have either direct or indirect action on the urinary system (Figure 15-2). The kidneys, urinary bladder, and ducts that carry urine work together to remove waste products from the circulatory system, to regulate blood pH and ion levels, and to maintain water balance. Strong pumping of the heart, good circulation through the vessels, and the full removal of waste products through

the urinary system are all needed to keep the body's fluids and electrolytes in balance.

ANTIANGINALS AND PERIPHERAL VASODILATORS

OVERVIEW

Narrowing or constriction of the smooth muscle in the small coronary arteries of the heart and the peripheral vascular system (vessels in the arms and legs) reduces the amount of blood carried to the heart and the peripheral tissues (Figure 15-3). When there is a lack of blood supply to bring oxygen and nutrients to the heart or to peripheral tissues, the pain of angina or peripheral vascular disease is felt.

ACTION

The heart receives its blood supply and oxygen from the coronary arteries. These small arteries are often plugged or damaged when the patient has angina or a heart attack. Blood may also be cut off from the coronary arteries if there is coronary vasospasm. Blockage or spasm causes cardiac angina when the heart muscle is without oxygen. Currently there are three major classes of drugs used in the medical management of angina. Nitrates (both short and long acting), β-blockers, and calcium channel blockers. Some other vasodilating agents (agents to open up the vessels) are used for increasing circulation in peripheral vascular disease. (Information about the use of beta blockers in treating angina by decreasing the oxygen demands of the heart and calcium channel blockers that may relieve angina by dilating the coronary vessels and reducing the work load of the heart can be found in the discussion of

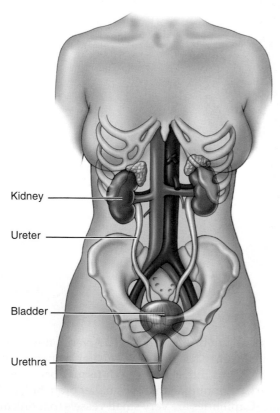

FIGURE 15-2 Urinary system.

Kidney

Ureter

Bladder

Urethra

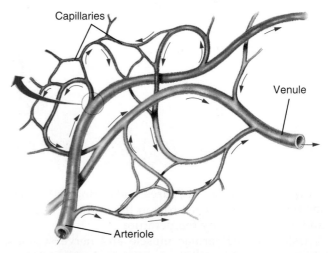

Microcirculation

Capillaries

Venule

Arteriole

FIGURE 15-3 Main components of the microcirculation. An arteriole supplies a capillary bed, which drains into a venule.

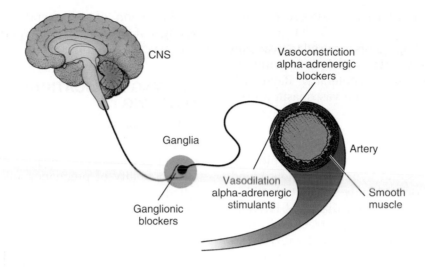

FIGURE 15-4 Site of action of peripheral vasodilators. *CNS*, Central nervous system.

antihypertensives and diuretics in the fifth section of this chapter.)

Nitrates

Nitrate products have a direct action on vascular smooth muscle and cause it to relax. This effect is felt in both the circulation in arteries and veins. Arterial relaxation reduces the pressures the heart has to pump against (afterload), whereas venous relaxation helps in pooling of venous blood, thereby decreasing the amount of blood returned to the heart (preload). These effects work together to decrease myocardial oxygen use. In addition, nitrates increase the use of the other small blood vessels in the heart (collaterals) so that there is better oxygen supply to the inner layers of the heart muscle.

Calcium Channel Blockers

Calcium is an electrolyte that helps move electrical impulses through cardiac tissue. Calcium channel blockers are drugs that help slow down the flow of calcium ions across the cell membrane, thus reducing the amount of calcium available for electrical impulse movement. The drugs in this group are used for a variety of actions. Some calcium channel blockers act directly on vascular smooth muscle to dilate (open up) coronary arteries and arterioles, which relieves anginal pain because more oxygen can go to the cardiac tissue. Other calcium channel blockers are used to reduce the response of the cardiac conduction system to electrical impulses and treat cardiac dysrhythmias. They are also used along with other drugs to treat hypertension. (See the sections on antidysrhythmics and antihypertensives for additional information on calcium channel blockers and beta-adrenergic blockers.)

Peripheral Vasodilators

Patients with occlusive arterial disease (blockage of the arteries that makes them smaller) have been treated with vasodilating drugs (drugs that help expand or open up the arteries), but with only limited success. These patients have decreased blood flow, which produces cold extremities, thin shiny skin, decreased hair growth on the legs, and the inability to walk without experiencing pain in their legs. Vasodilator drugs relax the smooth muscles of peripheral arterial blood vessels and help lead to better circulation to the arms and legs (Figure 15-4).

USES

Rapid-acting nitrates (such as amyl nitrite, sublingual nitroglycerin, and sublingual or chewable isosorbide dinitrate) are used mostly to relieve pain in acute angina. The long-acting nitrates and topical, transdermal, transmucosal, and oral sustained-release nitroglycerin products are used to prevent or treat anginal attacks when they are likely to occur (for example, with exercise) and to reduce the severity and frequency of anginal attacks. They are also used to reduce the work of the heart in cases of MI and in chronic heart failure; and for relief of gallbladder, gastrointestinal (GI), urethral, and bronchial smooth muscle pain.

It is not always clear if it is safe to use nitroglycerin in patients with acute MIs. When it is used in patients with recent MIs, the transdermal patch systems work best, but patients must be closely evaluated. Intravenous (IV) nitroglycerin is used to control severe angina in an acute MI and also to control acute pain during procedures on the heart, such as cardiac catheterization. This IV nitroglycerin requires careful monitoring of the patient in a cardiac care or critical care unit due to the possibility the medicine may cause a severe drop in blood pressure.

Peripheral vasodilating agents are used to treat pain in the legs caused by problems such as intermittent claudication, arteriosclerosis obliterans, Raynaud's disease, nocturnal leg cramps, and vasospasm caused by blood clots.

ADVERSE REACTIONS

There are many common adverse reactions to nitrates, including flushing, postural hypotension (low blood pressure when a person suddenly stands up), tachycardia (rapid heartbeat), confusion, dizziness, fainting, headache, light-headedness, vertigo (feeling of dizziness or spinning), weakness, drug rash, localized pruritus (itching), local burning in the mouth, nausea, and vomiting.

Some of these cardiac preparations contain tartrazine, a chemical that may cause an allergic type of reaction with symptoms similar to asthma. Patients who are allergic to aspirin have a greater chance of reacting to tartrazine.

When nitrate products are used, high doses may cause violent headaches. All nitrates should be given with care to patients with a recent history of stroke or cerebrovascular accident, because these conditions cause widening of the cerebral arteries.

Peripheral vasodilating agents may cause dizziness, headache, weakness, tachycardia, flushing, postural hypotension, dysrhythmias, confusion, severe rash, nervousness, tingling, and sweating. Some side effects disappear within a few weeks if they are mild and if the patient can keep taking the medication.

 Clinical Goldmine

Tolerance to Nitrates

Tolerance to nitrates may develop over time with repeated use. If the patient develops tolerance to one nitrate, it is likely that tolerance to other nitrates (cross-tolerance) will develop. Alternative coronary vasodilators may have to be used.

DRUG INTERACTIONS

Nitrates increase the effects of atropine-like drugs and tricyclic antidepressants and decrease the effects of all choline-like drugs. The action of anticholinergic drugs and antihistamines may be made stronger. Nitrates should not be taken at the same time as prazosin because of the possibility of a significant interaction. Taking alcohol, beta blockers, antihypertensives, narcotics, and vasodilators with nitrates and nitrites (especially amyl nitrite) may produce severe hypotension (low blood pressure) and cardiac collapse. Nitrates may antagonize (interfere with) the vasopressor actions of sympathomimetic drugs. A cold environment or the use of tobacco reduces the action of nitroglycerin.

The action of peripheral vasodilating agents is stronger if used with antihypertensives and alcohol and may cause hypotension.

❖ NURSING IMPLICATIONS AND PATIENT TEACHING

■ Assessment

Learn as much as possible about the health history of the patient. Ask about heart disease, other health problems, the possibility of pregnancy, allergies, smoking, and whether the patient is taking other drugs that may cause interactions. Get a full description of the angina pain.

■ Diagnosis

What other problems does this patient have that may interfere with treatment? For example, is the patient overweight? Does he or she smoke? What is the patient's understanding of what is happening? What is the patient's nutritional status and what dietary habits does the patient have? Is there any problem with the patient's kidneys?

■ Planning

Many times angina may be reduced or controlled if the patient makes lifestyle changes. This might include stopping smoking, limiting alcohol, limiting salt (sodium), increasing physical exercise, losing weight, eating a balanced diet rich in fruits and vegetables with lots of potassium and magnesium, avoiding dietary saturated fats, reducing stress, and treating other diseases such as hypertension and hyperlipidemia. Some patients who have the coronary arteries blocked may be candidates for surgery (coronary arterial bypass grafts or percutaneous transluminal coronary angioplasty) to reduce the symptoms. Medications are also an important part of treatment.

In reviewing the medicines that might be ordered, refer to the information in Table 15-1, which compares the action of various nitrate products. Nitrates are readily absorbed under the tongue, from nasal spray, through the skin, and orally, but products taken orally are rapidly changed in the liver to inactive products. The half-life for nitroglycerin given sublingually (under the tongue) is only 1 to 4 minutes. Newer forms of the medication can be applied directly to the skin or used as a patch, allowing nitrates to pass directly into the bloodstream, thus reaching the heart before being destroyed by the liver.

■ Implementation

Review Chapter 10 for the ways to administer different types of nitroglycerin products.

• Transmucosal nitroglycerin tablets should not be chewed or swallowed. The patient should put the tablet inside the cheek or under the lip, and let it slowly dissolve.

Table 15-1   Comparison of Nitrate Products

PRODUCT	ONSET	DURATION	PREPARATION
Agents for Acute Angina			
Amyl nitrate (Vaporole)	Short-acting 10-30 seconds; repeat 3-5 minutes		Inhalation
isosorbide dinitrate (Dilatrate SR, Isordil, Sorbitrate, Titradose)	2-3 min	1-2 hr	Sublingual/chewable May take 5-10 minutes before activities that may cause pain. Take every 5 minutes × 3 doses in 15 minutes for acute pain.
nitroglycerin ★ (Nitrostat, Nitro-Dur, NitroTime, Nitro-Bid, Nitrolingual pump spray)	1-3 min	3-5 min	Sublingual
	1-2 min	4-6 hr	Transmucosal
	Immediately	5-10 min	Intravenous, translingual
Agents for Angina Prophylaxis			
isosorbide dinitrate	45-60 min	8 hr	Oral
	Slow	12 hr	Sustained release, PO
isosorbide mononitrate (Ismo, Imdur, Monoket)	45-60 min	6 hr	Oral, sustained release
nitroglycerin ★ (Nitro-Time, Nitro-Bid, MiniTran, Nitro-Dur)	24-45 min	3-8 hr	Sustained release, PO
	30-60 min	3-7 hr	Topical ointment
	30-60 min	8-10 hr	Transdermal Patch. Remove for 12 or 24 hr to reduce development of tolerance.
Ranolazine (Ranexa ER)	Variable	Variable	Extended release product. Do not take with grapefruit.

PO, By mouth.
★ Indicates "Must-Know Drugs," or the 35 drugs most prescribers use.

Table 15-2   Peripheral Vasodilating Medications

GENERIC NAME	TRADE NAME	USE	MOST COMMON OR SERIOUS ADVERSE EFFECTS
hydralazine	Apresoline	Essential hypertension, CHF from high afterload	Angina, tachycardia, peripheral neuritis, blood dyscrasias, constipation, paralytic ileus, nausea, vomiting, diarrhea

CHF, Congestive heart failure.

Nitrate headaches often go away with a lower dose and analgesics. As the patient continues to take the nitroglycerin product, these headaches will gradually stop.

Table 15-2 provides a list of peripheral vasodilating medications.

■ Evaluation

The drug should be stopped if blurred vision or dry mouth occurs. If the patient says that some of the sustained-release medication is being passed in the stool, it is likely that food moves through the patient's GI tract too fast to allow the drug to be absorbed. Such patients may need to switch to transdermal or sublingual medication.

Older adult patients may have postural hypotension with these drugs and need to be watched very carefully. They may need to have someone with them when they take the medication.

The patient must learn the uses and limits of the nitrate being taken, understand the schedule of when to take the drug, and be given information about when to call for help if chest pain does not go away after taking the drug. There are many important things to learn about giving this medication by its various routes. A person who has been using a nitrate for a long time should not stop taking the drug suddenly as this may cause more angina.

Clinical Pitfall

Anginal Attacks

For acute angina, the patient should put one tablet under the tongue as soon as the pain begins. The medication should not be chewed or swallowed; it should be left to dissolve under the tongue. The patient should lie down and rest. If the pain is not relieved within 3 to 5 minutes, a second pill may be taken. If the pain is not relieved within another 3 minutes, a third pill may be taken. If the pain is still not relieved, the patient should chew an aspirin to help reduce blood clotting and be taken to an emergency room immediately to be evaluated for acute MI.

Clinical Pitfall

Patient History of Chronic Heart Failure

The antidysrhythmic drugs often cause or worsen chronic heart failure or urinary retention. Patients with a past history of heart failure should be watched carefully.

■ Patient and Family Teaching

Tell the patient and family the following:

- Nitroglycerin is very fragile and chemically breaks down rapidly; sunlight speeds up this process. Even under the best conditions, these drugs lose their strength 3 months after the bottle has been opened. The patient will need a new prescription every 3 months, and any old drugs should be thrown away. There was a time when a burning feeling under the tongue could tell the patient if nitroglycerin medication was still good, but this is no longer true. Medication that is still active produces a throbbing headache. If the patient fails to feel the throbbing in the head, usually the medication has lost its potency (strength).
- The headache usually lasts no longer than 20 minutes and may be relieved with analgesics. The patient should rest for 10 to 15 minutes after the pain is relieved. The physician should be notified if blurred vision, persistent headache, or dry mouth occurs.

Lifespan Considerations
Older Adults

NITROGLYCERIN

Nitroglycerin is an active product that deteriorates when exposed to light. It is readily absorbed by cotton, plastic, or cardboard packaging. Nitroglycerin should be dispensed in a dark-colored glass bottle, and patients should be cautioned not to transfer tablets to other containers. Storing nitroglycerin tablets in the refrigerator prolongs the activity of the pills beyond 3 months.

- The medication should be taken on an empty stomach when possible.
- The patient must not drink alcoholic beverages while taking nitrate products.
- The topical ointment tube should be kept tightly closed. Store nitroglycerin in the refrigerator.
- Patients using inhalant medication should take it only when lying or sitting down. Because this is a product that will catch fire easily, the patient must not smoke and should avoid using the drug around fire or sparks.
- The topical ointment should be spread in a thin layer on the skin, using an applicator and a ruler. The ointment should not be rubbed or massaged into the skin. The patient should wash off any medication that might have gotten on the hands.
- For transdermal application, the patient should select a hairless spot (or clip hair) and apply the adhesive pad to the skin. Washing, bathing, or swimming does not affect this system. If the pad does come off, it should be discarded and a new one placed on a different site.
- For patients who may have developed tolerance to the drug, stopping the drug for several days may be long enough to make the body sensitive to it again. The smallest possible dose should be taken to reduce the risk of tolerance. Some patients have been instructed to apply the patch in the morning and remove it at night. However, as the ability of the heart to provide circulation is often at its lowest point in the early morning hours, this is when many MI's develop—so removing the patch is NOT a good idea.
- The patient should keep a record of every anginal attack, the number of pills taken, and any side effects. The patient should bring this record to each visit to the health care provider.
- The patient should use nitroglycerin when anginal attacks are likely; taking the medication before the activity may prevent or reduce the degree of pain.
- This medication is only part of the therapy for angina. The patient should try to avoid things that cause pain (stress, heavy exercise, overeating, and smoking), reduce calorie intake if weight loss is desirable, and develop a program of regular and sensible exercise.
- The patient should not eat large amounts of foods that stimulate the heart (e.g., coffee, tea, caffeinated soft drinks, chocolate).
- This medication must be kept out of the reach of children and others for whom it is not prescribed.
- In the hospital, the patient's blood pressure should be taken before giving sublingual nitroglycerin and also between doses. Nitroglycerin may cause hypotension. Because the coronary arteries receive their blood supply during diastole, hypotension also decreases the blood flow to the coronary arteries, thus

making the blood pressure even lower if the patient is having an MI. In the hospital, the nurse should remove any nitroglycerin (NTG) patches before performing cardioversion or defibrillating a patient.

ANTIDYSRHYTHMICS

☀ OVERVIEW

A person with heart disease or other diseases, or nutritional or congenital problems that may affect heart muscle, is at risk of developing irregular beating of the heart, or cardiac **dysrhythmia**. Because the term *dysrhythmia* (irregular rhythm) explains what happens to the patient better than the older term *arrhythmia* (without rhythm), it is now commonly used. Dysrhythmias may be fast or slow, with an irregular or regular pattern. The most common causes of dysrhythmias are irritation to the heart tissue after the patient has suffered an MI, fluid and electrolyte imbalances, problems with diet, hypoxia (reduced blood oxygen), and reactions to drugs.

The middle layer of the heart wall, or **myocardium**, is made up of special muscle cells. These muscle cells work together under the direction of a special group of nerve fibers called the **pacemaker**, which located in the sinoatrial (SA) node. The pacemaker cells direct the rest of the cardiac cells by sending electrical impulses through a special nerve system known as the *cardiac conduction system*. These impulses cause atrial and ventricular contraction (pumping). A person's heart rate is governed by how fast the pacemaker cells direct the heart to pump and by how fast this information is spread through the heart. The usual path of information flow begins in the SA node, passes through the atrium to the atrioventricular (AV) node, through the bundle of His, through the right and left bundle branches, and out through the Purkinje fibers of the myocardium. When the electrical impulse has spread along this pathway, the heart will contract, forcing blood out into the arteries. After a brief rest, the cycle will begin again. This is called **normal sinus rhythm**.

The electrical message directing the heart to contract depends on a special balance of electrolytes (such as calcium and sodium) in the cardiac tissues and on good function of the cardiac conduction system. This electrical message is what is recorded on the **electrocardiogram (ECG)**. Figure 15-5 illustrates the conduction system of the heart and the ECG pattern that it makes.

When the cells in the conduction system do not have enough oxygen or are destroyed or damaged through disease, or when the electrolytes are not present in the right balance, irregular heart action is found. Some patients may describe very slow, regular or irregular heartbeats; some patients may have fast, irregular heartbeats. Some individuals may only feel a

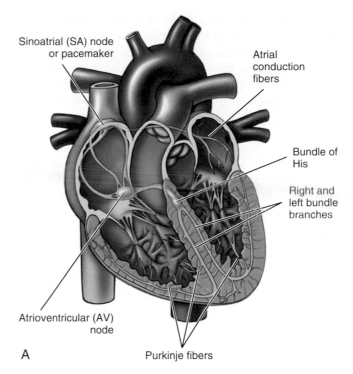

Sinoatrial (SA) node or pacemaker

Atrial conduction fibers

Bundle of His

Right and left bundle branches

Atrioventricular (AV) node

Purkinje fibers

A

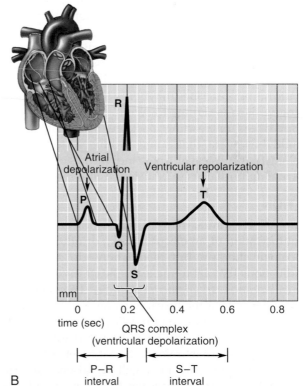

Atrial depolarization

Ventricular repolarization

R

P

Q

S

T

mm

0   0.2   0.4   0.6   0.8

time (sec)   QRS complex (ventricular depolarization)

P–R interval

S–T interval

B

FIGURE 15-5 A, Conduction system of the heart. **B,** Normal electrocardiogram showing one cardiac cycle.

little dizzy or report that their heart has "skipped a beat." Sometimes patients have no symptoms; sometimes the symptoms are life threatening. The nurse may feel an irregular pulse or hear the irregularity with the stethoscope. The exact type of irregular rhythm can only be determined by taking an ECG. The dysrhythmia is often classified by its location and type of rhythm abnormality produced, for example, atrial tachycardia. Outside the hospital, some patients may wear a heart monitor strapped to their chest, or inside the hospital, they may be placed in a coronary care unit so they may be closely watched. The goal of any treatment plan or therapeutic regimen is for the patient's heart to regain a normal rate and rhythm.

Research has confirmed that some individuals have a gene that places them at risk for sudden death. The problem occurs when there is lengthening or prolongation of the QT interval measured by the ECG. The problem is known as Long QT (LQT) Syndrome and is a disorder of cardiac repolarization caused by alterations in the transmembrane potassium and sodium currents. Congenital LQT is a disease of transmembrane ion-channel proteins. Six different genes might cause this problem and many members of a family may have the same problem. Single cases of the disease occur as a result of spontaneous gene mutations. The acquired causes of LQT include drugs, electrolyte imbalance, marked bradycardia, cocaine, organophosphorus compounds, subarachnoid hemorrhage, myocardial ischemia, protein sparing fasting, autonomic neuropathy, and human immunodeficiency virus disease. There are a great many drugs which might provoke this problem in at risk patients, including many cardiac and central nervous system (CNS) drugs. A complete list of those drugs which these patients should not be prescribed may be found at www.sads.org/living-with-sads/Drugs-to-Avoid. When studying about drugs or reading package inserts, the nurse should be aware that some products are found to prolong the QT interval. These individuals often require internal defibrillators to be inserted into their heart.

ACTION

Many dysrhythmias require placing of a pacemaker, administration of an electric shock, or other nonpharmacologic therapy. But medications do play a role. Medications that act to make the heart rhythm normal are called *antidysrhythmic medications.* They act on the individual cells of the heart. Each individual heart cell might be thought of as a gun. With each heartbeat, the cardiac muscle cell (gun) has to get ready to shoot (fire), fire, and then reload. As one cell discharges (fires), it triggers the next cell to discharge. After passing the electrical message to the next cell, each conduction cell must rest (reload) before it can pass another electrical signal. Antidysrhythmic drugs affect the cells that are beating (firing) irregularly by acting on each of these phases of cell activity. Dysrhythmic medications are classified by the stage at which they affect the cellular action potential. These include:

- **Class I drugs** (quinidine, procainamide, disopyramide):
  - These drugs are sodium channel blockers. They lengthen the **effective refractory period** (the time

period during which the cells cannot release or discharge their electrical activity [slow the reloading of the cell]) of atrial and ventricular myocardium (heart muscle) by slowing the fast inward current caused by the sodium electrolyte.
  - Make the heart less excitable. Overall, the result is to slow the rate of the impulse conduction through the heart.
- **Class II drugs** are beta blockers, such as propranolol, esmolol, and acebutolol, which reduce sympathetic excitation to the heart (affect the loading of the cell).
- **Class III drugs** are potassium channel blockers (such as amiodarone) that lengthen the **action potential duration**, or the length of time it takes for one cell to fire and recover (slow the firing).
- **Class IV drugs** are calcium channel blockers (such as verapamil) that selectively block the ability of calcium to enter the myocardium and prolong the effective refractory period (or resting period) in the AV node (affect the reloading of the cell).
- There is also a miscellaneous antidysrhythmic drug category that includes digitalis and other well-known and effective drugs.

USES

The cause of the dysrhythmia will determine which drug will be most effective in correcting it. The two basic actions within the heart that cause dysrhythmias are: (1) increased sensitivity of electrical cells in the heart, resulting in irregular or early **ectopic beats** (the cell fires before it should); and (2) electrical activity moving through abnormal conduction pathways (the trigger that causes the cell to fire does not always work properly). For example, a block of the sinus or AV node pacemakers force the heart to use a different pathway than usual. The amount of medication that can be given for these dysrhythmic drugs has a very small range. If too much is given, the dose may be toxic and add to the problems of the heart.

There are now many dysrhythmic drugs on the market. Only a few of the most commonly used drugs are described here. Two drugs that are often used to treat rapid and irregular dysrhythmias are quinidine and procainamide. These drugs are chemically different, but both act to quiet the myocardial cells and make them less excitable and less likely to fire. This not only decreases the heart rate but also stops some of the extra or irregular beats. These drugs were once the mainstay of dysrhythmia therapy but new drugs now have less significant side effects.

Bretylium is another drug that used to be in greater use to slow the conduction rate of the electrical impulse in the ventricular muscle. This drug also acts to slow the release of norepinephrine, a powerful chemical in the cardiac cells, so the heart muscle beats more slowly.

Disopyramide slows the depolarization of the cardiac cells. **Depolarization** is the movement of electrolytes into and out of the cell as it gets ready to send another electrical message. Under the influence of disopyramide, the heart rate is slowed because each cell is slower in recovering from sending the message to the next cell (the reloading time takes longer).

Lidocaine IV is a drug that was formerly widely used. The electrical impulse sent to the cardiac muscle must be of certain strength, or it cannot pass along the conducting nerve fibers. Lidocaine increases the strength of the impulse. A drug that affects the rate of rhythmic movements, such as the heartbeat, is called a **chronotropic** drug. A **dromotropic** drug influences the velocity (speed) of the passage of an electrical impulse in nerve or cardiac muscle fibers.

A diseased heart may have many electrical impulses trying to move at the same time, but some impulses are very weak. By increasing the strength the impulse must reach before it may be conducted, many weak impulses will be screened out, and the overall heart rate will be slower.

Adenosine is a powerful drug that slows the conduction through the AV node and decreases how rapidly the SA node will fire. An IV injection to end serious atrial tachycardia may cause the heart to stop beating for several seconds when a very rapid heartbeat is changed to normal (normal sinus rhythm). Although this drug has only a 10-second half-life, this pause in the heart beat is very upsetting for patients, who often refuse to take it more than once. Some institutions may use benzodiazepines at the same time to help the patients relax during this procedure.

Digoxin is used primarily to treat heart failure but also plays a role in treating fast dysrhythmias such as atrial fibrillation or tachycardia. It slows the heart rate by slowing how fast the SA node fires and slowing conduction through the AV node. It also strengthens the contraction of the heart. Toxic levels of this medication also cause dysrhythmias. (See cardiotonics in a later section.) Other drugs that affect heart activity are the beta-adrenergic blockers, of which propranolol (Inderal) and metoprolol (Lopressor) are the most well known. Drugs in this category act very much like quinidine, but they also decrease the response of the heart muscle to epinephrine and norepinephrine (other chemical neurotransmitters) by blocking the stimulation of the heart's beta receptors. (Again, the reloading of the cell is affected.)

It is clear that many of the antidysrhythmic drugs are so powerful that they should only be used in critical care units where the patient may be closely monitored. Some of these drugs are given as an IV injection followed by an IV solution filled with the medication. As the patient's condition becomes more stable, some drugs may be changed to other antidysrhythmic drugs that are better for long-term therapy.

Table 15-3 lists drugs that may commonly be used in the treatment of acute and chronic dysrhythmias.

ADVERSE REACTIONS

Most drugs given to control dysrhythmias may also cause other dysrhythmias. All patients receiving these drugs should have their heart carefully monitored by ECG for any change.

Quinidine is an older drug that is still in use in some hospitals and parts of the world, although it has many adverse effects. It may cause cardiac dysrhythmias, hypotension, diarrhea, tinnitus, headache, vertigo, confusion, delirium, disturbances in vision, and abdominal pain. Toxic effects are called *cinchonism*, and the patient will complain of tinnitus,

---

Table 15-3 Acute Treatment and Chronic Prophylaxis of Dysrhythmias

DYSRHYTHMIA	TYPE OF TREATMENT INDICATED*	
	ACUTE	CHRONIC PROPHYLAXIS
Sinus tachycardia (rarely treated)	propranolol ★	propranolol ★
Premature atrial contractions (usually in patients with history of atrial fibrillation)	digoxin ★	digoxin ★, quinidine, disopyramide, procainamide, propranolol ★
Premature ventricular contractions (multifocal, on vulnerable part of T wave, or in symptomatic patient)	Lidocaine ★ procainamide	quinidine, disopyramide, procainamide, digoxin ★, propranolol ★
Atrial flutter/atrial fibrillation	Cardioversion: digoxin ★	digoxin ★, propranolol quinidine, disopyramide, procainamide, verapamil ★
Paroxysmal supraventricular tachycardia	Carotid massage; cardioversion: propranolol ★, digoxin ★, verapamil ★, adenosine	propranolol ★, digoxin ★, quinidine, disopyramide, procainamide, verapamil ★

*Listed in order of suggested use.

★ Indicates "Must-Know Drugs," or the 35 drugs most prescribers use.

light-headedness, headache, fever, vertigo, nausea, vomiting, and dizziness. The first time the patient takes the medicine, a test dose should be given to check for quinidine syncope—a condition in which the body reacts to quinidine by reducing blood flow to the brain, producing syncope (light-headedness and fainting), loss of consciousness, and sometimes death.

See Table 15-3 for common adverse effects.

DRUG INTERACTIONS

Quinidine's effect is increased by potassium and is reduced by hypokalemia. Verapamil actions are stronger when used at the same time as digitalis and beta blockers. Beta blockers have many interactions with other drugs, and the nurse should read about every other drug the patient is taking when a beta blocker is prescribed.

❖ NURSING IMPLICATIONS AND PATIENT TEACHING

▪ Assessment

Learn everything possible about the patient's health history, including any drug allergies, other drugs being taken that may cause drug interactions, and other medical problems, including factors such as hypoxia (reduced blood oxygen), acid-base imbalance, increased or decreased potassium, or drug toxicity. It is good practice to always take an apical heart rate with any patient that may have an arrhythmia by placing the stethoscope in the left chest cardiac area. Some irregular heart rates are very weak and are difficult to accurately feel with a radial pulse.

▪ Diagnosis

Does the patient have other health problems that will affect therapy? Does the patient drink lots of caffeine? Smoke? Exercise? Is the patient overweight?

▪ Planning

An ECG should be obtained before medications are started. This will determine the status of the heart before treatment so that changes can be seen if treatment is helpful.

▪ Implementation

Vital signs must be taken before giving any antidysrhythmic medication. The nurse often has the responsibility of monitoring any changes that might develop in blood pressure or pulse while initial thrapy is given. Hospitalized patients often continue their antidysrhythmic medications when they go home, so the nurse might take advantage of every opportunity to teach patients about these medications and be prepared to answer questions.

Table 15-4 presents information about the antidysrhythmics.

▪ Evaluation

If the patient's heart is not being watched with a cardiac monitor, the results from ECGs must be closely followed to see any changes. Electrolyte levels and other laboratory data should also be obtained.

▪ Patient and Family Teaching

Tell the patient and family the following:
- The patient must take this medication exactly as ordered and not skip doses or double the dose.
- Some people have side effects from these drugs. The patient should report any new or distressing symptoms to the nurse, physician, or other health care provider, especially any sudden weight gain, trouble breathing, or increased coughing.
- The patient must return regularly for checkup visits to the physician or other health care provider to see how the medicine is affecting heart function.
- The patient must not take any other drugs before consulting with the health care provider to make sure the combination is safe. This includes aspirin, laxatives, cold and sinus products, or other over-the-counter (OTC) drugs.

ANTIHYPERLIPIDEMICS

OVERVIEW

Cholesterol and other fatty acids are called *lipids*. The body needs a certain amount of cholesterol and triglycerides, which are both normal and vital parts of blood plasma. Like other lipids, they are not soluble in liquid, so they are carried in the plasma by linking to lipoproteins (albumin and globulins). Lipoproteins are described by how thick or dense they are ("high-density lipids" and "low-density lipids"). The four major types of lipoproteins are as follows:

1. *Chylomicrons.* These are the largest and lightest of the lipoproteins. They are formed from the absorption of dietary fat in the intestine and are mostly triglycerides. Chylomicrons are normally present in plasma for only 1 to 8 hours after the last meal, and they make the plasma look cloudy. If a tube of blood from a fasting patient shows a thick layer of fat or cloudy plasma after several hours, the patient may have an inability to handle dietary fat.

2. *Very-low-density lipoproteins (VLDLs).* These are made up of large amounts of triglycerides that were made in the liver and are called *pre-beta lipoproteins.* The pre-beta form is a carrier state for moving triglycerides that have been produced in the liver into the plasma. Nearly all the triglycerides in plasma that are not in chylomicrons are considered to be VLDLs.

3. *Low-density lipoproteins (LDLs).* When VLDLs break down and link with cholesterol and protein, very

Table 15-4   Antidysrhythmics

GENERIC NAME	TRADE NAME	USES	ADVERSE REACTIONS
Class I Drugs			
A			
disopyramide	Norpace, Napamide	Treat ectopic ventricular dysrhythmias	Constipation, urinary hesitancy, headache, dry mouth, blurred vision, nausea dizziness, headache, and fatigue
procainamide	Procanbid Pronestyl Pronestyl SR	PVCs, ventricular tachycardia, atrial fibrillation, and PAT	Anorexia (lack of appetite), rash, pruritus, nausea, severe hypotension, and ventricular dysrhythmias
quinidine (sulfate or gluconate or polygalacturonate)	Duraquin Quinaglute, Quinidex	PACs, PVCs, PAT, atrial flutter, and atrial fibrillation	Tinnitus, disturbed vision, headache, nausea, and dizziness
B			
lidocaine ★ (without preservatives)	Xylocaine	Life-threatening ventricular dysrhythmias	Bradycardia, drowsiness, hypotension, light-headedness, convulsions tinnitus (ringing in the ears), blurred or double vision, bradycardia (slow heartbeat), and hallucinations
mexiletine	Mexitil	Symptomatic ventricular dysrhythmias	GI distress, tremor, light-headedness, incoordination, and hepatic and hematologic effects
Phenytoin	Dilantin	Unlabeled use for dysrhythmias	
Tocanide	Tonocard	Usually reserved for serious ventricular arrhythmias	
C			
flecainide	Tambocor	Usually reserved for serious ventricular dysrhythmias	
propafenone	Rythmol Rythmol SR	Life-threatening ventricular dysrhythmias	Dizziness, unusual taste, AV block, nausea, and vomiting
D			
moricizine (does not belong to A, B, or C category, but shares some characteristics of each)	Ethmozine	Severe ventricular dysrhythmias	May provoke other dysrhythmias.
Class II Drugs: Beta Blockers (see section on antihypertensives)			
acebutolol	Sectral	Ventricular tachycardia	Bradycardia and dizziness
esmolol	Brevibloc	Supraventricular tachycardia	Bradycardia and dizziness
propranolol ★	Inderal Pronol	Cardiac dysrhythmias, migraine, angina, MI, and pheochromocytoma	Bradycardia, dizziness, vertigo, rash, bronchospasm, hyperglycemia, hypertension, visual disturbances, fatigue, chest pain, arthralgia (joint pain), and pruritus

Continued

Table 15-4   Antidysrhythmics—cont'd

GENERIC NAME	TRADE NAME	USES	ADVERSE REACTIONS
Class III Drugs			
amiodarone	Cordarone Pacerone	Life-threatening ventricular dysrhythmias	GI distress, CNS symptoms, and photosensitivity (abnormal response to exposure to sunlight); pulmonary fibrosis
bretylium	Bretylol	Usually reserved for life-threatening ventricular dysrhythmias; IM form available	
dofetilide	Tikosyn	Used to convert atrial fibrillation/atrial flutter and maintain normal sinus rhythm	May precipitate other fatal dysrhythmias.
ibutilide	Corvert	atrial fibrillation or flutter	
sotalol	Betapace Sorine	Life-threatening ventricular tachycardia	Life-threatening ventricular tachycardia
Class IV Drugs Calcium Channel Blockers			
verapamil ★	Calan Isoptin Verelan Isoptin SR	Supraventricular tachydysrhythmias	Cardiac dysrhythmias, CHF, and hypotension It forms a cloudy mixture that cannot be injected if it is mixed in the same syringe or bottle with sodium bicarbonate or nafcillin.
Miscellaneous Drugs for Dysrhythmias			
adenosine	Adenocard	Supraventricular tachycardia	Facial flushing and shortness of breath
Digoxin	Lanoxin	Used primarily in atrial dysrhythmias.	

AV, Atrioventricular; *CHF,* congestive heart failure; *CNS,* central nervous system; *GI,* gastrointestinal; *IM,* intramuscular; *MI,* myocardial infarction; *PAC,* premature atrial contraction; *PAT,* paroxysmal atrial tachycardia; *PVC,* premature ventricular contraction.
★ Indicates "Must-Know Drugs," or the 35 drugs most prescribers use.

little triglyceride is left. What remains is then called *beta lipoprotein.* Approximately 75% of the cholesterol in plasma is moved in this form. High serum levels of LDLs indicate cholesterol levels that are higher than the body needs. Patients with high LDL levels are at high risk for developing atherosclerosis.

4. *High-density lipoproteins (HDLs).* These small, dense lipoproteins are called *alpha lipoproteins* and contain very small parts of triglycerides. They are mostly made up of protein and cholesterol. They serve as the "vacuum cleaners" of the tissues, clearing out excess cholesterol. They may prevent atherosclerotic activity by blocking uptake of LDL cholesterol by vascular smooth muscle cells.

Chylomicrons and VLDLs are seen as triglyceride-rich lipoproteins, whereas LDLs and HDLs are viewed as cholesterol-rich lipoproteins. These two lipoproteins differ in several respects, including their cholesterol transporting activities. Simply stated, LDLs move cholesterol from the liver to peripheral tissues, and HDLs remove cholesterol from the periphery and transport

it to the liver. Figure 15-6 shows the normal physiology of lipoprotein transport. Chylomicrons are the largest and least dense of the lipoproteins; as size decreases and density increases, the next type is the VLDLs (pre-beta lipoproteins), then the intermediate-density lipoproteins (IDLs, or broad beta lipoproteins), then the LDLs (beta lipoproteins), and finally the HDLs (alpha lipoproteins, the smallest and most dense).

The high blood lipid levels may be caused by problems in moving lipids (lipid transport) or chemical breakdown (metabolism) of lipids. **Hyperlipidemia** is the term used to describe high levels of lipoproteins in the blood. This may mean high amounts of triglycerides, high amounts of cholesterol, or both. These high levels may be classed according to Types I through V. Some of these types are genetic; some respond to drug or dietary treatment; and some are more likely to cause atherosclerosis. It is important to determine the type of hyperlipidemia the patient has (Figure 15-7),

Atherosclerosis in the coronary arteries causes coronary heart disease (CHD). The coronary arteries that

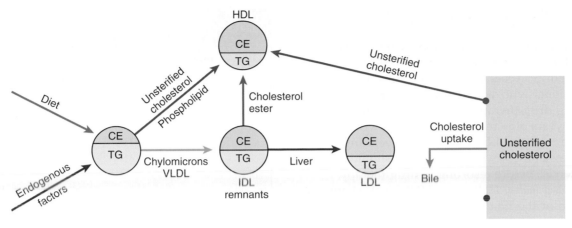

FIGURE 15-6 Normal pathway of lipid metabolism. *CE*, cholesterol esters; *HDL*, high-density lipoproteins; *IDL*, intermediate-density lipoproteins or remnants; *LDL*, low-density lipoproteins; *TG*, triglycerides; *VLDL*, very-low-density lipoproteins.

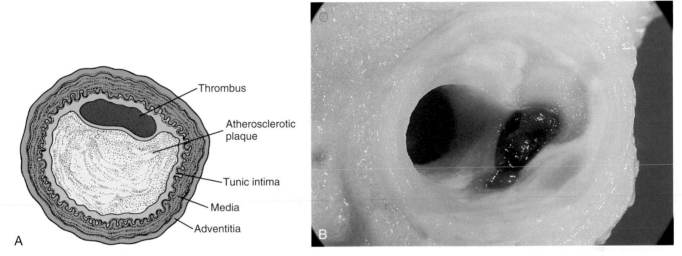

FIGURE 15-7 **A,** Occlusion of an atherosclerotic coronary artery by a thrombus. **B,** Plaque disruption. The cap of the lipid-rich plaque has become torn, and a thrombus has formed, mostly inside the plaque.

feed and nourish the heart become smaller because the inner wall of the arteries are narrowed as they fill with *plaques,* or patches of atherosclerotic tissue. Although the narrowing of the coronary artery may decrease the blood supply to the heart, it is only when a plaque is broken or torn, and platelets cling to the torn area and produce a blockage, that the blood supply is decreased enough to cause a heart attack. When the heart does not get enough blood to its muscle cells, those cells experience pain (angina) and then those cells die. This is called **myocardial infarction (MI)**, or heart attack. When the physician or nurse practitioner looks in the patient's eyes with the ophthalmoscope, they may see plaque in the linings of the arteries in the eyes. If there is plaque in the arteries of the eyes, then there are likely atherosclerotic plaques throughout all the arteries in the body and might be present before the patient shows any symptoms. These areas of plaque that lead to the lack of oxygen in the blood may also lead to cerebrovascular disease

(including stroke), peripheral ischemia (lack of oxygenated blood in the legs caused by problems in the circulation of the legs), and renovascular hypertension (high pressures and damage in the kidneys). Research suggests that high blood LDL cholesterol levels lead to CHD. There is an opposite link between HDLs and CHD risk—that is, high levels of HDL cholesterol are viewed as protecting the patient against CHD. This is why LDLs are sometimes called "bad cholesterol" and HDLs are called "good cholesterol." Evaluation of LDL and HDL levels is of primary importance, because research has now shown that lowering serum lipids or cholesterol can help reduce the risk of atherosclerotic disease. There are many people with high lipid and cholesterol levels that place them at risk for CHD. These lipid levels can often be lowered through diet, exercise, and lifestyle changes and the use of medications.

Guidelines for the diagnosis and treatment of hyperlipidemia are issued and regularly updated by the

National Cholesterol Education Program. These guidelines emphasize the following:

- *Establish therapy based on risk of CHD.* Those who have CHD, men older than 45 years old, and women older than 55 years old are now considered high-risk patients who would benefit from cholesterol-lowering drug therapy. Young adult men (younger than 35 years old) and premenopausal women with elevated total and LDL cholesterol levels are at risk, regardless of their overall health, but should try diet and exercise before resorting to drug therapy.
- *Take a closer look at HDL levels.* HDL levels should be recorded at the first cholesterol test and should be noted when choosing a cholesterol-lowering therapy. Higher HDL levels (>60 mg/dL) may in fact be a negative CHD risk factor; that is, patients with higher HDL levels are at lower risk for CHD.
- *Have some form of physical activity (which raises HDL levels and lowers triglycerides) daily.*
- *Lose and then keep weight at the best recommended level. Obesity is a major risk factor for cardiovascular disease.*
- *Eat a healthy diet, which includes keeping intake of saturated fat to 7% of total calorie intake; keeping cholesterol intake to less than 200 mg/day; and eating whole grains, vegetables, and fruits so that total dietary fiber is 10 to 25 g/day.*

Many times activity and diet will help achieve the proper blood lipid levels. The recommended laboratory values for all patients include:

- Total cholesterol level less than 200 mg/dL
- LDL cholesterol less than 100 mg/dL
- HDL cholesterol between 40 and 59 mg/dL
- Triglycerides less than 150 mg/dL

Both exercise and diet therapy are important and should always be a part of the treatment plan. If changing the diet and exercise alone does not produce the needed changes, drug therapy may also be offered. Five classes of drugs are used to treat hyperlipidemia: hydroxymethylglutaryl coenzyme A (HMG-CoA) reductase inhibitors, the fibric acid derivatives, bile acid sequestrants, selective cholesterol absorption inhibitors, and niacin. A list of the usual diet and drug therapy regimens in the various types of hyperlipidemias is provided in Table 15-5.

ACTION

HMG-CoA Reductase Inhibitors or Statins

The HMG-CoA reductase inhibitors are the first choice drugs used to treat hyperlipidemia. They are the most costly drugs for treating hyperlipidemia, but patients also tolerate them best, and they are highly effective at lowering LDL levels. The ability of the six drugs in this class to lower LDL levels can be roughly ranked in the following order, with the most powerful drug first: rosuvastatin, atorvastatin, simvastatin, pravastatin, lovastatin, and fluvastatin. Adverse effects are similar for all six of these agents. A switch from one drug to

Table 15-5	Diet and Drug Therapy for the Hyperlipidemias	
TYPE	**DIET**	**DRUGS**
I	Low fat; no other restrictions	None is effective
IIa	Low cholesterol, low in saturated fats; increased intake of polyunsaturated fats	HMG-CoA reductase inhibitors, bile acid sequestrants, nicotinic acid
IIb	Same as above	HMG-CoA reductase inhibitors, bile acid sequestrants, gemfibrozil, nicotinic acid, clofibrate, fenofibrate
III	Low cholesterol, low calorie, low in saturated fats; high protein	Nicotinic acid, gemfibrozil, clofibrate, fenofibrate
IV	Low carbohydrate, low alcohol, low cholesterol, low calorie; maintain protein intake	Gemfibrozil, nicotinic acid, clofibrate, fenofibrate
V	Low fat, low carbohydrate, low alcohol; high protein	Gemfibrozil, nicotinic acid, clofibrate, fenofibrate

HMG-CoA, Hydroxymethylglutaryl coenzyme A.

another may be needed if adverse reactions occur. Liver function tests (LFTs) should be monitored in patients taking these products.

Fibric Acid Derivatives

Gemfibrozil and fenofibrate are the preferred drugs of this class because they are more effective and have fewer adverse effects compared with some other drugs. Both are highly effective at lowering triglycerides and increasing HDL levels, but have little effect on lowering LDL levels. Gemfibrozil and fenofibrate are well tolerated but can cause liver toxicity and cholelithiasis (gallstones).

Bile Acid Sequestrants

These drugs increase cholesterol excretion and reduce LDL levels. They do this by forming an insoluble compound with bile salts and thus increasing bile loss through the feces (stool). This loss of bile, which would normally be recycled through the liver and bowel, causes increased oxidation of cholesterol to form bile. This results in a decrease in LDL plasma levels and a decrease in serum cholesterol levels (Figure 15-8). These drugs are usually used to treat type II **hyperlipoproteinemia** and are mostly used for

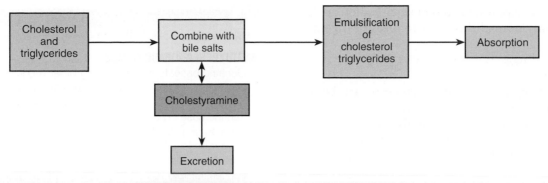

FIGURE 15-8 Mechanism of action of bile acid sequestrants.

lowering LDL levels. They are the only antihyperlipidemics that increase triglyceride levels. Patients may not be willing to use these drugs because of adverse GI effects such as constipation, bloating, and nausea. Both of these resin agent drugs are equally effective. Because they remain in the bowel and are not absorbed, there is no need to do tests to watch for adverse effects. They may also bind to other drugs and interfere with their absorption.

Niacin or Nicotinic Acid

Niacin is one of the most effective antihyperlipidemics at lowering triglyceride levels and increasing HDL levels and is similar to the bile acid sequestrants in its ability to lower LDL levels. The main limit to the use of niacin is its adverse effect of flushing (red color in the face and neck), although patients generally develop an ability to tolerate this problem with continued use. Flushing occurs shortly after the drug is taken and can be reduced by taking aspirin (30 minutes before) and increasing the niacin dosage very slowly over 3 to 4 weeks from 500 to 1000 mg three times daily. Niacin reduces glucose tolerance and may cause hyperuricemia (high uric acid levels), so it should be used with caution in patients with diabetes or gout. It remains the cheapest antihyperlipidemic and is probably underused in practice.

Selective Cholesterol Absorption Inhibitors

Ezetimibe is the first agent in this new category of drugs. This drug stays in the intestinal wall and acts on the intestinal epithelial cells to partially limit the absorption of cholesterol from food and from other sources in the body.

ADVERSE REACTIONS

All these medications may affect liver function, and the physician will be monitoring LFTs regularly. Also be aware of the following:

- Cholestyramine and colestipol hydrochloride may cause constipation.
- Lovastatin (Mevacor) should not be given to pregnant women.

DRUG INTERACTIONS

Because these drugs act by binding, giving the drug with other medications may cause those drugs to be bound to the product. Cholestyramine, colestipol, and gemfibrozil may make warfarin anticoagulants more effective. Therefore, the health care provider should make sure the patient knows when to take the medications and the nurse should help the patient remember that they can't all be taken at the same time.

Normal absorption of fat-soluble vitamins may be reduced with bile acid sequestrants, and the patient may show symptoms of vitamin deficiency if the dosage is at a high level or the drugs are taken for a long time. Watch for bleeding problems that may result from hypoprothrombinemia caused by vitamin K deficiency. Normal fat digestion may be disturbed. Some patients, especially very young or small patients, are more likely to develop hyperchloremic acidosis because of the chloride anion exchange.

These drugs delay or reduce the absorption of many important drugs and hormones. If the patient has been placed on a regular dose of any of these drugs, and then bile acid sequestrant therapy is discontinued, toxic levels of the other drugs may develop. This is especially important to consider in connection with digitalis therapy. These products may also produce mild increases of common electrolytes measured in the blood.

❖ NURSING IMPLICATIONS AND PATIENT TEACHING

■ Assessment

Learn as much as possible about the health history of the patient, including any allergies, other medications that are being taken that may lead to drug interactions, diet, other things the patient has done to try to reduce cholesterol levels, and the possibility of pregnancy.

■ Diagnosis

Does this patient have other problems that will interfere with this therapy? Does the patient have a family history that causes anxiety about early death? Does the patient have problems with exercise, diet, or stress that make it more difficult to follow the treatment plan?

▪ Planning

Encourage weight reduction when necessary, because obesity increases the risk of cardiovascular damage. The patient must be taught about the long-term nature of this disease and the need for lifelong diet changes. The nurse's ability to work with the patient, win confidence, be aware of reactions, and provide encouragement will be important in gaining compliance with diet, medication, and lifestyle changes that may save the patient's life. Frequent return visits to the health care provider will be necessary, so the nurse may have many chances to offer support and reinforcement.

▪ Implementation

If antihyperlipidemic drugs are taken for a long period, extra or supplemental oral or intramuscular doses of vitamins A, D, and K may be needed.

- Bile acid sequestrant preparations should be taken three times a day before meals. (Although there is no evidence that taking these drugs more than twice daily is helpful or therapeutic, the patient should get in the habit of taking the medication with each meal as a part of the total dietary change.) These drugs come as a powder that will need to be added to a liquid. They may be taken with milk, water, juice, or carbonated beverages; made into gelatin; or put into soups, cereals, or fruits with high moisture content, such as applesauce, nectars, fruit cocktail, or pineapple. The packet or a level scoopful of the powder should be added into a full glass or bowl. Allow the powder to dissolve slowly, without stirring, for at least 1 minute (stirring makes lumps). Once dissolved, the patient should stir it, make sure it is well mixed, and then drink it all. The container should be rinsed with water and this rinse swallowed as well so the patient gets all the medication in each dose.

Table 15-6 provides a summary of antihyperlipidemics.

Statin medications are often taken in the evening as the body makes higher amounts of cholesterol at night. Atorvastatin and rosuvastatin can be taken at any time of the day.

▪ Evaluation

- The patient may have constipation or hemorrhoids. Use of a high-bulk diet and a laxative may allow the patient to stay on the drug plan. The patient should be watched carefully to prevent serious constipation and impaction. To decrease constipation, the patient should eat a high-bulk diet (fruit, raw vegetables, bran) and drink at least 2 quarts of fluid per day.

Lifespan Considerations
Older Adults

ANTIHYPERLIPIDEMIC DRUGS

- Geriatric patients may be taking other medications in addition to antihyperlipidemia medications. Be aware that diuretics such as hydrochlorothiazide and chlorthalidone can increase cholesterol levels by 10% and beta blockers such as propranolol and estrogen may increase triglyceride serum levels by 25% to 50%.
- Dietary modifications and recommendations are vital to a successful lipid-reduction program. When goals cannot be met by diet alone, drug therapy may be prescribed.
- Constipation, a common (sometimes severe) side effect, has been reported in geriatric patients taking cholestyramine and colestipol. Encourage the patient to increase daily fluid intake to help reduce the irritation to the mouth and constipating effects of this drug.
- The antihyperlipidemic drugs should be administered before or with meals (follow the manufacturer's instructions) because these drugs are generally not effective if they are not administered with food. Lovastatin is often given with dinner to obtain its maximum beneficial effects, because the highest rate of cholesterol production occurs from midnight to 5 AM.

Modified from McKenry LM, Tessier E, Hogan MA: *Mosby's pharmacology in nursing*, ed 22, St Louis, 2006, Mosby.

Table 15-6   Common Antihyperlipidemics

GENERIC NAME	TRADE NAME
HMG-CoA Reductase Inhibitors—"Statins"	
atorvastatin Ca ★	Lipitor
fluvastatin	Lescol
lovastatin	Mevacor
pravastatin	Pravachol
rosuvastatin	Crestor
simvastatin	Zocor
Fibric Acid Derivatives	
gemfibrozil	Lopid
fenofibrate	Tricor, Lipofen
Bile Acid Sequestrants	
cholestyramine	Questran, Prevalite
colestipol	Colestid
colesevelam	Welchol
Niacin	
Nicotinic acid (niacin)	Niaspan, Niacor, Niac
Selective Cholesterol Absorption Inhibitors	
ezetimibe	Zetia

★ Indicates "Must-Know Drugs," or the 35 drugs most prescribers use.

If the patient takes high doses of niacin it may cause liver damage or gout. Instruct the patient to watch for any symptoms of these problems.

▪ Patient and Family Teaching

Tell the patient and family the following:

- The patient should take the medication as ordered and not change the dose or stop taking it without telling the nurse, physician, or other health care provider.
- The most important thing that can be done in learning to live with this problem is to follow the special diet. Lowering dietary intake of cholesterol and saturated fats, reducing calories, and increasing fluids and fiber content are very helpful. The patient should follow the diet that lists the foods that should and should not be eaten.
- The patient should take any other medicine 1 hour before or 4 to 6 hours after taking antihyperlipidemics. This is because these medicines are like glue and will delay the absorption of other drugs if taken at the same time.
- Some patients experience side effects from these drugs. The patient must tell the nurse, physician, or other health care provider if any new or troublesome symptoms occur, especially frequent stomach upset, constipation, gas, bloating, heartburn, nausea, vomiting, or bleeding of any type.
- The patient should keep this medication out of the reach of children and all others for whom it is not prescribed.

CARDIOTONICS

 ## OVERVIEW

Cardiotonics are drugs that have a positive inotropic action that make the heart beat stronger and slower. Cardiotonics that make composed of the *cardiac glycosides* (glycosides are sugar-containing substances made from plants); the phosphodiesterase inhibitors; and dobutamine, which is used occasionally in end-stage heart failure to increase myocardial contractility in a dose-dependent manner. The major cardiac glycoside is the digitalis preparation digoxin that has been used for many years.

ACTION

All cardiotonics have the following two actions:

1. They increase the strength or force of the contraction (or pumping) of the heart muscle (myocardium). This is considered a positive inotropic action.
2. They slow the heart rate. This is considered a negative chronotropic effect.

The overall result of these two actions is to increase the cardiac output. This is important in hearts that have become weakened and ineffective in pumping because of age or disease and where chronic heart failure has developed.

The normal heart pumps oxygenated blood from the left ventricle out through the body. If the heart is weak, less oxygenated blood can be pumped out with each contraction or beat of the heart.

When cardiac output (the amount of blood pumped out with each heartbeat × the heart beat) decreases, other organs are affected. For example, the brain reacts to receiving less blood by making us feel dizzy, drowsy, or less alert. The lungs are not as effective and the patient may have a productive cough or feel short of breath. The kidneys become less effective at removing waste products, electrolytes, and extra water from the bloodstream. This extra fluid may then pool in the spaces between cells or organs or in other dependent tissues like the hands and feet (**edema**). The patient may have rapid weight gain because of this fluid. Sometimes the heartbeat itself becomes irregular or too fast. As the body attempts to deal with these changes, over time, the heart may enlarge, develop murmurs or abnormal heart sounds, and the blood pressure may increase or a more rapid heart rate or rhythm may develop. These actions may place further strain on the heart. We call these symptoms of weak or inadequate heart muscle actions chronic or **congestive heart failure (CHF)** (Table 15-7). The specific therapy for heart failure depends on the severity of the problem causing the failure.

Heart failure may also be seen in patients who have had heart attacks or who have high blood pressure or diabetes. Cardiac glycosides have been used to treat heart failure and dysrhythmias for many years. Phosphodiesterase inhibitors (that prevent the inactivation of the intracellular cAMP and cGMP) are used in very ill patients and dobutamine (a beta 1 adrenergic stimulant) is used occasionally. Now angiotensin-converting enzyme (ACE) inhibitors have become the preferred drugs for treating heart failure and protecting the kidneys from damage. Diuretics are also used to relieve symptoms of heart failure by reducing blood volume.

Table 15-7	Symptoms of Congestive or Chronic Heart Failure
ORGAN AFFECTED	**SYMPTOMS**
Brain	Dizzy, less alert
Heart	Enlarged heart, murmurs or abnormal heart sounds, dysrhythmias
Lungs	Productive cough, shortness of breath
Kidneys	Edema of tissues of hands and feet
General	Rapid weight gain, weakness, lethargy (sleepiness)

Beta-adrenergic blockers are also used in combination with other drugs to slow the progression of heart failure. These other products are discussed in the section on antihypertensive agents. Cardiac glycosides are the drugs that licensed practical and vocational nurses need to know the most about.

Increasing the Strength of Myocardial Contraction

The first action of the cardiotonic drugs is to increase the strength of each heartbeat or the force of the contraction. The stronger heartbeat pumps more blood and increases the cardiac output. This effect of the drug is called a **positive inotropic action**. As more blood reaches the brain, lungs, kidneys, and other tissues, the signs of inadequate heart action decrease or go away (Figures 15-9 and 15-10).

Slowing Heart Rate

The second action of the cardiotonic drugs is to slow the heartbeat. They do this by: (1) slowing down the rate at which the pacemaker in the SA node begins the electrical cycle; and (2) by slowing the rate at which that information is passed through the rest of the heart. (See the discussion of cardiac conduction in the "Antidysrhythmics" section of this chapter.)

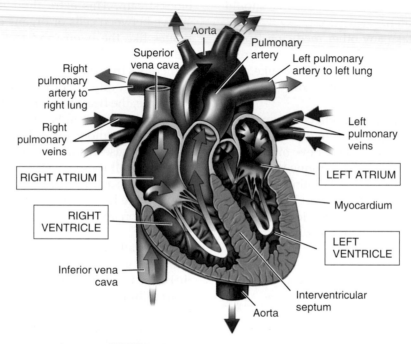

FIGURE 15-9 Internal anatomy of the heart.

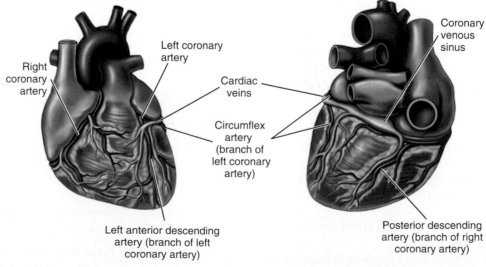

FIGURE 15-10 Coronary arteries.

USES

Cardiotonics are used to treat heart failure and rapid or irregular heartbeats such as atrial fibrillation, atrial flutter, and (sometimes outside the hospital) frequent premature ventricular contractions or paroxysmal atrial tachycardia.

ADVERSE REACTIONS

Cardiotonics are very powerful and can act as poisons on the heart. Thus a patient taking this drug must be closely watched. Phosphodiesterase inhibitors and dobutamine are given to critically ill hospitalized patients who are always carefully monitored. Older adult patients frequently use digitalis, and they are at particular risk of problems if they use it with other drugs.

Many things may happen that make even a safe dose of digitalis harmful to a patient. When a patient begins to show toxic or harmful reactions from too much medication, **digitalis toxicity** has developed. The symptoms of digitalis toxicity may begin slowly and are often easy to overlook. These symptoms include dysrhythmias (such as bradycardia, bigeminal VPCs, AV Node block, excessive fatigue, confusion, blurred vision, yellow-green vision, anorexia, nausea, and vomiting) and other vague symptoms.

 Clinical Goldmine

Medication Amounts

The amount of digitalis medicine that is helpful (therapeutic) and the amount that is harmful (toxic) are very close together. Sometimes it is hard to tell if the patient needs more medicine or has too much.

Treatment of digitalis toxicity begins by stopping the drug and beginning treatment of symptoms, as needed.

DRUG INTERACTIONS

Beta-adrenergic blocking agents, calcium gluconate, calcium chloride, succinylcholine, and verapamil increase both the therapeutic and the toxic effects of cardiotonics.

Cholestyramine reduces the therapeutic effects.

Any medication that changes the electrolyte balance may also lead to digitalis toxicity.

 Clinical Goldmine

Cardiotonics

Digitalis is one of the most common medicines. Because these drugs may reach toxic levels very quickly, it is important for the nurse to closely watch the patient receiving these drugs.

❖ NURSING IMPLICATIONS AND PATIENT TEACHING

▪ Assessment

Before beginning the medication, check the patient for the following:
1. History of nausea, vomiting, diarrhea, weakness, shortness of breath, confusion, or depression.
2. Presence on physical examination of muscle weakness, confusion, hypertension, bradycardia, tachycardia, dysrhythmias, abnormal heart sounds or murmurs, unusual lung sounds produced during inspiration or expiration, cyanosis (blue color to the skin), peripheral edema, or distended jugular veins. The patient should also be weighed.
3. Abnormal laboratory results may be found with ECGs, chest x-ray studies, complete blood cell counts, serum enzymes, serum electrolytes, and renal and hepatic studies.

▪ Diagnosis

What other problems does this patient have that interfere with therapy? Is the patient overweight? Anxious? Unwilling to accept having cardiac problems?

▪ Planning

Know about two different types of dosages for patients taking digoxin: 1) the initial **digitalizing dose** (or loading dose); and 2) maintenance (regular daily) doses. More frequent and higher digitalizing doses are given when a patient begins taking digoxin so that a specific level of medication can be reached in the blood. When the amount of drug in the patient's blood reaches the desired level, smaller maintenance doses are given once a day to maintain the blood level. How fast the desired drug level is reached is based on the dosage, the diagnosis of the patient, and many other factors.

 Memory Jogger

Safety Alert

Because these medications lower the patient's heart rate, the nurse should always take the patient's apical heart rate with a stethoscope before giving these drugs. This safety measure is essential to avoid overdosage with these drugs.

▪ Implementation

Before giving each dose of a cardiotonic drug, the apical pulse rate (using a stethoscope and listening to the chest) should be taken for 60 seconds. In an adult, if the apical pulse rate is less than 60, the medication should not be given until the nurse has discussed the low rate with the health care provider and the provider has decided whether it should be given. If there are any symptoms of digitalis toxicity or if the patient's condition has worsened since the last time the medication was given, the nurse notifies someone in

Table 15-8   Cardiotonics

GENERIC NAME	TRADE NAME	USES	SERIOUS ADVERSE REACTIONS
Cardioglycoside:			
digoxin ★	Lanoxin	Atrial flutter, atrial fibrillation, PAT, CHF	Digitalis toxicity (see text)
Phosphodiesterase Inhibitors			
inamrinone	Amrinone	For the short-term management of CHF patients who can be closely monitored and have not responded to digitalis	Ectopic activity of the heart, GI distress, hypersensitivity (allergy) reactions, and hepatotoxicity (damage to the liver)
milrinone	Primacor	CHF—short term	Ventricular dysrhythmias
Miscellaneous Product			
dobutamine		Beta-1 selective inotrope. Short-term treatment of cardiac decompensation	Ectopic activity, hypotension, tachycardia, and hypertension

CHF, Congestive heart failure; *GI,* gastrointestinal; *PAT,* paroxysmal atrial tachycardia.
★ Indicates "Must-Know Drugs," or the 35 drugs most prescribers use.

authority if they believe that the dose should not be given, so that a decision might be made.

Table 15-8 gives a summary of cardiotonic medications.

■ Evaluation

A big risk for patients taking a cardioglycoside is the chance they will get too much drug and have digitalis toxicity. Changes from the first time the patient is seen should be written down in the patient record. Vital signs, including daily weights, are very important to record. Patients with other lung, GI, kidney, or central nervous system (CNS) problems, patients taking many other medications (especially diuretics and electrolytes), and confused patients who are not eating or drinking well are all at risk for digitalis toxicity.

The nurse is alert to any changes in the patient that may suggest the patient has developed digitalis toxicity. The earliest symptom of digitalis toxicity is often extreme fatigue. Almost 100% of patients also experience anorexia. Other signs include nausea and vomiting, difficulty with reading (which may appear as visual alterations such as green and yellow vision, double vision, blurred vision, or seeing spots or halos), headaches, dizziness, weakness, confusion, depression, increased nervousness, and diarrhea. Digitalis toxicity may cause life-threatening dysrhythmias, such as bradycardia, tachycardia, and irregular rhythms.

The health care provider will order blood tests to measure the serum blood digitalis level. The serum level of digoxin that is needed to help the patient (be therapeutic) is 0.5 to 2 ng/mL (nanograms per milliliter), and the toxic serum level is 2.5 ng/mL. Digoxin has a rapid onset and a short length of action.

Episodes of digitalis toxicity may be treated with digoxin immune Fab (Digibind), which has antigen-binding fragments that come from specific antidigoxin antibodies. This product may save lives, but it requires careful monitoring of the patient's vital signs and potassium levels and special plans for slowly reducing the amount of drug that is given to avoid causing other life-threatening events.

Lifespan Considerations
Pediatric

DIGITALIS

- Digitalis is reported to be a leading cause of accidental toxicity in children.
- Individualized dosing based on weight or body surface area with very close monitoring is necessary, especially in premature and immature infants.
- Early signs of toxicity in infants and children may include a slow apical heart rate (less than 80 beats/min in children; less than 100 beats in infants) and irregular heart rhythms.

Modified from McKenry LM, Tessier E, Hogan MA: *Mosby's pharmacology in nursing,* ed 22, St Louis, 2006, Mosby.

Lifespan Considerations
Older Adults

DIGITALIS

- Older adults often have a reduced tolerance for this drug. Thus lower doses may be ordered. If there are changes in the patient that affect how much the patient exercises, if he or she become dehydrated or kidney function changes, or if he or she has diarrhea or is using laxatives, the amount of digitalis absorbed may change.
- Many of the adverse effects of digitalis are easy to ignore. Patients may not realize fatigue is an adverse effect.
- Decreased libido, gynecomastia (enlargement of the breasts in men), and breast tenderness have been reported in men.

■ Patient and Family Teaching

The patient usually continues to take this medication after discharge from the hospital. Tell the family and patient the following:

- The patient or a dependable family member must be taught to look for the same things the nurse, physician, or other health care providers have been watching. This may require teaching the patient or family member how to take the pulse. Ask on more than one occasion for a demonstration of the technique. Before discharge, make certain the patient and family know what to do when the pulse is less than 60 beats/min in adults, with higher rates for infants and children.
- The patient should tell the nurse, physician, or other health care provider if lack of appetite, nausea, vomiting, diarrhea, unusual weakness, fatigue, vision changes, depression, confusion, or dizziness occurs.
- The medication must be kept in a safe place, away from animals or small children.
- The medication must not be stopped unless the patient is told to stop by the nurse, physician, or other health care provider. It is very important that the patient does not run out of medicine. The nurse, physician, or other health care provider should be called if the patient has no medication.
- It is important to keep office visits with the nurse, physician, or other health care provider so that changes in the patient's health can be determined. The patient should have laboratory tests done as soon as possible when they are ordered.
- The patient should not take other prescription drugs or OTC drugs without the approval of the nurse, physician, or other health care provider. Some drugs interfere with the action of cardiotonic drugs and may cause very serious problems.
- The patient should take the medication at the same time every day, as directed by the nurse, physician, or other health care provider; digitalis products are usually taken after meals.
- The patient should wear a MedicAlert bracelet or necklace or have other emergency identification indicating the medication being taken.
- The patient taking cardiotonic drugs may be advised to eat foods rich in potassium. Good sources of potassium include bananas and citrus fruits, dried fruits, dried beans and lentils, and all-bran cereal.

ANTIHYPERTENSIVES, DIURETICS, AND OTHER DRUGS AFFECTING THE URINARY TRACT

OVERVIEW

Hypertension is a disorder in which the patient's blood pressure is elevated above normal values for his or her age. Research has shown that blood pressures of more than 140/90 mm Hg are associated with accelerated vascular damage of the heart, the brain, and the kidneys, leading to an increased risk of early death. Lowering the blood pressure to less than 120/90 mm Hg has been demonstrated to dramatically reduce the chance of MI, stroke, and other target organ damage. Primary hypertension (or essential hypertension) accounts for 80% to 90% of all cases of high blood pressure, but in most cases the cause is unknown. In some cases, high blood pressure results from another disease or other problem and is then called secondary hypertension.

Approximately 40 million people in the United States have hypertension, a disorder that cannot be cured but can be controlled. Risk factors for hypertension include increasing age, black race, male sex, family history of hypertension, obesity, diabetes mellitus, hypercholesterolemia, smoking, and previous history of vascular disease.

ACTION

Many types of drugs are available to treat hypertension. The drug selected for use depends on the severity of the disease. The drugs act at many sites in the body and through several different ways (Figure 15-11). These drugs fall roughly into the following five main categories:

1. *Diuretics* indirectly reduce blood pressure by producing sodium and water loss and lowering the tone or rigidity of the arteries. Most diuretics act by blocking sodium reabsorption in the nephron.
2. *Adrenergic antagonists or blockers* are nervous system stimulants and inhibitors that assist in lowering cardiac output and/or peripheral resistance.
3. *Renin-angiotensin–related drugs* affect the renin-angiotensin system of the kidney. ACE inhibitors act on the renin-angiotensin system to promote a decrease in the work of the heart (vascular afterload and preload) through vasodilation (vascular opening) when angiotensin II is inhibited. Angiotensin II receptor antagonists block the vasoconstrictive (narrowing) and aldosterone-secreting effects of angiotensin II by selectively blocking the binding of angiotensin II to angiotensin receptors in many tissues.
4. *Direct-acting vasodilators* lower the pressure in the vessels of the arms and legs, or the *peripheral resistance*.
5. *Calcium channel blocking agents* reduce peripheral resistance (in the arms and legs) through smooth muscle relaxation and vasodilation.

Because each of these five drug categories works in a different manner and is also useful in treating problems other than hypertension, the action of each drug category is discussed separately. Figure 15-9 shows the different places where these antihypertensive medications may act.

Many of these drugs can be mixed together to produce a new combination drug with many actions. Some of these products combine potassium-sparing and potassium-losing drugs. These drugs may be good for some patients (they do not need to take so many

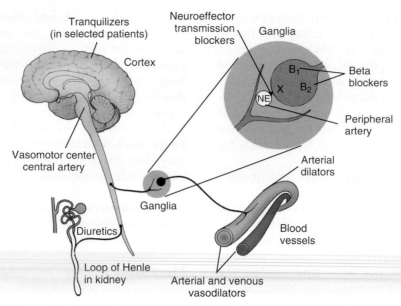

FIGURE 15-11 Sites of action for antihypertensive medications. *NE,* norepinephrine.

pills), but the ability to increase or decrease one of the drugs in the combination product to meet the specific needs of a patient is lost.

Diuretics

The action of all diuretics is to increase fluid loss from the body. Diuretics have been the main drugs used in antihypertensive therapy for the past 40 years and they are the first-line drugs used in many patients who have mild to moderate hypertension. They are popular because they work quite well, are quite safe, are well tolerated, and are not very expensive. Diuretics may be classed into four related groups: thiazides (for example, chlorothiazide and hydrochlorothiazide), the thiazide-like sulfonamides (for example, metolazone, and indapamide), loop diuretics (for example, furosemide and bumetanide), and the potassium-sparing diuretics (for example, amiloride, triamterene, and spironolactone). The most-effective diuretics are those that work at the loop of Henle.

Thiazides and Sulfonamide Diuretics. Thiazides and sulfonamide diuretics are the most commonly used class of diuretics and they have similar actions. They work to prevent the reabsorption of sodium and chloride through direct action on the end of the ascending loop and the beginning of the distal tubule of the loop of Henle in the distal kidney tubule (Figure 15-12). They act to block sodium and chloride reabsorption and slightly limit carbonic anhydrase. Their long half-life may lead to the loss of large amounts of potassium.

The thiazides also act directly to dilate the smooth muscles in the arterioles, the smallest vessels in the arterial system. Because the arterioles are made larger,

the heart does not have to pump so hard to get blood into them. This helps keep blood pressure lower. Thiazides also work to promote reabsorption of calcium, which may make them good for use in older adults with osteoporosis.

Lifespan Considerations
Pregnant and Postpartum Women

Thiazide diuretics may not be taken during pregnancy or when a mother is breastfeeding, because of risk to the neonate.

Lifespan Considerations
Older Adults

DIURETICS

* Older adult patients are more susceptible to the development of the adverse reactions of postural hypotension, impaired mentation, hypokalemia (except with potassium-sparing diuretics), and increased serum glucose levels.
* Lower doses of diuretics are advised in the older adult population, with dosage increases based on the patient's individual therapeutic response and the development of adverse reactions.
* Patients taking diuretics must be observed for symptoms of potassium loss. This is often seen when the patient develops muscle weakness and other symptoms of dehydration. Many patients require potassium replacement while taking diuretics and digitalis.
* When a diuretic is to be discontinued, it is recommended that the drug be reduced gradually to avoid the development of serious edema.

From McKenry LM, Tessier E, Hogan MA: *Mosby's pharmacology in nursing,* ed 22, St Louis, 2006, Mosby.

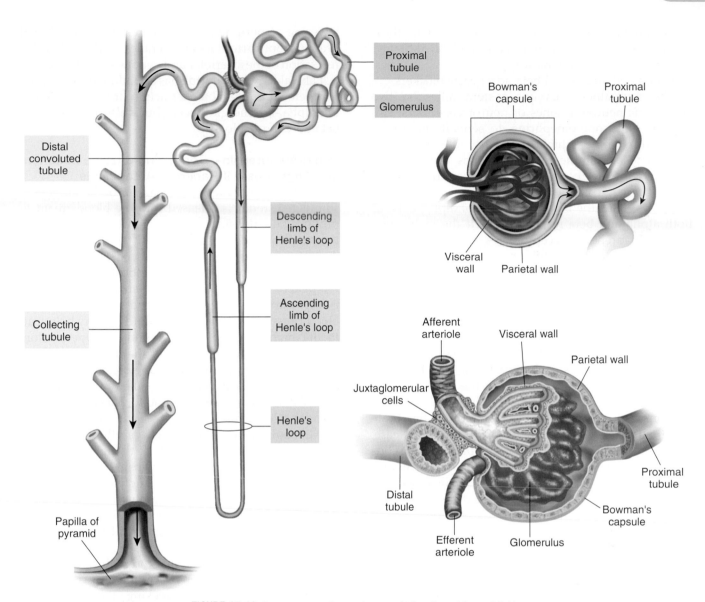

FIGURE 15-12 Components of a nephron and direction of flow of fluid.

Loop Diuretics. Loop diuretics act by blocking active transport of chloride, sodium, and potassium in the thick ascending loop of Henle. They are very effective drugs. These drugs often work well in patients with very low glomerular filtration rates, because they are so efficient in limiting the reabsorption of sodium. The peak diuretic effect is much greater for loop diuretics than that seen with any other type of diuretic. They are often used in patients with kidney disease and to treat CHF, cirrhosis of the liver, and kidney diseases in which a powerful diuretic is required.

Fluid Balance

In understanding fluid and electrolyte balance, a good rule to remember is that water tends to follow sodium; thus, with sodium loss, water also is pulled out and lost through the urine.

Potassium-Sparing Diuretics. Potassium-sparing diuretics increase the excretion of water and sodium, but save potassium. These drugs act by binding at receptor sites in the distal renal tubular cell nucleus, resulting in changes in the creation of proteins that affect the exchange of sodium and potassium. These drugs are used in patients with kidney disease, in older adult patients with poor kidney function who have hypokalemia, or in those patients with the risk for having hypokalemia, often because of treatment with other medications such as digitalis. (Refer to Figure 15-12 for a review of the different parts of the kidney nephron.)

Adrenergic Inhibitors
Adrenergic inhibitors are also divided into five different categories of drugs:
1. Beta-adrenergic blockers
2. Central adrenergic inhibitors

3. Peripheral adrenergic antagonists (most of these drugs are now off the market in the United States)
4. Alpha$_1$-adrenergic inhibitors
5. Combined alpha- and beta-adrenergic blockers

The sympathetic nervous system relies on two adrenergic neurohormones or neurotransmitters, epinephrine and norepinephrine, to send its messages. These adrenergic inhibitors occupy the adrenergic receptors so that the neurohormones cannot make contact with the receptors, thus preventing stimulation. Adrenergic nerve fibers have either alpha or beta receptors. Thus the blocking can be of alpha, beta, or both alpha and beta receptor sites. If the medication blocks all adrenergic receptor sites, we say it is *nonselective* in its blocking. Alpha receptor blockers are an important drug group.

Beta Blockers. Beta blockers are classed into two groups: nonselective and selective beta antagonists. The nonselective agents block both beta$_1$ and beta$_2$ sites. The selective beta$_1$ blocking agents stop the action of the beta$_1$ receptors of the heart, but they have less influence on the beta$_2$ receptors of the bronchi in the lung. There are no selective beta$_2$ inhibitors.

Nonselective beta blockers: (1) reduce the heart rate and the force of contraction, (2) prevent renin release, and (3) slow the outflow of sympathetic nervous system messages from the brainstem to the vasomotor center telling the body to narrow the blood vessels and increase the heart rate. Because these drugs block both beta$_1$ and beta$_2$ impulses, they have a wide range of side effects.

Central Adrenergic Inhibitors. Central adrenergic inhibitors stimulate peripheral alpha-adrenergic receptors. They cause brief vasoconstriction and then stimulate the presynaptic alpha$_2$-adrenergic receptors in the centers in the brainstem that coordinate cardiovascular function. As a result of this, the total number of sympathetic nervous system messages from the brain is decreased, leading to vascular relaxation and lower blood pressure.

Peripheral Adrenergic Antagonists. Peripheral adrenergic antagonists work as adrenergic neuron blocking agents that prevent sympathetic nervous system vasoconstriction by limiting norepinephrine release from storage sites in the neurons and by using up all the norepinephrine at nerve endings. When vascular smooth muscle is relaxed, total peripheral resistance to blood flow is decreased. Because of the many side effects of these drugs, most have been removed from the market in the United States.

Alpha$_1$-Adrenergic Inhibitors. Alpha$_1$-adrenergic inhibitors work through selective blocking of postsynaptic alpha-adrenergic receptor sites, leading to a lowering of peripheral vascular resistance and blood pressure. Both arterioles and venules are dilated by this relaxation of the arteriolar and venous smooth muscles.

Labetalol hydrochloride has a combination of alpha- and beta-adrenergic blocker action. It works as selective alpha$_1$-adrenergic blocker, but is also a nonselective beta-adrenergic blocker.

Renin-Angiotensin—Converting Enzyme Inhibitors *and* Angiotensin II Receptor Antagonists

When the juxtaglomerular apparatus of the kidneys is stimulated, renin is released into the bloodstream to produce angiotensin I. Angiotensin I is then changed to angiotensin II in the liver and the lungs by ACE. Angiotensin II is a powerful vasoconstrictor that acts on the adrenal cortex to increase aldosterone secretion. If a patient is in shock, this renin-angiotensin reaction is important in saving sodium and water to keep the blood pressure up, but at other times, it may help lead to the high blood pressure found in hypertension. Figure 15-13 shows a review of the renin-angiotensin system. It is also known that angiotensin-converting enzymes also form chemicals called angiotensin III and IV that also have weak inhibitor function and play a minor role in this process.

Although we do not know everything about the action of ACE inhibitors, they are thought to stop the change of angiotensin I to angiotensin II by preventing the action of ACE in the plasma and vascular endothelium. There may be other complex actions of these drugs that also help reduce blood pressure. ACE inhibitors are not to be given to pregnant women in the second and third trimesters.

Angiotensin II receptor antagonists block the vasoconstrictor and aldosterone-secreting effects of angiotensin II by selectively blocking the binding of angiotensin II to the angiotensin receptor found in many tissues. ACE inhibitors often produce a cough in patients. Angiotensin II antagonists do not produce cough.

Vasodilators

Vasodilators reduce systolic and diastolic blood pressure by direct relaxation of arteriolar smooth muscle, thus lowering peripheral vascular resistance. The exact way these drugs work is not known, but they appear to block calcium from moving through the cell membrane.

Calcium Channel Blocking Agents

Calcium channel blocking agents selectively limit the passage of extracellular calcium ions through specific ion channels of the cell membrane in cardiac, vascular, and smooth muscle cells. This causes a lowered peripheral vascular resistance and a fall in systolic and diastolic blood pressure. These drugs are now commonly used to decrease blood pressure.

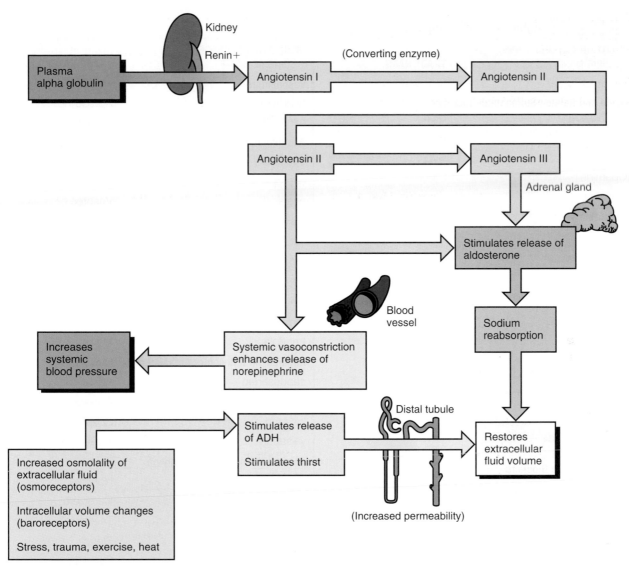

FIGURE 15-13 Physiologic effects of renin-angiotensin system. *ADH,* Antidiuretic hormone.

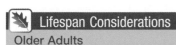

Lifespan Considerations

Older Adults

CALCIUM CHANNEL BLOCKERS

- Older adults are more susceptible to these agents and the side effects of increased weakness, dizziness, fainting episodes, and falls.
- Although nitroglycerin (or other nitrates) may be taken at the same time as these agents, the patient should be advised to report any increase in frequency or intensity of angina attacks to the health care provider.
- Nicotine may reduce the effectiveness of these agents; reduction or avoidance of tobacco products is advisable.
- Alcohol consumption may result in hypotensive episodes in some patients. Whenever possible, the use of alcohol should be avoided.
- These agents should not be suddenly stopped because severe rebound angina attacks may result; gradual drug withdrawal is required.

From McKenry LM, Tessier E, Hogan MA: *Mosby's pharmacology in nursing,* ed 22, St Louis, 2006, Mosby.

USES

Antihypertensives and diuretics (Table 15-9) are used alone or in combination to decrease elevated systolic and diastolic blood pressure. *Blood pressure* may be defined as pressure of the blood against the walls of the various vessels. The blood pressure is highest at the moment the ventricles contract (systole), because the heart has to push very hard to get the blood out into the circulation. This is called *systolic pressure.* Pressure during ventricular relaxation is known as *diastolic pressure* and is the pressure at the lowest part of the cardiac cycle. These pressures are written as a fraction, with the systolic as the numerator (the number on top of the fraction) and the diastolic as the denominator (the number on the bottom of the fraction). Respected clinical studies suggest that it is beneficial to use a combination of diet, drug therapy, and reduction of risk factors to treat hypertension. The therapeutic goal in the hypertensive patient is to reduce the blood

Table 15-9 Antihypertensive Agents

MEDICATION CATEGORY AND GENERIC NAME	TRADE NAME	MEDICATION CATEGORY AND GENERIC NAME	TRADE NAME
Diuretics		**Vasodilators**	
Thiazide and Related Sulfonamide Diuretics		hydralazine	Apresoline
chlorothiazide	Diuril	minoxidil	Loniten
hydrochlorothiazide	HydroDIRUIL, Microzide	**Ace Inhibitors**	
chlorthalidone	Hygroton	benazepril	Lotensin
indapamide	Lozol	captopril	Capoten ★
metolazone,	Zaroxolyn Mykrox	enalapril	Vasotec
Loop Diuretics		fosinopril	Monopril
bumetanide	Bumex	lisinopril	Zestril
furosemide	Lasix	moexipril	Univasc
torsemide	Demadex	perindopril	Aceon
Potassium-Sparing Agents		quinapril	Accupril
amiloride	Midamor	ramipril	Altace
spironolactone	Aldactone	trandolapril	Mavik
triamterene	Dyrenium	**Angiotensin II Receptor Antagonists or Blockers**	
Adrenergic Inhibitors		candesartan	Atacand
Central Adrenergic Inhibitors		irbesartan	Avapro
clonidine	Catapres, Duraclon	losartan	Cozaar
guanabenz	Wytensin	valsartan	Diovan
methyldopa	Aldomet	**Calcium Channel Blocking Agents**	
Alpha1-Adrenergic Blockers		amlodipine	Norvasc
doxazosin	Cardura	diltiazem	Cardizem
prazosin	Minipress	eprosartan	Teveten
terazosin	Hytrin	felodipine	Plendil
Beta-Adrenergic Blockers		isradipine	DynaCirc
atenolol	Tenormin	nicardipine	Cardene
betaxolol	Kerlone	nifedipine	Procardia ★
bisoprolol	Zebeta	nisoldipine	Nisocor, Sular
metoprolol	Lopressor, Toprol XL	olmesartan	Benicar
nadolol	Corgard	telmisartan	Micardis
propranolol)	Inderal ★	verapamil	Calan ★
Combined Alpha- and Beta-Adrenergic Blocker			
carvedilol	Coreg		
labetalol	Normodyne, Trandate		

★ Indicates "Must-Know Drugs," or the 35 drugs most prescribers use.

pressure to normal or near normal with few adverse effects. Reduction of both systolic and diastolic pressure has been associated with decreased risk of damage to the vascular tissues of the heart, kidneys, brain, eyes, and other organs, or **end-organ damage**.

The patient with hypertension may have no symptoms or may complain of not feeling well in general. Headaches, frequently associated with hypertension, are often produced by stress, tension, or other reasons, rather than being related to high blood pressure, unless very severe blood pressure elevations are present. In cases of secondary hypertension, there may be reports of getting up at night to go to the bathroom (nocturia), history of renal trauma (producing renal artery stenosis), or a family history of hypertension.

Hypertension is classified according to the stages listed in Table 15-10. The choice of antihypertensive drug depends on many factors: how severe the hypertension is, the presence of **compelling indications** (other diseases for which a specific class of antihypertensives

| Table 15-10 | Classification and Management of Blood Pressure for Adults |

			INITIAL DRUG THERAPY	
BP CLASS	SYSTOLIC BP (mm HG)	DIASTOLIC BP (mm HG)	WITHOUT COMPELLING INDICATION	WITH COMPELLING INDICATION
Normal	<120	and <80	None indicated	Drugs for compelling indications
Prehypertension	120-139	or 80-89		
Stage 1 HTN	140-159	or 90-99	Thiazide-type diuretics for most; ACEI, ARB, BB, CCB, or combination may be considered	Drug(s) for compelling indications
				Other antihypertensive drugs (diuretics, ACEI, ARB, BB, CCB)
Stage 2 HTN	>160	or >100	Two-drug combination for months (usually thiazide-type diuretic and ACEI or ARB or BB or CCB)	As needed

ACEI, Angiotensin-converting enzyme inhibitors; *ARB,* angiotensin II receptor blockers; *BB,* beta blockers; *BP,* blood pressure; *CCB,* calcium channel blockers; *HTN,* hypertension.

| Table 15-11 | Management of Hypertension Based on Risk Stratification |

BLOOD PRESSURE STAGES (MM HG)	RISK GROUP A (NO RISK FACTORS AND NO TOD/CCD)	RISK GROUP B (AT LEAST ONE RISK FACTOR, NOT INCLUDING DM; NO TOD/CCD)	RISK GROUP C (TOD/CCD AND/OR DM, WITH OR WITHOUT OTHER RISK FACTORS)
High-normal (130-139/85-89)	Lifestyle modification*	Lifestyle modification	Drug therapy†
Stage 1 (140-159/90-99)	Lifestyle modification (up to 12 mo)	Lifestyle modification (up to 6 mo)	Drug therapy
Stages 2 and 3 (>160/>100)	Drug therapy	Drug therapy	Drug therapy

DM, Diabetes mellitus; *TOD/CCD,* target organ damage/clinical cardiovascular disease.
*Should be adjunctive therapy for all patients recommended for pharmacologic therapy.
†For those patients with heart failure, renal insufficiency, or diabetes.

has been shown to improve the patient's condition), the use of other drugs, and the patient's willingness to accept the mild but unavoidable side effects that may develop.

The Joint National Committee on the Prevention, Detection, Evaluation, and Treatment of High Blood Pressure has indicated how the antihypertensive drugs should be used for initial therapy and when and what additional drugs are to be used (Table 15-11). The treatment plan starts with lifestyle modifications, then a single mild agent, gradually increasing the dosage, and then adding drugs from other drug categories to bring the diastolic blood pressure under control. The drug effects are balanced in this approach to take advantage of different kinds of drug action. (See treatment algorhythm, Figure 15-14).

Stage I: Lifestyle Changes
Before starting drug therapy for patients with hypertension, a lot of effort should be made to help patients reduce their risk factors. Lifestyle changes to help

patients lose weight; increase physical activity; and reduce fat, salt, and calories in the diet are helpful in lowering blood pressure. Behavior change to assist them to stop smoking and reduce alcohol intake is also important.

Stage II: Drug Therapy
The drug of choice in starting antihypertensive therapy is an oral thiazide—or thiazide-like sulfonamide drug—or an adrenergic beta blocker. Other drugs are added if needed, based on how the patient responds to the first drug. Most thiazides or beta blockers are effective when given once a day. The drug is started at a low dosage and increased as needed until the maximum dose is reached. In many cases, one of the drugs by itself will reduce the diastolic blood pressure to the desired level. Because these drugs commonly produce hypokalemia, a potassium supplement may also be required. Loop diuretics are used when hypertension is severe and the blood pressure must come down quickly. An

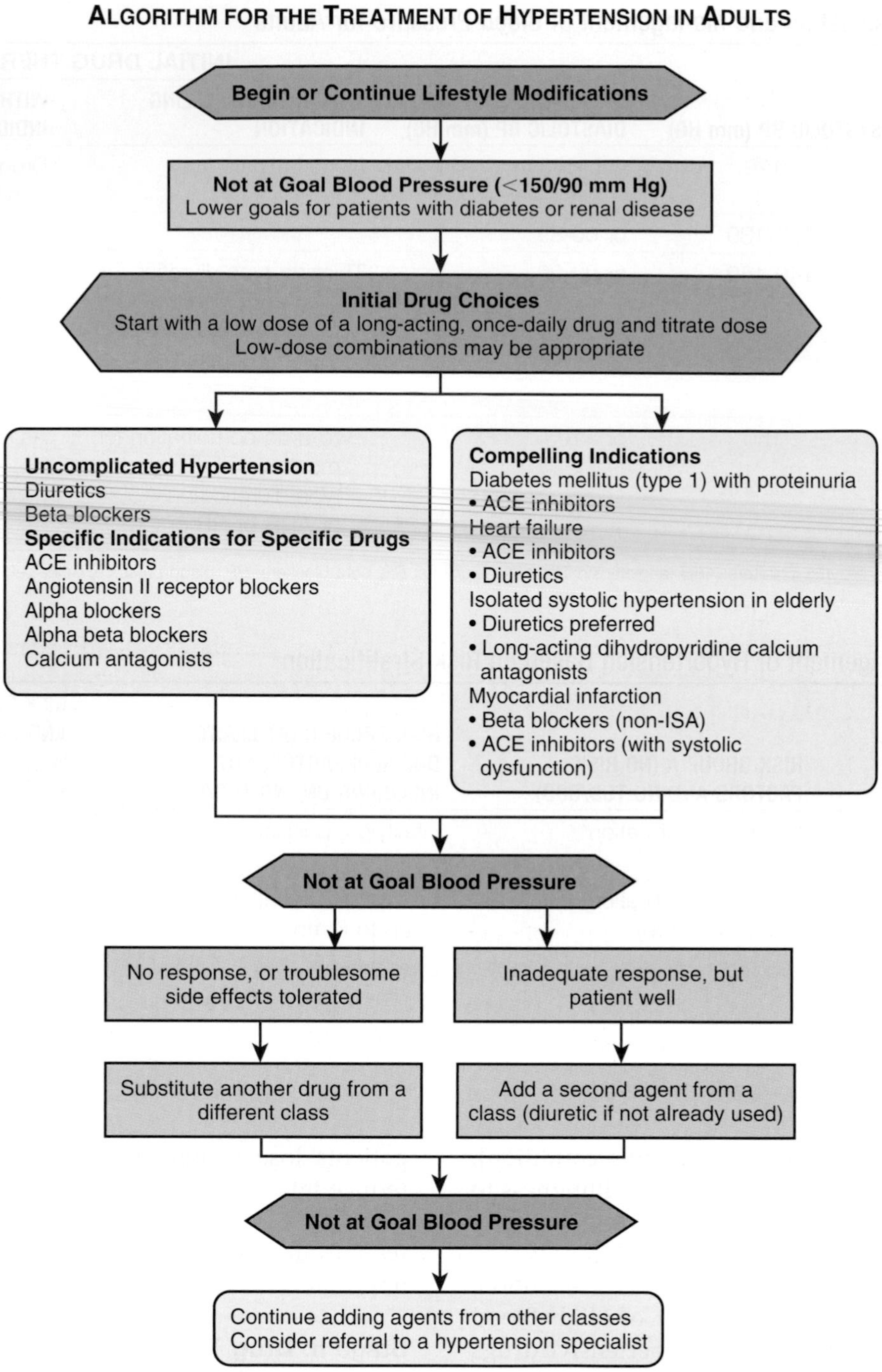

ALGORITHM FOR THE TREATMENT OF HYPERTENSION IN ADULTS

Begin or Continue Lifestyle Modifications

Not at Goal Blood Pressure (<150/90 mm Hg)
Lower goals for patients with diabetes or renal disease

Initial Drug Choices
Start with a low dose of a long-acting, once-daily drug and titrate dose
Low-dose combinations may be appropriate

Uncomplicated Hypertension
Diuretics
Beta blockers
Specific Indications for Specific Drugs
ACE inhibitors
Angiotensin II receptor blockers
Alpha blockers
Alpha beta blockers
Calcium antagonists

Compelling Indications
Diabetes mellitus (type 1) with proteinuria
• ACE inhibitors
Heart failure
• ACE inhibitors
• Diuretics
Isolated systolic hypertension in elderly
• Diuretics preferred
• Long-acting dihydropyridine calcium
  antagonists
Myocardial infarction
• Beta blockers (non-ISA)
• ACE inhibitors (with systolic
  dysfunction)

Not at Goal Blood Pressure

No response, or troublesome
side effects tolerated

Inadequate response, but
patient well

Substitute another drug from a
different class

Add a second agent from a
class (diuretic if not already used)

Not at Goal Blood Pressure

Continue adding agents from other classes
Consider referral to a hypertension specialist

FIGURE 15-14 Treatment regimen for hypertension. *ACE,* Angiotensin-converting enzyme; *ISA,* intrinsic sympathomimetic activity.

antiadrenergic agent may be added to the treatment plan if the maximum doses of diuretics or beta blockers fail to lower the blood pressure to the desired level. These two categories of drugs work well together to bring down blood pressure and lower the chance of side effects, and they are better than using an antiadrenergic agent alone. There are a variety of antiadrenergic drugs, so the patient can try different combinations to find the ones that work best. The patient should move on to the next level of drug treatment only if a drug regimen fails to adequately control blood pressure. It should be noted that beta blockers seem to be less effective in black and much older adult patients. Captopril is another drug that seems to be less effective in black patients.

Other drugs that might be added to the therapeutic plan are vasodilators. Vasodilators are most effective when used with a beta-adrenergic blocking agent to control the rapid heartbeat that often results from lowering peripheral resistance.

Table 15-12	Antihypertensive Drug Classes used in other Diseases					
COMPELLING INDICATION	DIURETIC	BETA BLOCKER	ANGIOTENSIN-CONVERTING ENZYME INHIBITOR	ALPHA RECEPTOR BLOCKER	CALCIUM CHANNEL BLOCKER	ALDOSTERONE ANTAGONIST
Heart failure	X	X	X	X	X	
Post MI	X	X	X			
High risk for CAD	X	X	X	X		
Diabetes	X	X	X	X	X	
Chronic kidney disease	X	X				
Recurrent stroke prevention	X	X				

Modified from National Heart, Lung, and Blood Institutes, National High Blood Pressure Education Program: *The Seventh Report of the Joint National Committee on the Prevention, Detection, Evaluation, and Treatment of High Blood Pressure,* Bethesda, MD, 2003, National Institutes of Health.
CAD, Coronary artery disease; *MI,* myocardial infarction.

There has been a lot of research on antihypertensive drugs in therapy in recent years; new drugs have entered the market and more research findings have been published. Some drugs are particularly helpful in certain conditions. Refer to Table 15-12 for drugs used in other diseases.

ADVERSE REACTIONS

Each category and each drug has many important adverse reactions. Hypokalemia and drowsiness are commonly seen, and many drugs produce impotence in men. Table 15-13 provides a list of the most common adverse reactions to the antihypertensive and diuretic drugs. For example, prazosin may cause severe syncope after the first dose, so the patient should take the first dose when someone else can be there. Potassium chloride (KCl) tablets may be irritating to the mouth and stomach if not taken with food. Antacids may help reduce this irritation.

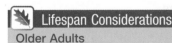

Lifespan Considerations
Older Adults

ANTIHYPERTENSIVES
- Geriatric patients are particularly likely to become light-headed and weak when taking these medications. The postural hypotension they experience places them at risk of falling when they rapidly change positions, such as getting up quickly from a chair or bed.
- The action of antihypertensive medications, especially beta blockers, plus other vascular changes in male hypertensive patients may cause impotence. These men may be reluctant to acknowledge they have this problem. Nurses should ask if men have trouble achieving or keeping an erection; a change in medication may help reduce this problem.

DRUG INTERACTIONS

Frequently a patient with high blood pressure has to take many different medicines because other medical problems exist. All of the antihypertensive drugs may have drug interactions. The nurse checks each drug the patient is taking; interactive effects that lower the blood pressure too much or make the blood pressure go even higher can occur.

Clinical Goldmine
Collecting Data

It is important to collect and record a good initial database (history, physical, and laboratory findings) to evaluate the progression of end-organ damage over the years.

❖ NURSING IMPLICATIONS AND PATIENT TEACHING

■ Assessment

Learn as much as possible about the health history of the patient. Although the cause for most high blood pressure is unknown, the health care provider will look for any disease that might also cause hypertension, such as Cushing disease, Addison disease, renal artery stenosis, coarctation of the aorta, or pheochromocytoma. The nurse will want to ask about whether the patient has other diseases, allergies, or medications that may affect antihypertensives and diuretics.

The number of drug side effects and problems that occur when hypertension is not treated effectively is high, and good record keeping is important in learning if the patient is getting well.

■ Diagnosis

Does the patient understand that high blood pressure medication may need to be taken for the rest of his or her life? Does the patient understand that to reduce

Table 15-13   Adverse Drug Effects of Antihypertensive and Diuretic Drugs

MEDICATION	SIDE EFFECTS	PRECAUTIONS
Diuretics		
Alpha-adrenergic blockers	"First-dose" syncope with prazosin; postural hypotension, weakness, palpitations, dizziness	Use cautiously in older adult patients because of hypotension.
Beta-adrenergic blockers	Bradycardia, insomnia, fatigue, sexual dysfunction, bizarre dreams, decreased HDL cholesterol	Not for use in patients with asthma, COPD, CHF, heart block, and sick sinus syndrome. Used with caution in patients with diabetes and peripheral vascular disease.
Central-acting adrenergic blockers	Drowsiness, fatigue, sexual dysfunction, dry mouth	Clonidine and guanabenz may produce rebound hypertension if abruptly stopped. Methyldopa may cause liver damage and a positive direct Coombs test.
Combined alpha- and beta-adrenergic blockers	Nausea, fatigue, dizziness, asthma, headache	Not for use in sick sinus syndrome or heart block; used with caution in CHF, bronchial asthma, COPD, and diabetes mellitus.
Loop diuretics	Same as for thiazides	Effective in chronic renal failure; caution with hypokalemia and hyperuricemia; may cause hyponatremia, especially in older adults.
Peripheral-acting adrenergic inhibitors	Sexual dysfunction, nasal congestion, postural hypotension, diarrhea, lethargy	Used very cautiously in older adult patients because of hypotension. Rauwolfia and reserpine are not to be given to patients with a history of mental depression.
Potassium-sparing agents	Hyperkalemia, sexual dysfunction, gynecomastia, mastodynia	Monitor fluid and electrolytes.
Thiazides and thiazide-related sulfonamides	Hypokalemia, hyperuricemia, glucose intolerance, hypercholesterolemia, sexual dysfunction	May be ineffective in renal failure; hypokalemia increases digitalis toxicity; hyperuricemia may precipitate acute gout.
Vasodilators		
Vasodilators	Headache, tachycardia, fluid retention	May produce angina in patients with coronary artery disease.
	Hydralazine may produce positive ANA	Lupuslike syndrome may occur with higher doses of hydralazine.
	Minoxidil may produce abnormal growth of hair, ascites (intraperitoneal pooling of large amount of fluid)	May cause or aggravate pleural and pericardial effusions.
Angiotensin-Converting Enzyme Inhibitors		
ACE inhibitors	Hyperkalemia, nonproductive cough (frequent)	Can cause neutropenia with autoimmune-collagen disorders. May cause proteinuria or reversible acute renal failure in patients with bilateral renal artery stenosis.
Calcium Channel Blocking Agents		
Calcium channel blockers	Headache, hypotension, nausea, dizziness, flushing, edema, constipation	Used with caution in patients with CHF or heart block; do not administer immediately after MI.

ACE, Angiotensin-converting enzyme; *ANA,* antinuclear antibody; *CHF,* congestive heart failure; *COPD,* chronic obstructive pulmonary disease; *HDL,* high-density lipoprotein; *MI,* myocardial infarction.

high blood pressure, lifestyle changes may be as important as medication? What factors does the patient have that will make therapy difficult?

■ Planning

Because there is no cure for high blood pressure, a lot of patient teaching and education is needed to help the patient understand what is happening and cooperate with successful treatment. Although taking the medication is important, it is also important to work on other things in the patient's life, such as removing risk factors and changing the diet.

■ Implementation

Many patients with hypertension do not feel sick, so they have a hard time being compliant with the treatment regimen. High blood pressure is a "silent disease" because it has no symptoms. Because patients may only have symptoms as a result of side effects from their medication, they may not want to take drugs. It is important to teach patients about what is really happening to them to help them understand their disease.

The high cost of antihypertensive drugs and the desire of patients to have control over their therapy lead many of them to explore the use of herbal medications to lower blood pressure. The Complementary and Alternative Therapies box describes some of the more common herbal products patients may use. Little standardized research has been done to discover whether herbal products are safe or effective.

Patients taking diuretics should avoid caffeinated beverages as the diuretic effect of caffeine plus their medications may cause them to become dehydrated.

Encourage patients to lose weight, lower sodium intake, avoid stress and emotional pressures, develop regular and reasonable exercise routines, and have hobbies or activities that make them feel good about themselves (improve self-esteem). Remind them that taking their medications is only a small part of the total treatment plan.

When taking loop or thiazide diuretics, the patient should eat or drink more potassium-rich foods such as citrus fruits; bananas; potatoes; dark, leafy vegetables; and nuts. If the patient is taking a potassium-sparing diuretics, he or she should avoid excessive quantities of these foods.

■ Evaluation

In addition to taking the patient's blood pressure, a good eye examination can tell if the patient's hypertension is well controlled. The blood vessels of the eye can be seen by looking through the pupil into the eye with an ophthalmoscope. By examining the fundus of the eye, it is possible to tell whether the blood pressure has been high, even if it is low when the patient is seen. Many parts of the body are damaged by high blood pressure: the heart, the lungs, the eyes, and the kidneys.

🔲 Complementary & Alternative Therapies

Hypertension

HERBAL PREPARATION	COMMENTS
Coleus	Potential interactions with anticoagulants, aspirin, NSAIDs, antiplatelet agents
Garlic	Potential interaction with anticoagulants, aspirin, NSAIDs, antiplatelet agents; may potentiate antihypertensives, antihyperlipidemics
Hawthorn	May interact with antidysrhythmics, antihypertensives, cardiac glycosides, ACE inhibitors, angiotensin II receptor blockers

Data from Krinsky DL, LaValle JB, Hawkins EB, et al: *Natural therapeutics pocket guide*, ed 2, Hudson, Ohio, 2003, Lexi-Comp, Inc.
ACE, Angiotensin-converting enzyme; *NSAIDs*, Nonsteroidal antiinflammatory drugs.

Ask if the patient has any complaints that might suggest problems in any of these areas (end-organ damage). Ask about side effects the antihypertensive medication might be producing. Men should always be asked about their sexual functioning, because impotence is often caused by these medications, and they may not share this information unless asked. They may not even realize sexual problems may be related to their medication.

■ Patient and Family Teaching

Tell the patient and family the following:
- The patient should take this medication exactly as ordered. If a dose is missed, it should be taken as soon as it is remembered, if it is within an hour or two of the scheduled time. If it is close to the next scheduled dose, the next dose should be taken at the regular time; the doses should not be doubled.
- The patient should take medication with a full glass of orange juice (unless not permitted by diet). Other potassium-rich foods should be eaten daily, including citrus foods (especially oranges and tomatoes), bananas, dried fruits, apricots, cantaloupe, watermelon, nuts, dried beans, beef, and fowl.
- The patient should know that taking the medication is only one part of the treatment plan. Getting rid of other risk factors is also important, such as losing weight (if overweight), lowering sodium intake, stopping smoking, increasing exercise, and avoiding extra stress and emotional pressures. The patient should avoid foods high in sodium, such as lunch meats, smoked meats, Chinese food, processed cheese, and snack foods. The patient should not salt food when cooking or add salt to food after it is cooked.
- Numerous side effects could occur from use of these drugs. The patient must notify the nurse, physician, or other health care provider of any new or uncomfortable symptoms that develop. Changing drugs

may be necessary. Good relationships among all those working to help the patient get better are important. It is very important for the patient to keep appointments and to want to come back for care.

- This medication must be kept out of the reach of children and others for whom it is not prescribed, because it is very dangerous for them. The patient should not leave it lying on night tables or low dressers where young children might take it accidentally.
- The goal of therapy is to help the patient feel as healthy as possible and to avoid any long-term problems. Many times there is not a cure and therapy may last a lifetime. Great improvements of many chronic diseases, including hypertension and obesity, have been made when the patient loses weight. It is important to keep taking the medicine, even when the patient feels well, and to keep seeing the health care provider regularly.
- Patients should wear a MedicAlert bracelet or necklace and carry a medical identification card saying they have high blood pressure and listing the drugs they are taking.

OTHER NONDIURETIC DRUGS USEFUL IN TREATING URINARY PROBLEMS

OVERVIEW

There are many problems that might produce urinary tract symptoms. Drugs used for these problems usually involve giving relief for symptoms. These include drugs used to treat urinary incontinence (wetting) and benign prostatic hyperplasia (BPH) and drugs for urinary tract analgesia (pain relief) and urinary tract infections.

ACTION AND USES

Drugs for Urinary Incontinence

Urinary incontinence is when patients wet themselves or leak urine, and this problem may have many causes. Medications used in treating this problem include some anticholinergics and antispasmodics, alpha-adrenergic agonists, estrogens, cholinergic agonists, and alpha-adrenergic antagonists. The anticholinergic agents stop contraction of the bladder and decrease the response of some of the bladder muscles. Antispasmodic drugs have a direct action on smooth muscle relaxation. Estrogen used either orally or vaginally may help restore urethral mucosa and increase vascularity, tone, and the ability of the urethral muscle to respond.

BENIGN PROSTATIC HYPERPLASIA

BPH is a noncancerous growth of the prostate gland frequently seen as men age; if this gland becomes large enough, it can cause voiding problems because the prostate puts pressure on the bladder and urinary sphincter. Drugs used in the management of BPH are the alpha$_1$-adrenergic receptor blockers (these have already been discussed for the treatment of hypertension). Tamsulosin (Flomax) is an alpha-adrenergic receptor blocker used only for the treatment of symptoms of BPH. Finasteride is also used for treatment of BPH. Use of these products either reduces the urgency to urinate or shrinks the prostate so that urine can pass more easily.

SHORT-TERM ANALGESIA

Phenazopyridine is a drug used to control pain in the urinary tract, usually from acute urinary tract infection. The agent may also be ordered following procedures on the urinary tract such as a cystoscopy or biopsy. This product is effective for only a couple of hours and so will require repeated administration.

❖ NURSING IMPLICATIONS AND PATIENT TEACHING

■ Assessment

Learn the history of the urinary problem to make certain the patient's symptoms are recorded correctly. The patient may be nervous about discussing these problems.

■ Diagnosis

Find out the reason why the medication is being given. Are the symptoms because of another problem, or do they represent the major problem? (Is there other gynecologic or genitourinary disease present?) Read any medical records kept by the patient about urinary incontinence or voiding problems. This may be helpful in learning the cause of the symptoms.

■ Planning

Teach the patient about what has caused the problem and how the medication will help.

■ Implementation

Sometimes the patient is asked to keep a bladder diary. If so, explain clearly how to keep the records about wetting accidents and why. Give the patient a lot of support so they will be compliant.

Drug action and uses, adverse effects, drug interactions, and important patient teaching points are given in Table 15-14.

■ Evaluation

All of these medications should reduce symptoms. Explain to patients how they will know when the medication is working. For medications related to BPH, explain that treatment may be required for weeks or months before symptoms go away.

Table 15-14 Miscellaneous Nondiuretic Drugs Used to Treat Urinary Problems

MEDICATION	ACTION AND USES	ADVERSE EFFECTS	DRUG INTERACTIONS	NURSING IMPLICATIONS AND PATIENT TEACHING
Drugs for Urinary Incontinence				
Anticholinergics/Antispasmodics				
flavoxate (Urispas)	Antispasmodic action for dysuria, nocturia, urgency, suprapubic pain, frequency, incontinence caused by detrusor instability, and hyperreflexia	Headache, confusion, nervousness, nausea, vomiting	Enhances anticholinergic effects of other anticholinergic drugs	Discuss anticholinergic effects with older patients, as they may pose a problem.
oxybutynin chloride (Ditropan)	Used to relieve symptoms associated with detrusor instability, hyperreflexia, or involuntary bladder contractions	Drowsiness, dry mouth, blurred vision, constipation; may aggravate symptoms of heart disease, hyperthyroidism, GI problems	May increase digoxin serum concentrations; may decrease action of haloperidol and enhance development of tardive dyskinesia (repeated involuntary muscle movements); avoid alcohol	Requires careful patient teaching concerning response and side effects; monitor clinical effectiveness through use of a bladder diary documenting voiding activity.
propantheline (Pro-Banthine)	Treats involuntary ureteral and bladder contractions by competitively blocking action of acetylcholine at postganglionic parasympathetic receptor sites	Dry mouth, constipation, urinary retention	Increases effect of narcotic analgesics, class I antidysrhythmics, antihistamines, phenothiazines, TCAs, corticosteroids, CNS depressants, beta blockers, amoxapine	Side effects more often seen and may cause problems in older patients.
tolterodine (Detrol)	For urinary frequency, urgency, and urge incontinence caused by bladder overactivity	Less dry mouth than with oxybutynin; dyspepsia, headache, constipation, dry eyes	None noted	Tolterodine should be avoided by patients with glaucoma, ulcerative colitis, megacolon, GI or urinary obstruction; should be used with care by individuals with BPH.
Cholinergic Agonist				
bethanechol chloride	Used in nonobstructive urinary retention	Hypotension, dizziness, flushing, sweating	With other cholinergics, additive cholinergic effects and toxicity may occur	Dosage highly individualized.

Continued

Table 15-14   **Miscellaneous Nondiuretic Drugs Used to Treat Urinary Problems—cont'd**

MEDICATION	ACTION AND USES	ADVERSE EFFECTS	DRUG INTERACTIONS	NURSING IMPLICATIONS AND PATIENT TEACHING
Drugs for Benign Prostatic Hyperplasia				
Alpha-Adrenergic Antagonists				
finasteride (Proscar)	Treats symptoms of BPH	Impotence, decreased libido, decreased volume of ejaculate, breast tenderness and enlargement, hypersensitivity reactions, including lip swelling and skin rash	None noted	May be taken with or without food; 6-12 mo of therapy may be required to assess response.
tamsulosin (Flomax)	Treats symptoms of BPH by selective inhibition of alpha$_1$A receptors	Postural hypotension, dizziness, somnolence, rhinitis, diarrhea, abnormal ejaculation	Potentiates other alpha-adrenergic blocking agents	Take at the same time every day, approximately ½ hr after eating; may take 2-4 wk before response is seen.
terazosin	Treats hypertension and provides superior action in treating BPH	Angina, blurred vision, constipation, diarrhea, orthostatic hypotension, syncope May have first-dose response of acute postural hypotension.	May reduce antihypertensive effects if given with NSAIDs. Antihypertensive effects of other drugs may result in acute postural hypotension.	Monitor for exaggerated hypotensive effects, particularly in geriatric patients or those with renal impairment.
Drug for Urinary Tract Analgesia				
Phenazopyridine (Pyridium)	Symptomatic relief of pain, burning, urgency, frequency associated with UTI	Headaches, rash, vertigo, GI disturbance, anaphylactic (shock)-like reactions	None noted	Stains the urine orange or red and may stain fabrics; notify doctor if jaundice (yellow color of skin or eyes) develops; available OTC.

BPH, Benign prostatic hypertrophy; *CNS,* central nervous system; *GI,* gastrointestinal; *NSAID,* nonsteroidal antiinflammatory drug; *OTC,* over the counter; *TCA,* tricyclic antidepressant; *UTI,* urinary tract infection.

■ Patient and Family Teaching

Tell the patient and family the following:

- The patient and family should learn the causes of urinary incontinence or BPH.
- The embarrassment some patients feel can be eased by talking about how common these problems are for patients.
- The patient should be given instructions about taking the medication with food or after meals.
- Patients may be asked to keep records to help show the results of treatment; these should be reviewed at each patient visit.
- The patient who is taking medication for urinary pain should know that the drug will change the color of urine. Patients should return for further treatment if symptoms return after they have taken all the medication.

FLUID AND ELECTROLYTES

OVERVIEW

Strong pumping of the heart, good circulation through the vessels, and the full removal of by-products through the urinary system are all needed to keep the body's fluid and electrolyte balance. Lack of body fluid may be due to inadequate intake, excess loss, or both. This imbalance may be treated by administration of fluids and electrolyte mixtures. The kidneys play the major role in how much fluid is present in the body and the number and types of electrolytes, acids, and bases. The kidneys work to make adjustments in fluid and electrolytes all the time. If the kidneys do not work properly, major changes may occur in fluids and electrolytes that may affect the body's ability to work.

ACTION AND USES

Patients taking diuretics should avoid caffeinated beverages as the diuretic effect of caffeine plus their medications may cause them to become dehydrated. There are two types of IV replacement fluids: (1) Crystalloid mixtures made of **fluid and electrolyte mixtures** that may be composed of water and calories in the form of carbohydrates, or with minerals and electrolytes such as sodium, potassium, chloride, calcium, and phosphorus. These solutions travel in the blood and then enter cells and tissue. As they replace missing fluid or electrolytes they help the kidneys so urine is produced. (2) Colloids such as plasma or volume expanders. These products contain large molecules or proteins that remain suspended in the blood and do not cross cell membranes but act to draw water molecules from the cells and tissues into the blood vessels as they increase osmotic pressure.

Many fluid and electrolyte solutions are given when oral food intake has been stopped or to prevent **dehydration** (loss of a large amount of water from the body tissues, along with loss of electrolytes), especially in patients with diarrhea. Causes of dehydration include vomiting, bowel obstruction (which causes a pooling of fluid and electrolytes), diarrhea, and fever (which increases the use of fluid and electrolytes). The body attempts to adjust to the reduced circulating volume by pulling in first extracellular fluid and then intracellular fluid. This causes an imbalance of both fluid and electrolytes that must be corrected.

Fluid and electrolytes may be given either orally or parenterally to prevent dehydration when oral intake is briefly halted and to replace moderate losses of fluids and electrolytes (Table 15-15 and Box 15-1).

The healthy body is able to make constant changes in kidney function, breathing, and heart rate, to keep it healthy. When the body is seriously ill, these balancing tasks do not occur well. Not only does the body need fluid, but a careful balance between acid and base must be maintained when patients are very ill. The amount of acid and base or alkalinity in the body is measured by its pH. Blood or body fluids that measure above 7.0 are called *basic* or *alkaline*. Those that measure below 7.0 are called *acidic*. The normal body pH is 7.35 to 7.45—a very narrow range. Movement either higher or lower than this pH range poses a threat to life. If the body pH is abnormally high or low, the cause must be identified and treated as soon as possible through use of IV fluids. If it is not restored to the normal range, the body will go into acidosis with

Table 15-15	Fluid and Electrolytes for Oral Administration
PRODUCT	**COMMENTS AND DOSAGE**
Oral Electrolyte Solutions	
Pedialyte	Dosage should be based on water requirements calculated on the basis of total body surface area for infants and young children. A general guide uses 1500 mL/m2 for maintenance during illness and 2400 mL/m2 for maintenance and replacement of mild to moderate fluid losses (as in diarrhea or vomiting). *Replacement in mild to moderate fluid losses: Children 5-10 years of age:* 1-2 quarts/day *Older children and adults:* 2-3 quarts/day
Salt Substitutes	
Adolph's salt substitute Morton salt substitute Neocurtasal NoSalt Nu-Salt	OTC preparations that can be used in both cooked and uncooked foods to make food more palatable for patients with sodium restrictions. These potassium chloride preparations come in a salt shaker dispenser and are used in amounts slightly less than normal amounts of NaCl. Note: Contraindicated in patients with severe kidney disease or oliguria. Long-term use may require iodine supplements in some patients.
sodium bicarbonate	Used as gastric, systemic, and urinary alkalinizer. May relieve symptoms of occasional overeating and indigestion. Usual adult dose 325 mg to 2 g 2-4 times daily. Daily maximum intake should not exceed 16 g.

NaCl, Sodium chloride; *OTC,* over the counter.

severe CNS depression or coma, or into CNS stimulation and convulsions with alkalosis. Neither extreme will allow the patient to live. If the patient is acidotic, sodium bicarbonate may be added to the fluid to help the patient achieve homeostasis, or the right balance. If the patient is alkalotic, ammonium chloride or sodium chloride with KCl may be added to fluids. So electrolytes are very important in keeping this balance.

Electrolytes are small, inorganic molecules with either a positive or negative charge. Positive charged molecules are called *cations;* negatively charged molecules are called *anions.* Laboratory testing will help determine what electrolytes need to be given and how much. Electrolyte solutions are especially useful in managing dehydration in infants caused by diarrhea.

Box 15-1	Fluid and Electrolytes for Parenteral Administration

- Products are available in a variety of concentrations, volumes, and combinations.
- See the physician or other health care provider's order and the package insert.

AMINO ACIDS
- Amino acid substrates with electrolytes in a variety of combinations.

CARBOHYDRATES
- Dextrose in water with 2.5% to 70% concentrations
- 5% or 10% alcohol in 5% dextrose infusions
- 10% fructose in water
- 10% invert sugar in water

ELECTROLYTES
- 0.2% to 5% sodium chloride solutions
- Potassium chloride or potassium acetate for injection
- Calcium chloride for injection
- Calcium gluconate for injection
- Calcium gluceptate for injection
- Calcium products—combined
- Magnesium sulfate or magnesium chloride for injection
- Sodium bicarbonate for injection
- Sodium lactate for injection
- Sodium acetate for injection
- Tromethamine for slow infusion
- Sodium phosphate for injection
- Potassium phosphate for injection
- Ammonium chloride for injection

TRACE METALS (FOR SLOW INFUSION)
- Zinc, copper, manganese, molybdenum, chromium, selenium, and iodine

Potassium is the major cation inside the cell. The normal range of potassium in the body is very small and even minor excess (hyperkalemia) or loss (hypokalemia) may cause serious problems. KCl solutions are given to correct hypokalemia. Sodium is the major electrolyte in the extracellular fluid. If there is an excess of sodium (hypernatremia) in the blood because it is not removed by the kidneys, IV fluids such as 5% dextrose with water may be given. Some diuretics also help remove sodium through the kidneys. If there is a lack of sodium (hyponatremia), it may be treated with solutions that include sodium chloride.

See Box 15-1 for a listing of the most common colloid and crystalloid products.

❖ NURSING IMPLICATIONS AND PATIENT TEACHING

Patients who are dehydrated need fluids. Water alone is often not adequate. Signs of dehydration include weight loss, dry skin, lack of sweat, dry mucous membranes, decreased urinary output, hypotension, tachycardia, and increased respirations. In infants, dehydration may also include sunken fontanelles and loss of skin turgor (strength and mass). Fluid and electrolytes are also required in the comatose or acutely ill patient who is unable to take oral substances for a long time.

Oral fluids are contraindicated when the patient has severe or continuing diarrhea or other major fluid loss that requires IV replacement or has vomiting that cannot be stopped. They should not be used in patients with intestinal obstruction or bowel perforation (opening), decreased renal function, or when the homeostatic mechanism of the body is damaged. IV fluids with replacement electrolytes are required.

The prescribed amount of fluid and electrolytes should be ordered by the health care provider and should not be exceeded. If the patient is still thirsty after taking the recommended dose, extra fluids in the form of water or other fluids that do not contain electrolytes might be ordered.

 Clinical Goldmine

Electrolyte Deficiency

Electrolyte deficiency may result if the patient increases intake of liquids with a low mineral content (such as drinking distilled water after vigorous exercise and sweating).

Get Ready for the NCLEX® Examination!

Key Points

- The major classes of cardiovascular medications are antianginals, peripheral vasodilators, antidysrhythmics, antihyperlipidemics, antihypertensives, cardiotonics, and diuretics. (Other miscellaneous drugs affecting the urinary tract are also included in the last section.)
- Each major class deals with an important part of the circulatory and renal systems.
- Cardiovascular medications are commonly used by patients, and the nurse has an important teaching job in helping the patient understand the proper storage and use of medications.

- In addition, a thorough understanding of the anatomy and physiology of the heart is important, because this will help in understanding both the cardiovascular problem and the action of the various medications.
- Electrolytes are given in the event that oral food intake has been suspended or to treat or prevent dehydration and electrolyte loss.

Additional Learning Resources

SG Go to the Study Guide for additional learning activities to help master this chapter content.

Get Ready for the NCLEX® Examination!—cont'd

evolve Go to the Evolve website (http://evolve.elsevier.com/Edmunds/ LPN/) for additional online resources.

Review Questions for the NCLEX® Examination

1. The patient is prescribed transmucosal nitroglycerin tablets. These tablets should be:
   1. chewed
   2. swallowed
   3. placed on the tongue
   4. placed inside the cheek

2. The patient has a history of acute angina. What is the most accurate information that he should be taught regarding how often he can take his nitroglycerin tablets?
   1. take 1 pill when pain is experienced; if there is no relief, take a second pill after 3-5 minutes; if pain is not relieved within 3 minutes, a third pill may be taken
   2. take 1 pill when pain is experienced; if there is no relief, take 2 pills after 3-5 minutes; if pain is not relieved within 3 minutes, 3 pills may be taken
   3. take 2 pills when pain is experienced; if there is no relief, take another pill after 3-5 minutes; if pain is not relieved with 3 minutes, another pill may be taken
   4. take 2 pills when pain is experienced; if there is no relief, take 2 more pills after 3-5 minutes; if pain is not relieved with 3 minutes, 2 more pills may be taken

3. The patient has been prescribed niacin. The nurse anticipates that the patient will have the most difficulty adjusting to the side effect of:
   1. hyperuricemia
   2. glucose tolerance
   3. flushing
   4. constipation

4. The patient has been placed on a antihyperlipidemic medication. The most appropriate time for him to take other medication while he is still ordered the antihyperlipidemic drug is:
   1. 4 hours before or 3-6 hours after taking the antihyperlipidemic drug
   2. 3 hours before or 2-4 hours after taking the antihyperlipidemic drug
   3. 2 hours before or 1-3 hours after taking the antihyperlipidemic drug
   4. 1 hour before or 4-6 hours after taking the antihyperlipidemic drug

5. The nurse is due to administer a dose of a cardiotonic drug. The highest priority nursing intervention prior to administration should be:
   1. count the radial pulse for 60 seconds
   2. assess the respiratory rate
   3. count the apical pulse for 60 seconds
   4. assess the temperature

Case Study

A 50-year-old black man comes to the clinic with a 1-week history of occipital headache that he describes as "a constant ache in the back of my head." The 650-mg Tylenol that he has taken regularly four to five times daily over the past week often has not cured his headache. Approximately 7 months ago, the patient was told that his blood pressure was "up" during a yearly employment physical. He has a history of asthma, gout, and angina. His father and sister have high blood pressure. His diet is high in fat and salt.

Physical examination: Blood pressure: right arm sitting, 160/105 mm Hg; left arm sitting, 162/104 mm Hg. The heart is not enlarged; there are no murmurs or abnormal rhythms. Apical pulse, 84 beats/min and regular.

1. Assuming the patient's blood pressure remained at the same level after two more blood pressure checks, what things specific to this patient should be considered before he is placed on antihypertensive medications?
2. What class of medication would initially most likely be of greatest help in controlling this patient's blood pressure with the fewest adverse reactions?
   a. Thiazide or loop diuretic
   b. Beta blocker
   c. Alpha blocker
   d. Centrally-acting agent
   e. Adrenergic neuron blocking agent
   f. Direct-acting vasodilating agent
   g. Angiotensin-converting enzyme inhibitor
   h. Calcium channel blocker
3. Which of the drugs listed in question 2 would not be indicated?
4. The physician orders hydrochlorothiazide 12.5 mg daily. What would the nurse tell the patient about this drug?
5. Assuming the drug as ordered was ineffective in reducing the patient's blood pressure after 4 weeks, what would be the next thing to be done to achieve adequate control of the blood pressure?

Drug Calculation Review

1. Procainamide (Pronestyl) IV bolus of 0.1 g has been ordered by the physician for a patient with frequent premature ventricular contractions. The vial is labeled 200 mg/mL. How many milliliters should the nurse prepare for this bolus?
2. Order: Proprananol (Indera)l 30 mg by mouth 4 times per day. Supply: Inderal 20 mg per tablet.
   Question: How many tablets of Inderal should be given with each dose?
3. Order: Furosemide (Lasix) 60 mg by gastrostomy tube daily. Supply: Lasix 20 mg/5 mL.
   Question: How many milliliters of Lasix should be given with each dose?

Get Ready for the NCLEX® Examination!—cont'd

Critical Thinking Questions

1. Ms. Henson, age 70, was admitted to the hospital yesterday with acute angina. She is a heavy smoker and says that most evenings she drinks either wine or beer with her dinner and coffee with dessert every night. Her physician prescribes sublingual nitroglycerin for anginal pain.
   a. Describe major points to teach this patient, especially regarding medication storage and administration and the results she may expect.
   b. Draw up a plan of action for teaching Ms. Henson.
   c. What should she do if she has taken three nitroglycerin tablets and continues to have pain.

2. Point out some key distinctions between class I, class II, class III, and class IV antidysrhythmics. Consult Table 15-4 if more information is required.

3. Explain the need for careful ECG monitoring of patients taking antidysrhythmic medications. What are the things the patient should know about every drug they take?

4. Identify nursing strategies and patient teaching points associated with bile acid sequestrants and antihyperlipidemic agents.
   a. Describe how to make these medications more palatable,
   b. Discuss methods for reducing unpleasant side effects,
   c. Discuss need for long-term medication and diet therapy
   d. Emphasize need for regular medical follow-up.

5. Develop a generalized, introductory patient teaching plan for the patient with recently diagnosed hypertension focusing on lifestyle modifications.
   a. Outline several short lessons to avoid overwhelming the patient with information.
   b. Stress what the patient can do, rather than focusing only on what the patient should not do.

6. Describe the signs and symptoms of heart failure. Why might some dysrhythmias cause heart failure?

7. Create a teaching plan for the patient taking digoxin or a drug that slows the patients pulse. Be sure to include the following elements:
   a. why the drug is needed,
   b. why it is important to take the drug regularly,
   c. what adverse effects to watch out for,
   d. how to take a radial pulse,
   e. what to do if the radial pulse is lower than 60 beats/min.

8. Using the information from Question 7, what types of nursing interventions might be used when a patient has signs and symptoms of digitalis toxicity.

9. Miss Green comes in for treatment of a urinary tract infection. She is in great pain, and the nurse practitioner orders phenazopyridine (Pyridium). What information does Miss Green need to know when she takes this product?

10. When getting a nursing history from a patient taking a newly prescribed diuretic, what information would be a priority? To obtain this information, what questions would be asked?

11. Referring to the data obtained in Question 10, what information would be emphasized in a teaching plan for this patient?

12. The nurse is asked to monitor a new patient, Ms. Falk, for dehydration. Review the signs and symptoms of dehydration. When is dehydration most likely to occur?

13. Ms. Falk has been told she needs fluid and electrolyte supplementation. Explain to her the reasons for such therapy and how it will help her.

Central and Peripheral Nervous System Medications

Objectives

1. Explain the physiologic processes of the central and peripheral nervous systems.
2. Identify the major classes of drugs that affect the central nervous system (CNS).
3. List different actions of antimigraine products.
4. Explain the major actions of drugs used to treat disorders of the CNS.
5. Identify the role of psychotropic drugs in psychotherapeutic intervention.
6. Compare and contrast different categories of medications used to treat mood disorders.
7. Evaluate medications used to help promote sleep.

Key Terms

acetylcholine (ăs-ě-tǐl-KŌ-lēn, p. 252)
adrenergic blocking agents (ăd-rěn-ĚRJ-ǐk, p. 253)
adrenergic fibers (ăd-rěn-ĚRJ-ǐk, p. 252)
anticholinergics (ăn-tǐ-kō-lǐn-ĚRJ-ǐks, p. 253)
autonomic (ŏ-tō-NŎM-ǐk, p. 252)
barbiturates (bär-BǏ-chŭ-rets, p. 259)
catecholamines (kăt-ě-KŌ-lǎ-mēnz, p. 253)
central nervous system (CNS) (SĚN-trŭl NŬR-vŭs SǏS-těm, p. 251)
cholinergic drugs (kō-lǐn-ĚRJ-ǐk, p. 253)
cholinergic fibers (kō-lǐn-ĚRJ-ǐk, p. 252)
hypnotic agent (hǐp-NŎT-ǐk, p. 293)
idiopathic (ǐd-ē-ō-PĂTH-ǐk, p. 257)
initial insomnia (ǐn-ĬSH-ǎl ǐn-SŎM-nē-ǎ, p. 293)

intermittent insomnia (ǐn-těr-MǏT-ěntǐn-SŎM-nē-ǎ, p. 293)
neurotransmitters (nŭr-ō-TRĂNS-mǐt-ěrz, p. 252)
norepinephrine (NŌR-ěp-ǐn-ĚF-rěn, p. 252)
Parkinson disease (PĂR-kǐn-sěnz dǐ-ZĚZ, p. 267)
parasympathetic (p. 252)
peripheral nervous system (PNS) (pě-RǏF-ěr-ǎ l, p. 252)
receptor (rē-SĚP-tŏr, p. 253)
sedative agent (SĚD-ǎ -tǐv, p. 293)
seizures (SĚ-zhŭ rz, p. 257)
somatic (sō-MĂT-ǐc, p. 252)
status epilepticus (STĂT-ŭsě p-ǐ-LĚP-tǐ-kŭ s, p. 260)
sympathetic (p. 252)
terminal insomnia (TŬR-mǐn-ǎl ǐn-SŎM-nē-ǎ, p. 293)

OVERVIEW

This chapter has six sections discussing drugs that act on various parts of the central nervous system (CNS) and the peripheral nervous system (PNS). Although many drugs are used in treating CNS diseases, the principles of drug usage, actions of the medications, and adverse reactions are very similar. The nurse will benefit from learning how these drugs are the same and how they are different for the various categories of drugs. Although narcotic and nonnarcotic analgesics are also CNS drugs, they will be discussed in Chapter 17.

The first section of this chapter explores antimigraine agents. The second section covers the medications used to treat various types of seizures. The third section discusses drugs for vertigo (feeling of dizziness or spinning), and the fourth section presents drugs used to treat Parkinson disease. The fifth section introduces all the psychotropic drugs and includes subsections dealing specifically with medications used to treat anxiety, depression, and psychosis. Lithium, a unique antimanic medication, is covered in this section. The sixth section discusses sedative-hypnotics and their use in anxiety and sleep disorders.

NERVOUS SYSTEM

The major structures of the nervous system include the brain, spinal cord, nerves, and sensory receptors (Figure 16-1). The nervous system regulates and coordinates the body's activities (including the senses), controls movement, and coordinates physiologic and intellectual functions.

The nervous system has two divisions, the central and the peripheral. The **central nervous system (CNS)**, made up of the brain and the spinal cord, is located within the cranial cavity of the skull and the vertebral

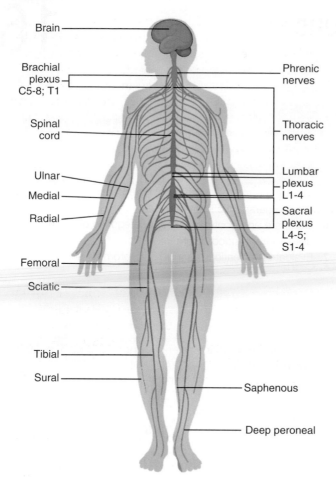

Brain

Brachial
plexus
C5-8; T1

Spinal
cord

Ulnar

Medial

Radial

Femoral

Sciatic

Tibial

Sural

Phrenic
nerves

Thoracic
nerves

Lumbar
plexus
L1-4

Sacral
plexus
L4-5;
S1-4

Saphenous

Deep peroneal

FIGURE 16-1 Central nervous system. *C,* Cervical; *L,* lumbar; *S,* spinal; *T,* thoracic.

canal of the spinal column. The **peripheral nervous system (PNS)** includes all nervous structures (ganglia and nerves) that lie outside the cranial cavity and the vertebral canal. These include the cranial and spinal nerves and the **sympathetic** division of the **autonomic** nervous system.

Pathologic conditions in the brain may produce either local or general symptoms; abnormalities in the peripheral system usually cause only local symptoms. Because the nerve and muscle systems are mixed together so closely, it is often difficult to tell if disease lies within the nerves or the structures activated by the nerves.

Although the drugs covered in this chapter focus on the actions of the CNS, or those actions controlled by the brain and spinal cord, many of these agents act through the PNS. The PNS produces changes or activity in the body through the nerves and chemicals of the motor nervous system and the autonomic nervous system as they carry out directions from the CNS.

Drugs act on the CNS and peripheral nerves by sending or transmitting information from the brain through chemical messengers or **neurotransmitters.** The neurotransmitter chemical is released at the end

of one neuron and passes across a small gap (the synapse) to activate the next neuron in the chain. At the end of the nerve chain, it stimulates an organ, smooth muscle, or gland to produce a physiologic response.

In the PNS, nerves of the **somatic** nervous system have voluntary control over skeletal muscle. Nerves of the autonomic nervous system provide involuntary control over organs and tissues of the heart muscles, and over smooth muscles and glands affecting the salivary glands and digestive tract, eyes, respiratory tract, and reproductive tracts. The action of the autonomic nervous system is very important to understanding the action of key drugs that act on this system.

The autonomic system works through two subdivisions—the sympathetic nervous system and the **parasympathetic** nervous system. These two systems work together in directing how most organs and glands work. The sympathetic system helps the body prepare for stressful situations by producing chemicals that will induce the "fight or flight" response. The parasympathetic nervous system provides the basic, routine maintenance of the body actions and has been called the "rest-and-digest response".

The nervous system is made up of small cells called *neurons.* The cells might be thought of as people standing in line passing a message to each other to do something. Instead of one person telling the next person the message, in the nervous system, a neurotransmitter chemical is released by the neuron which crosses the space or synapse between the two messengers (neurons) and is received by the receptor neuron on the other side. Then that neuron messenger turns to the next neuron cell to send the message forward until the final message is received, perhaps to affect skeletal muscle that will move the hand.

There are a variety of neuron transmitters that carry these messages. The two major neurotransmitters in the body are **norepinephrine,** which acts on the sympathetic nerves, and **acetylcholine,** which acts on the parasympathetic nerves. There are several other important neurotransmitters, especially in the brain. Nerve fibers that release norepinephrine are called **adrenergic fibers.** Nerve fibers that release acetylcholine are called **cholinergic fibers.** Most organs in the body are influenced by both types of fibers, which have opposite effects. For example, adrenergic activity speeds up the heart rate, and cholinergic activity slows it down. It is possible to compare this system to a car that is influenced by an accelerator and a brake. It is very important to understand these concepts because many drugs look or act like neurotransmitters and they act to help or block the action of neurotransmitters.

There are several names for the types of drugs that act on the nervous system. Because autonomic drugs either block or stimulate either the sympathetic or parasympathetic nervous systems, these autonomic drugs are classified based on their actions. These drugs have been called by several different names as, over time, research reveals more information about them.

- Drugs that stimulate the sympathetic nervous system. Drugs that produce effects in the body similar to those produced by norepinephrine are called adrenergic receptor agonists, or *sympathomimetic drugs*. These drugs are also referred to as **catecholamines**. There are three naturally occurring catecholamines in the body: norepinephrine, which is secreted from nerve terminals; epinephrine, which is secreted from the adrenal medulla; and dopamine, which is found at selected sites within the brain, kidneys, and gastrointestinal (GI) tract. These chemicals produce the flight-or-fight response.
- Drugs that stimulate the parasympathetic nervous system. Those drugs whose action is similar to acetylcholine are called **cholinergic drugs**, acetylcholine receptor agonists, or *parasympathomimetic drugs.* These drugs produce the rest-and-digest response.
- Drugs that block the actions of the parasympathetic nervous system. Agents that block the release of acetylcholine and inhibit cholinergic activity are called **anticholinergics**, acetylcholine receptor antagonists, or cholinergic blockers. The actions of these drugs are the opposite of those of the parasympathomimetics.
- Drugs that block the sympathetic nervous system. Agents that block the release of epinephrine and norepinephrine and inhibit the adrenergic system are called **adrenergic blocking agents** or adrenergic receptorantagonists. The actions of these drugs have actions opposite to those of the sympathomimetics.

These basic terms are used throughout this chapter. Remembering these terms and definitions will help in understanding drug actions.

When neurotransmitters release their chemicals, the chemicals are targeted to act at certain parts of the body. Each neurotransmitter has a certain chemical shape (like a key), which produces an action only when it "fits into" a specific **receptor** (lock) for that chemical.

Acetylcholine (cholinergic) receptors are classified as either muscarinic (which stimulate smooth muscle and gland secretions and decrease the heart rate and force of heart contraction) or nicotinic (which stimulate smooth muscle and gland secretions). Norepinephrine (adrenergic) receptors are identified as alpha 1 (provides for constriction of blood vessels and dilation of pupils); alpha 2 (blocks norepinephrine release); beta 1 (increases heart rate and force of contraction and release of renin); and beta 2 (blocks smooth muscle action). Note that when stimulated, alpha receptors often have the opposite effect of beta receptors on the heart, blood vessels, GI tract, or eye muscles. The text often refers to a medication as having *alpha* or *beta* properties. For example, some medications are called *beta blockers* because of their selective action in blocking only the beta-adrenergic effects in the body.

Many of the drugs discussed in the following sections act on more than one type of receptor. Each agent acts differently, making it possible for certain drugs to be given for specific actions without many adverse reactions. It should be clear that if dosages are exceeded, many receptors may be overly stimulated, causing widespread and serious effects. Thus accuracy in giving the right amount of drug and at the proper time is very important in giving these drugs safely.

SYMPATHOMIMETIC DRUGS

Adrenergic agonists or sympathomimetic drugs produce chemicals involved in the fight-or-flight syndrome and have many of the same effects as the anticholinergics. Some of the drugs have been developed so that they act specifically on either the alpha or beta subreceptors. This makes their actions more focused and predictable.

The effects of these drugs depend on which adrenergic subreceptors are stimulated. Some act very selectively, for example, on drying secretions in the nose. Other drugs act primarily on the heart or to help bronchodilation in the lungs. Thus these drugs may have specific uses prior to surgery, with specific heart problems, or asthma. Other drugs may stimulate more than one type of adrenergic receptor and so are considered nonselective. Thus product information may say that drugs act on both beta 1 and beta 2 receptors or both alpha 1 and beta 2 receptors. This should help the nurse anticipate what these drug actions might be.

Because of the variability in drug actions, many of these drugs are discussed in other relevant chapters in the book. Only a few of the most common sympathomimetics are listed in Table 16-1, along with their receptors.

ADRENERGIC AGONISTS OR BLOCKERS

The actions of the sympathetic nervous system are blocked by adrenergic blocker medications. These agents are common and are used in the treatment of hypertension. The actions of adrenergic blockers are quite specific and this makes them very useful. They are used primarily in blocking the effect on beta 1 receptors only present in the heart, or blocking receptors in vascular smooth muscle in small arteries, causing vasodilation and reducing blood pressure. Other beta blockers are nonselective so they block both beta 1 and beta 2 receptors. These drugs usually have more side effects. A list of these drugs and their primary receptor subtype is in Table 16-1. A more complete

Table 16-1 Selected Sympathomimetics and Adrenergic Drugs

DRUG	TRADE NAME	RECEPTOR SUBTYPES	USE
Sympathomimetics			
Albuterol	Proventil, Ventolin	Beta 2	Asthma treatment
dobutamine	Dobutrex	Beta 1	Heart stimulant
dopamine	Intropin	Alpha 1 and beta 1	Treatment of shock
epinephrine ★	Adrenalin, Primatene	Alpha and beta	Comes in variety of forms to treat asthma, shock, cardiac arrest
isoproterenol	Isuprel	Beta 1 and beta 2	Comes in variety of forms to treat heart failure, asthma, dysrhythmias
metaproterenol	Alupent	Beta 2	Used to treat asthma attacks and maintenance
metaraminol	Aramine	Alpha 1 and beta 1	Used to treat shock
norepinephrine	Levarterenol, Levophed	Alpha 1 and beta 1	Used to treat shock
oxymetazoline	Afrin	Alpha	Topical OTC product to treat nasal congestion
phenylephrine	Neo-Synephrine	Alpha	Topical OTC product to treat nasal congestion
pseudoephedrine	Sudafed	Alpha and beta	Topical OTC product to treat nasal congestion
ritodrine	Yutopar	Beta 2	Slow uterine contractions and reduce risk of abortion
salmeterol	Serevent	Beta 2	Used to treat nasal congestion and asthma
terbutaline	Brethine	Beta 2	Used to treat asthma
Adrenergic Blockers			
acebutolol	Sectral	Beta 1	Used for treating dysrhythmias, angina, hypertension
atenolol	Tenormin	Beta 1	Used for treating hypertension and angina
carteolol	Cartrol	Beta 1 and beta 2	Used in treatment of glaucoma and hypertension
carvedilol	Coreg	Alpha 1, beta 1, and beta 2	Used in treating hypertension
doxazosin	Cardura	Apha 1	Used in treating hypertension
esmolol	Brevibloc	Beta 1	Used in treating hypertension
metoprolol	Lopressor	Beta 1	Hypertension, heart failure, MI
nadolol	Corgard	Beta 1 and beta 2	Used in treating hypertension
phentolamine	Regitine	Alpha	Used in severe hypertension
prazosin	Minipress	Alpha 1	Used in treating hypertension
propranolol ★	Inderal	Beta 1 and beta2	Used in dysrhythmias, angina, hypertension, treatment of migraines
sotalol	Betapace	Beta 1 and beta 2	Used in dysrhythmias
terazosin	Hytrin	Alpha 1	Used in treating hypertension
timolol	Blocadren, Timoptic	Beta 1 and beta 2	Used in treating angina, hypertension, glaucoma

MI, Myocardial infarction; OTC, over the counter.
★ Indicates "Must-Know Drugs," or the 35 drugs most prescribers use.

discussion of these drugs and their uses in hypertension is found in Chapter 15.

PARASYMPATHETIC DRUGS

Parasympathomimetic drugs that produce the rest-and-digest responses act like the parasympathetic chemicals in the body. The action of these drugs is difficult to limit to a small part of the body and they have many adverse effects. Thus there are only a small number of these drugs and they are used carefully for specific neurologic problems. For example, bethanechol (Urecholine) is a direct-acting agonist and neostigmine (Prostigmin) is a reversible cholinesterase inhibitor. Both are used to help contract the muscles in the ureters or bladder when treating for urinary retention. Physostigmine (Antilirium) and pilocarpine (Isopto Carpine) are commonly used to treat glaucoma by reducing intraocular pressure. Pyridostigmine (Mestinon) is a drug used only for the treatment of myasthenia gravis, a relatively uncommon neurologic problem.

ANTICHOLINERGIC DRUGS

Anticholinergic drugs mimic the fight-or-flight response. These drugs are commonly used for their autonomic function in the treatment of many respiratory and GI disorders. The drugs increase heart rate, dilate pupils, dry secretions, and dilate the bronchi of the respiratory tract. The usefulness of these drugs is limited because of their adverse effects—primarily producing a rapid heart rate and causing urine release to be blocked in older men who have enlarged prostate glands. Some of the newer medications have fewer side effects than older drugs in this category.

Examples of common anticholinergics are atropine and glycopyrrolate (Robinul) that are used prior to anesthesia to dry up secretions, to increase heart rate in some arrhythmias, and dilate the pupils in assessment of some eye problems. Glycopyrrolate also has been used in the treatment of peptic ulcers and irritable bowel syndrome, along with Propantheline (Pro-Banthine) and dicyclomine (Bentyl). Cyclopentolate (Cyclogyl) is also used to dilate pupils. Ipratropium (Atrovent) is used in treating asthma, oxybutynin (Ditropan) is used in treating urinary bladder urgency and incontinence, and scopolamine (Hyoscine, Transderm-Scop) is used not only for treating irritable bowel syndrome, but also has a central effect in controlling motion sickness and alcohol withdrawal symptoms. Many of these drugs have significant interactions when given with other medications. The more important of these medications will be discussed as relevant drugs in other chapters.

ANTIMIGRAINE AGENTS

OVERVIEW

Headaches are a common problem seen in primary care patients. Tension headaches that occurs when stress causes the muscles of the head and neck to tighten are successfully treated with over-the-counter (OTC) drugs such as acetaminophen (Tylenol), ibuprofen (Advil, Motrin), naproxen (Aleve, Naprosyn), or aspirin.

Migraine headaches are more serious and complex headaches in which the patient feels throbbing or pulsating pain, often made worse by noise or bright light. These headaches are often triggered by specific products (like monosodium glutamate in some foods), food additives, chocolate, red wine, and caffeine. A warning sign or aura that a migraine headache is developing might occur when the patient has changes in vision, hearing, taste, or smell. These headaches might also produce nausea, vomiting, and severe fatigue. These migraine headaches are treated with a variety of different drugs and may also be prevented by some types of medicines (prophylactic medicine).

Antimigraine agents block nerve impulses in the receptors of the sympathetic nervous system and so may be used for either prevention or treatment. The ergot alkaloids used in the treatment of vascular headaches are adrenergic-blocking agents. Treatment medications should be given as soon as the pain begins. Other medications can be taken to prevent migraines from occurring (prophylactically).

ACTION

There are two commonly used classes of drugs used in migraine treatment: (1) ergot alkaloids; and (2) triptans. Both of these drug classes stimulate serotonin (5-hydroxytryptamine [5-HT]) and affect the many serotonin receptor subtypes found throughout the CNS. There are a variety of other anticonvulsant, antidepressant, beta-adrenergic blockers, or calcium channel blockers that may be used to treat severe migraines. Riboflavin (Vitamin B_2) and feverfew are alternative therapies some have found to be effective.

The process that produces migraine headaches is thought to be local dilation of the blood vessels in the cranium or the release of sensory neuropeptides through nerve endings in the trigeminal system. The vascular 5-HT receptor is present on the human basilar artery and in the vessels of human dura mater. Use of the 5-HT, or serotonin, receptor antagonists results in cranial vessel constriction (narrowing) and blocking of neuropeptides that cause inflammation, which happens at the same time the patient feels the relief from migraine headache. Some of these products also cross the blood-brain barrier, produce central activity on the trigeminovascular system, and stop nerve depolarization at peripheral sites in the cranium.

Additionally, adrenergic-blocking agents dilate the veins in smooth muscle tissue in the peripheral vascular system, reducing cerebral blood flow and arterial pulsing, which reduces headache pain. Other actions include dilation of veins in the uterus, an increase in uterine contractions (oxytocic effect), and a decrease in blood pressure.

USES

Antimigraine agents are used in both the prevention and treatment of vascular headaches. They relieve the pain of vascular headaches by narrowing dilated cerebral arteries. OTC drugs such as ibuprofen or aspirin are usually started first. If these drugs are not helpful, triptans such as sumatriptan (Imitrex) are used. The triptans come in a variety of forms, including injection and inhalation, so that if the patient has nausea or vomiting, he or she may still take the drug. The action of 5-HT agonists is not affected by whether or not the person with the migraine has an aura or by the length of the attack, sex or age of the patient, relationship to menstrual periods, or the use of other common migraine prevention drugs. Ergot alkaloids like ergotamine (Ergonal) are used if triptans are not effective, although less commonly. Ergot alkaloids are also used for pregnant women for oxytocic (labor-inducing) and other smooth-muscle spasmogenic effects. They are not used in early pregnancy as they are pregnancy category X drugs.

ADVERSE REACTIONS

Adverse reactions to antimigraine agents in general include heart murmurs, brief tachycardia (rapid heartbeat), confusion, depression, dizziness, drowsiness, fixed miosis (constriction) of the pupil of the eye, paresthesias (numbness and tingling) in the toes, weakness (especially in legs), nausea and vomiting, leg cramps, localized pruritus (itching) and edema (fluid buildup in the body tissues), and neutropenia of the blood. Symptoms of overdosage include numb, cold, pale extremities; constant muscle pain, even at rest; decreased or absent arterial pulses; drowsiness; confusion; depression; convulsions; hemiplegia; and fixed miosis. Because of the potential for 5-HT agonists to cause coronary vasospasm, patients with ischemic heart disease or other major cardiovascular disease, or uncontrolled hypertension (high blood pressure) should not use these products.

DRUG INTERACTIONS

When antimigraine agents are used with other vasoconstrictors, vasoconstriction may be increased. The 5-HT agonists may not be used within 24 hours of taking an ergotamine-containing preparation and may not be used at the same time with monoamine oxidase (MAO) inhibitor therapy, selective serotonin reuptake inhibitors (SSRIs) serotonin/norepinephrine reuptake inhibitors (SNRIs), lithium (given for depression), and many other drugs. Some of the different triptans cannot be used within 24 hours of each other because of drug interactions.

❖ NURSING IMPLICATIONS AND PATIENT TEACHING

■ Assessment

Learn as much as possible about the overall health history of the patient, as well as the history of headaches (whether tension, migraine, or cluster). Find out whether there are factors that might affect the patient's use of antimigraine drugs (e.g., coronary artery disease or conditions in which a sudden change in blood pressure may be dangerous).

The patient may have a history of migraine headaches, vascular headaches, or headache pain of a periodic, throbbing, severe nature. The pain may be one-sided (unilateral) and commonly felt over one eye. Photophobia (sensitivity to light) and sensitivity to sound may be present, as well as nausea and vomiting. A family history of vascular headaches or history of motion sickness as a child, series of headaches in clusters, history of hypertension, a food allergy, or use of birth control pills may be present. The headache may have been relieved or eased by sleeping, vomiting, or drinking a caffeinated drink.

Ask whether the patient uses any herbal products or vitamins to control headache or migraines, because some of these products may interact adversely with other drugs, including nonsteroidal antiinflammatory drugs (NSAIDs). The Complementary and Alternative Therapies box summarizes herbal preparations the patient may be using and their drug interactions. The nurse may observe signs of sweaty hands and feet, scalp tenderness, autonomic dysfunction (such as miotic pupil), red eye, and unilateral nasal congestion.

Potential Drug-Drug Interactions with Complementary and Alternative Therapies

Headache

PRODUCT	COMMENTS
Feverfew	Potential interaction with anticoagulants, aspirin, NSAIDs, antiplatelet agents
Ginkgo	Potential interaction with anticoagulants, aspirin, NSAIDs, antiplatelet agents; may interact with MAO inhibitors, acetylcholinesterase inhibitors
White willow	Potential interaction with aspirin, anticoagulants, methotrexate, metoclopramide, phenytoin, probenecid, spironolactone, valproic acid, NSAIDs, antiplatelet agents

Data from Krinsky DL, LaValle JB, Hawkins EB, et al: *Natural therapeutics pocket guide*, ed 2, Hudson, Ohio, 2003, Lexi-Comp, Inc.

▪ Diagnosis

In addition to the medical diagnosis, what other symptoms does this patient have that require nursing action? Are there needs for patient education, nutrition information, and quiet time away from people? Sometimes identifying the migraine triggers leads to the diagnosis of other emotional or physical problems.

▪ Planning

Ergot alkaloids increase uterine contraction and may be harmful to the pregnant patient. These migraine medications are slowly and incompletely absorbed from the GI tract. Traces of ergotamine remain in various tissues; this accounts for its long-lasting and toxic actions.

▪ Implementation

Patients who have had migraines often have a regimen they follow that helps bring relief. These behaviors often include isolating themselves in a dark, quiet room, use of icepacks on head, and avoiding food. If migraine agents are used at the onset of an attack, the ability of the drugs to relieve migraine pain and symptoms is increased. If the patient's pain is relieved after an intramuscular (IM) injection of 1 mL (0.5 mg) of ergotamine, the diagnosis of vascular headaches is confirmed.

Antimigraine products are available in oral, sublingual, parenteral, and rectal forms, and as a solution for inhalation. Many factors, including whether the purpose of the agent is to prevent or to treat migraine, influence which form will be best tolerated and most effective.

Oral and rectal preparations are absorbed slowly and incompletely from the GI tract. To speed up this absorption, caffeine is included with oral and rectal preparations of ergot alkaloids. Persons who are vomiting and cannot tolerate oral preparations are given rectal forms of the agent. Inhalant methods are preferred by some patients. Sublingual tablets are more quickly absorbed than either rectal or oral preparations. IM and subcutaneous preparations are commonly used, but absorption is often incomplete and slow.

A list of important dosage information about antimigraine products is presented in Table 16-2.

▪ Evaluation

When evaluating the patient with recurrent migraines, determine if the drug is helping. There should be a decrease in number and severity of migraine headaches. To determine if overdosage, toxicity, or adverse reactions are developing, monitor the patient's blood pressure in standing, sitting, and lying positions and check for peripheral pulses.

Long-term use of migraine agents can lead to acute overdosage or chronic toxicity because of the wide variability in their absorption, metabolism, and excretion. Because patients often treat themselves, they may not realize that they are overdosing.

Abruptly stopping any of the agents used to treat migraines after long-term use can result in rebound (or new-onset) migraine headaches; therefore, they should be stopped very slowly.

▪ Patient and Family Teaching

Tell the patient and family the following:
- The patient should take the medication as ordered and not increase the dosage without talking to the nurse, physician, or other health care provider, because acute poisoning or overdosage may result.
- The patient should not take these medications along with alcohol or other CNS agents.
- The patient should dress warmly and not allow the arms and legs to get cold after taking tryptan or ergot medications.
- The nurse, physician, or other health care provider should be contacted immediately if numbness, coldness of extremities, or pain in the legs during walking occurs.
- Oral antimigraine agents, such as the f-HT blockers, may produce stomach upset. The medication should be taken with milk or meals, if possible, to decrease this effect.
- Common side effects of antimigraine agents include headache, nausea, vomiting, diarrhea, dizziness, and light-headedness when rapidly changing positions.
- After taking this drug, the patient should lie down immediately in a quiet, dark room to help obtain relief of symptoms. Soft music or relaxation techniques may also benefit the patient.
- The health care provider should be contacted immediately if more than 8 mg of oral ergotamine (Ergonal) is needed to relieve migraine pain.
- Ergot drugs should not be used by a patient who suspects she is pregnant because of the risk to the fetus.

ANTICONVULSANTS OR ANTIEPILEPTIC DRUGS

OVERVIEW

Seizures are sudden muscle contractions that happen without conscious control. They are a symptom of abnormal and excessive electrical discharge in the brain. A variety of diseases and disorders can produce seizures. High temperatures in infants and children may provoke seizures. One of the most common causes of chronic sand recurring seizures is epilepsy, which is frequently of an unknown cause (**idiopathic**). Head injury, brain tumor, stroke, meningitis, temperature

Table 16-2   Antimigraine Preparations

GENERIC NAME	TRADE NAME	COMMENTS
Serotonin (5-HT) Receptor Agonists		
almotriptan	Axert	For acute treatment of migraine and prevention.
eletriptan	Relpax	Used for acute treatment, as well as prophylaxis. Older adults may be particularly sensitive and have hypotension. May cause angina or MI.
frovatriptan	Frova	Used for acute treatment, as well as prophylaxis. Produces tachycardia.
naratriptan	Amerge	Single doses taken with fluid are typically effective in relieving acute pain. If headache returns or patient has only partial response, dose may be repeated in 4 hr. Higher doses do not produce better results.
rizatriptan benzoate	Maxalt	Comes as a tablet or an orally disintegrating tablet that does not require liquid but must not be opened until just before dosing.
sumatriptan succinate ★	Imitrex	Comes PO, SC injection, or intranasal spray.
zolmitriptan	Zomig	Break tablet in half for initial dose. Repeat in 2 hr if headache returns. Use care in patients with liver dysfunction. Also comes as nasal spray.
Ergotamine Derivatives		
dihydroergotamine ★	DHE 45 Migranal	An alpha-adrenergic blocking agent with pharmacologic and toxic properties similar to ergotamine used to treat migraine headaches. The drug causes cerebral vasculature to constrict, but it does not have an oxytocic effect and can be used during pregnancy.
ergotamine	Ergomar	An alpha-adrenergic blocking agent that exerts direct vasoconstriction on cranial blood vessels, relieving pulsations thought to be responsible for vasoconstriction. Dependence on ergotamine may develop, necessitating gradual withdrawal from this product.
Combination products	Cafergot	Cafergot is a combination of ergotamine, caffeine, and other products used to treat migraine and vascular headaches. Caffeine is included in these products to increase absorption of ergot alkaloids. Small amounts of belladonna alkaloids and barbiturates may also be included to control nausea and produce sedation. Comes PO or suppository.
Other Migraine Prophylaxis Products		
Beta-Adrenergic Blockers		
atenolol	Tenormin	Also used in treatment angina and hypertension.
metoprolol	Lopressor	Also used in treatment angina and hypertension. Comes in sustained-release and IV forms.
propranolol HCl	Inderal	Also used in treating cardiac dysrhythmias.
timolol	Blocadren	Also used for treatment glaucoma, angina, and hypertension.
Calcium Channel Blockers		
nifedipine	Procardia	Also used for treatment of angina and hypertension. Available in sustained-action product.
nimodipine	Nimotop	Used following strokes to improve neurologic statue; unlabeled use in preventing migraines.
verapamil HCl	Calan	Unlabeled use in preventing migraines.
Tricyclic Antidepressants		
amitriptyline	Elavil	Unlabeled use in preventing migraines.
imipramine	Tofranil	Also used to control bedwetting in children and alcohol or cocaine dependence. Many side effects.
Miscellaneous Agents		
valproic acid	Depakote	Also used for absence or mixed generalized seizures and mania.
methysergide	Sansert	Similar to ergotamine.

5-HT, 5-Hydroxytryptamine; *IV,* intravenous; *MI,* myocardial infarction; *PO,* by mouth; *SC,* subcutaneous.
★ Indicates "Must-Know Drugs," or the 35 drugs most prescribers use.

elevation, and poisoning, especially from excessive alcohol intake or drugs, are also common causes of seizure activity. *The most frequent cause of a seizure is the failure to take medication to control previously diagnosed seizure activity.* It is estimated that as many as 10% of all people will have a seizure during their lifetime, although this percentage may rise as more people abuse drugs. The diagnosis of epilepsy often has legal consequences, which vary among states, including restriction of driver's licenses and restriction from operation of heavy machinery or doing other activities that require alertness. It is obvious how it might be a problem if someone were driving a car or big truck and suddenly had a seizure.

The terms *epilepsy, convulsions,* and *seizures* are commonly used to mean the same thing, although they each have a slightly different medical meaning. A variety of terms have been used over the years to describe types of seizures, including *grand mal (tonic-clonic), petit mal (absence), psychomotor, myoclonic, atonic,* and *jacksonian.* More recently, there has been agreement to group seizures into two broad categories, *generalized* or *focal,* based on their clinical presentation and electroencephalographic (EEG) patterns. This chapter uses both terms.

Sometimes surgery or dietary treatment may be used to control symptoms in a patient with a seizure disorder. More commonly, epileptic seizures are treated with medication. The goal of this type of therapy is to suppress or reduce the number of patient seizures.

ACTION

A number of drugs control seizures through depression or slowing of abnormal electrical discharges in the CNS. These products work in a variety of ways. There is usually one drug that is more effective than another for a patient, depending on the type of seizure activity. Patients with newly diagnosed and acute seizure disorders are often started on parenteral injection therapy; when seizure activity has come under control, oral therapy is started.

There are five major anticonvulsant or antiepileptic drug (AED) groups: barbiturates, benzodiazepines, hydantoins, succinimides, and γ-aminobutyric acid (GABA) analogues (Figure 16-2). A list of anticonvulsants and their uses is presented in Table 16-3. In addition to prescription medications, patients and families sometimes try a variety of supplements and herbal products to treat seizure disorders. The Complementary and Alternative Therapies box provides a list of common herbal products and drug interactions important for patients to know.

USES

Barbiturates, which have a long duration of action, are an important category of prescription anticonvulsants and are used for their sedative effect on the brain. They

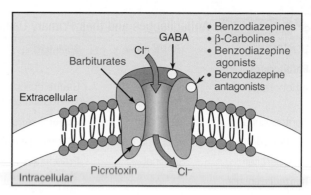

FIGURE 16-2 The GABA receptor depicting the membrane-associated protein composed of five subunits, the CL-channel, and relative location of binding sites for GABA, benzodiazepines, barbiturates, and picrotoxin.

Complementary and Alternative Therapies

Epilepsy

PRODUCT	COMMENTS
Bitter melon	Potential interactions with insulin, oral hypoglycemics
Ginkgo	Potential interaction with anticoagulants, aspirin, NSAIDs, antiplatelet drugs; may interact with MAO inhibitors, acetylcholinesterase inhibitors
Gymnema	Potential interactions with insulin, oral hypoglycemics

Data from Krinsky DL, LaValle JB, Hawkins EB, et al: *Natural therapeutics pocket guide,* ed 2, Hudson, Ohio, 2003, Lexi-Comp, Inc.

may be used in combination with medications from the other three groups. Benzodiazepines are useful with some problems but also have a lot of serious adverse effects. Hydantoins have a wide range of uses, and phenytoin (Dilantin) is by far the most commonly used anticonvulsant. Succinimides are used to control petit mal seizures. GABA analogs have wide use for many types of seizures. Each of these five groups, along with a variety of other newer miscellaneous anticonvulsants, are discussed in this section.

Because of the variety of drugs and the many possible side effects, the choice of an anticonvulsant tends to be a trial or experiment for each patient. When seizures are not stopped with one drug, another may be added, or the first drug may be stopped and another product used instead.

BARBITURATES

ACTION

Barbiturates are CNS depressants. They act primarily on the brainstem reticular formation, reducing nerve impulses that go to the cerebral cortex. Barbiturates depress the respiratory system and slow the activity of nerves and muscles (smooth, skeletal, and cardiac).

	Table 16-3	Antiepileptics and their Primary Uses	
GENERIC NAME	**TRADE NAME**	**COMMENTS**
Barbiturates		
amobarbital	Amytal	Status epilepticus, acute convulsive episodes; also used for preoperative sedation and insomnia, preoperative anxiety and sedation
pentobarbital	Nembutal	General seizure, reduce ICP in head trauma; preoperative sedation, insomnia
phenobarbital ★	Phenobarbital	All forms of epilepsy, status epilepticus, severe recurrent seizures, eclampsia
secobarbital	Seconal	Preoperative sedation; insomnia
Benzodiazepines		
clonazepam	Klonopin	Petit mal, myoclonic seizures
clorazepate	Tranxene	Focal seizures
diazepam ★	Valium	All forms of epilepsy, status epilepticus, severe recurrent seizures, tetanus
lorazepam	Ativan	Used for all seizures except febrile seizures
Hydantoins		
fosphenytoin	Cerebyx	Status epilepticus
phenytoin	Dilantin Phenytek	Used for partial seizures, status epilepticus
Succinimides		
ethosuximide	Zarontin	Absence atonic seizures and myoclonic seizures
methsuximide	Celontin	Absence seizures; adjunct therapy in mixed seizures
phensuximide	Milontin	Absence seizures
GABA Analogs		
tiagabine	Gabatril	Inhibits uptake of GABA into presynaptic neurons, prolonging GABA action; used for adjunctive therapy in adult partial seizures
Other Drugs		
acetazolamide	Diamox	Absence seizures, metabolic alkalosis in mechanically ventilated patients, altitude sickness
carbamazepine	Tegretol	Status epilepticus, partial seizures
gabapentin	Neurontin	Partial seizures in adults, children
lamotrigine	Lamictal	Partial seizures in adults, children
levetiracetam	Keppra	Partial seizures in adults, children
oxcarbazepine	Trileptal	Partial seizures in adults, children
primidone	Mysoline	Grand mal, psychomotor, focal seizures in adults and children
topiramate	Topamax	Adjunctive therapy for partial-onset seizures in adults, children
valproic acid	Depakene Depakote	Used for all types of seizures

GABA, γ-Aminobutyric acid.
★ Indicates "Must-Know Drugs," or the 35 drugs most prescribers use.

Barbiturates also raise the seizure threshold, or the level of electrical activity that must be produced before a seizure will occur. Barbiturates may be short-acting, intermediate-acting, or long-acting.

USES

Long-acting barbiturates are used as anticonvulsants to control and prevent grand mal seizures. They are sometimes used if other drugs do not help to treat status epilepticus, a condition in which a series of severe grand mal seizures occur one after another without stopping. They may also be used to treat seizures caused by tetanus, fever, or drugs.

ADVERSE REACTIONS

Adverse reactions to barbiturates include worsening of symptoms of certain organic brain disorders in older adult patients, dizziness, drowsiness, hangover, headache, lethargy (sleepiness), paradoxical restlessness or excitement, unsteadiness, photosensitivity (abnormal

Lifespan Considerations
Pediatric

ANTICONVULSANTS

- The young patient (younger than age 23) is more susceptible to gingival hyperplasia, especially with phenytoin (Dilantin) therapy. Gingivitis, or gum inflammation, usually starts during the first 6 months of drug therapy, although severe hyperplasia is unlikely with dosages of less than 500 mg/day. A dental program of teeth cleaning and plaque control begun within 7 to 10 days of initiating drug therapy helps to reduce the rate and severity of this condition.
- Coarse facial features and excessive body hair growth are more frequently reported in young patients on dilantin.
- Chronic use of clonazepam (Klonopin) may result in impaired physical or mental functions in the developing child. This may not become apparent until years later.
- Impaired school performance is reported with long-term, high-dose hydantoin (Dilantin) therapy (especially at high or toxic serum levels).
- Children receiving valproic acid (Depakene), especially those younger than 2 years old or those receiving multiple anticonvulsant drugs, are at a greater risk for serious hepatotoxicity. This risk decreases with advancing age.

Modified from McKenry LM, Tessier E, Hogan MA: *Mosby's pharmacology in nursing*, ed 22, St Louis, 2006, Mosby.

Lifespan Considerations
Older Adults

ANTICONVULSANTS

- Because much seizure activity in older adults is associated with use of drugs for other diseases or problems, (e.g., cerebrovascular disease, dementia, etc.), treatment often includes evaluation of nonantiepileptic drug therapy as part of good care. Cerebrovascular accident or stroke risk may be considerably higher in older clients with new-seizures compared with other older individuals.
- Older individuals are at greater risk for fractures. Antiepileptic medications increase the risk for the patient to have fractures of the hip and other bones. Older patients are more susceptible to carbamazepine-induced confusion or agitation, atrioventricular heart block, syndrome of inappropriate antidiuretic hormone, and bradycardia than younger patients. If a rash develops with the use of phenytoin (Dilantin), notify the prescriber immediately and discontinue taking the drug.
- Debilitated patients or persons with renal or liver disease have a greater risk of developing toxicity with the AEDs. Lower doses will help to avoid adverse effects.
- The older adult population tends to metabolize anticonvulsants more slowly; thus drug accumulation and toxicity may occur. Monitor closely, because dosage adjustments (lower doses) may be necessary.
- Serum albumin levels may be lower in geriatric patients, resulting in decreased protein binding of drugs such as phenytoin (Dilantin) and valproic acid (Depakene). Monitor closely, because lower drug doses may be necessary.
- Administer intravenous (IV) doses at a rate slower than the recommended rate for an adult. The rate of administration of phenytoin to older adult patients should be 5 to 10 mg/min, up to a maximum of 25 mg/min.

Modified from McKenry LM, Tessier E, Hogan MA: *Mosby's pharmacology in nursing*, ed 22, St Louis, 2006, Mosby.

response to exposure to sunlight), rash, diarrhea, nausea, hepatitis with jaundice, vomiting, anemia, decreased platelet counts, unusual bleeding or bruising, urticaria (hives), joint and muscle pains, tolerance (increased resistance to the drug caused by repeated use), and withdrawal symptoms due to physical dependence when discontinued.

In cases of acute overdose, the patient may show exaggerated CNS depression, slow, shallow respirations, miosis, tachycardia, areflexia (absence of reflexes), shock, or coma. Death may occur as a result of cardiorespiratory failure.

DRUG INTERACTIONS

Because barbiturates act through the P450 enzyme system to speed up the metabolism of some drugs in the liver, they reduce the activity of anticoagulants, corticosteroids, and digitalis preparations. MAO inhibitors may increase the depressant effects of the barbiturates. There may be significant additive effects if barbiturates are used along with alcohol, antihistamines, benzodiazepines, methotrimeprazine, narcotics, and tranquilizers.

BENZODIAZEPINES

ACTION

Benzodiazepines are CNS depressants. Their exact mechanism of action is not known, but they are thought to act on the hypothalamus and limbic system of the brain, decreasing the vasopressor response and increasing the arousal threshold. Benzodiazepines suppress the electrical spike-and-wave brain discharge in seizures and decrease the frequency, amplitude, duration, and spread of the discharge in minor motor seizures.

USES

Benzodiazepines are used to treat partial seizures and also to treat Lennox-Gastaut syndrome (petit mal variance) and for patients who have failed to respond to succinimide drugs such as ethosuccinimide (Zarontin). Three benzodiazepines are approved for use as anticonvulsants. Diazepam (Valium) is used intravenously to control seizures and is the drug of choice for treatment of status epilepticus. Clonazepam (Klonopin) is used for oral treatment of petit mal seizures in children, and clorazepate (Tranxene) is used with other antiepileptic agents to control partial seizures.

ADVERSE REACTIONS

Adverse reactions to benzodiazepines include hypotension (low blood pressure), shortness of breath, difficulty focusing or blurred vision, confusion, drowsiness, flushing (red color in the face and neck), headaches, light-headedness, paradoxical reactions (excitement, stimulation, hyperactivity), slurred speech, sweating, anorexia (lack of appetite), bitter taste, dry mouth, diarrhea, heartburn, nausea, vomiting, pruritus, rash, joint pains, and burning eyes.

Overdosage may produce marked drowsiness, weakness, impairment of stance and gait, confusion, and coma.

DRUG INTERACTIONS

Alcohol, other sedatives and hypnotics, antidepressants, anticonvulsants, and narcotics may produce additive sedative effects if used with benzodiazepines. Some combinations of anticonvulsants may result in an antidepressant effect or provoke additional seizures.

HYDANTOINS

ACTION

Hydantoins act primarily on the motor cortex, where they stop the spread of seizure activity by blocking neuronal sodium and calcium channels. This stabilizes the nerve cell against hyperexcitability and reduces the maximal activity of brainstem centers responsible for the tonic phase of grand mal seizures. It also has an antiarrhythmic property.

USES

Hydantoins are used to treat tonic-clonic and psychomotor seizures. Sometimes they are used to treat status epilepticus, migraine, and trigeminal neuralgia. They are also used in some nonepileptic psychotic patients.

ADVERSE REACTIONS

Adverse reactions to hydantoins include ataxia (poor coordination), dizziness, drowsiness, hallucinations, inattentiveness, nystagmus (rhythmic movement of the eyes), ocular disturbances, poor memory, slurred speech, constipation, nausea, vomiting, blood cell disturbances, purpura (bruising), acnelike eruptions, gingival hyperplasia (overgrowth of gums), lupus erythematosus, hepatitis with jaundice, and lymph node hyperplasia. Hydantoins are also teratogenic-category D (producing changes in the fetus). Overdosage may produce ataxia, coma, dysarthria, hypotension, nystagmus, and unresponsive pupils.

DRUG INTERACTIONS

Hydantoin drug interactions are frequent and often substantial. Even when given alone, the drug requires careful monitoring of the patient. It is very important to see the patient regularly when it is used with any other medication or vitamins because the dose that prevents seizure is very close to the toxic dose. It may also alter the results of various laboratory tests.

SUCCINIMIDES

ACTION

Succinimide-type anticonvulsants raise the seizure threshold in the cortex and basal ganglia, making seizures less likely and reduce response at the nerve synapse to some specific types of nerve stimulation.

USES

Succinimides are used to control absence seizures.

ADVERSE REACTIONS

Adverse reactions to succinimides include dizziness, headaches, hiccups, hyperactivity, lethargy, mood or mental changes, rashes, blurred vision, photophobia (intolerance to light), anorexia, abdominal pain, diarrhea, nausea, vomiting, urinary frequency, vaginal bleeding, blood cell changes, alopecia (hair loss), muscular weakness, systemic lupus erythematosus, disturbances of sleep, inability to concentrate, mental slowness, and night terrors.

DRUG INTERACTIONS

If these drugs are used with other anticonvulsants, they can result in increased sex drive (libido) or increased frequency of tonic-clonic seizures. Bone marrow–depressing drugs used with succinimides can result in significant and fatal blood dyscrasias or conditions.

γ-AMINOBUTYRIC ACID ANALOGS (GABA)

ACTION

The mechanism of action for GABA analogs is not clearly understood. All of these drugs are chemically unrelated but they all increase the actions of GABA, which is an inhibitory neurotransmitter. It is thought that they might slow the sodium channel, helping to stabilize the neuronal membranes. Some of the newer GABA analogs also increase the action of GABA, block voltage of sodium channels, antagonize glutamate, and modulate calcium channels.

USES

Although relatively new drugs, GABA analogs are used in the treatment, along with other antiepileptic drugs, for simple partial, complex partial, secondarily generalized, generalized tonic-clonic, and absence seizures. These medications are also used in treating peripheral neuropathy, post-herpatic neuralgia, and fibromyalgia.

ADVERSE REACTIONS

Adverse reactions include GI disturbances; weight gain; irregular menses; alopecia; pruritus; rashes, including erythema multiforme; photosensitivity; hair loss; anxiety; mood problems; tremor; and nervousness. Drowsiness and ataxia that are dose-dependent may also be seen. Inattention, anorexia, paresthesias, and renal stones may also be produced by some drugs.

DRUG INTERACTIONS

Increased CNS depression may occur when valproic acid is administered with other CNS depressants, including other anticonvulsants and alcohol. These drugs interact with many other CNS drugs and may increase or decrease their blood levels. This is particularly true of phenytoin. It is advisable to monitor serum concentrations of any other anticonvulsants being used with these drugs to prevent overdosage.

OTHER DRUGS

A variety of other products that are chemically unrelated have been in use for years in the treatment of seizures. New products continue to be developed in efforts to obtain better seizure control with reduced side effects. These products and their uses are listed in Table 16-3. All of these products have widespread usage for many different neurologic problems. Some also have other indications. For example, Valproic Acid (Depakote) is widely used in patients with bipolar symptoms and for migraine headaches.

 Memory Jogger

Drug Dependence

Dependence can develop with indiscriminate use, and abrupt withdrawal is dangerous. These drugs must be carefully monitored and the patient must return for evaluation regularly.

❖ NURSING IMPLICATIONS AND PATIENT TEACHING

■ Assessment

Learn as much as possible about other drugs currently being taken that may produce drug interactions. Ask about other anticonvulsants, response to anticonvulsants taken in the past, hypersensitivity (allergy), and the possibility of pregnancy. Cardiac, respiratory, hepatic, or renal diseases are contraindications or precautions to the use of anticonvulsants.

■ Diagnosis

For patients who are just starting on an antiseizure medication, find out what particular fears or concerns they have, as well as specific learning deficits. The diagnosis of these problems will help the nurse develop an appropriate nursing care plan to meet those needs. If the patient has alcohol and drug abuse problems, there may be problems with drug withdrawal, legal issues, or difficulties with compliance that will need to be part of the care plan.

■ Planning

Older adult or weakened patients may be more sensitive to barbiturates and should be started on lower dosages. These patients are more likely to have hangover, confusion, and delirium.

Several of the anticonvulsant medications may produce blood dyscrasias or systemic lupus erythematosus. Benzodiazepines are changed by the liver into long-acting forms that may remain in the body for 24 hours or more and produce increased sedation; liver function may be affected with long-term use. In addition, there is a risk of congenital malformations and neonatal depression with most anticonvulsants, if used during pregnancy.

■ Implementation

Barbiturates are legally controlled substances. They should not be given to patients with a history of abuse or addiction. Barbiturates should not be given to patients in pain, because these drugs may worsen the pain. When barbiturates are given parenterally, use great caution to avoid accidentally allowing the medicine to infiltrate tissues, because serious ischemia or gangrene could result. One of the major problems with this whole class of drugs is that they cause respiratory depression. This side effect has caused clinicians to turn to other drugs as they have become available.

When benzodiazepines are used in patients who have a mixed type of seizure activity, the drugs may increase or cause the onset of generalized tonic-clonic seizures. These drugs should also be used with caution in patients with poor or reduced renal function. Stopping the drugs quickly can produce status epilepticus.

The dosage of benzodiazepines is individualized for each patient, depending on the patient's response. The onset of action is about for oral medicine is 30 to 60 minutes, and the effects last 7 to 8 hours. The drug should be given 15 to 30 minutes before bedtime. Older adult or weakened patients should receive reduced dosages of all anticonvulsants. It is important to very slowly increase or decrease dosages.

Oral phenytoin (Dilantin) suspension is often difficult to give accurately. The oral suspension should be shaken well before being given, and the liquid should not be frozen. Chewable tablets should not be used for once-a-day treatment.

Subcutaneous or perivascular (around the veins) injection of hydantoins should be avoided because of the highly alkaline nature of the solution. Hydantoins

Clinical Goldmine

Oral Dilantin Therapy

There are two types of oral Dilantin therapy: "prompt" and "extended" capsules. Capsules labeled "extended" are given only once a day. Capsules labeled "prompt" are given two or three times a day. Giving the wrong type of therapy could result in either undermedication or overmedication.

should be administered very slowly when given intravenously.

Talk to the patient and family about the chance of brief but short-term personality changes with phensuximide therapy. These should be reported to the nurse, physician, or other health care provider if they occur.

Once the patient is seizure-free with a particular drug, changing to phenytoin (Dilantin) products should be avoided. All dosages must be determined for the individual. The dosage for children is usually larger by weight than for adults. The patient is usually given a single dose within the therapeutic range, and then the amount is gradually increased until the seizures are controlled and the serum levels are stable, or until symptoms of overdosage or toxicity indicate that no further increases can be made.

Table 16-4 provides a list of important information about anticonvulsants, including dosages. A variety of miscellaneous anticonvulsants are also available. See Tables 16-2 and 16-3 for brief information about those products. Felbamate (Felbatol) has been used for partial seizures and Lennox-Gastaut syndrome. Enough cases of aplastic anemia and hepatic failure have developed from use of this drug that it carries a warning regarding its use.

■ Evaluation

It takes several weeks before the success of an anticonvulsant dosage plan can be seen. The therapeutic effects should be monitored. Note seizure pattern and change. Note whether or not the sedation is a problem. Blood levels may be needed to see if the drug dosage is in the therapeutic range.

The patient's compliance should be followed in regard to the amount of and times the drug is taken, any pattern of abuse, and drinking of alcohol. In addition, the patient should be asked about any paradoxical reactions and evaluated for tolerance, dependence, withdrawal, and toxicity. Liver toxicity is indicated by jaundice (yellow color of skin, eyes, and mucous membranes), rash, and sore throat.

The patient should keep a record of any seizures, with information about the time, length, characteristics, and reaction.

Complete blood cell counts and liver function tests should be followed as a baseline and repeated on a set schedule for patients on long-term barbiturate therapy.

Tolerance is usually related to the total amount of drug received. Dependence and withdrawal symptoms may occur if these drugs are used for very long periods. If the patient has been taking the drug for a long time, the drug should not be discontinued quickly.

Hydantoins are metabolized at various rates by patients; therefore, be alert to symptoms of toxicity. The patient should avoid alcohol while taking most anticonvulsants.

Adverse effects are common in long-term therapy. Gum overgrowth around the teeth (hyperplasia) is a typical finding with phenytoin (Dilantin) and may cause distress to the patient and family. The patient and family must be educated about how to prevent and treat this problem.

Memory Jogger

Oral Hygiene

Hydantoins may be associated with overgrowth of gum tissue in the mouth. The importance of good oral hygiene, especially of gums, should be emphasized to patients taking phenytoin (Dilaintin).

■ Patient and Family Teaching

Tell the patient and family the following:
- The patient should be aware that problems with tolerance, dependence, and addiction may occur with anticonvulsant medications.
- The patient should take the medication exactly as prescribed and not discontinue taking it, even if feeling well and having no seizures. If a dose is forgotten, it should be taken as soon as it is remembered if it is within 1 to 2 hours of the regular dosage time. If it is later than 2 hours, the patient should skip the dose and take the next dose at the regular time. Double doses should not be taken. The regular medication schedule should be continued.
- This medication should be kept in a locked cabinet or out of the reach of children and all others for whom the drug is not prescribed. The medication should not be shared with anyone.
- Barbiturates may cause drowsiness, and the patient must be cautious when driving, using hazardous machinery, or performing tasks that require alertness.
- Some medications produce daytime sedation that may interfere with the patient's job or home and childcare responsibilities.
- Sometimes the medication causes respiratory depression. Family should be alerted to watch for very slow breathing or pauses in breathing,

Table 16-4   Antiepileptics

GENERIC NAME	TRADE NAME	COMMENTS
Barbiturates		
Long Acting		
phenobarbital ★	Luminal Phenobarbital	Give IM in large muscle mass, because injection is very painful. Give slowly IV. Some forms come in sustained-release capsules. Onset in 1 hr, effective for 16 hr.
Benzodiazepines		
clonazepam	Klonopin	*Give initial doses.* After 4-9 days, dosage may be increased by 0.5-1.5 mg/day every 3 days until seizures stop or until side effects prevent any further increase. Whenever possible, give in 3 equally divided doses; if this is not possible, give the largest dose before bedtime.
clorazepate	Tranxene	
diazepam ★	Valium	Comes PO, sustained-release capsules, and IV. Parenteral therapy: Inject IV medication slowly only into large veins, 1 min for each 5 mg. May cause respiratory arrest if this is exceeded.
Hydantoins		
fosphenytoin	Cerebyx	Continuously monitor ECG and vital signs.
phenytoin ★	Dilantin	Monitor blood levels carefully. Watch for adverse neurologic effects.
Succinimides		
phensuximide		Shake suspension well before pouring. Take drug with meals to decrease gastric discomfort. Efficacy of the drug decreases with long-term use.
Miscellaneous Anticonvulsants		
acetazolamide	Diamox	
carbamazepine	Tegretol	
gabapentin	Neurontin	Add-on therapy for patients older than 12 yr. Effective.
lamotrigine	Lamictal	Consult package insert for complex dosing instructions.
topiramate	Topamax	
valproic acid	Depakene	

ECG, Electrocardiogram; *IM*, intramuscular; *IV*, intravenous; *PO*, by mouth.
★ Indicates "Must-Know Drugs," or the 35 drugs most prescribers use.

particularly if the patient seems heavily asleep and unresponsive. This is a problem requiring immediate attention.

- The health care provider should be notified immediately if the patient experiences any rash, fever, unusual bleeding, bruising, sore throat, jaundice, or abdominal pain. Some people experience side effects or adverse effects while taking these drugs, so the health care provider should be notified of any new or uncomfortable symptoms.
- The patient may have excessive dreaming when barbiturates are discontinued; this should lessen each night.
- Tablets and capsules should be kept in a dry, tightly closed container.
- Elixirs should be kept in a tightly closed, brown, glass bottle.
- A hangover feeling may sometimes be experienced the day after taking a benzodiazepine. It is dangerous to drink alcohol within 24 hours after taking this drug. The patient who takes this medication must not drink any alcohol.
- Smoking may decrease the length of time benzodiazepines are effective.
- Succinimides such as ethosuximide (Zarontin) may be taken with food or milk to decrease stomach upset.
- The liquid form of ethosuximide (Zarontin) should be shaken well before the dose is measured.
- The patient should maintain good oral hygiene: brushing teeth and gums with a soft toothbrush twice daily and rinsing the mouth well is important. The patient should see a dentist every 6 months; this is especially true if the patient is taking phenytoin (Dilantin).
- The patient should wear a MedicAlert bracelet or necklace or other identification that states the medical problem and the medication being taken.
- Succinimide agents may make the urine appear pink, red, or reddish brown.

- Chewable tablets must be chewed or crushed before they are swallowed.
- When undergoing any kind of surgery, including dental work, patients should alert the dentist, nurse, physician, or other health care provider that they are taking anticonvulsant medication.
- The use of antiepileptics is not advised in pregnancy. The patient and the health care provider should discuss questions about the patient becoming pregnant.
- The patient should keep regular follow-up appointments with the health care provider; this is essential to evaluate reactions to anticonvulsants.

 Memory Jogger

Alert Regarding Staying with the Same Brand

The patient must not change the brands or dosage forms unless ordered to do so by the nurse, physician, or other health care provider. Not all brands of these medications are the same so they cannot be substituted for each other (they are not interchangeable). This means that prescriptions for a particular brand of medication will be written by the provider. Once a patient's seizures are controlled with a certain brand, the patient should continue to receive that brand. This is important for the patient to discuss with his or her pharmacist and they should be asked to make sure their medicines are the same each time the prescription is filled.

ANTIEMETIC-ANTIVERTIGO AGENTS

OVERVIEW

Antiemetic or antivertigo agents are used to prevent and treat motion sickness and the nausea and vomiting that occur with anesthesia and surgery or cancer treatment. They are also used to treat severe, intractable (cannot be stopped by the usual treatment methods) vomiting and hiccups.

ACTION

The vomiting center of the brain may be stimulated by many factors: drugs, metabolic disorders, radiation, motion, gastric irritation, and vestibular neuritis. Vomiting is produced by direct action on the vomiting center of the brain, by indirect action through stimulation of the chemoreceptor trigger zone, and through increased activity of chemical neurotransmitters. Nausea and vomiting resulting from motion are probably caused by impulses to the vestibular network of the labyrinth system of the ear, which is located near the vomiting center. The impulses are conducted to the vomiting center by cholinergic nerves. Thus drugs that inhibit cholinergic nerve impulses should be effective in treating motion sickness.

USES

Antidopaminergic agents such as chlorpromazine (Thorazine) and prochlorpromazine (Compazine) are used almost exclusively to control nausea and vomiting. Selected first generation H1 blocker antihistamine/ anticholinergic medications are used to control motion sickness. Meclizine (Antivert) and dimenhydrinate (Dramamine) are the only products used to control acute vertigo. 5-HT$_3$ antagonists such as ondansetron (Zofran) are routinely used prophylactically in patients expected to have nausea (e.g., patients undergoing chemotherapy).

ADVERSE REACTIONS

Drowsiness or sedation is the most common side effect of the anticholinergics, but tolerance to this reaction usually develops with long-term therapy. Patients may also feel dry mouth, stuffy nose, blurred vision, constipation, urinary retention, and other anticholinergic reactions.

DRUG INTERACTIONS

The sedative effect of some antiemetic medications is increased (or potentiated) by other CNS depressants. Anticholinergic antiemetics can increase the anticholinergic side effects of many other drugs. The drug interactions may vary, depending on the type of antiemetic-antivertigo drug, but would be similar to other anticholinergic or antidopaminergic products. (See the earlier discussions about anticholinergic and antidopaminergic actions at the beginning of this chapter.)

❖ NURSING IMPLICATIONS AND PATIENT TEACHING

▪ Assessment

Learn as much as possible about the health history of the patient, including episodes of motion sickness, extrapyramidal reactions caused by antipsychotic therapy, labyrinthitis, vertigo, Meniere disease, radiation therapy, or diabetes. Nausea and vomiting are common adverse reactions to drug therapy and may occur after taking almost any medication.

Find out whether the patient has a history of allergy, is currently using drugs that would cause drug interactions (especially MAO inhibitors), or is pregnant. In all cases, the underlying cause of vomiting, nausea, or vertigo should be found. In women of childbearing years, the possibility of pregnancy should always be considered. These drugs should not be used for treating morning sickness, because many drugs are not safe for the fetus.

Peppermint and ginger have been used in the treatment of motion sickness and nausea. Ask patients about the use of these herbs, because ginger has the potential to interact with anticoagulants, aspirin,

NSAIDs, antiplatelet agents, and cardiac glycosides (digoxin).

▪ Diagnosis

For patients who have been vomiting for a long time or who have vertigo, other problems may develop. Is the patient dehydrated? Getting enough good food? Are there problems related to work or family because of the patient's vomiting? Explore these areas to determine if there are problems that require action.

▪ Planning

Antiemetic and antivertigo agents should be used with extreme caution in patients doing tasks that require them to be mentally alert, because some of these products produce drowsiness. These agents are not recommended for use in children, because they may contribute to the development, the misdiagnosis, or the severity of symptoms in Reye syndrome, a brain encephalopathy that is often fatal in children.

Vomiting is often an important diagnostic clue and may point to a serious underlying problem. The cause of the vomiting or nausea should be found so that the best treatment can be given to get rid of the problem. Antiemetic drugs should not be the only form of therapy in cases of nausea or vomiting. Attempts to maintain hydration, restore electrolyte balance, and reduce other symptoms should be made.

Lifespan Considerations
Pediatric

ANTIEMETIC AGENTS
Pediatric patients with chickenpox, CNS infections, measles, dehydration, gastroenteritis, or other acute illnesses are at special risk for adverse reactions and possibly Reye syndrome. Avoid use of phenothiazine (Phenergan) antiemetic therapy in such patients.

Modified from McKenry LM, Tessier E, Hogan MA: *Mosby's pharmacology in nursing*, ed 22, St Louis, 2006, Mosby.

▪ Implementation

All phenothiazine derivatives (chlorpromazine [Thorazine], prochlorperazine [Compazine] and promethazine [Phenergan]), turn the urine pink or reddish brown. They also may produce photosensitivity, so the patient should avoid exposure to sunlight. Antiemetic and antivertigo agents generally come in tablets, sustained-release capsules, and concentrates for oral use. For patients who are vomiting or so nauseated they are unable to take oral medications, injection or suppository forms are usually given.

The dose should be as low as possible, and therapy should be stopped as soon as possible. IV preparations should be reserved for severe cases in patients in the hospital. Medications given IM should be switched when the patient can tolerate oral agents.

Table 16-5 summarizes important information about antiemetic-antivertigo agents.

▪ Evaluation

The nurse should monitor for therapeutic effectiveness and side effects.

▪ Patient and Family Teaching

Tell the patient and family the following:
- The patient should take this medication as instructed by the health care provider and not double the dosage or alter the medication schedule.
- If the drug is taken for motion sickness, the patient should take it 30 to 60 minutes before departure and 30 minutes before meals thereafter.
- While taking these drugs, the patient should not drive, operate dangerous machines, or do anything that requires alertness.
- The patient should not take any other medications without the knowledge of the nurse, physician, or other health care provider. It is especially important for the patient to avoid other CNS depressants, including alcohol, because of the sedative effect.
- Although some patients get very sleepy while taking these medications, this is usually a brief problem and will disappear if they keep taking the drug.
- This medication should be kept out of the reach of children and others for whom it is not prescribed. Overdosage of this medication may be toxic.

ANTIPARKINSONIAN AGENTS
OVERVIEW

Parkinson disease is a chronic disorder of the CNS. The cause is unknown, but it is thought to involve an imbalance in chemical neurotransmitters within the brain. Problems seem to stem from too much acetylcholine and not enough dopamine in the basal ganglia. Medicine for Parkinson disease is designed to replace dopamaine, as well as to control symptoms. Common symptoms are fine muscle tremors while they are at rest, slowness of movement, rigidity, muscle weakness, a characteristic shuffling, forward-pitched gait, and resulting changes in posture and balance. Patients often develop dementia as time progresses. There is no known cure for Parkinson disease. Treatment goals are designed to relieve symptoms and maintain movement and activity of the patient.

Table 16-5 Antiemetic and Antivertigo Agents

GENERIC NAME	TRADE NAME	COMMENTS
Antidopaminergics		
Phenothiazines		
chlorpromazine	Thorazine	A phenothiazine derivative used to control nausea and vomiting and to treat intractable hiccups.
prochlorperazine ★	Compazine	A phenothiazine derivative used to treat vomiting. Available PO, sustained-release tablets, and IM.
promethazine	Phenergan	A phenothiazine derivative used to treat motion sickness and prevent and control nausea and vomiting associated with surgery and anesthesia. Caution: subcutaneous injection may cause tissue necrosis; intraarterial injection may produce gangrene of the extremity.
		Motion sickness: Adults: 25 mg 30-60 min before travel, repeat 8-12 hr later PRN. On succeeding days, take 25 mg on arising and again before the evening meal.
		Nausea and vomiting: Available PO, IM, IV, or suppository and topical cream. IV medication should be given to hospitalized patients only.
		Preoperatively, may give equal doses of promethazine and a barbiturate or narcotic and an atropine-like drug.
Other		
metoclopramide	Octamide Reglan	Give before meals and at bedtime.
Anticholinergics		
Antihistamines		
dimenhydrinate	Dramamine	Antiemetic and antivertigo agent used in motion sickness, in radiation sickness, or following anesthesia. Appears to depress motion-induced stimulation of the labyrinthine structures; may alter blood counts.
diphenhydramine ★	Benadryl Genahist	Antihistamine that blocks histamine receptors on peripheral effector cells. Has anticholinergic, antitussive, antiemetic, and sedative properties. With IV use, blood pressure should be carefully monitored.
meclizine	Antivert	Antiemetic, anti-motion-sickness, and antivertigo agent with anticholinergic properties. Motion sickness: 50 mg 1 hr before departure; repeat q24h PRN.
Other		
dronabinol	Marinol	Antiemetic primarily used for nausea and vomiting from chemotherapy. Give 5 mg/m^2 1-3 hr before the administration of chemotherapy, then every 2-4 hr after chemotherapy is given, for a total of 4-6 doses/day. May be increased by 2.5 mg/m^2 if dose is ineffective and no side effects have occurred. Use cautiously, because disturbing psychiatric symptoms develop with higher dosages. Also used as an appetite stimulant.
phosphorated carbohydrate solution	Emetrol (OTC)	Hyperosmolar carbohydrate solution that relieves nausea and vomiting by direct local action on the wall of the GI tract, reducing small muscle contraction. Used as antiemetic or for motion sickness.
		Morning sickness: 15-30 mL on arising, and repeat every 3 hrs or when nausea threatens.
scopolamine	Transderm-Scōp	Comes as a transdermal patch, which is placed behind the ear and releases medication at a constant rate over a 3-day interval. The transdermal mechanism allows for lower dosage and produces fewer adverse anticholinergic effects than the oral forms. Scopolamine is used to control motion sickness in adults. Many contraindications.
		Motion sickness: 0.24-0.8 mg PO 1 hr before anticipated travel. Long-term therapy: Apply 1 patch behind ear at least 4 hours before the antiemetic effect is desired; replace every 3 days for continued therapy.

Table 16-5 Antiemetic and Antivertigo Agents—cont'd

GENERIC NAME	TRADE NAME	COMMENTS
trimethobenzamide	Tigan	Antiemetic that inhibits the chemoreceptor trigger zone in the medulla; used to control nausea and vomiting. Drug has been linked to the development of Reye syndrome in children. Give deep IM; solution is highly irritating to tissues.
5-HT Receptor Antagonists		
dolasetron	Anzemet	*Controlling nausea and vomiting associated with chemotherapy:* Give within 1 hr before chemotherapy. Lower dosages may be given to control postoperative vomiting.
granisetron	Kytril	Used for prevention of nausea and vomiting associated with initial and repeat courses of chemotherapy.
ondansetron	Zofran	Used in controlling nausea and vomiting associated with chemotherapy. See package insert for complex dosing instructions. May be given IV, suppository, solution, or tablet.

5-HT, 5-Hydroxytriptamine; *GI,* gastrointestinal; *IM,* intramuscular; *IV,* intravenous; *OTC,* over the counter; *PO,* by mouth; *PRN,* as needed.
★ Indicates "Must-Know Drugs," or the 35 drugs most prescribers use.

ACTION

The two main actions of the antiparkinsonian agents are to: (1) block the uptake of acetylcholine at postsynaptic muscarinic cholinergic receptor sites; and (2) elevate the functional levels of dopamine in motor regulatory centers. These drugs exert a wide range of effects on all the tissue affected by the autonomic nervous system, including the eyes, respiratory tract, heart, GI tract, urinary bladder, nonvascular smooth muscle, exocrine glands, and CNS. Antiparkinsonian agents reduce muscle tremors and rigidity and improve mobility, muscular coordination, and performance.

USES

Antiparkinsonian agents are anticholinergic and dopaminergic drugs used to control the symptoms of Parkinson disease. Amantadine (Symmetrel) was originally introduced as an antiviral agent for the prophylaxis of Influenza A but was unexpectedly found to cause improvement in symptoms. The patient may achieve good control of symptoms for a while with these drugs but patients develop tolerance to the drugs, requiring frequent readjustment of doses and medications.

ADVERSE REACTIONS

Dopaminergic agents may produce dysrhythmias (irregular heartbeats), muscle twitching, psychotic reactions, rigidity, diarrhea, epigastric distress, GI bleeding, nausea, vomiting, blurred vision, alopecia, bitter taste, hot flashes, rash, and urinary retention.

Anticholinergic agents may cause postural hypotension (low blood pressure when a person suddenly stands up), tachycardia, agitation, confusion, depression, headache, memory loss, muscle cramping, constipation, vomiting, diplopia (double vision), increased intraocular pressure, decreased sweating, flushing, dry mouth, and skin rash.

Early signs of toxicity in the patient taking dopaminergic agents include muscle twitching and blepharospasm (eyelid spasms). Overdosage is a common phenomenon, particularly with long-term drug therapy. It is recognizable because the patient experiences a sudden onset of progressively worsening parkinsonian symptoms. These drugs should be tapered gradually.

DRUG INTERACTIONS

Common drug interactions differ, according to whether the preparation is an anticholinergic or a dopaminergic agent. These drugs commonly interact with many types of medications; product information must be closely studied. These patients often take antipsychotics, which have the potential to interact with these antiparkinson drugs. Two herbal products, ginkgo and grape seed, are commonly used to treat symptoms of Parkinson disease. The Complementary and Alternative Therapies box summarizes these products and their drug interactions.

❖ NURSING IMPLICATIONS AND PATIENT TEACHING

■ Assessment

Learn as much as possible about the health history of the patient, including hypersensitivity; drugs currently being taken that may produce drug interactions; asthma, renal, liver, and cardiovascular disease and epilepsy; other contraindications for the drug; and the possibility of pregnancy.

The patient may have a history of Parkinson disease, drooling, or difficulty with coordination and walking. The patient may be taking an antipsychotic drug; with long-term use, these drugs can cause tardive dyskinesia, with symptoms similar to those of Parkinson disease. The patient may be middle-aged or an older adult and may have tremors at rest that are made worse by emotional stress. The arms may fail to move when walking, with rigidity first occurring in the proximal musculature, and the patient may be unable to perform activities of daily living.

■ Diagnosis

These patients frequently have other problems as a result of their medical diagnosis. Ataxia (staggered walking) frequently leads to falls and soft-tissue and bone injuries. They may have breakdown of the skin, poor hygiene, poor nutrition, or other problems related to immobility or difficulty walking, cooking, and so on. Their intelligence and ability to understand may be underestimated when they are unable to communicate well. They are frequently angry, depressed, and lonely. If the nurse is willing to spend the time learning to communicate with the patient, they will gain a clear picture of the multitude of problems relevant to the patient.

Complementary and Alternative Therapies

Parkinson Disease

PRODUCT	COMMENTS
Ginkgo	Potential interaction with anticoagulants, aspirin, NSAIDs, and antiplatelet agents; may interact with MAO inhibitors and acetylcholinesterase inhibitors.
Grape seed	Potential interaction with anticoagulants, aspirin, NSAIDs, antiplatelet agents, and methotrexate.

Data from Krinsky DL, LaValle JB, Hawkins EB, et al: *Natural therapeutics pocket guide*, ed 2, Hudson, Ohio, 2003, Lexi-Comp, Inc.

■ Planning

There is a wide variety of medications given for Parkinson's disease and medications are frequently changed as patients develop tolerance to them. See Table 16-6 for details about specific agents. Anticholinergic agents are contraindicated for persons with known hypersensitivity, acute narrow-angle glaucoma, asthma, history of epilepsy, peptic ulcer disease, and skin lesions. Persons on CNS stimulants, those exposed to rubella (measles), those with acute psychoses, those with a history of melanoma, or patients receiving MAO inhibitor therapy should not take these medications. These drugs are known to aggravate many other diseases and must be used with caution.

The anticholinergics and some dopaminergics must be withdrawn slowly, because many of these drugs have a long half-life. When withdrawing one preparation and beginning a new preparation, the new drug should be started in small doses and the old drug should be withdrawn gradually. These agents are usually initiated at the lowest dosage possible, and the dosage is increased gradually until the maximum therapeutic effect has been obtained.

■ Implementation

These drugs are available in tablets, sustained-release capsules, syrup, and elixir. They are generally well absorbed from the GI tract. Peak blood levels of carbidopa-levodopa (Sinemet), one of the main treatment drugs, are achieved in 1 to 6 hours, depending on the route of administration and the type of drug administered, except for the sustained-release capsules, which reach peak plasma blood levels in 8 to 12 hours. Sustained-release capsules are not recommended for initial therapy, because they do not allow enough flexibility in dosage regulation. IV injection of anticholinergics can cause hypotension and incoordination.

Although dopamine cannot cross the blood-brain barrier, levodopa can move into the brain, where it is converted into dopamine. However, levodopa alone becomes less effective over time, and side effects are related to the dose. Therefore carbidopa and levodopa are often administered together, usually as a fixed-combination product (Sinemet). Carbidopa is added to prevent peripheral breakdown of levodopa and reduce the overall dose of levodopa required.

If this combination drug is administered after levodopa therapy, the levodopa should be discontinued at least 8 hours before initiating therapy with carbidopa-levodopa. The carbidopa-levodopa combination should be substituted at a dosage level that provides 25% of the previous levodopa dose. When the fixed-combination dose is excessive, carbidopa can be given separately with levodopa so that each drug can be titrated individually.

Table 16-6 summarizes the important medications used to treat Parkinson disease.

■ Evaluation

Long-term use of dopaminergic and anticholinergic agents often leads to akinesia (loss of movement), tardive dyskinesia (abnormal and involuntary movements especially of the lower face), and dystonia (impairment of muscle tone). To reverse these effects, the dosage is likely to be reduced to the minimum effective level and very slow and careful changes in dosages made as necessary to avoid overmedication.

Numerous laboratory tests may be altered by these medications; this should be taken into account when monitoring patient status.

■ Patient and Family Teaching

Tell the patient and family the following:
• The patient should take any of the prescribed medications exactly as ordered by the nurse,

Table 16-6   Antiparkinsonian Drugs

GENERIC NAME	TRADE NAME	COMMENTS
Anticholinergic Drugs		
benztropine	Cogentin	Contains anticholinergic and antihistamine properties. Pharmacologically, drug inhibits excessive cholinergic activity in striatal fibers. Used to treat extrapyramidal symptoms (except tardive dyskinesia) induced by antipsychotic agents. IM injection provides rapid (15 min) relief from acute dystonic reactions. Oral doses of the drug are cumulative; therefore therapy should begin with a low dose and increase gradually at 5- to 6-day intervals as necessary. Used for parkinsonian symptoms and drug-induced extrapyramidal side effects.
biperiden	Akineton	Blocks central cholinergic receptors, restoring balance between cholinergic and dopaminergic activity in basal ganglia. IV or IM administration may produce incoordination. Used for parkinsonian symptoms and drug-induced extrapyramidal side effects.
diphenhydramine ★	Benadryl	Blocks receptors on peripheral effector cells. Used in idiopathic parkinsonism treatment.
trihexyphenidyl	Artane	Exerts direct inhibitory effect on the parasympathetic nervous system. Decreases rigidity, but most other symptoms improve to some degree.
Dopaminergic Drugs		
amantadine	Symmetrel	This drug enhances release of dopamine from presynaptic nerve endings. Drug has no anticholinergic activity. Used for parkinsonian symptoms and drug-induced extrapyramidal side effects.
bromocriptine	Parlodel	Directly stimulates dopamine receptors in corpus striatum; especially helpful in patients who are beginning to deteriorate or develop tolerance to levodopa.
carbidopa	Lodosyn	Used with levodopa to slow the breakdown of levodopa; has no therapeutic action itself. Used when treatment requires separate titration of each drug.
carbidopa-levodopa	Sinemet–10/100 Sinemet–25/100 Sinemet–25/250 Sinemet–50/200	Fixed-combination antiparkinsonian agent used in all types of treatment of Parkinson disease. Composed of both carbidopa and levodopa. Tablet strength indicated by numbering (mg carbidopa/mg levodopa). For patients not receiving levodopa: 1 tablet (10/100 or 25/100) 3 times daily initially; increased by 1 tablet daily until a maximum of 8 tablets is given. For patients receiving levodopa, levodopa must be discontinued at least 8 hr before initiating therapy with this product. Administer 1 tablet (25/250) 3 to 4 times daily to patients previously requiring 1500 mg or more of levodopa each day.
entacapone	Comtan	Used as adjunct to carbidopa-levodopa to treat patients with idiopathic Parkinson disease who experience the signs and symptoms of end-of-dose "wearing-off." Given as 200-mg tablet with each carbidopa-levodopa dosage.
levodopa	Dopar Larodopa	A metabolic precursor of dopamine. Enters CNS by crossing blood-brain barrier and is converted to dopamine.
selegiline	Eldepryl Carbex	Irreversible MAO inhibitor. Usual dose 5 mg at breakfast and lunch; allows carbidopa-levodopa dosages to be reduced.
tolcapone	Tasmar	May cause hallucinations and tardive dyskinesia. Give without food and always as adjunctive therapy to carbidopa-levodopa therapy.
Dopamine Receptor Agonists, Nonergot		
pramipexole	Mirapex	Binds with high affinity to dopamine D_3 receptors. May stimulate dopamine receptors in the striatum. Follow precise dosing schedule in package insert.
ropinirole	Requip	Follow precise dosing schedule listed in package insert.

CNS, Central nervous system; *IM,* intramuscular; *IV,* intravenous; *MAO,* monoamine oxidase.
★ Indicates "Must-Know Drugs," or the 35 drugs most prescribers use.

physician, or other health care provider. Clinical improvements are cumulative and may take 2 to 3 weeks, so the patient should not stop taking the medication unless advised to do so by the health care provider.

- Antiparkinsonian agents should be taken after meals to avoid stomach upset.
- The patient taking levodopa (Larodopa) should avoid taking vitamin preparations with vitamin B_6 (pyridoxine) as the vitamin accelerates the inactivation of the drug. If the paient takes levodopa-carbadopa (Sinemet), this interaction does not exist.
- The nurse, physician, or other health care provider should be contacted immediately if parkinsonian symptoms become suddenly worse, if intermittent winking or muscle twitching occurs, or if abdominal pain, constipation, distention, or urinary problems occur.
- Common side effects include dry mouth, dizziness, drowsiness, and GI symptoms. Some patients experience dizziness or light-headedness, especially as they move from lying to standing positions. The patient should avoid driving or tasks requiring alertness or rapid changes of movement.
- The patient's urine, sweat, and saliva may darken after exposure to air.
- The patient should avoid overexertion during hot weather.
- Periodic eye examinations are necessary when taking anticholinergic drugs.

 Clinical Goldmine

Controlling Adverse Effects

Most of the drugs used to treat Parkinson's Disease have numerous possible adverse effects associated with them. Decreasing the dosage of many of these products can control the numerous adverse effects of these drugs. When this is not possible, the prescribed drugs often need to be changed. The nurse should be especially watchful for the development of adverse side effects and report them immediately.

PSYCHOTHERAPEUTIC AGENTS

OVERVIEW

Many of the drugs introduced in the following subsections act on more than one type of neuroreceptor. Each agent acts differently, making it possible for certain drugs to be given for specific actions without many adverse reactions. It should be clear that if dosages are exceeded, many receptors may be excessively stimulated, causing widespread and serious effects.

❖ ANTIANXIETY AGENTS

Anxiety is a common problem associated with many medical and surgical conditions, as well as a primary symptom in many psychiatric disorders. Anxiety is a normal human emotion, but when it is felt too frequently or interferes with a person's ability to perform activities of daily living, it is considered abnormal. There are a number of disorders associated with anxiety. Anxiety creates subjective feelings of helplessness, indecision, worry, apprehension, and irritability. Patients may complain of headache, gastric distress, and inability to concentrate. It may also produce objective symptoms of restlessness, tremor, constipation, diarrhea, nausea, and muscle tension. Insomnia is one of the most common problems associated with anxiety.

Specific regions of the brain produce symptoms of anxiety. There are a number of strategies that are used to prevent, control, or treat anxiety. When anxiety is so severe that it must be treated with medication, antianxiety medications such as benzodiazepines are used to reduce some of the symptoms. They do not prevent the anxiety, because the feelings or problems that produce the anxiety are still there. These are the products commonly referred to as tranquilizers. Some other medications such as the SSRIs act at the level of the brain to prevent feelings of anxiety. In general, antianxiety medication should be used for only a short time until other remedies can be found. It is especially important to view the use of these medications as a short-term solution because of the potential for addiction of these agents.

The major products used today for anxiety are the benzodiazepines, accounting for approximately 75% of the antianxiety prescriptions written today. Although benzodiazepines have a variety of uses, there are particular drugs in this category that are used primarily for treating anxiety. These drugs are intended primarily for short-term treatment of anxiety or related insomnia. Other antianxiety agents are briefly included in this discussion.

The other drugs used for treating anxiety are categorized as nonbezodiazepine antianxiety agents. These include buspirone (BuSpar), doxepin (Sinequan), and hydroxyzine (Hypan and Vistaril).

ACTION

Benzodiazepines are thought to act at the limbic, thalamic, and hypothalamic levels of the CNS, producing a calming effect.

USES

Benzodiazepines such as alprazolam (Xanax) and diazepam (Valium), as well and nonbenzodiazepines, are used to relieve anxiety, tension, and fears that occur by themselves or as the result of illness. Other indications include management of delirium tremens after alcohol withdrawal; premedication for surgical and endoscopic procedures or electric cardioversion; treatment of convulsive disorders (diazepam only); and relief of muscle spasm.

ADVERSE REACTIONS

Adverse reactions to antianxiety agents include hypotension, tachycardia, clumsiness, confusion, depression, drowsiness, fatigue, headache, insomnia, paradoxical reactions (excitement, hallucinations, agitation, hostility, or rage), syncope (light-headedness and fainting), unsteadiness, visual disturbances, weakness, anorexia, constipation, difficulty swallowing, dry mouth, hiccups, jaundice, nausea, vomiting, urinary retention, blood cell changes, pruritus, skin rash, joint pain, and unexplained sore throat and fever.

Overdosage may produce sleepiness, confusion, coma, diminished reflexes, and hypotension. Tolerance is easily developed.

DRUG INTERACTIONS

Giving benzodiazepines along with any of the following substances may increase the effect of either agent: alcohol; anesthetics; MAO inhibitors; or CNS depressants such as antihistamines, barbiturates, phenothiazines, narcotics, sedatives, tranquilizers, hypnotics, anticonvulsants, or tricyclic antidepressants (TCAs). Caffeinated products and excessive cigarette smoking can antagonize (decrease) the anxiolytic (antianxiety) effect of these drugs. Herbal products are also often used by patients to treat stress and anxiety. The Complementary and Alternative Therapies box summarizes herbal preparations the patient may be using and their drug interactions.

Complementary and Alternative Therapies

Stress and Anxiety

PRODUCT	COMMENTS
Chamomile	No reported toxicities
Kava kava	Potential interactions with ethanol and CNS depressants
St. John's wort	Potential interactions with antidepressants (including SSRIs, tricyclics, MAO inhibitors), narcotics, other CNS depressants, reserpine, and digoxin
Valerian	Increased effect and toxicity with CNS depressants, sedative-hypnotics (barbiturates), antidepressants, anxiolytics, and antihistamines

Data from Krinsky DL, LaValle JB, Hawkins EB, et al: *Natural therapeutics pocket guide*, ed 2, Hudson, Ohio, 2003, Lexi-Comp, Inc.

❖ NURSING IMPLICATIONS AND PATIENT TEACHING

▪ Assessment

Learn as much as possible about the health history of the patient, including hypersensitivities, underlying systemic disease (especially pulmonary, cardiac, liver,

or renal disease; epilepsy or seizures; myasthenia gravis; mental illness; and drug abuse or dependence), possibility of pregnancy, breastfeeding, or whether the patient is currently taking any medications (both prescribed and OTC) that may produce drug interactions. These conditions are contraindications or precautions to the use of antianxiety agents.

Memory Jogger

Benzodiazepines

The patient should be given the smallest dosage possible to reduce the risk for overdose, particularly in those patients with a history of drug addiction or dependence.

The patient may have a history of feelings of apprehension, uncertainty, fear, an unpleasant state of tension, a sense of impending doom, insomnia (inability to sleep), irritability, hypersensitivity to stress, difficulty in concentrating, or nightmares.

▪ Diagnosis

In addition to the medical diagnosis, what other problems does the patient experience? Does he or she have family support, or is he or she isolated and lonely? Is the patient able to work and take care of daily needs, or is the patient incapacitated with anxiety? Does the patient have to drive long distances or do careful, precision work that requires steady muscles and nerves?

▪ Planning

Older adult patients (older than age 60) and those with chronic illnesses may require a decreased initial dosage and may need careful monitoring of individual response before changes in dosage are made. These drugs are potentially harmful in the elderly if the patient is not closely supervised. Benzodiazepines generally have a long half-life and can have cumulative effects. Patients with a history of seizures or epilepsy should have their dosages of benzodiazepines tapered slowly.

▪ Implementation

Administering the benzodiazepines during or immediately after meals decreases the incidence of GI side effects. The manufacturers' instructions for diluting and slowly injecting parenteral medications should be followed to prevent the possibility of severe respiratory depression and failure.

Patients with anxiety are often depressed and depressed patients may have anxiety. Because both conditions are so commonly seen together, patients should be questioned and observed for suicidal tendencies.

Treatment with antianxiety agents should proceed slowly in older adults, the debilitated, those with limited pulmonary reserve, and those in whom a hypotensive episode might precipitate heart problems.

Clinical Pitfall

Benzodiazepines

Benzodiazepines are stored in adipose (fat) tissue, which increases their half-life or the time that they are in the body. This makes these drugs dangerous, particularly for older patients for whom the symptoms of overdosage are often severe.

Table 16-7 summarizes important dosage information about antianxiety medications.

▪ Evaluation

Mental alertness, cognitive functions, and physical abilities may be impaired with the use of antianxiety agents. These drugs should be given in conjunction with counseling or psychotherapy for maximum benefit.

Abrupt termination of these agents may cause delayed withdrawal symptoms (up to 1 week later) of abdominal or muscle cramps, vomiting, diaphoresis (sweating), tremor, or convulsions. Tapering the dosage for patients on long-term therapy helps prevent this problem.

Take the patient's blood pressure lying, sitting, and standing to monitor for hypotensive changes.

Alternatives for coping with stress and change should be discussed with the patient. For example, increased regular physical activity, muscle relaxation exercises, and participation in hobbies may be helpful.

▪ Patient and Family Teaching

Tell the patient and family the following:
- The patient should take this medication exactly as ordered and not stop taking the medication

Table 16-7 Antianxiety Medications

GENERIC NAME	TRADE NAME	COMMENTS
Benzodiazepines		
alprazolam	Xanax	Action peaks in 1-2 hr; half-life 12-15 hr. Effectiveness and safety in children younger than the age of 18 have not been determined. Give reduced dosage in older adult or debilitated patients.
chlordiazepoxide	H-Tran Librium	Peak levels in 1-4 hr; half-life 5-30 hr. Food or antacids slow absorption. Injection IV must be very slow to avoid producing respiratory arrest. Give reduced dosage in older adult or debilitated patients.
clorazepate	Tranxene	Peak effect in 60 min; half-life 2 days. Some reports indicate a fall in hematocrit with long-term use. Can be given once each day. Give reduced dosage in older adult or debilitated patients.
diazepam ★	Valium	Peak blood levels reached within 1-2 hr; half-life 20-50 hr. Anxiety and management of convulsive disorders. Also used for skeletal muscle spasm. Give reduced dosage in older adult or debilitated patients.
lorazepam	Ativan	Action peaks in 2½ hr; half-life 10-15 hr. Patients may experience withdrawal manifested as insomnia 2 or 3 nights after cessation of therapy. IM injection used as a preanesthetic agent for adults only. Also given IV for sedation and relief of anxiety. Used for anxiety and insomnia. Give reduced dosage in older adult or debilitated patients.
oxazepam	Serax	Peak blood levels at 2-4 hr; half-life 5-20 hr. Low incidence of toxicity. Used for anxiety. Give reduced dosage in older adult or debilitated patients.
Nonbenzodiazepine Antianxiety Agents		
buspirone	BuSpar	Approved for short-term use in anxiety disorders. Mechanism of action unknown; chemically unrelated to other antianxiety medications.
doxepin	Sinequan	For oral concentrate, do not mix with grape juice.
hydroxyzine	Hy-Pam Vistaril	Antihistamine for symptomatic relief of anxiety, especially in psychoneurosis. Also has analgesic activity that may be helpful in relieving pruritus caused by allergies. Medication may be used preoperatively for surgery or obstetric patients to permit decrease in narcotic dosages, reduce anxiety, and control emesis. Product also helps control acutely disturbed or hysterical patients. For IM use only. Caution: subcutaneous, intraarterial, or IV use may produce tissue necrosis and hemolysis.

IM, Intramuscular; *IV,* intravenous.
★ Indicates "Must-Know Drugs," or the 35 drugs most prescribers use.

unless advised to do so by the nurse, physician, or other health care provider. If a dose is forgotten, it should be taken as soon as it is remembered, if it is within 1 to 2 hours of the regular dosage time. If it is later than 2 hours, the patient should skip the dose and take the next dose at the regular time. The patient should not double the dosage. The patient must keep regular appointments with the nurse, physician, or other health care provider so that progress can be checked and side effects of the drug can be monitored.

- Antianxiety agents can cause dizziness, lightheadedness, drowsiness, and unsteadiness. They may decrease the patient's ability to think or react clearly and quickly. The patient should not drive, operate hazardous machinery, or perform activities requiring alertness until response to the drug has been determined. These symptoms often disappear after the patient has taken the medication for several weeks. Additionally, the patient should change to sitting or standing positions slowly to minimize these symptoms and prevent falls.
- The patient should notify the nurse, physician, or other health care provider if any new or troublesome symptoms occur while taking this medication (e.g., ulcers or sores in the mouth, hallucinations, feelings of confusion, difficulty sleeping, skin rash, jaundice, bradycardia [slow heartbeat], difficulty with breathing, sore throat and fever, unusual nervousness, excitement, irritability, depression, or eye pain).
- This medication must be kept out of the reach of children and all others for whom it is not prescribed.
- The nurse, physician, or other health care provider should be informed if the patient begins taking any new prescription or nonprescription drugs. Many different medications have interactions with antianxiety agents; therefore the health care provider may want to increase or decrease the dosage.
- The patient should not drink any alcohol while taking this medicine.
- The patient should be aware that cigarette smoking and the use of caffeinated beverages (coffee, tea, cola) can decrease the effect of antianxiety agents.
- Benzodiazepines are not intended for use by pregnant women. If the patient is pregnant or breastfeeding, or if the patient should become pregnant while taking this medicine, the nurse, physician, or other health care provider should be informed immediately.
- This drug may be habit forming; the patient should use it for the least time possible.

❖ ANTIDEPRESSANTS
OVERVIEW

Depression, whether mild or so severe that it interferes with activities of daily living, has been recognized for centuries. Most people have days when they feel "down" or "blue." Sometimes people have good reasons to be depressed. But intense and prolonged inability to interact with others, go to work, and keep up with the activities of daily life represent more significant depression. Sometimes hormones, substance abuse, or medications taken for other problems may produce depression. There may be a family history of depression, as some conditions seem genetic. There are several different categories of depression including milder dysthymic disorder, major depressive disorder, and bipolar disorder. Many types of therapy have been explored, but only in the last 30 years have medications been discovered that significantly help improve a patient's mood without extensive side or adverse effects from each drug. Although all medications are equally effective in treating depression if they work, not all patients respond to all medications and patients may experience different side effects with each drug. So if a patient does not respond to one drug, there are many more drugs which might be tried to see which has the best antidepressant effect and the fewest side effects. Research has demonstrated that the best treatment for severe depression involves both psychotherapy and medication.

There are now several new categories of drugs that are used in treating depression. These drugs elevate the mood by affecting neurotransmitters in the brain, primarily norepinephrine and serotonin (Figures 16-3 and 16-4). MAO inhibitors were initially used to treat other diseases. The antidepressant effect was discovered as an unexpected side effect of that therapy. They were then used to treat depressed patients until TCA therapy became available in the 1960s. MAO inhibitors are now ordered primarily when tricyclic therapy is unsatisfactory. In the last few years, a number of other drugs have entered the field for treatment of depressed patients, including several that act on serotonin or norepinephrine reuptake. Each of these groups is discussed separately.

All antidepressants now carry a black box warning detailing the risk of suicide in children and adolescents who are taking medications. The antidepressants may cause young adults to become suicidal, so the benefit must be weighed against the risk of increased suicidality. Patients taking these medications must be observed closely for clinical worsening, suicidality, or unusual changes in behavior, particularly within the first few months of starting therapy or when dosage changes.

None of these drugs should be abruptly stopped by the patient. Care must be taken to teach the patient about gradually reducing the drugs as directed by

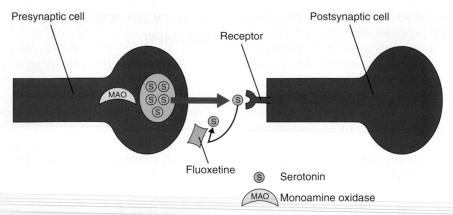

Presynaptic cell

Postsynaptic cell

Receptor

Fluoxetine

Ⓢ Serotonin

MAO Monoamine oxidase

FIGURE 16-3 Normal release, reuptake, and destruction of the monoamine transmitters.

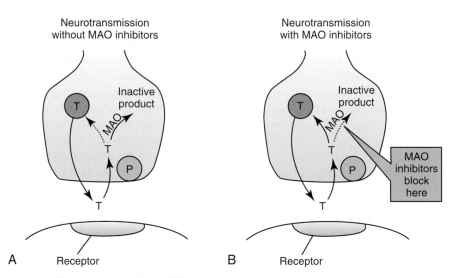

Neurotransmission
without MAO inhibitors

Neurotransmission
with MAO inhibitors

Inactive
product

Inactive
product

MAO
inhibitors
block
here

A   Receptor

B   Receptor

FIGURE 16-4 Mechanism of action of monoamine oxidase inhibitors. A, Under normal conditions, most of the norepinephrine or serotonin that undergoes reuptake into nerve terminals is inactivated by MAO. Inactivation keeps the right amount of transmitter within the nerve terminal. B, MAO inhibitors prevent inactivation of norepinephrine and serotonin, thereby there is more transmitter available for release. Release of supranormal amounts of transmitter intensifies transmission. (MAO = monoamine oxidase, P = uptake pump; T = transmitter [norepinephrine or serotonin]).

the health care provider when the drug is to be discontinued.

TRICYCLIC ANTIDEPRESSANTS

ACTION

The antidepressant effect of tricyclics is not completely understood. It is thought that tricyclic antidepressants (TCAs) potentiate the effects of or inhibit the uptake of norepinephrine andserotonin (biogenic amines) by the presynaptic neuronal membrane in the CNS, thereby increasing the concentration of these biogenic amines at the synapse.

USES

TCAs are used primarily to relieve the symptoms of severe depression that has internal biologic causes (endogenous depression). They may also be used to treat mild depression caused by factors in the patient's

life (exogenous or reactive depression), which is not self-limiting and does not interfere with usual activities of daily living. They are less commonly used for bipolar disorders as adjunctive or additional therapy.

ADVERSE REACTIONS

Adverse reactions to TCAs include dysrhythmias, postural hypotension, confusion, headache, drowsiness that lasts a long time, constipation, nausea, vomiting, blood dyscrasias, fever, photosensitivity, pruritus, skin rash, muscle twitching, tremors, urinary hesitancy or retention, altered liver function tests, blurred vision, and nervousness.

Overdosage may initially produce stimulation of the CNS, resulting in irritability, agitation, hallucinations, delirium, twitching, hypertonia, hyperreflexia, nystagmus, hyperpyrexia (very high body temperature), hypertension, and seizures (more commonly seen in children). This initial CNS stimulation is followed by CNS depression, causing drowsiness, areflexia, hypothermia (abnormally low body temperature), hypotension, dysrhythmias, respiratory depression, coma, or cardiorespiratory arrest.

DRUG INTERACTIONS

TCA increase the CNS depressant effect of alcohol and other CNS depressants, particularly ethchlorvynol (Placidyl). The effects of anticonvulsants may be decreased when used with TCAs. The antihypertensive effects of guanethidine (Ismelin) and clonidine (Catapres) may be blocked when used with most TCAs, with the exception of doxepin (Sinequan). There may be a reduction in the antidepressant effect of tricyclics and an increase in their side effects when used concurrently with estrogen, including oral contraceptives containing estrogen. An increased incidence of cardiac dysrhythmias has been found with concurrent use of thyroid medication and TCAs. Severe hypertension or hyperpyrexia may result when TCAs are used with MAO inhibitors or sympathomimetics.

❖ NURSING IMPLICATIONS AND PATIENT TEACHING

■ Assessment

Learn as much as possible about the health history of the patient; allergy, disease, and other medications the patient may currently be taking, including OTC preparations, must be considered. Many diseases present contraindications or precautions for the use of tricyclic drugs. Patients may be taking herbal remedies to help with symptoms of depression. The Complementary and Alternative Therapies box provides a summary of herbal products and their drug interactions.

Complementary and Alternative Therapies

Depression

PRODUCT	COMMENTS
St. John's wort	Potential interaction with antidepressants (including SSRIs, tricyclics, MAO inhibitors), narcotics, other CNS depressants, reserpine, and digoxin
Ginkgo	Potential interaction with anticoagulants, aspirin, NSAIDs, antiplatelet agents, MAO inhibitors, and acetylcholinesterase inhibitors

Data from Krinsky DL, LaValle JB, Hawkins EB, et al: *Natural therapeutics pocket guide*, ed 2, Hudson, Ohio, 2003, Lexi-Comp, Inc.

Patients experiencing clinical depression may have a history of insomnia, early morning awakening, anorexia, constipation, loss of motivation, and fatigue. They may express feelings of hopelessness and pessimism, say negative things about themselves, respond slowly to questions, and have slowed motor movements, decreased facial expression, and stooped posture. Assess these patients thoroughly for any suicidal feelings.

■ Diagnosis

What problems does the depressed patient have that necessitate nursing intervention? Does the patient eat, bathe, and dress appropriately? Has contact with other people been cut off? Is the patient unable to work? Any of these problems may be addressed once the therapeutic effects of antidepressant medication have eased the patient's immediate crisis.

■ Planning

If the patient has taken any antidepressant drugs before, get a careful history about what medications they took and their response, including any adverse effects. TCAs should not be given if the patient has a history of hypersensitivity to a TCA. A patient who is hypersensitive to one type of tricyclic will likely be sensitive to all tricyclics (cross-sensitivity). Patients with a history of recent myocardial infarction, narrow-angle glaucoma, or severe hepatic or renal failure also should not take these drugs. TCAs should be used very carefully with MAO inhibitors. Discuss the importance of contraception with women of childbearing age who are taking TCAs.

Antidepressants may cause patients with bipolar disorder to go into the manic phase of their illness; exaggerated symptoms of paranoid ideation and schizophrenia may develop in patients who have these disorders. The prescribing health care provider may need to reduce the dosage of the TCA or add a medication to reduce anxiety.

Antidepressants are started in low doses which are increased slowly until the depression is relieved or adverse effects develop. Prescriptions are often given for only the smallest but reasonable amount of antidepressant because the patients should be regarded as potentially suicidal. Patients should be observed taking their pills so they cannot save them up and take them all at one time.

■ Implementation

It is often difficult to determine the most appropriate dose for the patient. The plasma concentrations of TCAs vary widely and may not correspond well with the dosage or therapeutic effects. Thus, the initial and maintenance dosages of these drugs must be carefully determined, based on the patient's age, physical health status, and response to the drug.

Patient's may experience drowsiness or sedation with the initial dose, especially when the patient is taking a tricyclic known to have moderate to strong sedative effects. Therefore TCA therapy will likely be started with a single bedtime dose, especially for

Table 16-8 Tricyclic Antidepressants

GENERIC NAME	TRADE NAME	COMMENTS
amitriptyline ★		Strong sedative effect, especially early in therapy. Should be taken at bedtime to decrease daytime drowsiness. Used to treat endogenous depression accompanied by anxiety.
doxepin	Sinequan	Has marked sedative effect, particularly during initial phase of therapy. Used to treat psychotic and psychoneurotic depression with associated anxiety and somatic symptoms. Oral concentrate should be diluted in milk, fruit juice, or water before administration.
imipramine	Tofranil	Used to treat endogenous depression; only tricyclic that is also used to treat enuresis in children.
nortriptyline	Aventyl	Used to treat endogenous depression.

★ Indicates "Must-Know Drugs," or the 35 drugs most prescribers use.

patients who are depressed and also have a sleep disturbance. Typically, the drug dosage is then adjusted or titrated to achieve the best response with the lowest dosage and minimal side effects. A maintenance dosage, administered in divided doses or as a single bedtime dose, may be continued for 6 months to 1 year. The patient should be reevaluated at this time to determine the course of therapy.

Table 16-8 summarizes the important information nurses should know about TCA medications.

▪ Evaluation

The desired antidepressant effect of the drug will usually occur within 3 to 4 weeks after therapy is initiated.

If a TCA is given in large doses or for a long time, the drug should be stopped by gradually reducing the dose over 4 to 8 weeks to avoid withdrawal symptoms of general listlessness, headache, and nausea.

▪ Patient and Family Teaching

Tell the patient and family the following:
- The patient should take this TCA medication exactly as ordered. It may be taken with food to avoid gastric distress. It may take up to 8 weeks before the patient begins to feel better. Therefore it is important to take the drug in the exact amount and frequency specified, even though the patient notices no changes initially.
- TCAs should never be stopped suddenly, because there could be an increase in symptoms, as well as nausea, headache, and feelings of listlessness. The patient must not stop taking the drug without talking to the nurse, physician, or other health care provider.
- TCAs may cause drowsiness or make the patient feel less alert than usual. If so, the patient should avoid driving or doing other activities that require alertness. This feeling should pass after the medication is taken for a short time. The patient should tell the health care provider if drowsiness or decreased alertness persists longer than 2 weeks and interferes with usual activities.
- Dryness of the mouth may occur when medication is first started. Chewing sugarless gum, sucking on hard candy, or rinsing the mouth frequently may help relieve the dryness.
- Some TCAs, particularly amitriptyline (Elavil), cause a red or pink color in the urine. This drug also causes photosensitivity and the patient should be warned about exposure to the sun.
- TCAs will increase the effects of alcohol, sleeping pills, and some medications for the relief of colds and hay fever. The patient should avoid alcohol and check with the health care provider before taking any other medications.
- TCAs are very powerful drugs and must be kept out of the reach of children and others for whom they are not prescribed. They should not be left on dressers or low bedside tables.
- Light-headedness, dizziness, or feelings of faintness occur in some people taking this drug, especially older people. To reduce this feeling, the patient should move slowly, especially when changing from a lying or sitting position to standing upright.
- A surgeon will generally require that TCAs are stopped several days before the patient has any surgery that requires anesthesia. The prescribing health care provider must develop a plan to gradually stop the medication in the correct way and evaluate when the patient should start taking the medicine again.
- The health care provider should be contacted if the patient develops any new or troublesome symptoms, especially the appearance of urinary retention, constipation, blurred vision, or excessive sleepiness.
- If the patient will be taking this medication for a long time, a MedicAlert bracelet or necklace or a wallet medical identification card listing this drug is advised.

MONOAMINE OXIDASE INHIBITORS (MAOIS)

ACTION

MAO is an enzyme found in the mitochondria of cells located in nerve endings and other body tissues such as the kidney, liver, and intestines. This enzyme normally acts as a catalyst by inactivating dopamine, norepinephrine, epinephrine, and serotonin (biogenic amines) and therefore regulating the intracellular levels of these neurotransmitters. MAO inhibitors block the inactivation of the biogenic amines, resulting in an increased concentration of dopamine, epinephrine, norepinephrine, and serotonin at neuronal synapses. The antidepressant effects of MAO inhibitors such as phenelzine (Nardil) or tranylcypromine (Parnate) are thought to be directly related to this increased concentration of biogenic amines.

Clinical Pitfall

MAO Inhibitors

MAO inhibitors may cause very dangerous reactions if taken with certain foods or beverages containing tyramines. The patient must not eat foods such as cheese, yogurt, sour cream, raisins, bananas, avocados, bean pods, chicken livers, or pickled herring and should avoid meat tenderizers and soy sauce. Only very small amounts of coffee, tea, cola drinks, and chocolate are permitted.

USES

MAO inhibitors are used to relieve the symptoms of severe reactive or endogenous depression that have not responded to TCA therapy, electroconvulsive therapy, or other modes of psychotherapy. Effects may be seen within days but the full antidepressant effect is often delayed for weeks. MAO inhibitors are considered second-line treatment for depression because of their serious adverse effects. MAO inhibitors are not approved for use in children.

ADVERSE REACTIONS

Adverse reactions to MAO inhibitors include postural hypotension, dysrhythmias, ataxia, drowsiness, hallucinations, headache, hyperactivity, insomnia, seizures, tremors, vertigo, anorexia, constipation, diarrhea, nausea, vomiting, fever, photosensitivity, skin rash, dysuria (painful urination), incontinence, blurred vision, dry mouth, edema, and impotence.

Overdosage produces mental confusion, restlessness, hypotension, respiratory depression, tachycardia, seizures, and shock, which may persist for 1 to 2 weeks.

DRUG AND FOOD INTERACTIONS

MAO inhibitors have many drug interactions. The potential for drug interactions differs between agents based upon the type of MAO inhibition that occurs.

Drugs that inhibit MAO A may interact with other serotonergic agents, causing a potentially fatal serotonin syndrome characterized by mental status changes, myoclonus, fever, and tremor. Therefore, concurrent use of MAO A inhibitors with medications such as SSRIs, meperidine, dextromethorphan, sumatriptan, and buspirone should be avoided. Conversely, MAO B inhibitors, such as selegiline, may interact with other dominergic drugs such as amantadine and bromocriptine.

MAOIs may potentiate the CNS depressant effect of alcohol, anesthetics, sedatives, hypnotics, and narcotics and may cause severe hypertension and hyperpyrexia. If they are used with anticonvulsants, they may cause a change in the seizure pattern of the patient, and the dosage of the anticonvulsant medication may have to be adjusted accordingly. The hypotensive effects of diuretics and antihypertensives may be enhanced when those agents are used with MAO inhibitors. The hypoglycemic effects of insulin or oral hypoglycemics may be enhanced by MAO inhibitors, and dosages may require adjustment accordingly. MAO inhibitors and tricyclic antidepressants are generally not used together because hyperpyrexia, severe convulsions, hypertensive crisis, and death may result. MAOIs should not be given with other MAOIs drugs.

Foods with more than 6 mg of tyramine per serving must be avoided: These include aged and mature cheeses, air-dried sausages (e.g., pepperoni), fermented soy products (soy and teriyaki sauce), sauerkraut, and all tap beers, to name a few.

Memory Jogger

Food and Beverage Interactions

Sudden and severe hypertension crisis can result when MAO inhibitors are used with the following foods and beverages, which are high in tyramine and other vasopressor amines: alcoholic beverages such as beer and wines (particularly sherry, hearty red wines, and Chianti), yeast extracts, meat tenderizers, soy sauce, beef or chicken liver, cured meats, dried or cured fish, sausage prepared with yeast, pickled herring, bean pods, figs, raisins, bananas, avocados, fava beans, sour cream, yogurt, and cheese. Concurrent use of MAO inhibitors and large amounts of caffeine-containing products (coffee, tea, cola, chocolate) can cause hypertension and cardiac dysrhythmias.

❖ NURSING IMPLICATIONS AND PATIENT TEACHING

■ Assessment

Learn as much as possible about the health history of the patient, including the presence of any diseases that may contraindicate the use of MAO inhibitors. The patient should be asked about other medications including OTC and herbal products (particularly

St John's Wort) currently being taken (especially TCAs) and the possibility of pregnancy. Also assess the level of the patient's depression and check for suicidal ideas.

■ Diagnosis

What other problems does the patient have as a result of this diagnosis? Is the patient able to understand the dietary restrictions that must be followed while taking these medications? What self-care assistance does the patient need? The nurse should focus on things to teach or learn about the patient that will provide encouragement and support in getting well.

■ Planning

The safe use of MAO inhibitors in pregnant patients or nursing mothers has not been established.

■ Implementation

MAO inhibitors are given only orally and are well absorbed by this route. The desired antidepressant effect of MAO inhibitors usually occurs within 1 to 4 weeks of drug therapy. If results are not obtained after this time, the patient will not be helped by continuing to take the drug. When improvement is noted during the first 4 weeks of drug therapy, the dosage will likely be reduced gradually over a period of several weeks until an effective maintenance dosage is reached. MAO inhibitors are usually not given in the evening because of their psychomotor stimulating effect, which may produce insomnia.

The maintenance dose of MAO inhibitors can be administered in either single or divided doses. MAO inhibitors should be discontinued at least 2 weeks before elective surgery. If emergency surgery is indicated, doses of narcotics and anesthetics should be reduced. All patients treated on an outpatient basis need to be closely monitored.

Information about MAO inhibitors is provided in Table 16-9.

■ Evaluation

All patients taking MAO inhibitors must be monitored for symptoms of orthostatic hypotension. If this occurs, the dosage of the drug may need to be reduced or the drug discontinued.

Patients who are agitated or who have schizophrenia may become more hyperactive. Bipolar patients may go into the manic phase of their illness; this is sometimes treated by stopping the drug for a brief period and then starting again at a lower dosage.

The effects of MAO inhibitors continue for approximately 2 weeks after the drug is stopped. Therefore patients who have been taking MAO inhibitors should avoid taking any drugs or eating any foods that are known to interact with MAO inhibitors for this 2-week period.

■ Patient and Family Teaching

Tell the patient and family the following:

- The patient needs to take this medication exactly as ordered by the prescribing health care provider. It may take up to 4 weeks before the patient begins to feel better. Therefore it is important to take the drug in the exact amount and frequency ordered even though the patient may notice no changes.
- MAO inhibitors can increase the effects of alcohol and other drugs such as narcotics, sleeping pills, and amphetamines. Alcohol (including beer and wine) should be avoided. The patient should check with the health care provider before taking any other prescription or OTC or herbal medications.
- The effect of MAO inhibitors continues for 2 weeks after the patient stops taking them. Therefore the patient must continue to avoid eating or drinking the previously specified foods or beverages during the 2-week period.
- The patient may experience light-headedness, dizziness, or a feeling of faintness, especially when getting up from a lying or sitting position. To reduce this feeling, the patient should move slowly when changing positions.
- MAO inhibitors may cause drowsiness or make the patient feel less alert than usual. If so, the patient should avoid driving or other activities requiring alertness.
- MAO inhibitors should be discontinued 2 weeks before the patient has any surgery that requires anesthesia. The health care provider must be informed if surgery is planned so that the drug may be stopped in the correct way.

Table 16-9   Monoamine Oxidase Inhibitors

GENERIC NAME	TRADE NAME	COMMENTS
tranylcypromine	Parnate ♣	Improvement in symptoms usually seen 1-3 wk after therapy is begun. Higher incidence of hypertensive reactions with this drug than with other MAO inhibitors. Used to treat endogenous depression.
phenelzine sulfate	Nardil ♣	For depressed patients clinically described as typical, non- endogenous or neurotic. Use in patients who have failed other drugs.

MAO, Monoamine oxidase.

- The nurse, physician, or other health care provider should be contacted immediately, or the patient should go to the hospital emergency room if fever, severe headache, nausea, vomiting, chest pain, or rapid heartbeat develops.
- MAO inhibitors are dangerous drugs that should be kept out of the reach of children and all others for whom they are not prescribed. These drugs must not be left sitting on a dresser or low bedside table.
- The patient should wear a MedicAlert bracelet or necklace or carry a medical identification card listing this medication.

SELECTIVE SEROTONIN REUPTAKE INHIBITORS, SEROTONIN/NOREPINEPHRINE REUPTAKE INHIBITORS AND OTHER MISCELLANEOUS ANTIDEPRESSANTS

ACTION

Since the beginning of the 1980s, a series of new antidepressant medications have been available. Some are chemically unrelated to one another, but all act in some way to prolong serotonin in the brain. Their differences are often in terms of side effects.

Among the selective SSRIs, several products have become very well known: Their antidepressant action is thought to be linked to their inhibition of CNS neuronal uptake of serotonin. These products are powerful and selective inhibitors of neuronal serotonin reuptake. Other medications have been developed that work by SNRIs or norepinephrine/dopamine reuptake inhibiton (NDRIs). Because these more focused products cause far fewer side effects than other antidepressant medications, they have become extensively used and are considered the drugs of choice in the treatment of depression.

There are also other antidepressant products that have an effect on serotonin uptake but that are chemically unrelated to the SSRIs, but are all tetracyclic compounds. Trazodone (Desyrel) and nefazodone (Serzone) are serotonin 2-agonists/blockers/serotonin reuptake inhibitors (SARIs/SSRIs)—A totally new classes of drugs. Nefazodone (Serzone) inhibits neuronal uptake of serotonin and norepinephrine, but the mechanism for this action is unknown.

Mirtazapine (Remeron) is an α_2 noradrenergic antagonist, another new drug class. Tetracyclic compounds enhance central noradrenergic and serotonergic activity through an unknown mechanism. They have different amounts of antagonistic activity toward alpha2 and5-HT2 receptors. These products inhibit the uptake of serotonin at the neuronal synaptosomes in the brain and enhance the behavioral changes caused by serotonin. The action of these drugs is more selective than that of other types of antidepressants. They have less effect on the cardiac conduction system than do tricyclic antidepressants, and they cause almost no CNS stimulation, which occurs frequently with MAO inhibitors.

USES

SSRI drugs are the drugs of choice for most depressive disorders due to their low adverse effect profile and for short-term treatment (less than 5 weeks) of outpatients with a diagnosis that is listed in the category of major depressive disorders in the fourth edition of the *Diagnostic and Statistical Manual of Mental Disorders.* They have also been used extensively for long-term therapy in patients with dysthymic depressive disorders and minor depressive episodes. Fluoxetine (Prozac) is the only SSRI approved for treating depression in the pediatric population and it is only given to those children older than 8 years of age.

Some of these antidepressant agents are approved to treat specific anxiety and eating disorders, assist in smoking cessation (bupropion [Wellbutrin]), or obsessive compulsive disorders.

ADVERSE REACTIONS

Adverse reactions to these drugs in general include dizziness, drowsiness, tachycardia, dysrhythmias, hypertension, hypotension, rash, pruritus, constipation, weight loss, nausea and vomiting, anorexia, weight gain, diarrhea, appetite increase, dyspepsia (stomach discomfort after eating), menstrual complaints, impotence, urinary frequency, dry mouth, headache, excessive sweating, tremor, sedation, insomnia, blurred vision, agitation, confusion, hostility, and disturbed concentration.

In nearly 4% of patients taking fluoxetine (Prozac), a rash develops with accompanying fever, leukocytosis, arthralgia (joint pain), edema, carpal tunnel syndrome, respiratory distress, lymphadenopathy, proteinuria, and mild transaminase elevation.

Trazodone (Desyrel) has also produced early menses, hematuria (blood in the urine), urinary frequency, and weight changes.

Patients who abruptly stop taking the medication may experience a sudden increase in dangerous symptoms. Patients must be taught to follow their health care provider's directions and gradually decrease the amount of medicine taken if the drug is to be stopped.

DRUG INTERACTIONS

If bupropion (Wellbutrin) is taken with levodopa, the chance of adverse effects increases. If bupropion is used with carbamazepine (Tegretol), cimetidine, phenobarbital, or phenytoin (Dilantin), the hepatic metabolism of the drugs may be increased. Acute toxicity may develop if bupropion is given with phenelzine (Nardil).

Fluoxetine (Prozac) increases the half-life of some drugs and may displace drugs bound to protein, such as warfarin and digitoxin, or be displaced by them. Concurrent use of trazodone (Desyrel) and antihypertensives can cause hypotension. There are many other isolated drug interactions. Trazodone (Desyrel) may increase the effects of alcohol, barbiturates, and other CNS depressants. The drug should be stopped as long as possible before general anesthesia because interactions are unknown.

Some antidepressants may cause cardiac repolarization problems shown by prolongation of the QT Interval on the electrocardiogram (ECG). These patients are at risk for sudden death. The more drugs the patients take, the more care should be shown to try to prevent drug interactions that might lead to this problem.

❖ NURSING IMPLICATIONS AND PATIENT TEACHING

■ Assessment

Learn as much as possible about the health history of the patient, including history of hypersensitivity, presence of seizure disorder, current or prior diagnosis of bulimia or anorexia nervosa (these patients tend to have more seizures when receiving bupropion [Wellbutrin]), or recent use of an MAO inhibitor. After stopping MAO inhibitor therapy, the patient should wait at least 14 days before starting bupropion (Wellbutrin).

■ Diagnosis

Determine what other problems this patient may be having as a result of depression. Assessment of deficits in nutrition, safety, and knowledge are important. What other problems does this patient have specifically? For a patient who has been taking the medication, side effects such as insomnia, impotence, and taste disorders may make the underlying depression worse. Evaluate the extent of side effects and the impact on the patient's ability to function.

■ Planning

The incidence of seizures in patients taking bupropion (Wellbutrin) is approximately four times greater than that in patients taking other antidepressant medications.

Fluoxetine (Prozac) has a relatively long half-life (2 to 3 days), and problems with liver or renal failure may prolong the drug's action in the body. There is growing evidence that this product may be useful in treating panic attacks, obsessive-compulsive disorders, and other psychiatric problems.

Dosage levels are individualized based on symptoms. Patients may need to keep a diary or journal to actually realize that they are feeling better. A stable amount of the drug in the blood may not be reached until 4 to 5 weeks after starting therapy. Fluoxetine (Prozac) stays in the body for weeks. This may be important when drug therapy must be stopped.

Trazodone (Desyrel) should not be used while the patient is having electroshock therapy.

■ Implementation

Patients on bupropion (Wellbutron) therapy should be watched for worsening of depressive symptoms, agitation, insomnia, and suicide risk. Be alert for seizure activity, because this drug has been linked to a risk for dose-related seizures at levels of more than 450 mg. Bupropion (Wellbutrin) has been known to produce unwanted changes in appetite, weight, and blood pressure (i.e., increase); monitor for these changes.

Additional important information about these medications is summarized in Table 16-10.

■ Evaluation

The desired antidepressant effect usually begins within 1 to 2 weeks after drug therapy is initiated and reaches its full effect within 4 weeks. The patient's level of depression should respond with an improvement in symptoms and attitude, and a return to the normal activities of daily living should be possible. Some patients who begin feeling better have enough emotional energy to commit suicide and family or friends should closely monitor patients for this possibility.

■ Patient and Family Teaching

Tell the patient and family the following:
- The patient should take these medications exactly as ordered by the prescribing health care provider. It is important that the patient continue to take the drug as ordered, even if no changes are experienced, because it may take up to 2 weeks before the patient begins to feel better.
- These drugs may produce a variety of side effects. Patients vary in their ability and willingness to tolerate these effects. They most frequently cause agitation and restlessness but may also interfere with sleep. In some individuals, these drugs can produce seizures. Because some of these medications cause sexual dysfunction, some male patients refuse to continue taking them. The health care provider must be contacted immediately if there are any problems that are new or troublesome.
- These drugs can cause drowsiness or make the patient feel less alert than usual. If so, the patient should avoid driving or doing other activities that require alertness. If drowsiness persists, the nurse, physician, or other health care provider should be contacted.
- These medications must be kept out of the reach of children and all others for whom they are not

Table 16-10   Selective Serotonin Reuptake Inhibitors and Other Miscellaneous Antidepressants

GENERIC NAME	TRADE NAME	COMMENTS
Selective Serotonin Reuptake Inhibitors		
citalopram	Celexa	For treatment of depression, alcoholism, panic disorder, premenstrual dysphoria, and social phobia.
escitalopram	Lexapro	Reassess after 8 wks of treatment.
fluoxetine ★	Prozac	Full antidepressant effect may not be seen for 4 wk. Lower dosage used in patients with renal or hepatic impairment, patients with multiple diseases or medications, and the elderly. Effective in reducing symptoms of premenstrual syndrome in women, panic attacks, and obsessive-compulsive disorders.
fluvoxamine	Luvox CR	
paroxetine	Paxil	
sertraline	Zoloft	
Miscellaneous Antidepressants		
Tetracyclic Compounds		
mirtazapine	Remeron	For treatment of major depressive disorder.
trazodone	Desyrel	If drowsiness occurs, a larger dose can be given at bedtime.
maprotiline	Maprotiline	For relief of anxiety associated with depression.
Unrelated Products		
bupropion ★	Wellbutrin	Instituted gradually to avoid producing seizures. May require addition of sedative-hypnotic in first week of therapy.
desvenlafaxine	Pristique	Comes as extended release tablet.
duloxetine	Cymbalta	May require prolonged duration of therapy.
nefazadone	Nefazadone	Has chemical structure unrelated to all other antidepressants. Has potential for serious drug interactions with many other drugs.
venlafaxine	Effexor	Take with food. Patients should taper off drug and not stop it suddenly.

★ Indicates "Must-Know Drugs," or the 35 drugs most prescribers use.

prescribed. The patient should wear a MedicAlert bracelet or necklace or carry a medical identification card listing the name of this medication. The patient should avoid alcohol while taking these medications.

- There are other precautions that should be taken for these psychotherapeutic agents as a whole depending upon the age of the patients. Some of these considerations are summarized in the following box.

Lifespan Considerations
Pediatric

PSYCHOTHERAPEUTIC AGENTS

- Buspirone has not been studied in persons younger than 18 years; therefore it is not recommended for use in that age group.
- Although diazepam (Valium) may be used in infants 6 months and older, this drug and other benzodiazepines should not be used to treat a hyperactive or psychotic child.
- The tricyclic antidepressants are usually not recommended for the treatment of depression in children younger than 12 years old. However, some agents, such as amitriptyline, desipramine, and imipramine, have been used in children older than the age of 6 for major depression. Several of these agents are also used in the treatment of enuresis and attention deficit disorder. Be aware that children are very sensitive to an acute overdose, which should always be considered very serious and potentially fatal. Adolescents often require a decreased dose because of their sensitivity to this drug category.

- All adolescents taking antidepressants must be closely monitored for suicidal ideation (persistent thoughts of taking one's own life), because research suggests this group is at higher risk for suicide than some other groups.
- Adverse effects reported in children receiving TCAs include changes in ECG patterns, increased nervousness, sleep disorders, complaints of tiredness, hypertension, and mild stomach distress.
- Children are at greater risk for neuromuscular or extrapyramidal side effects (such as, tremor, slurred speech, akathisia, anxiety, distress, paranoia, and bradyphrenia), especially dystonias (involuntary muscle spasms). Monitor closely if antipsychotic agents are administered.
- Lithium may decrease bone density or bone formation in children. If this drug is prescribed, patients' serum levels should be monitored closely and signs of toxicity reported.

Modified from McKenry LM, Tessier E, Hogan MA: *Mosby's pharmacology in nursing,* ed 22, St Louis, 2006, Mosby.

Lifespan Considerations
Older Adults

PSYCHOTHERAPEUTIC AGENTS

- The older adult population tends to have higher serum levels of the antipsychotic and antidepressant drugs because of changes in drug distribution resulting from a decrease in lean body mass, less total body water, less serum albumin, and usually an increase in body fat. Therefore these patients require a lower drug dose and a more gradual drug-dose titration than those of the average adult patient.

- Geriatric patients are more prone to have orthostatic hypotension, anticholinergic side effects, extrapyramidal side effects, and sedation. They should be carefully evaluated before starting antipsychotic agents. If such potent medications are necessary, close supervision and the lowest dose possible are recommended.

- The older adult patient generally should receive half the recommended adult dose of benzodiazepines. The patient with organic brain syndrome should receive only 33% to 50% of the usual adult dose, with increases in dosage at 7- to 10-day periods. When clinical improvement is noted, attempts at tapering and discontinuing the drug should be instituted.

- TCAs may cause increased anxiety in the geriatric patient. If the patient has cardiovascular disease, the use of the TCAs increases the risk of dysrhythmias, tachycardia, stroke, congestive heart failure, and myocardial infarction.

- In older clients with dementia, the treatment of behavioral disorders with atypical (second-generation) antipsychotic medications is associated with increased mortality.

Modified from McKenry LM, Tessier E, Hogan MA: *Mosby's pharmacology in nursing,* ed 22, St Louis, 2006, Mosby.

✤ ANTIPSYCHOTIC DRUGS
OVERVIEW

Severe mental illness such as schizophrenia, psychotic depression, mania, or organic brain syndrome have no identifiable cause and require long term therapy with antipsychotic drugs. These medications are used initially to sedate, or slow the patient down, thereby reducing some of the psychotic symptoms. This allows other therapy to be used. Antipsychotic medications have many side effects and require constant monitoring. Psychotic symptoms may change over time, requiring constant adjustment of medication. Psychotic symptoms, particularly those associated with schizophrenia, are labeled as either positive because they add on to normal behavior (delusions, disorganized thoughts or speech, hallucinations), or negative because they subtract from normal behavior (lack of interest, failure to respond, no motivation, nothing provides pleasure). Monitoring of these symptoms helps in choosing the best medications to give.

Antipsychotic drugs are powerful drugs with significant actions and side effects. They are grouped into three broad categories:

1. The phenothiazines, such as chlorpromazine (Thorazine);
2. The nonphenothiazines, including haloperidol (Haldol), loxapine (Loxitane), and molindone (Moban). These two categories make up the first generation or conventional antipsychotic agents and are quite effective in treating positive symptoms but also cause extrapyramidal effects and many other side effects that interfere with patient acceptance.
3. The second generation of drugs or atypical antipsychotic drugs include a variety of unrelated drugs and a new class of drugs, the dopamine system stabilizers. All these new drugs have a lower adverse risk profile, especially a lower risk of extrapyramidal symptoms and tardive dyskinesia and are more effective in treating negative symptoms while also dealing with positive symptoms. The newer atypical drugs tend to cost much more than conventional drugs.

All antipsychotic agents act by blocking the action of dopamine in the brain. Because they are from different chemical groups, however, these drugs work at different sites in the brain and also produce side effects on different body systems. The major categories will be presented separately. The atypical antipsychotics have become the standard of care in the treatment of schizophrenia and associated psychotic disorders and in treating various other psychiatric conditions such as bipolar disorder. They may also be used in treatment of obsessive-compulsive disorder, aggression due to dementia, post-traumatic stress disorder, psychosis in Parkinson's disease, and borderline personality disorder. Chlorpromazine (Thorazine) is the prototype antipsychotic from which all other antipsychotic potencies are compared.

FIRST GENERATION OR CONVENTIONAL ANTIPSYCHOTIC DRUGS—PHENOTHIAZINES AND NONPHENOTHIAZINES

ACTION

The conventional phenothiazine antipsychotics first came into the market and, while somewhat effect in treating psychophrenia, had many side effects. It was disappointing for clinicians to find that the nonphenothiazines that were introduced later also had many side effects. They did offer some treatment options for patients.

The three major actions of both the phenothiazine and nonphenothiazines are as follows:

1. Blocking dopamine at the postsynaptic receptor sites in the brain, thus increasing the metabolism of dopamine. The drugs also decrease the uptake of

norepinephrine and serotonin. In the CNS, these drugs decrease the level of cyclic adenosine monophosphate (AMP), particularly in areas of the brain that control emotion and behavior. These changes are thought to produce the antipsychotic effects of the phenothiazines.

2. Reducing sensory stimulation of the reticular activating system in the brainstem, thereby producing a sedative effect.
3. Dopamine blockade in the chemoreceptor rigger zone may account for the antiemetic effect of many antipsychotics.

USES

Conventional antipsychotics such as chlorpromazine (Thorazine), thioridazine (Mellaril), and promazine (Prozine) are used primarily for reducing or relieving the symptoms of acute and chronic psychoses, including schizophrenia, schizoaffective disorders, and involutional psychosis. The nonphenothiazine class thioxanthene is preferred for use in psychotic patients who are withdrawn or are exhibiting retarded behavior. Clinical evidence has shown that patients with certain types of apathetic psychosis respond well to this drug. Haloperidol (Haldol) may be injected and is often used in calming patients with dementia.

ADVERSE REACTIONS

Adverse reactions to phenothiazines and nonphenothiazines include severe extrapyramidal symptoms which may not be reversible: psueoparkinsonism, dystonic reactions (severe spasms, particularly of back muscles, tongue and facial muscles), akathiasia (constant pacing and compulsive movements), tardive dyskinesia (bizarre tongue and face mvoements such as lip smacking an chewing movements). Additionally, the drugs may cause, postural hypotension, tachycardia, confusion, drowsiness, hyperactivity, insomnia, amenorrhea, gynecomastia (enlargement of the breasts in men), hyperglycemia (high blood sugar level), hyperreflexia, tardive dyskinesia, blood cell abnormalities, contact dermatitis, photosensitivity, constipation, dry mouth, dyspnea (uncomfortable breathing), incontinence, nasal congestion, opaque deposits on the cornea and lens, and urinary retention. Production of a severe agranulocytosis has prevented Clozapine (Clorazil) from becoming a first line treatment drug.

In general, the nonphenothiazine agents cause less sedation and fewer anticholinergic side effects than phenothiazine products, but cause an equal or even greater incidence of extrapyramidal symptoms. Therapy with these products and other CNS depressants must be carefully watched because of potential additive effects.

Haloperidol (Haldol) produces orthostatic hypotension, drowsiness, tardive dyskinesia, blurred vision, breast engorgement, constipation, decreased libido, dry mouth, impotence, nausea, and vomiting.

Overdosage produces exaggerated CNS depression, coma, or severe hypotension, and extrapyramidal symptoms, seizures, or cardiac dysrhythmias may appear.

DRUG INTERACTIONS

Phenothiazines taken concurrently with CNS depressants (alcohol, barbiturates, narcotics, and anesthetics) may increase and prolong the effects of either the CNS depressant or the phenothiazine. The effects of MAO inhibitors and TCAs are increased when they are taken at the same time as phenothiazines, and antacids and antidiarrheal drugs reduce the absorption rate. The effects of many other drugs and the results of laboratory tests are altered by phenothiazines and thioxanthenes.

Haloperidol (Haldol) increases the CNS depressant effects of alcohol, barbiturates, opioids, and anesthetics, and may produce severe hypotension when taken with antihypertensive drugs or epinephrine.

Some of these products have been implicated in causing changes in cardiac repolarization as shown by prolongation of the QT interval on the ECG. This problem places the patient at sudden risk. Any patient taking several antidepressant-antipsychotic medications should be closely monitored for any alteration in ECG.

❖ NURSING IMPLICATIONS AND PATIENT TEACHING

■ Assessment

Learn as much as possible about the health history of the patient, including the presence of hypersensitivity to any phenothiazines (because cross-sensitivity occurs); the history of cardiac, respiratory, or blood diseases; current use of other medications; and the possibility of pregnancy. These conditions are either contraindications or precautions to the use of phenothiazines and nonphenothiazines.

The patient may have a history of emotional unrest, agitation, paranoid ideas, hallucinations (visual, auditory, or tactile), delusions, inability to think clearly, severe mood swings, and inability to cope with reality. Patients may or may not talk about paranoid thoughts and often have difficulty paying attention and responding to things going on around them. They may not give appropriate answers to questions, and behavior, dress, and general appearance may not be appropriate.

■ Diagnosis

What other needs does this patient have? Safety? Nutrition? Does the patient have a support system of family or friends?

Table 16-11 Antipsychotic Medications

GENERIC NAME	TRADE NAME	COMMENTS
First Generation—Conventional Antipsychotics		
Phenothiazines and Phenothiazine-Type Drugs		
Aliphatic Phenothiazines		
chlorpromazine	Thorazine	Traditional phenothiazine product, popular and inexpensive. Used in psychotic disorders to control the manic phase of manic-depressive reactions, preoperatively for restlessness, to treat behavioral problems of children who are combative, or for hyperactive children with excessive motor activity.
promazine	Promazine	Used primarily to manage psychotic disorders. Oral medication usually preferred.
Piperazine Phenothiazines		
fluphenazine	Prolixin	Also used for dementia; comes IM or SQ
perphenazine	Trilifon	Also used for dementia; for nausea in IM and IV
trifluoperazine	Stelazine	Also for dementia; available only IM
prochlorperazine	Compazine	Also as antiemetics. Comes in a variety of delivery systems.
Piperdine Phenothiazines		
mesoridazine	Serentil	Strong sedative. Also used for dementia, anxiety, hyperactivity, and alcohol dependence
thiordazine	Mellaril	Strong sedative; used for moderate to severe depression
First Generation Conventional Nonphenothiazine Antipsychotic Medications		
Thioxanthene Derivative		
thiothixene	Navane ✦	Monitor the patient for early signs of tardive dyskinesia and jerky movements, particularly of the hands.
Phenylbutylpiperadines		
haloperidol	Haldol	Used to calm demented or manic patients
Miscellaneous Conventional Nonphenothiazines		
chloroprothixene	Taractan	Strong sedative effects; available in IV form
loxapine succinate	Loxitane	Also used for dementia
molindone	Mobane	Has either sedative or stimulating effect, insomnia
primozide	Orap	Anticholinergic effects increased; Tardive dyskinesia if abruptly stopped. Also used for Tourette's syndrome

IM, Intramuscular; *IV*, intravenous; *SQ*, subcutaneous.

■ Planning

Phenothiazines and nonphenothiazines are not recommended for use in pregnant women or nursing mothers.

Patients with severe asthma, emphysema, or acute respiratory infections (especially children) may have slowing of respiration as a result of the CNS depressant effects of phenothiazines. Phenothiazines may also depress the cough reflex, putting a patient who is vomiting in danger of aspirating.

■ Implementation

Phenothiazines can be taken either orally or parenterally. The oral form is fairly well absorbed, but the absorption rate will be slowed if the drug is taken with antacids or antidiarrheal agents.

Most nonphenothiazines are only available orally.

Stomach upset from the oral form of phenothiazines can be reduced or avoided by taking the drug with bland food or 8 ounces of water. Additional information about these medications is listed in Table 16-11.

■ Evaluation

The desired antipsychotic effects of phenothiazines may take several weeks to appear after therapy is started. The beginning dose should be the lowest recommended amount, according to the individual's tolerance and the severity of psychosis, until the psychotic symptoms are controlled. The dosage of phenothiazines that controls the patient's symptoms will likely be maintained for 2 to 3 weeks and then gradually reduced until the lowest effective maintenance dosage is reached. Phenothiazines given in large doses or for a long time should be discontinued by gradual reduction over several weeks to avoid symptoms of dyskinesia (difficulty in movements of the body), nausea, vomiting, dizziness, and trembling.

The patient should have a complete eye examination by a specialist, including inspection of the internal structures and the lens, to establish baseline data.

■ **Patient and Family Teaching**

Tell the patient and family the following:

- The patient should take this medication exactly as ordered and continue to take the drug in the exact amount and frequency specified, even if not starting to feel better. It may take several weeks before any changes occur.
- Phenothiazines and nonphenothiazines can increase the effects of alcohol, sleeping pills, and many other prescribed medications. The patient should avoid alcohol and should check with the nurse, physician, or other health care provider before taking any other prescribed or OTC drugs.
- Phenothiazines and nonphenothiazines may cause drowsiness or make the patient feel less alert than usual, particularly when first taking the medicine. If so, the patient should avoid driving or doing other activities that require alertness. The patient should talk with the nurse, physician, or other health care provider if drowsiness or decreased alertness continues.
- Light-headedness, dizziness, or feelings of faintness occur in some people taking phenothiazines. To reduce these feelings, the patient should move slowly when changing from a lying or sitting position.
- Some people taking phenothiazines become more sensitive to the sun. To avoid sunburn, the patient should use a sunblock and limit exposure to the sun or sunlamps.
- Patients taking this drug in liquid form should avoid contact of the medicine with the skin or clothes, because it can cause irritation.
- Gastric distress caused by the medication may be reduced by taking the drug with food, milk, or 8 ounces of water. The patient should not take any antacids or antidiarrheal medicine within 1 hour of taking the drug.
- If the drug comes in a bottle with a medicine dropper, the patient should measure the prescribed dose as marked on the dropper and then dilute it in a glass of water or juice.
- Dryness of the mouth may occur when the patient starts taking this drug. Chewing gum, sucking on hard candy, or rinsing the mouth frequently may help relieve this dryness.
- Phenothiazines may make the patient perspire less than usual. Therefore the patient should avoid becoming overheated in hot and humid weather or when exercising.
- The health care provider should be contacted immediately if urinary retention, change in vision, sore throat with fever, muscle spasms, trembling or shaking (particularly of hands), skin rash, jaundice, small uncontrollable movements of the tongue, or other new or troublesome symptoms develop.

- This medication must be kept out of the reach of children and all others for whom it is not prescribed.
- Patients taking these drugs should wear a Medic-Alert bracelet or necklace and carry a medical identification card stating the name of the medication.

SECOND GENERATION OR ATYPICAL ANTIPSYCHOTICS

A variety of chemically unrelated products have more recently come on the market to help in treating psychotic patients. The newest addition to this category is a new class of medication called dopamine system stabilizers.

ACTION

The mechanism of action for these products is often not precisely understood but they are thought to act by blocking several different receptor types in the brain. Aripiprazole (Abilify) is the new dopamine system stabilizer. It is thought to be a partial dopamine agonist (whereas other antipsychotic agents are full dopamine agonists) and thus has a targeted mechanism of action.

USES

These atypical antipsychotic drugs have a broad spectrum of action, controlling both positive and negative symptoms of schizophrenia and have now become the drugs of choice for treating psychoses. These drugs are now used primarily in the treatment of schizophrenia.

The new dopamine system stabilizer apripiprazole (Abilify) shows both negative and positive symptoms of schizophrenia are reduced by this drug. Motor side effects appear to be less of a problem than with other antipsychotics with low incidence of extrapyramidal effects. Overall efficacy appears to be similar to haloperidol (Haldol) and risperidone (Risperdal) in schizophrenia. It has been approved for use in schizophrenia and as adjunctive treatment in major depressive disorder in adults, and in treatment of acute manic or mixed episodes of bipolar I disorder. It has been approved by the Food and Drug Administration as an adjunctive therapy to lithium or valproate (Depakote) in bipolar I disorder and for the treatment of irritability associated with autistic disorder. Some indications are approved for children and adolescents; some indications are reserved for adults.

ADVERSE REACTIONS

These drugs do not cause extrapyramidal side effects when taken at therapeutic doses. Although there are fewer side effects with these drugs, most cause weight gain and may cause obesity. Some of these agents may alter glucose metabolism and increase the risk for development of type 2 diabetes. Risperidone (Risperdal) may cause decreased sex drive in men and women and menstrual disorders and osteoporosis in women.

The antipsychotic medications in general have been found to cause changes in cardiac repolarization as measured by a prolonged QT interval on the ECG. This places the patient at risk for sudden death. These patients should have their ECGs closely monitored. Some patients know that they have a gene that increases their risk for LQT syndrome and there are some drugs that these patients should not be given. When studying about drugs or reading package inserts, the nurse should be aware that some products are found to prolong the QT interval. A complete list of those drugs which these patients should not be prescribed may be found at www.sads.org/living-with-sads/Drugs-to-Avoid.

Aripiprazole has fewer side effects than many other current antipsychotics. Common effects include vomiting, somnolence, and tremor. Overdoses may produce acidosis, aggression, atrial fibrillation, bradycardia, coma, confusional state, convulsions, depressed level of consciousness, hypertension, hypotension, lathery, ECG disturbances, respiratory arrest, status epilepticus. Patients may experience increase in anxiety and headache.

Some of the major features of these products are briefly presented in Table 16-12.

DRUG INTERACTIONS

Many of these drugs have the same interactions as the phenothiazine drugs. One of the most widely used drugs, haloperidol (Haldol) interacts with many drugs. It may block the action of centrally acting antihypertensives. It's action may be decreased by aluminum- and magnesium-containing antacids, levodopa, lithium, phenobarbital, phenytoin, rifampin, and beta blockers.

Table 16-12   Second Generation or Atyical Antipsychotic Medications

DRUG	ACTION	ADVERSE REACTIONS	DRUG INTERACTIONS
Nonphenothiazine Antipsychotic Medications			
clozapine (Clozaril) ♣	Increased affinity for 5-HT receptors; acts on several neurotransmitters, including antagonism of some dopamine receptors.	Life-threatening agranulocytosis (very low number of white blood cells)	Increases effect of digoxin and warfarin; may decrease effects of other highly protein-bound drugs.
olanzapine (Zyprexa)	Increased affinity for 5-HT receptors; acts on several neurotransmitters, including antagonism of some dopamine receptors.	CNS stimulation	Carbamazepine decreases concentrations; interferes with cytochrome P-450 system.
quetiapine (Seroquel)	Increased affinity for 5-HT receptors; acts on several neurotransmitters, including antagonism of some dopamine receptors.	May produce cataracts with long-term use; may increase cholesterol level. Lengthens ECG Q-T interval in some patients.	Increased levels when given with phenytoin; cimetidine decreases clearance and thus increases serum level.
risperidone (Risperdal)	Increased affinity for 5-HT receptors; acts on several neurotransmitters, including antagonism of some dopamine receptors.	Lengthens ECG Q-T interval in some patients; elevated prolactin level; causes agitation, anxiety, headache, insomnia, constipation, dyspepsia, and rhinitis.	Use with clozapine decreases clearance of risperidone.
ziprasidone (Geodon)	Acts on several neurotransmitters.	Lengthens ECG Q-T interval in some patients and may produce lethal dysrhythmias.	Take medication with food.
Dopamine System Stabilizers			
Aripiprazole (Abilify)	Partial dopamine agonist	Many side effects including lengthening of ECG QT-interval; increased risk of suicide.	Patient should not stop taking suddenly. Watch for development of high blood glucose, cardiac problems, changes in consciousness or neurologic function, and weight.

5-HT, 5-Hydroxytriptamine; *CNS*, central nervous system; *ECG*, electrocardiogram.

Aripiprazole is metabolized by liver enzymes and so has the potential to interact with many different types of drugs. The patient should be monitored very closely when aripiprazole is taken with other drugs because the action of aripiprazole may be increased or decreased or the other drug absorption may be increased or decreased.

❖ NURSING IMPLICATIONS AND PATIENT TEACHING

▪ Assessment

Care should be taken to collect a detailed psychiatric history and a thorough drug history about past and current drugs and the patient's reaction to taking them.

▪ Diagnosis

Does the patient have other problems that might interfere with taking this drug such as dehydration, confusion? When these drugs are used in psychotic patients, patient symptoms may become worse, with development of agitation, irritability, unusual changes in behavior, or suicidality.

▪ Planning

Use with caution in patients with preexisting hypotension or cerebrovascular disease, cardiac disease, heart failure, history of heart attack, angina, and some arrhythmias. The patient should have a baseline ECG taken before beginning this medication. Because of high risk of suicide in some of these patients, prescriptions should be written for the smallest quantity of tablets possible to reduce the risk of overdose. Safety of the drug during pregnancy and breastfeeding has not been established. Patient should have baseline weight and blood sugar levels recorded to use in following up response to the drug.

▪ Implementation

Encourage the patient and family to watch for any changes in behavior or symptoms and report them promptly. These drugs should not be stopped abruptly. Patients should avoid extremes of cold or heat, as the drug may affect the area of the brain responsible for temperature regulation and patients could develop heat stroke.

▪ Evaluation

High blood sugars and seizures have both been seen in patients who take these medications. Drowsiness has also been a common problem and may interfere with driving or operating machinery or other tasks that require mental alertness. This drug has a black box warning regarding increased risk of suicide, particularly in adolescents. Behavior should be closely monitored and any suspicious behavior reported.

ANTIMANIC MOOD STABILIZERS AND CNS AND NON-CNS STIMULANTS

Mood stabilizers are used in patients with manic-depressive disorder or psychosis to limit the extremes of both the depression and manic episodes and also to decrease the mood switches back and forth. These drugs seem to have a calming effect on the brain. But sometimes patients have a need for CNS stimulation. This is most often seen in patients with attention-deficit/hyperactivity disorder (ADHD). The drugs in these two categories have different actions and uses, but both act to modify the brain action so patient behavior is more normal.

ANTIMANIC MOOD STABILIZERS

ACTION

Lithium is the primary drug used to treat patients in manic states. Some other antiseizure drugs are also used for mood stabilization. The exact mechanism of lithium action is not known. The mood-stabilizing effect of the drug may be attributed to its ability to alter sodium transport at the nerve endings, inhibit cyclic AMP formation in nerve cells, and enhance the uptake of serotonin and norepinephrine by nerve cells, thus increasing the inactivation of these neurotransmitters. It has no sedative, depressant, or euphoric actions, making it unique from all other psychiatric drugs.

USES

Lithium is specifically used for patients with bipolar disorder (manic-depressive psychosis) who are in an acute manic phase. It also may be used to prevent recurrent episodes of mania in the bipolar patient.

ADVERSE REACTIONS

Adverse reactions to lithium include dysrhythmias, hypotension, ataxia, coma, dizziness, drowsiness, motor retardation, restlessness, slurred speech, tinnitus (ringing in the ears), pruritus, rash, abdominal pain, anorexia, diarrhea, vomiting, urinary incontinence or retention, polyuria (excretion of a large amount of urine), albuminuria, blurred vision, hyperglycemia, hypothyroidism, leukocytosis, and weight gain.

Overdosage may produce toxicity which will present as diarrhea, vomiting, muscle weakness, drowsiness, and ataxia.

 Clinical Pitfall

Lithium Monitoring

There is a very narrow therapeutic window for lithium, and careful monitoring of blood levels is required to avoid toxic overdosages or toxicity, which can threaten the life of the patient.

DRUG INTERACTIONS

Use of lithium with diuretics can lead to lithium toxicity. There are many significant drug interactions with various medications. No other medication should be taken by the patient without the knowledge and approval of the health care provider.

❖ NURSING IMPLICATIONS AND PATIENT TEACHING

▪ Assessment

Learn as much as possible about the health history of the patient, including the presence of hypersensitivity, underlying disease, the possibility of pregnancy, and other medications being used. These conditions may be contraindications or precautions to the use of lithium.

The patient may have a history of excessive talkativeness, restlessness, hyperactivity, aggressiveness, and perhaps ideas of being very important, talented, or powerful.

▪ Diagnosis

What other problems does this patient have that might influence the effectiveness of the medication? If the patient becomes dehydrated, grows excitable and forgets to take the medication on a regular basis, or dislikes the effects of lithium and believes it is not needed, this may result in significant treatment problems.

▪ Planning

Lithium is not safe for use in pregnant patients and breastfeeding mothers. If a patient receiving lithium becomes pregnant, especially during the first trimester, the drug needs to be stopped because it may cause birth defects.

Older adult patients are often more sensitive to lithium toxicity. It is important to start these patients on lower doses and monitor the therapeutic and adverse effects closely while increasing dosage.

▪ Implementation

Make sure the patient has adequate hydration (enough fluids) and that electrolytes are balanced during lithium therapy.

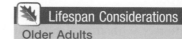

Lifespan Considerations
Older Adults
LITHIUM

Lithium is more toxic in the geriatric patient. Lower lithium dosages, a lower serum lithium level, and very close monitoring are critical in this age group. Older adults are more prone to CNS toxicity, lithium-induced goiter, and clinical hypothyroidism than the average adult. Generally, excessive thirst and polyuria may be early side effects of lithium toxicity that are frequently seen in older adults.

Modified from McKenry LM, Tessier E, Hogan MA: *Mosby's pharmacology in nursing*, ed 22, St Louis, 2006, Mosby.

Table 16-13 summarizes the important information the nurse needs to know about lithium.

▪ Evaluation

The therapeutic blood level of lithium is relatively close to the toxic level, so the serum lithium level must be monitored on a regular basis. Blood should be drawn 12 hours after the dose of lithium is given. Monitoring should be carried out every few days during the initial therapy and then at least every 2 months after the patient is stabilized. The therapeutic serum lithium level is 1 to 1.5 mEq/L in most laboratories. At each patient visit, observe for therapeutic effects and monitor the patient's mental and emotional status.

Lithium is better tolerated when the patient is in an acute manic stage than in a stage in which symptoms of mania have decreased. The dosage of lithium may have to be adjusted according to the patient's symptoms and the lithium blood serum levels.

Patients who develop diarrhea or become ill and do not eat are at increased risk of toxicity, and their condition should be followed closely.

▪ Patient and Family Teaching

Tell the patient and family the following:
- The patient should take this medication exactly as ordered. It is important to continue to take the drug in the exact amount and frequency ordered, even if the patient does not begin to feel better,

Table 16-13	**Mood Stabilizer Medications**	
GENERIC NAME	**TRADE NAME**	**COMMENTS**
lithium	Carbolith ♦ Eskalith Lithane ♦ Lithonate	Lithium administered orally is rapidly absorbed in the GI tract. The desired effect of lithium may take 1 to several weeks to occur. Lithium is excreted by the kidneys, with a half-life of approximately 24 hr in a healthy adult, but in the older adult patient, half-life may be increased to 36 hr; therefore lower dosages are indicated for this group. Lithium excretion is inhibited in the presence of low serum sodium levels. The therapeutic serum level of lithium is 1-1.5 mEq/L. Lithium is not recommended for children younger than 12 years of age. Used to treat acute phase of mania and for prophylaxis.

GI, Gastrointestinal.

because it may take several weeks before any changes occur. Gastric upset caused by the medication may be reduced by taking the drug with milk or food.

- Because the serum lithium levels can become in the toxic range if the patient takes too much lithium or becomes dehydrated, the patient should avoid activities that cause excessive sweating (strenuous exercise, sunbathing, hot tub baths) and things that produce excessive urination (consuming large amounts of caffeine in coffee, tea, or cola drinks). The nurse, physician, or other health care provider should be contacted if the patient becomes ill or does not feel well.
- Some patients taking lithium experience side effects, but these are usually mild and disappear with time. The nurse, physician, or other health care provider should be notified of any new or troublesome symptoms, such as vomiting, nausea, shakiness, trembling, jerky movements of arms or legs, or generalized weakness.
- The patient will need to have the level of the drug in the blood (serum lithium levels) measured frequently so that the drug can be kept at the proper level and side effects may be reduced. The patient will need these blood tests every few days when beginning treatment, and then every 1 to 2 months.
- This medication must be kept out of the reach of children and others for whom it is not prescribed.
- The patient on lithium therapy should wear a MedicAlert bracelet or necklace and carry a medical identification card stating the name of the drug.

CNS AND NON-CNS STIMULANTS

Over the years an increasingly large number of children who have trouble completing tasks and paying attention have been identified with ADHD. They have increased motor activity, which gets children in trouble when they cannot sit still in school, cannot stay on task, talk constantly, interrupt others, and are always "wiggling, poking, and moving". There may be aggressive behavior, impulsivity, and anxiety, all of which may make it difficult for these children to learn or creates behavior problems when they can't interact with other children in a normal way. These children are easily distracted, have trouble remembering, do not follow instructions properly, cannot complete long or complex tasks, and may have sleep disturbances. It may take several years for some children to be accurately diagnosed—usually girls are diagnosed later than boys.

Some adults now recognize that attention deficit disorder (ADD) is a problem that they have had since childhood and are seeking treatment for the same problems. In adults, the primary symptoms include restlessness, depression, anxiety, or even manic like behavior. They may have mood swings that are similar to bipolar depression disorder. All of these symptoms have usually contributed to struggles in educational, employment, and social situations that have created poor self-esteem. This may in turn lead to introverted behaviors causing people to pull away and isolate themselves from others.

ACTION

The cause of ADD or ADHD is not clearly identified, so treatment is been difficult. It is now believed that the hyperactivity may be related to a deficit or dysfunction of neurotransmitters in the brain—particularly dopamine, norepinephrine, and serotonin in the reticular activating system of the brain. The drugs used to treat ADHD are mostly CNS stimulants that increase activity in specific areas of the brain to heighten alertness and help them focus better. The drugs do this by increasing norepinephrine release in some pathways of the reticular activating system. They also directly stimulate the release of dopamine in areas of the brain responsible for concentration. These drugs have some potential for addiction and so most are classified as Schedule II drugs.

Another non-CNS stimulant drug, atomoxetine (Strattera) is approved for treating ADHD. Although the exact mechanism of action is not clear, it is classed as a selective norepinephrine reuptake inhibitor—thus it is not an addictive or Schedule II drug.

The two categories of drug therapy appear to be equivalent in efficacy but patients may respond better to one than the other.

USES

These drugs are limited to treatment of ADD and ADHD.

ADVERSE REACTIONS

These CNS stimulants are associated with a wide variety of symptoms that make some children reluctant to take them. These include anorexia, abdominal pain, depression, dizziness, nausea, nervousness, and weight loss. Common adverse effects of atomoxetine includes headache, cough, decreased appetite, upper abdominal pain, and insomnia.

 Clinical Pitfall

CNS Stimulant Monitoring

These patients must be closely monitored for paradoxical hyperactivity—actually causing the symptom that is trying to be controlled. Trying to determine if the patient needs more medicine or less medicine is often a difficult challenge.

DRUG INTERACTIONS

These drugs interact with many other drugs and may decrease the effectiveness of anticoagulants and anticonvulsants. Use with some other drugs may increase the adverse effects. CNS stimulants should not be given with MAO inhibitors.

❖ NURSING IMPLICATIONS AND PATIENT TEACHING

▪ Assessment

Learn as much as possible about the health history of the patient, including the presence behavioral or social problems related to ADHD. The patient may have a history of excessive talkativeness, restlessness, hyperactivity, and aggressiveness.

▪ Diagnosis

What other problems does this patient have that might influence the effectiveness of the medication? Does the patient have a support system to help him or her take the medicine—particularly if the patient is a child?

▪ Planning

Some patients experience anorexia. While dosing depends on specific agents, drugs should be given after meals to reduce the appetite suppressant symptoms. Insomnia is a common side effect of CNS stimulants, as well as of ADHD itself. Drugs should be taken at least 6 hours before bedtime to reduce the risk of sleep problems. These drugs are pregnancy category C drugs and Schedule II controlled substances. Is there any suggestion of previous drug addiction? Because this drug has the potential for addiction or patients may develop tolerance to the drug when used for a long time, periodic drug-free "holidays" are recommended to help clear the patient's system of the drug.

Due to high potential for abuse, parents should keep these drugs in a locked cabinet to prevent the patient from taking the drugs to give to or sell to people at school.

Some children like taking the drugs because they feel more in control of themselves. They may even remind their parents when they need to take the drugs. This feeling of control might be encouraging to children.

▪ Implementation

Avoid taking these drugs with caffeine products, which may produce increased stimulation.

These drugs must be taken on a regular basis. They may also require that the patient take them for several months before an adequate evaluation can be made about the adequacy of their effects. Thus patients should be encouraged to keep regular appointments for drug evaluation.

Table 16-14 summarizes the important information needed to know about drugs for ADHD.

▪ Evaluation

Changes in dosages are usually based on long-term changes in patient behavior. CNS stimulants may increase blood pressure and this should be monitored regularly. Height and weight should be monitored in children with long-term therapy because of the potential for changes in body metabolism.

▪ Patient and Family Teaching

Tell the patient and family the following:
- The patient should take this medication exactly as ordered. It is important to continue to take the drug in the exact amount and frequency ordered, even if the patient does not begin to feel better, because it may take several weeks before any changes occur. Gastric upset caused by the medication may be reduced by taking the drug with milk or food.

Table 16-14   CNS and Non-CNS Stimulants

GENERIC NAME	TRADE NAME	COMMENTS*
CNS Stimulants		
d- and l-amphetamine racemic mixture	Adderall	High potential for abuse. Used for narcolepsy (daytime sleep disorder).
dextroamphetamine	Dexedrine	Used only for short-term treatment. Produces severe anorexia and insomnia. May prolong QT interval on ECG.
methamphetamine	Desoxyn	Commonly abused.
methylphenidate	Ritalin	Controls attention deficit better than hyperactivity. Most widely used drug for ADHD.
pemoline	Cylert	Used with other drugs rather than alone.
Non-CNS Stimulants		
atomoxetine	Strattera	Inhibits reuptake of norepinephrine.

ADHD, Attention-deficit/hyperactivity disorder; *CNS*, central nervous system.
*Many of these drugs have not been approved for use in children younger than 3 or 6 years old. Consult prescribing information for safety recommendations.

- Parents should keep medicine in a locked cabinet and watch for symptoms of dependence (i.e., taking more than ordered or more frequently).
- Side effects should be monitored and reported.

SEDATIVE-HYPNOTIC MEDICATIONS

OVERVIEW

Sedatives help calm and reduce anxiety in a patient. Hypnotics induce drowsiness and promote both sleep and an inability to remember. Both medications are often used in the hospital to help patients relax and produce sleep before anesthesia or medical testing procedures such as EEG. They are also used to treat patients with insomnia (inability to sleep) caused by mental and physical stress.

Sleep is a normal cyclic process that involves varying levels of unconsciousness from which a patient may be aroused. Normal sleep produces relaxation and relief from stress. Although individual patterns vary, each time a person sleeps, four stages occur in a cycle for varying lengths of time. Stages I and II are very light stages of sleep, during which the person may be easily aroused. Stage III is a transition to stage IV, the period of deepest sleep in which basic vital signs slow and the body totally relaxes. It is this period of sleep that makes people feel very refreshed. Approximately every 90 minutes, a period of body arousal is reached, which is often superimposed on stage I or stage II of sleep. This is called *paradoxical sleep* because instead of relaxing, the body is more active. It is also called *REM time* because dreaming is common, as demonstrated by rapid eye movements (REM). This is an important part of sleeping, when the unconscious mind works out anxieties and tensions. When people do not have enough REM time each night, they feel anxious and tired.

ACTION

At times, people may be unable to sleep because of stresses or anxiety. Difficulty falling asleep is termed **initial insomnia**. The inability to stay asleep is termed **intermittent insomnia**, and **terminal insomnia** refers to early awakening with an inability to return to sleep. Terminal insomnia is often associated with depression.

If warm baths, warm drinks, appropriate temperature, and bedding changes do not help the patient relax, a medication may be prescribed on a short-term basis. A **sedative agent** is a medication that relaxes the patient and so may lead to sleep. A **hypnotic agent** actually induces drowsiness and promotes sleep in the patient. Whether a medication acts as a sedative or a hypnotic is often determined not by the drug, but by the dosage used, with smaller dosages producing sedative effects and larger dosages producing hypnotic effects.

 Clinical Goldmine

Sedative-Hypnotic Medications

Although most sedative-hypnotic medications increase the sleeping time, many of them produce a feeling of lethargy or a "hangover" feeling in the morning. Even a few doses of the medication may reduce the occurrence and length of REM time, making the patient feel irritable and tired on waking.

The ideal medication would reproduce the normal sleep pattern for the patient; the patient would sleep an appropriate length of time, have no side or adverse effects, and wake up feeling rested and relaxed with no risk of developing drug dependency. Unfortunately, no ideal medication exists.

Postmedication "hangover" from reduced REM time often leads the patient to feel they haven't slept "well" and may increase their desire for more medicine so that the patient may have a refreshing sleep. This pattern may result in dependency or abuse.

Once a patient has taken sedative-hypnotics, the normal sleep patterns may not return for several weeks. During that time, an increased period of REM will be seen, as if the body is trying to "catch up" for missed time. This may produce long, vivid, or frightening dreams.

USES

Barbiturates are CNS depressants used for a variety of medical problems. All barbiturates act primarily on the brainstem reticular formation, reducing nerve impulses to the cerebral cortex. Barbiturates also depress the respiratory system and the activity of nerves and muscle (smooth, skeletal, and cardiac), thus producing relaxation and sleep.

Barbiturates are used for short-term treatment of anxiety, agitation, and insomnia caused by transient psychosocial stresses. They are also prescribed at times when rest is mandatory, such as before surgery. Large doses of short-acting barbiturates can produce surgical anesthesia (see the third section of this chapter).

The main action of benzodiazepines is CNS depression. Although the exact mechanism is not known, they are thought to act on the hypothalamus and limbic system of the brain, decreasing the vasopressor response and increasing the arousal threshold. They are used as hypnotic agents to treat insomnia. The therapeutic objective is to prevent insomnia and restore normal sleep patterns. Benzodiazepines are used in patients with acute or chronic medical problems who require restful sleep or sedation (see the third section of this chapter for more detail).

The nonbarbiturate-nonbenzodiazepine sedative-hypnotics include a variety of chemically unrelated medications, as well as the GABA receptor agonists such as eszopiclone (Lunesta), zolpidem (Ambien), and zalepion (Sonata). All produce some effects on

REM sleep, and most have a potential for tolerance and habituation and so are schedule IV drugs. Many may produce rebound REM. Ramelteon (Rozerem) is a little different in that it stimulates melatonin, the body's normal chemical to produce sleep, so it has no addictive properties.

ADVERSE REACTIONS

Nonbarbiturate-nonbenzodiazepine sedative-hypnotics may produce drowsiness, decreased emotional reaction, dullness, distortion of mood, impaired coordination, hypersensitivity, lethargy, headache, muscle or joint pain, and mental depression. A feeling of "hangover" commonly occurs with their use.

DRUG INTERACTIONS

Nonbarbiturate-nonbenzodiazepine sedative-hypnotics increase the sedative effects of CNS depressants, including sleeping aids, analgesics, anesthetics, tranquilizers, alcohol, and narcotics. Chloral hydrate may increase the anticoagulant effects of warfarin.

❖ NURSING IMPLICATIONS AND PATIENT TEACHING

▪ Assessment

Learn as much as possible about the health history of the patient, including any medications the patient may be taking that may produce drug interactions, other barbiturates the patient is taking (sometimes these are present in bronchodilators or antispasmodics), response to barbiturates taken in the past, or hypersensitivity. Sedative-hypnotics are not considered safe in pregnancy. Determine whether there are any underlying diseases that would represent contraindications to the use of sedative-hypnotics. The Complementary and Alternative Therapies box summarizes herbal preparations patients may be using to induce sleep and their potential to interact with other drugs.

Complementary and Alternative Therapies

Insomnia

PRODUCT	COMMENTS
Valerian	May cause increased effect or toxicity with CNS depressants, sedative-hypnotics (particularly barbiturates), antidepressants, anxiolytics, and antihistamines
Kava kava	Potential interactions with ethanol, CNS depressants (particularly benzodiazepines, antidepressants, and sedative-hypnotics)
Passion flower	Potential interactions with antianxiety agents, antidepressants, hexobarbital, hypnotics, and sedatives
Chamomile	Effects may be addictive with CNS depressants.
Melatonin	Excessive dosages may cause morning sedation or drowsiness

Data from Krinsky DL, LaValle JB, Hawkins EB, et al: *Natural therapeutics pocket guide*, ed 2, Hudson, Ohio, 2003, Lexi-Comp, Inc.

▪ Diagnosis

What are the underlying problems that require use of a sedative? Does the patient have physical or emotional concerns that could be the cause of these problems?

▪ Planning

In general, if sedative-hypnotics are used for more than 1 week, they may cause further disturbances in the sleep cycle and rebound insomnia. Hypothermia may occur with the use of barbiturates. Alcohol can increase the sedation produced by these drugs and depress vital brain functions.

 Lifespan Considerations
Pediatric

SEDATIVE-HYPNOTICS

Young children are more susceptible to the CNS depressant effects of the benzodiazepines. In neonates, profound CNS depression may result because of the lower rate of drug metabolism by the immature liver.

Paradoxical reactions have been reported in children on barbiturate therapy.

Modified from McKenry LM, Tessier E, Hogan MA: *Mosby's pharmacology in nursing*, ed 22, St Louis, 2006, Mosby.

 Lifespan Considerations
Older Adults

SEDATIVE-HYPNOTICS

The sedative-hypnotics are particularly hazardous in older adult patients. Reductions in urinary clearance and accumulation of drug in adipose tissue may prolong the half-life of many of these drugs to a dangerous length. For example, the half-life of flurazepam (Dalmane) can increase to 100 hours, thus increasing the potential for overdosage.

- Sleep latency increases even though REM and stage 4 sleep may be absent in the older client. Sleep disturbance is a frequent concern of older adults.
- Evaluate the individual for preexisting health conditions, because various illnesses, such as arthritic pain, hyperthyroidism, cardiac dysrhythmia, and paroxysmal nocturnal dyspnea, may alter sleep patterns.
- Hypnotics should be reserved to treat acute insomnia and when prescribed, they should be limited to short-term or intermittent use to avoid the development of tolerance and dependency.
- A hypnotic with a short duration of action is preferred. When longer-acting hypnotics are given, daytime sedation, ataxia, and memory deficits may result.
- Encourage the older client to use nonpharmacologic approaches to promote sleep.
- Be aware that older adults, children, and persons with CNS dysfunction may experience a paradoxical reaction (CNS stimulation) to hypnotics and antihistamines.

Modified from McKenry LM, Tessier E, Hogan MA: *Mosby's pharmacology in nursing*, ed 22, St Louis, 2006, Mosby.

Table 16-15   Benzodiazepine Sedative-Hypnotic Medications

GENERIC NAME	TRADE NAME	COMMENTS
estazolam		Intermediate-acting oral benzodiazepine. Similar to flurazepam, but has fewer side effects.
flurazepam	Dalmane	Flurazepam can be used for a longer time (effective for 28 nights) and has less REM rebound than some other hypnotics. Markedly suppresses stage IV, increases stage II sleep. Hypnotic. Less likely to cause rebound insomnia and tolerance than other drugs.
lorazepam	Ativan	This antianxiety agent is generally used for mild or transient situational stress. It is used parenterally as a preanesthetic medication. Mild anxiety or insomnia, preanesthesia medication, and sedation.
quazepam	Doral	
temazepam	Restoril	Induces sleep in 20-40 min. Hypnotic: Give PO before bedtime; in elderly or debilitated patients lower dosage is adequate.
triazolam	Halcion	Used primarily for short-term treatment of insomnia or early morning awakening.

PO, By mouth; *REM,* rapid eye movement.

Flurazepam (Dalmane) is increasingly effective on the second or third night of consecutive use. For one to two nights after the drug is stopped, both the amount of time before the patient falls asleep and the total awake time may still be decreased.

Barbiturates and benzodiazepines are Schedule IV controlled substances. The patient may develop dependence if these drugs are used indiscriminately, and abrupt withdrawal is dangerous.

▪ Implementation

I general, sedative-hypnotics should be given 15 to 30 minutes before bedtime. Table 16-15 summarizes important information regarding benzodiazepine sedative-hypnotics.

Use great caution when parenterally administering barbiturates to avoid intraarterial injection or extravasation, because serious ischemia or gangrene could result. Barbiturates may worsen a patient's pain.

Geriatric or debilitated patients should receive lower-than-recommended dosages of barbiturates.

All barbiturates exhibit the same sedative-hypnotic effect, but they differ in time of onset, duration, and potency. Onset and duration are determined by the lipid solubility of the particular drug. Therapy typically begins with the lowest possible effective dose and is adjusted upward according to the individual patient's response. Patients given barbiturates should be closely monitored for untoward effects. Table 16-16 presents a comparison of different barbiturates used for sedation and hypnosis. As these drugs produce respiratory depression, benzodiazepines are usually preferred.

There are a variety of other drugs whose primary use may be for other indications, but which also have sedative-hypnotic effects and may be useful in selected situations. Table 16-17 summarizes the nonbarbiturate-nonbenzodiazepine sedative-hypnotics.

Table 16-16   Barbiturate Sedative-Hypnotic Medications*

DRUG	ONSET OF ACTION (MIN)	DURATION (HOURS)
Long-Acting		
phenobarbital (Barbital) ★	60	10-16
Intermediate-Acting		
butabarbital (Butisol)	30	6-8
Short-Acting		
pentobarbital (Nembutal)	30	3-6
secobarbital (Seconal)	15-30	3-6

*Sedative dose is less than hypnotic dose
★ Indicates "Must-Know Drugs," or the 35 drugs most prescribers use.

▪ Evaluation

Benzodiazepines are transformed by the liver into long-acting forms that may remain in the body for 24 hours or more and produce increasing sedation. Liver function may be impaired with long-term use. The onset of action is approximately 30 to 60 minutes; the effects last 7 to 8 hours. Sedative-hypnotics should always be discontinued slowly in people who have been on long-term therapy. Tolerance is usually proportional to the total amount of the drug received. Barbiturates are controlled substances, so attempts should be made to avoid giving them to patients with a history of abuse or addiction.

▪ Patient and Family Teaching

Tell the patient and family the following:
- Sedative-hypnotics are only for short-term use. Sometimes tolerance, dependence, or addiction develops with these drugs.
- The patient should take the medication exactly as prescribed.

Table 16-17	Non-Benzodiazepine Non-Barbiturate Sedative-Hypnotic Medications*	
GENERIC NAME	**TRADE NAME**	**COMMENTS**
Chloral Derivatives		
chloral hydrate	Aquachloral	Effective in 30-60 min and lasts 4-8 hr. Has a very disagreeable taste and causes gastric irritation; should be taken after meals; elixir may be taken in water, juice, or soda.
Miscellaneous		
zolpidem	Ambien	Approved for short-term use only.
eszopiclone	Lunesta	Approved for short term use only.
ramelteon	Rozerem	Avoid taking medication after high-fat meal.
zaleplon	Sonata	Do not take for longer than 7 to 10 days.

*Sedative dose is less than hypnotic dose.

- The medication should be kept out of reach of children and all others for whom it is not prescribed.
- A hangover feeling may sometimes be experienced the day after taking the medication. The patient should avoid any driving or activities that require alertness until all drowsiness has disappeared.
- It is dangerous for the patient to drink alcohol within 24 hours after taking this drug.
- Smoking may decrease the length of time the drug helps the patient sleep.
- The patient should avoid drinking beverages containing caffeine for at least 4 hours before taking the medication because it reduces the ability of the drug to produce sleep.
- Some people experience side effects while taking this drug, so the health care provider should be notified if any new symptoms appear, such as rash, fever, unusual bleeding, bruising, pain sore throat, jaundice, or abdominal pain.
- The patient may develop excessive dreaming when the drug is stopped; this should lessen each night.
- Tablets and capsules should be kept in a dry, tightly closed container. Elixirs should be kept in a tightly closed brown glass bottle.
- If using this drug primarily to relax or to promote sleep, the patient should investigate alternative methods of relaxation to help reduce the need for medication.

Get Ready for the NCLEX® Examination!

Key Points

- CNS medications include analgesics, antimigraine agents, seizure medications, antiemetics, antivertigo medications, antiparkinsonian agents, antipsychotics, and sedative-hypnotics.
- It is important to understand how nerves transmit information from the brain through chemical neurotransmitters and how these medications interact with the body.
- Neurotransmitters fit into receptors in various parts of the body to act on them, and many CNS drugs act on more than one type of receptor.
- Each agent acts differently.
- It is extremely important for the nurse to administer dosages carefully, because serious adverse reactions are possible if dosages are exceeded.

Additional Learning Resources

SG Go to the Study Guide for additional learning activities to help master this chapter content.

evolve Go to the Evolve website (http://evolve.elsevier.com/Edmunds/ LPN/) for additional online resources.

Review Questions for the NCLEX® Examination

1. The nurse notes that the patient has been ordered the sympathomimetic drug Terbutaline (Brethine). The nurse anticipates that the patient most likely experiences symptoms of:
   1. shock
   2. cardiac arrest
   3. asthma
   4. dysrhythmias

2. The nurse reviews the patient's medications and finds that he is being treated with the adrenergic blocker carvedilol (Coreg). The nurse anticipates that the patient's medical history will include a diagnosis of:
   1. angina
   2. hypertension
   3. glaucoma
   4. migraines

Get Ready for the NCLEX® Examination!—cont'd

3. The nurse is caring for a patient who is being treated with the serotonin (5-HT) receptor agonist drug zolmitriptan (Zomig). The patient is experiencing difficulty swallowing the medication. An alternative method of administering the medication could be to give it by:

   1. nasal spray
   2. topical ointment
   3. intradermal injection
   4. subcutaneous injection

4. The patient is a pregnant adult who is experiencing migraine headaches. The best choice of a medication to treat such headaches during pregnancy will be:

   1. ergotamine (Ergomar)
   2. nimodipine (Nimotop)
   3. verapamil HCL (Calan)
   4. dihydroergotamine (DHE 45)

5. The nurse is caring for a 12-year-old boy who is experiencing bedwetting. The nurse notes that the physician has written an order to the patient to receive:
   1. amitriptyline (Elavil)
   2. imipramine (Tofranil)
   3. valproic acid (Depakote)
   4. timolol (Blocadren)

Case Study

Mrs. Jane Michner, a 65-year-old widow, was admitted 2 weeks ago with a fractured hip. She has a 6-year history of Parkinson disease. Her hip is healing well, but she is having difficulty learning to walk with crutches. This has made her very depressed, and she is concerned about how she will manage when she returns home. She has also developed symptoms of a urinary tract infection, a problem she has had repeatedly. She is currently receiving:

- ascorbic acid (vitamin C): 1 g PO 4 times daily
- levodopa (Larodopa): 1 g PO 3 times daily with meals
- nitrofurantoin (Macrodantin): 100 mg PO 3 times daily

1. Why is Mrs. Michner taking ascorbic acid?
2. What special information does the nurse need to give Mrs. Michner about her antiparkinsonian medications?
3. Several days after admission, Mrs. Michner develops a maculopapular eruption of the skin all over her trunk. What is the likely cause of this problem?

4. What medication class are the drugs Mrs. Michner might take to treat the urinary tract infection?
5. The health care provider starts Mrs. Michner on imipramine HCl (Tofranil) 20 mg PO twice daily. Why was this drug ordered? What does the patient need to know about it?
6. Does Mrs. Michner have any contraindications to the use of imipramine HCl?

Drug Calculation Review

1. The health care provider orders valproic acid (Depakote) at 15 mg/kg/day PO. The patient weighs 150 lb today. What will be the daily dose in milligrams of this antiseizure medication for this patient?

2. Order: Dilantin 200 mg by gastrostomy tube twice a day. Supply: Dilantin 125 mg/5 mL.
   Question: How many milliliters of Dilantin are needed for each dose?

3. Order: Lorazepam (Ativan) 0.5 mg IV push stat. Supply: Lorazepam 2 mg/mL.
   Question: How many milliliters of lorazepam is needed?

Critical Thinking Questions

1. Describe the properties of antimigraine products that differentiate them from other nonnarcotic analgesics.
2. With antianxiety agents, how would the nurse distinguish signs of overdosage from adverse reactions? What patient data would the nurse need to obtain to make this distinction?
3. What nonpharmacologic suggestions could the nurse make to patients to assist them with management of their insomnia? Why are antihistamines often used in place of sedative-hypnotics for older adult patients?
4. Antiemetics, among other CNS-acting medications, should not be taken with any other drugs or substances that act on the CNS because of the increased risk of sedative effects. What would the nurse assess for in a hospitalized patient admitted to the hospital unit for observation for oversedation?

Medications for Pain Management and Anesthesia

Objectives

1. Explain why there are so many rules about how opioids and related analgesic drugs may be given.
2. Compare and contrast drug tolerance and drug addiction.
3. List behavior that would make the nurse believe a patient is addicted to a drug.
4. Evaluate different forms of opioid agonists and opioid agonist-antagonists in their ability to control pain.
5. List medications commonly used for the treatment of moderate to severe pain.
6. Identify common methods of local and regional anesthesia.

Key Terms

acute pain (ă-KYŪT PĂN, p. 299)
addiction (ă-DĬK-shŭn, p. 300)
anesthesia (ANN-ess-THEE-zee-uh, p. 309)
chronic pain (KRŎN-ĭk PĂN, p. 299)
dependence (dē-PĔN-dĕns, p. 300)
hydration (hī-DRĀ-shŭn, p. 306)

miosis (mī-Ō-sĭs, p. 300)
opioids (Ō-pē-ŏydz, p. 298)
pain (PĂN, p. 299)
tolerance (TŎL-ŭr-ŭns, p. 300)
withdrawal symptoms (p. 300)

OVERVIEW

There are many nerve paths that carry the sensation of pain from an injured part of the body to the brain. This means that there are several different places to block the feeling of pain. Some feelings of pain may be treated by exercise, heat, ice, or other methods. Some pain is so severe that it requires drug treatment. There are now a wide range of drugs used in controlling pain. The most common drugs for mild pain relief include over-the-counter analgesics such as aspirin and acetaminophen. (These drugs are described separately in Chapter 18 because they also have actions other than pain reduction.) Many of the drugs used for treating severe pain are opioids. (An **opioid** is any substance that produces stupor associated with analgesia, and are used to treat severe pain.) Natural opioids come from opium, which comes from unripe seed capsules of the poppy plant. Opium contains many chemicals, including morphine and codeine. (Heroin is diacetylmorphine, which chemically breaks down into morphine.) Opioid medications interact with specific receptors in the brain and spinal cord to reduce pain. There are also nonopioid analgesics that produce moderate pain relief for conditions not severe enough to require an opioid.

In addition to natural opioids, artificial or synthetic opioids have been developed. It was hoped that many of these new drugs would not be as addictive as morphine, but this was not so. However, these new drugs are useful for pain management and to reverse the effects of opioids. Many of these new drugs are made by changing morphine chemically. Morphine is the basic chemical from which the synthetic opioid analgesics hydrocodone, hydromorphone, and oxycodone have developed. Other classes of synthetic opioids are made of different chemicals but have actions similar to morphine.

Analgesics used in pain management are classified according to their mechanism of action. Opioids are classified as agonist, partial agonist, or agonist-antagonist medications. The term *agonist* means "to do"; the term *antagonist* means "to block." An agonist drug binds with the receptors to activate and produce the maximum response of the individual receptor. A partial agonist produces a partial response of this type. An opioid agonist-antagonist drug produces mixed effects, acting as an agonist at one type of receptor and as a competitive antagonist at another type of receptor. This information is key to understanding the rest of the chapter. Refer back here if needed.

The mechanism of action for opioids is determined by where they bind to specific opioid receptors inside and outside the central nervous system (CNS). There are six types of opioid receptors (delta, epsilon, kappa, mu [types one and two], and sigma). These receptors are responsive to the opiates (have opiate receptors) in each of these areas that interact with autonomic nervous system nerves that carry pain messages (including the release of neurotransmitters), and this interaction produces changes in the person's reaction to pain. Some opioids block a particular receptor; others stimulate a particular receptor. Although analgesia can occur with the stimulation of delta, epsilon, and kappa receptors, most action occurs at the mu and kappa receptors. Mu receptors produce analgesia, respiratory depression, sedation, euphoria, decreased gastrointestinal (GI) motility, and constricted pupils (miosis). These mu receptors may also lead to physical dependence. Kappa receptors produce analgesia, sedation, and are also associated with decreased GI motility and miosis. Sigma receptors seem to produce mostly unwanted effects.

 Memory Jogger

The opioid medications for treatment of acute and chronic pain may be summarized as:

- Opioid agonists act in the CNS (spinal cord, brain stem, reticular formation, thalamus, and limbic system) and interact with the autonomic nervous system nerves to change the person's reaction to pain.
- Opioid agonist-antagonists act through the level of the limbic system in the brain and with chemicals at specific nerve sites to decrease pain perception.
- Nonopioid (centrally acting) analgesics also act at the level of the brain to control mild or moderate pain. Some other nonopioid analgesics may act locally or regionally.

Morphine is the main opioid agonist drug with which all other pain management drugs are compared (Table 17-1). It is used a great deal in acute care and also in hospice settings for dying patients who have severe pain. Codeine, hydrocodone (Hydromet), and oxycodone (OxyContin) are often used in combination with acetaminophen in the outpatient setting. Hydromorphone (Dilaudid) is very potent (with regard to the number of milligrams that are equivalent to morphine) and is only used for treating severe pain not relieved by morphine. It comes as a powder for compounding as well as a tablet.

Opioid agonist-antagonist drugs may be preferred over opioid agonists for use in patients in the community because their risk for abuse is less. A common drug, pentazocine (Talwin) which is estimated to be about 1/6 as potent as morphine has limited use because of its CNS toxicity. In efforts to limit the abuse of these drugs, the federal government created many regulations that describe who may prescribe or administer opioids. Nurses learn and follow these rules. The nurse may have responsibility for keeping opioids in a safe place, typically a locked cabinet, and account for their use in the hospital or nursing home setting.

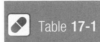

	Table 17-1	Equivalent Doses of Opioid Analgesics Compared with Morphine 10 mg PO and IM

ANALGESIC	ORAL DOSE (MG)	PARENTERAL DOSE (IM) (MG)
morphine ★	60 single dose; 30 repeated doses	10
morphine (MS Contin) ★	60	
hydromorphone	7.5	1.5
fentanyl	NA	0.1
codeine ★	200	130
hydrocodone	30	NA
levorphanol	4	1-2
oxycodone	15-20	NA
meperidine	300	75-100
methadone	10-20	5-10

Modified from Brunton L, Lazo L, Parker K, editors: *Goodman and Gilman's pharmacological basis of therapeutics*, ed 11, New York, 2005, McGraw-Hill. *IM*, Intramuscular; *IV*, intravenous; *NA*, not applicable.
★ Indicates "Must-Know Drugs," or the 35 drugs most prescribers use.

This chapter is divided into three sections. The first section deals with opioid agonist analgesics. The second section presents opioid agonist-antagonist analgesics. Nonopioid (centrally acting) combination drug analgesics are presented in the third section.

PAIN AS A PROCESS

Pain is defined by the International Association for the Study of Pain as an unpleasant sensation or emotion that produces or might produce tissue damage. Pain is always subjective; that is, pain is something the patient feels and that cannot be felt or measured by someone else.

Researchers believe four things are required for pain to occur:

1. An unpleasant stimulus affects nerve endings and sets off electrical activity.
2. The nerve endings carry the unpleasant stimulus along the nerves through electrical signals to the spinal cord, using different types of nerve fibers. Different types of fiber carry different types of pain signals.
3. The signals go to the brain.
4. A feeling of pain develops that includes behavioral, psychologic, and emotional factors. **Acute pain** is usually related to an injury, such as recent surgery, trauma, or infection, and ends within an expected time. **Chronic pain** is any pain that continues beyond the usual course of an acute injury process. Persons

with cancer-related pain or chronic disorders (for example, arthritis, post Shingles) are the majority of people with chronic pain. This type of pain may interfere with activities of daily living and many people spend all their time just trying to find ways to cope with the pain.

Anxiety, depression, fatigue, and other chronic diseases may increase the perception of pain. Activities designed to distract the patient, create positive attitudes, or provide support may reduce the perception of pain. There are many nondrug methods for doing this. Some of these activities might involve listening to music, massage therapy, cold or hot packs, hydrotherapy, acupuncture, biofeedback, relaxation therapy, art therapy, hypnosis, therapeutic touch, Qigong or Reiki energy therapies, or use of transcutaneous electrical nerve stimulation (TENS) units. Sometimes pain requires nerve blocks or surgical intervention to relieve pain on nerves or structures.

TOLERANCE, DEPENDENCE, AND ADDICTION

Tolerance is a drug-related problem that is seen when the same amount of drug produces less effect over time. In the case of pain, more drug is needed for relief. **Dependence** is a state in which the body shows withdrawal symptoms when the drug is stopped or a reversing drug or antagonist is given. **Withdrawal symptoms** are changes in the body or mind, such as nausea or anxiety, that occur when a drug is stopped or reduced after regular use. Tapering off (slowly taking less of the drug) can reduce withdrawal symptoms. Psychologic dependence, or **addiction**, is the desperate need to have and use a drug for a nonmedical reason and patients have a limited ability to control their drug use. Tolerance and dependence result from regular use of an opioid for a certain length of time and should not be confused with or labeled as addiction. Addiction is a problem; however, a patient in pain should not be denied pain relief because of fear of addiction. All opioid drugs have the potential to cause tolerance and dependence when taken on a long term basis. This is not the same as abuse.

OPIOID AGONIST ANALGESICS

OVERVIEW

Drugs called *opioid agonist analgesics* are thought to prevent painful feelings in the CNS (in the substantia gelatinosa [gray matter] of the spinal cord, brain stem, reticular formation, thalamus, and limbic system). (See Chapter 16 for additional information on receptors and neurotransmitters in the CNS.) Figure 17-1 demonstrates how opioids act on neurons.

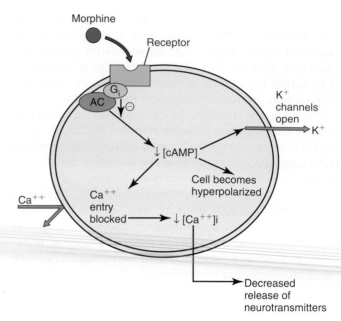

FIGURE 17-1 Mechanism of action of opioids on neurons. Opioids bind to three types of opioid receptors: mu, kappa, and delta receptors. They produce analgesia primarily by activating mu receptors. However, they also engage with and activate kappa and delta receptors, producing other effects, such as sedation and vasomotor stimulation. When morphine or another narcotic analgesic binds to opioid receptors, activation occurs. The receptors send signals to the enzyme adenyl cyclase (AC) to slow activity by way of G proteins (Gi). Decreased adenyl cyclase activity causes less cyclic adenosine monophosphate (cAMP) to be produced. As a secondary messenger substance, cAMP is important for regulating cell membrane channels. A reduced cAMP level allows fewer potassium ions to leave the cell and blocks calcium ions from entering the cell. This ion imbalance—especially the reduced intracellular calcium level—ultimately decreases the release of neurotransmitters from the cell, thereby blocking or reducing pain impulse transmission.

ACTION

Opioid agonists bind to opioid receptors. The opioid action of the drug in the CNS is shown through pain relief (analgesia), sleepiness, euphoria (feeling of well-being), unclear thinking, slow breathing, **miosis** (the pupil of the eye constricts or gets smaller), slowed peristalsis (slowing of the action of smooth muscle in the bowel) causing constipation, reduced cough reflex, and hypotension (low blood pressure).

USES

Opioid agonist analgesics are used to treat moderate to severe acute pain and chronic pain. They may be used preoperatively to treat pain from injury or other diseases processes; for people who are addicted to opioids (methadone only); for constant cough (codeine); postoperatively for pain; and for labor.

These products are also commonly available as combination products along with medications such as acetaminophen, aspirin, caffeine, and barbital. These allow a small dose of opioid to be combined with other chemicals to relieve symptoms or calm the patient.

ADVERSE REACTIONS

Adverse reactions to opioid agonist analgesic drugs include bradycardia (slow heartbeat), hypotension, anorexia (lack of appetite), constipation, confusion, dry mouth, euphoria (excessive happiness), fainting, vomiting, pruritus (itching), skin rash, slow breathing, and shortness of breath. Overdosage may cause bradypnea (very slow breathing, with a rate less than 12 breaths/minute); irregular, shallow breathing; sedation; coma; miosis; cyanosis (blue color to the skin); gradual drop in blood pressure; oliguria (reduced ability to form and pass urine); clammy skin; and hypothermia (abnormally low body temperature). Chronic overdosage symptoms seen in drug abusers include very small pupils, constipation, mood changes, and reduced level of alertness. For IV drug users, there may also be skin infections, pruritus, needle scars, and abscesses. Respiratory rate and sleepiness are the variables most closely watched for signs of overdosage.

DRUG INTERACTIONS

The CNS depressant effects of opioid agonist analgesics may be increased by the use of other opioid agonist analgesics, alcohol, antianxiety agents, barbiturates, anesthetics, nonbarbiturate sedative-hypnotics, phenothiazines, skeletal muscle relaxants, and tricyclic antidepressants. Opioids act with many other medications to increase or decrease their effects. It is important to identify other medications that the patient is taking prior to starting opioid analgesics.

❖NURSING IMPLICATIONS AND PATIENT TEACHING

■ Assessment

Before a patient can be effectively helped with pain relief, it is important to determine the cause of the pain. Some organizations have called for pain assessment to be the fifth vital sign, but this is not universally accepted. Do not simply administer drugs prescribed for pain without understanding the source of the particular pain. Even in a patient with terminal cancer, evaluate each new pain for a specific cause that may be specifically treated. For example, bone pain can often be managed by radiation. Table 17-2 lists the classifications of pain and their characteristics.

When assessing pain, ask the patient to describe the pain. Learn the history of the pain, including when it started, where it is, what it feels like, how often it occurs, and what makes it worse or relieves it. Accept that patients have pain when they say they have it at the intensity level they say it is. Use a pain scale to make the assessment more objective. In addition to what patients say, the nurse may also

Table 17-2	Classification of Pain	
CATEGORY	**CHARACTERISTICS**	**EXAMPLE**
Nociceptive	Somatic Well localized Dull, aching, or throbbing	Laceration, fracture, cellulitis, arthritis
Visceral	Poorly localized Continual aching Referred to dermatomal sites that are distant from the source of the pain	Subscapular pain arising from diaphragmatic irritation; right upper quadrant pain arising from stretching of liver capsule
Neuropathic	Shooting or stabbing pain superimposed over a background of aching and burning	Postherpetic neuralgia, postthoracotomy neuralgia, poststroke pain, trigeminal neuralgia, diabetic polyneuropathy

Modified from McKenry LM, Tessier E, Hogan MA: *Mosby's pharmacology in nursing*, ed 22, St Louis, 2006, Mosby.

sometimes see changes in their breathing, blood pressure, and pulse, as well as tense muscles, sweating, and pupil reaction. Also, they may be restless, crying, or moaning.

Learn as much as possible about other parts of the health history, such as whether the patient has a history of allergic or adverse reaction to morphine or related drugs, past ability to deal with pain, and whether there is any reason to think opioid abuse might become a problem.

The Agency for Health Care Policy and Research Clinical Practice Guidelines include the following principles of pain assessment (*A-A-B-C-D-E-E*):

Ask about pain regularly. Medication is to be given regularly and is more effective if it is given before the patient is in severe pain and begging for medication. There is acceptance that addiction is generally not a concern, especially for patients with chronic pain or terminal illness.

Assess pain systematically. Use pain intensity scales (Figures 17-2 and 17-3).

Believe the patient and family in their reports of pain and what relieves it.

Choose pain-control options appropriate for the patient, family, and setting. The health care provider who makes this decision should be aware of the wishes of the family and individual.

Deliver interventions in a timely, logical, and coordinated fashion.

Empower patients and their families.

Enable them to control their course to the greatest extent possible.

Lifespan Considerations
Pediatric
PAIN MEASUREMENT

Pain measurement scales exist to help evaluate how much pain the patient is feeling. Children experience pain in the same way as adults. Sometimes they have more difficulty communicating their pain, so providers need to be alert. A pain scale using smiling or frowning faces may help assess a child's pain (see Figure 17-2).

■ Diagnosis

Are there reasons the patient should not use these medications? Are there risk factors for their use? Is the nurse aware of other things that might pose a problem for a patient taking these medications? Report any problems discovered to the registered nurse or physician.

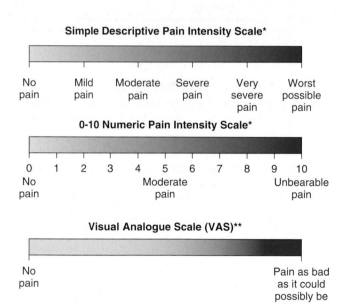

Simple Descriptive Pain Intensity Scale*

No pain | Mild pain | Moderate pain | Severe pain | Very severe pain | Worst possible pain

0-10 Numeric Pain Intensity Scale*

0 1 2 3 4 5 6 7 8 9 10
No pain — Moderate pain — Unbearable pain

Visual Analogue Scale (VAS)**

No pain — Pain as bad as it could possibly be

* If used as a graphic rating scale, a 10-cm baseline is recommended.
** A 10-cm baseline is recommended for VAS scales.

FIGURE 17-2 Pain measurement scales.

■ Planning

Whenever possible, pain treatment should begin with simple and nonopioid analgesics and supportive pain-relief measures first. These measures are described later.

Remember that pain relief is best if the drug is given before the patient has intense pain.

The main problem in using opioids, especially when the patient is at home where they control their own medicines and not in a hospital, is the risk of physical and psychologic addiction or dependence for the patient. Use caution when opioids are given to older adults, to pregnant women, to physically weak patients, to patients in shock or those who have consumed alcohol, and to children or newborns.

Clinical Pitfall
Opioid Agonist Analgesics

Pain is often a key symptom that helps identify the patient's problem. Opioid agonist analgesics reduce pain, so it is sometimes hard to determine what is wrong with the patient. Opioid agonist analgesics, as well as any CNS depressants, should not be used in persons with increased pressure in their eyes (intraocular pressure), head injury, or loss of consciousness, because the action of the drugs may worsen these conditions.

Lifespan Considerations
Older Adults
OPIOIDS

Older adult patients are more susceptible to the CNS and constipation side effects of opioids because of their ability to affect the CNS and to decrease GI motility. Usually these patients should be placed on a bowel regimen with a stimulant laxative, such as senna, when opioids are started. Older adult patients should be on lower doses of opioids, and drugs like tramadol (Ultram) and methadone must be used with caution.

Many times, patients are afraid to take opioids for pain because they fear addiction. Risk for addiction is decreased in the presence of severe pain. Talk to patients about such fears and help them understand that when taken as directed, opioids can be both safe and effective.

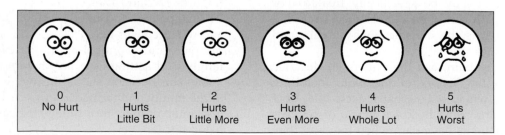

0 No Hurt | 1 Hurts Little Bit | 2 Hurts Little More | 3 Hurts Even More | 4 Hurts Whole Lot | 5 Hurts Worst

Brief word instructions: Point to each face using the words to describe the pain intensity. Ask the child to choose face that best describes own pain and record the appropriate number.

FIGURE 17-3 Wong-Baker FACES Pain Rating Scale.

Nonpharmacologic treatment of pain can be used alone or in combination with medications. This type of treatment includes patient education, management of anxiety and depression, cognitive-behavioral therapy, and appropriate exercise and activity. Complementary and alternative medicine (CAM) therapies may be helpful, although there is little scientific evidence to support the use of chiropractic manipulation, homeopathy, and spiritual healing. Heat, ice, massage, topical analgesics, acupuncture, and TENS may provide relief alone or in combination with analgesic medications. Guided imagery and distraction are especially good in pediatric patients.

▪ Implementation

Because these drugs are often abused, there are many rules related to giving opioid analgesics. The nurse should learn and follow the laws that tell what to do when giving opioid agonist analgesics. The Controlled Substances Act of 1970 (see Chapter 3) classified the opioid agonist analgesics by their potential for abuse. The rules are strict to help prevent people from easily abusing these drugs.

Once the opioid agonist analgesic is metabolized by the body, pain returns, and the patient may then complain of even more pain. This is why these patients often need regular doses of medication before the actions of the previous dose are gone. To prevent respiratory depression (severe slowing of breathing) from the opioids, the drugs should also be given no less than 2 hours before a baby is delivered or before surgery.

The cough reflex is reduced by many of the opioid analgesics. This may be a problem in patients with lung disease. Opioid analgesics may also produce a faster heart rate in patients who have a particular heart rhythm problem. These drugs may also make convulsions worse in people who have seizures. Opioids may be given orally or rectally, by injection into the muscle, the subcutaneous tissue, directly into the vein, or by epidural or intrathecal (spinal) administration. Sometimes the health care provider also prescribes a range of medicine that might be given. The amount of pain felt by the patient will help the nurse determine the dose of the opioid and how it should be given. Intermittent or patient controlled infusion of opioids into the bloodstream may be required when the patient has pain from terminal cancer or has some other chronic condition that causes severe pain. (Review materials in Chapter 10 related to the patient controlled analgesia [PCA] in hospitalized patients.)

The specific information for the opioid agonist analgesics is listed in Table 17-3. A selection of the opioid analgesic combination products are also listed in Table 17-4.

▪ Evaluation

Usually, oral opioid agonist analgesics begin to take effect in 15 to 30 minutes. The time needed for opioids injected into the tissue to take effect may vary depending on the route of administration. This is because of differences in the ability of these drugs to be metabolized, which causes differences in how fast the body can absorb them. Opioids given by mouth are much less effective than those given by injection because much of the medicine is destroyed by the stomach acid. However, oral opioid agonist analgesics produce pain relief for a longer time. Following institutional policies, intravenous (IV) opioids may be given in small doses by PCA by the patient or nurse through IV tubing.

The dose of the opioid agonist analgesic depends on the severity of the pain experienced by the patient, the patient's response to the pain and the medication, and the nature of the illness. In the past, many patients had pain because the dose of medication was not high enough. In the last 10 years, higher doses have been recommended for treating patients with cancer or chronic pain. The new guidelines suggest much higher doses at more frequent intervals and for longer times than previous guidelines. The doses for such patients are much higher than preoperative doses or postoperative doses for acute pain.

The patient who receives any type of opioid analgesic should be checked at regular, frequent intervals. Because opioid agonist analgesics may slow the respiratory rate and decrease the cough and sigh reflexes, patients who have had surgery, especially those who have smoked for a long time, may develop areas where the lungs do not inflate well (atelectasis) or collect fluid and develop pneumonia.

In both the hospital or out patient office, the nurse has the chance to assess each patient's behavior while taking the drug. For example, the patient may be unable to stop taking the drug, may make frequent requests for the drug, or may use more than one health care provider or office. These behaviors may be signs of dependence, abuse, or addiction.

Opioid agonist analgesics are metabolized by the liver, and any unused chemicals leave the body through the kidneys; 90% of most opioids are passed with the urine in first 24 hours.

▪ Patient and Family Teaching

Tell the patient and family the following:
• The patient should take this medication as ordered by prescribing health care provider and not change the dosage. For acute pain it is most effective when taken before the patient has severe pain. For more chronic pain, the patient should gradually make an effort to wait for longer periods of time between doses. The patient should write down the time when

Table 17-3 Opioid

GENERIC NAME	TRADE NAME	COMMENTS
Opioid Agonists		
alfentanil HCl	Alfenta	Individualized dosage used in maintenance of anesthesia.
codeine ★	Codeine Phosphate, Codeine Sulfate	Classified as Schedule II drug.
hydrocodone	Duragesic Hycodan	Respiratory depressant effects of fentanyl are particularly dangerous; have resuscitation equipment nearby.
	Sublimaze	Given preoperatively.
hydromorphone	Dilaudid	Potent synthetic compound that maximizes analgesic effects and minimizes some of the common side effects of morphine; hydromorphone has 7-10 times the analgesic action of morphine.
		Adults: Give IM, SQ, PO, or rectal suppository.
levorphanol	Levo- Dromoran	Used to relieve moderate to severe pain; often used preoperatively to reduce apprehension and to prolong analgesia. Relatively longer onset of action than other opioid agonist analgesics.
		May also be given by slow IV injection.
meperidine	Demerol	Schedule II drug; synthetic opioid analgesic with less potency than morphine; each dose of syrup should be taken in one-half glass of water, because if undiluted, it can exert a topical anesthetic effect on mucous membranes.
		Give IM, PO, or SQ.
methadone	Dolophine	Schedule II drug; synthetic opioid analgesic used primarily in detoxification, treatment, and maintenance of heroin addicts or for severe pain. When drug is used for severe pain, it is administered IM. Drug is highly addictive. When used for heroin addicts for more than 3 wk, methadone moves from a treatment phase to a maintenance phase.
morphine ★	Duramorph MS Contin	Schedule II drug; primary opioid analgesic used for relief of severe pain. Morphine is the opioid analgesic against which all others are compared. Also produces sedation and euphoria when pain is present. Traditionally used for preoperative sedation and postoperative analgesia. Morphine is more effective against dull, continuous pain than sharp, spasmodic pain. IV medication should be given slowly over a 4- to 5-min period. Protect drug from light and freezing.
opium combinations	Opium tincture	Schedule II drug. Opium tincture is equivalent to 1% morphine. Avoid confusing these two medications.
	Paregoric	Paregoric is equivalent to 0.04% morphine. Paregoric is used for cramps, diarrhea, and teething pain in infants (as a topical application to gums).
oxycodone	OxyContin, Oxycodone	These agents are similar in action and structure but are not identical; they are opium alkaloids and are morphine-like in action.
oxymorphone	Numorphan	Give IV or rectal.
Opioid Antagonists		
nalmefene HCl	Revex	Used for postoperative opioid depression or overdose.
naloxone HCl	Narcan	Used for postoperative opioid depression or overdose.
naltrexone HCl	ReVia	Has longer effect than Naloxone. Used for alcohol or opioid dependence.

Table 17-3   Opioid—cont'd

GENERIC NAME	TRADE NAME	COMMENTS
Opioid Agonist-Antagonists		
buprenorphine	Buprenex	Available in SQ, epidural, and rectal forms.
butorphanol	Stadol	Onset of action in 10 min after IM injection and almost immediately after IV injection. Respiratory depressant effect is similar to that of morphine, is dose related, and is easily reversed with naloxone. Available in IV and intranasal forms. Used for obstetric analgesia, renal colic, and cancer pain.
nalbuphine	Nubain	Onset in 15 min, duration 3-6 hr. This product tends to be more expensive than other agonist-antagonist products.
		Adults: 10 mg SC, IM, or IV, repeated q3-6h prn; not to be given more than 20 mg in 1 dose or more than 160 mg/day.

IM, Intramuscular; *IV*, intravenous; *PO*, by mouth; *prn*, as needed; *SQ*, subcutaneous.
★ Indicates "Must-Know Drugs," or the 35 drugs most prescribers use.

Table 17-4   Selected Opioid-Analgesic Combination Products

TRADE NAME	CHEMICAL COMPONENTS
Acetaminophen with Codeine	Codeine, acetaminophen
ASA with Codeine Compound	Codeine, aspirin (ASA)
Empirin with Codeine	Codeine, aspirin
Fiorinal with Codeine	Codeine, aspirin, caffeine, butalbital
Percocet	Oxycodone, acetaminophen
Percodan	Oxycodone, aspirin
Phenaphen-650 with Codeine	Codeine, acetaminophen
Tylox	Oxycodone, acetaminophen
Vicodin, Lortab	Hydrocodone bitartrate, acetaminophen

ASA, Acetylsalicylic acid.

the medication was last taken to prevent taking too much medication by accident.

- If the patient is not feeling a lot of pain, other methods for treating the pain should be used whenever possible, i.e., distraction, heat, cold, etc.
- The patient should not take any other medications without telling the health care provider. Alcohol increases the effect of the medication, and taking both of them together may cause a problem with thinking and breathing.
- Some patients have side effects or adverse effects from this drug, such as dizziness, light-headedness, nausea, drowsiness, sweating, flushing (red color in the face and neck), or stopping of the cough reflex. The patient or family should report any new or troubling symptoms to the nurse, physician, or other health care provider.
- The patient taking this medicine should not operate heavy machinery, drive, or perform tasks that require alertness.
- The patient should prevent constipation by increasing fluid intake and adding extra fiber to the diet.
- The patient should get up slowly from lying or sitting positions to decrease feelings of light- headedness and should avoid standing in one position for long periods.
- When taking the first doses of opioids, the patient should lie down for a short period to prevent nausea.
- This medication must be kept locked up to prevent use by otherss for whom it is not prescribed. All extra medication should be thrown away when there is no longer any need for it; it should not be kept for another time.

OPIOID AGONIST-ANTAGONISTS

OVERVIEW

Opioid agonist-antagonists are strong drugs that act through the CNS, possibly at the limbic system. They act with other chemicals at specific nerve sites.

ACTION

Drugs in this category have different sites of action, but they usually act like morphine in producing analgesia, euphoria, and respiratory depression. Some drugs may compete with other opioids. Thus they may produce withdrawal symptoms in patients who are dependent on opioids, but they are also less likely to be abused than pure opioid agonists.

USES

Opioid agonist-antagonists are used mostly for the relief of moderate to severe pain. They are also used in the injectable form for preoperative analgesia and for pregnant women during active labor. These drugs may be better than opioids for use in patients outside the hospital. Tramadol (Ultram) is an agonist-antagonist in common use in office practice that has a unique dual mechanism action as a mu-opioid receptor agonist and a weak inhibitor of norepinephrine and serotonin reuptake.

The specific information for opioid agonist analgesics is listed in Table 17-3.

ADVERSE REACTIONS

Adverse reactions to opioid agonist-antagonists include bradycardia, hypertension (high blood pressure) or hypotension, tachycardia (rapid heartbeat), changes in mood, blurred vision, confusion, dizziness, headache, weakness, nervousness, nystagmus (rhythmic movement of the eyes), syncope (light-headedness and fainting), tingling, tinnitus (ringing in the ears), tremor, unusual dreams, pruritus, rash, hardening of the soft tissue from swelling, stinging on injection, ulcers, anorexia, abdominal cramps, constipation, diarrhea, dry mouth, dyspepsia (stomach discomfort after eating), nausea, vomiting, low production of white blood cells, dyspnea (uncomfortable breathing), flushing, speech difficulty, and either the urge to urinate or difficulty urinating. Overdosage may produce sedation and respiratory depression.

 Clinical Goldmine

Narcan

Because there is a very real danger of overdosage of opioids, it is important to know about a drug called naloxone (Narcan). This drug is an opioid antagonist that may be used to reverse overdoses of opioids (whether taken by accident or on purpose). Narcan is shorter acting than opioids. If it is given, the nurse must watch for an increase in the opioid symptoms (rebound) when Narcan wears off.

DRUG INTERACTIONS

Alcohol and drugs that slow the actions of the body (depressants) should be used with caution with opioids because of the risk for increased CNS depression.

❖ NURSING IMPLICATIONS AND PATIENT TEACHING

■ Assessment

Learn as much as possible about patients' health history, including the presence of lung, liver, or kidney disease; pregnancy or breastfeeding; recent heart attack; or clues that they might have emotional problems or might have problems with drug dependency or drug misuse. These conditions may be contraindications or precautions to the use of opioid agonist-antagonist analgesics.

The individual's subjective experience of the pain and his or her pain tolerance should be determined. A history of the pain, including when it started, where it is located, what it feels like, how bad it is, and things that make it worse or make it better should be obtained. The nurse may see that the patient has tensed muscles, shallow breathing, changes in blood pressure or pulse, sweating, changes in reaction of the pupils, or restlessness, crying, or moaning. Use a pain scale to classify pain before, during, and after giving pain medication.

■ Diagnosis

Are there any other problems in addition to the medical diagnosis that will affect the patient's response to these drugs? Is the patient frightened? Are there concerns about blood loss, ability to breathe, safety, and whether tissues are dry (**hydration**)? Any problems discovered should be reported to the registered nurse or physician.

■ Planning

Opioid agonist-antagonists should be used with caution in patients who have emotional problems or in those who have a history of drug abuse. Because both physical and emotional dependence may occur, these drugs should be given to such patients only when they can be carefully watched and given only in limited amounts.

Opioid agonist-antagonists should not be given to patients with head injury, because the nurse will need to be able to monitor how the patient acts without the confusing effects of the medication. It has not been established whether it is safe to use these drugs in children or in pregnant women (other than during labor). Because these drugs tend to cause slowed breathing, they should be used very carefully in patients with breathing problems (especially asthma), obstructive breathing conditions, and cyanosis. Pain is an important finding that helps clinicians figure out what is wrong with the patient. For example, abdominal pain from appendicitis. These patients should not have pain medication until it is determined what is wrong with the patient.

Opioid agonist-antagonists may produce withdrawal symptoms in patients who have developed dependence. These products may also cause seizures, especially in patients with known seizure disorders.

Patients who take combination drug products may have adverse effects or develop problems due to any of the drugs used in the medications.

■ Implementation

All of these opioid agonist-antagonists are available in injectable form, but only pentazocine (Talwin) is available in oral form. These medications should be given by intramuscular (IM) injection because subcutaneous injection may damage tissues.

When frequent injections are needed, give each dose in a different site to avoid damaging the tissues. (Refer to Figure 10-15, which shows a typical injection rotation plan.)

For acute pain, one to two tablets or capsules of opioids combined with other medications are given every 4 to 6 hours. Table 17-3 presents a review of opioid agonist-antagonist medications.

■ Evaluation

Monitor the patient to determine whether relief from pain has been achieved and whether any adverse effects have developed as a result of the medicine. If the patient starts seeing things that are not there (hallucinations), or becomes confused or consciousness is reduced, the medication should be stopped.

Watch the patient's behavior for signs for dependence. For example, the patient may be unable to stop taking the drug, may want the drug all the time, or may try to get the drug from multiple physicians or hospitals.

■ Patient and Family Teaching

Tell the patient and family the following:
- The patient should take this medication as ordered by the prescribing health care provider and not change the dosage. Even though this product has a risk for addiction, it is most effective when taken before the patient has severe pain.
- As the patient begins to feel better, other methods for pain relief should be used whenever possible.
- Some patients have side effects from these drugs, such as drowsiness, nausea, vomiting, dizziness, blurred vision, sweating, dry mouth, headache, and confusion. The patient should report any new or troubling symptoms to the nurse, physician, or other health care provider.
- The patient should avoid working with heavy machinery, driving, or tasks that require alertness after taking this medication.
- This medicine must be kept out of the reach of children and others for whom it is not prescribed.

NONOPIOID (CENTRALLY ACTING) ANALGESICS AND COMBINATION ANALGESIC DRUGS

OVERVIEW

Nonopioid (centrally acting) analgesics are drugs that act at the level of the brain to control mild or moderate pain. Many times, small amounts of opioids are included, along with analgesics such as acetaminophen or aspirin, for treatment of minor acute pain.

ACTION AND USES

Nonopioid (centrally acting) analgesics are a small group of miscellaneous drugs. Many of these are used primarily to relieve mild to moderate pain. (See Table 17-5 for a selected listed of these drugs.)

Many of the nonopioid-analgesics are combination drugs that include other chemicals that also work on the pain centers of the CNS. These drugs may contain acetaminophen, aspirin, and caffeine, combined with opioids such as codeine, oxycodone, or hydrocodone. Some combination agents also contain a form of barbiturate (butalbital), which is added for its sedative (calming) effects. Caffeine, a plant extract, has mild brain, lung, and heart stimulant effects, as well as some diuretic activity. It has no analgesic properties, but it is used to treat some types of headaches. Opioids and barbiturates are legally defined as controlled substances, so there are many rules about how they are prescribed.

Combination drugs are used for the relief of moderate to severe pain of an acute origin, such as postoperative or dental pain when a tooth is pulled. They are often ordered when the patient leaves a hospital or when the patient is not in a hospital. These drugs are addictive and should be used for only a brief time. Table 17-6 lists common nonopioid combination products used for analgesia.

There are many different combination products. The dosages and formulations often change. Consult a drug formulary for the latest information.

ADVERSE REACTIONS

Adverse reactions to nonopioid analgesics include the same adverse effects found with the drugs that make up the combinations. Thus, each drug combination

Table 17-5	Nonopioid Centrally Acting Analgesics	
GENERIC NAME	**TRADE NAME**	**COMMENTS**
clonidine	Duraclon	Give 30 mcg/hr for continuous epidural infusion.
tramadol	Ultram	Give PO.

PO, By mouth.

Table 17-6	Selected Nonopioid Analgesic Combination Products
TRADE NAME	**CHEMICAL COMPONENTS**
Anacin	Aspirin, caffeine
Bromo-Seltzer	Acetaminophen, sodium bicarbonate, citric acid
Equagesic	Aspirin, meprobamate
Excedrin	Aspirin, acetaminophen, caffeine
Fiorinal	Aspirin, caffeine, butalbital
Vanquish	Aspirin, acetaminophen, caffeine, antacids

will have its own adverse effects profile. Many of these products are considered quite safe with mild symptoms that include nausea, vomiting, and increased risk of GI bleeding. High doses may be involved with agitation, anxiety, tinnitus, and kidney damage depending upon the products involved.

DRUG INTERACTIONS

Nonopioid analgesics have CNS depressant effects that add to those of other depressants, including alcohol. Each product interacts with other drugs, although these products have fewer chemical interactions than opioids.

❖ NURSING IMPLICATIONS AND PATIENT TEACHING

■ Assessment

Learn as much as possible about the patient's health history, including whether the patient has any respiratory or hepatic disease, or is pregnant or breastfeeding. In addition, look for clues that the patient has emotional problems or has had problems with drug dependency or drug misuse. These conditions may be contraindications or precautions to use of nonopioid analgesics.

Determine the patient's feelings about the pain and its history, including when it started, where it is located, what it feels like and how severe it is, and things that make it worse or make it better. The nurse may also see that the patient has tensed muscles, changes in breathing, sweating, change in pupils, restlessness, crying, or moaning, as well as changes in blood pressure and pulse rate. How well the patient can accept pain should be determined. Use a pain scale to grade the intensity of the patient's pain.

■ Diagnosis

What other problems does the patient have that might interfere with the action of this medication? Are there concerns about moving around, sensory awareness, or level of alertness?

■ Planning

Do not give nonopioid analgesics, including phenothiazines, to patients who are allergic to the products they contain. Always ask the patient about drug allergies before giving a medication.

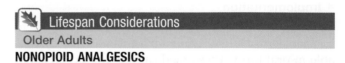

Lifespan Considerations
Older Adults

NONOPIOID ANALGESICS

Older adult and weakened patients may react more strongly to many nonopioid analgesics. These patients should not engage in activities that require them to be alert while taking these drugs, because the medication may slow down their ability to respond quickly.

■ Implementation

These drugs are available in a variety of forms. Many of these products the patient will take by themselves at home.

■ Evaluation

Check the patient regularly and frequently to determine the response to the drug. If the patient seems confused, look for symptoms of overdosage. Patients who have emotional problems, who have abused drugs in the past, or who may not take their medicine properly should not be given these medications.

Because of the risk of hepatotoxicity in former alcoholics using acetaminophen, watch for any sign of alcohol abuse.

■ Patient and Family Teaching

Tell the patient and family the following:
- The patient should take the medication as ordered by the prescribing health care provider and not change the dosage. Although these drugs have a risk for addiction, they are most effective when taken before the patient has severe pain.
- As the patient begins to feel better, other methods for reducing pain should be used whenever possible.
- Some patients have side effects from these drugs, such as dizziness, sleepiness, nausea, and vomiting. The patient may also note a feeling of lightheadedness, especially when getting up from lying down, so the patient should stand up slowly to stop this feeling. The patient should tell the nurse, physician, or other health care provider about any new or troublesome symptoms.
- The patient should not operate any heavy machinery, drive, or perform tasks for which he or she needs to be alert while taking this medication.
- This medication must be kept out of the reach of children and others for whom it is not prescribed.

DRUGS FOR ANESTHESIA

When a part of the body or the total body can be made numb and unresponsive to pain, this is known as **anesthesia**. If the loss of sensation is only a very small part of the body, we call it *local anesthesia*. Dental procedures or minor surgery are examples. This type of anesthesia may be produced by topical application of a medication or by injecting the medication into the skin (infiltration). Regional anesthesia achieves loss of sensation in a larger area by deadening a nerve that would carry pain (nerve block), and injection of medicine into the spinal canal or epidural areas controls pain sensations in a particular area.

Local anesthetics interrupt pain and motor sensation by blocking the movement of sodium ions into neurons. The length of this activity is usually short but can be increased by adding other medications to the injection. The local anesthetics are classified by their chemical structures as either amides or esters. Amides are most commonly used because they have fewer side effects and a longer duration of action. Adverse effects to local anesthetics are uncommon but some people may be allergic to the drug or the preservatives that might be added to the medication. Sometimes patients with heart disease are particularly sensitive and have longer systemic effects, such as anxiety, restlessness, hypotension, or irregular heartbeats, caused by local anesthetics if they contain epinephrine (adrenaline); Common local anesthetics that might be used are listed in Table 17-7.

General anesthesia is produced when the body is unconscious and unresponsive. Patients may be heavily sedated or conversely, may have received a paralytic agent so they cannot move or breathe and must be intubated. Patients not only do not feel pain, they cannot move, talk, or breathe by themselves. An anesthesiologist or nurse anesthetist must be there to help them breathe and to monitor their vital signs. General anesthesia is usually produced by giving IV medication or by having patients breathe a gas through their mouth and nose.

Many drugs may be given along with general anesthesia for different purposes. These include cholinergic agents to dry up respiratory secretions, opioids to help control pain, neuromuscular blocking agents to paralyze the muscles so the respiratory tube may be inserted and to prevent movement and intestinal protrusion during abdominal surgery. Drug combinations help the patient go quickly to sleep and progress to very deep relaxation so that surgical procedure is possible. The anesthesia provider makes sure the patient does not become too deeply anesthetized and decreases risk to the patient. Nitrous oxide is a gas used in obstetrics or dentistry or for short medical procedures. It may also be used with other more potent inhaled gases. Other anesthetics involve use of volatile liquids that

Table 17-7	Selected List of Local Anesthetics
DRUG	**COMMENTS**
articaine (Septanest)	Very long duration. Good for nerve blocks.
benzocaine (Americaine, Solarcaine)	Topical OTC anesthesia used for sunburn and minor abrasions
bupivacaine (Marcaine)	Used in epidural anesthesia
dibucaine (Nupercaine)	Used in topical or spinal anesthesia.
etidocaine (Duranest)	Used in nerve blocks, procedures, and epidural and spinal anesthesia.
lidocaine (Xylocaine)	Most popular agent used for topical, procedures, nerve block, and epidural and spinal anesthesia.
mepivacaine (Carbocaine)	Used for nerve block and epidural anesthesia; intermediate duration
procaine (Novocain)	Short duration ester used in procedures, nerve blocks, and epidural and spinal anesthesia.
prilocaine (Citanest)	Used for procedures, nerve block, and epidurals; intermediate duration.
tetracaine (Pontocaine)	Ester used for long duration in topical and spinal anesthesia.

OTC, Over the counter.

are converted to gases for the induction (beginning) and maintenance of general anesthesia. Halothane (Fluothane) is the best-known volatile liquid, although it is not used as much now because newer products are safer; desflurane, enflurane, isoflurane, methoxyflurane, and sevoflurane are others that might be used. Methoxyflurane is often used in labor because it is the least likely to suppress uterine contractions.

Many drugs may be given prior to gas anesthesia to help relax the patient and reduce pain. Some of these preoperative drugs are those mentioned earlier in this chapter. Other IV drugs are given at the same time as inhaled anesthetics so that the dose of the inhaled drug can be reduced. This helps reduce the possibility of serious side effects. These IV drugs used as anesthetics include benzodiazepines, barbiturates, and opioids. Table 17-8 briefly identifies other IV drugs that might be used for anesthesia; however, more detailed information is provided in Chapter 16 and earlier in this chapter.

What do licensed practical and vocational nurses (LPNs/LVNs) need to know about anesthesia? LPNs/LVNs may be asked to find medication for physicians

Table 17-8 Selected Other Drugs Used with Anesthetics

INTRAVENOUS ANESTHETIC AGENTS	SELECTED DRUGS
Barbiturate and barbiturate-like agents	Etomidate, methohexital sodium, propofol, thiopental sodium
Benzodiazepines	diazepam, lorazepam, midazolam HCl
Opioids	alfentanil HCl, fentanyl, remifentanil, sufentanil
Others	ketamine
ADJUNCTS TO ANESTHESIA	SELECTED DRUGS
Barbiturates and barbiturate-like agents	amobarbital, butabarbital sodium, pentobarbital, secobarbital
Cholinergic agent	bethanechol
Dopamine blockers	droperidol, promethazine
Neuromuscular blockers	succinylcholine
Opioids	alfentanil, fentanyl, remifentanil, sufentanil

to use to inject and produce local or regional anesthesia. They may occasionally give IM or prepare IV preoperative medications. But primarily LPNs/LVNs may hear the surgeons or anesthesiologists discussing general anesthesia or read about other IV medications that were given during surgery.

The role of the nurse for a patient going to surgery is primarily to monitor the patient and try to calm him or her. Patients are often frightened when going to surgery. If the patient has a history of fainting (hypotensive episode) when IV lines are started or if he or she is having an elective procedure for which anesthesia will be required, the anesthesiologist should know this so he or she will be able to watch for it. What previous nursing research has shown is that if patients are given good information about the procedure or surgery—where they will go, who will be with them during surgery, how long surgery will take, and how long they will be in the recovery room—that the incidence of nausea, vomiting, anxiety and pain are reduced.

Get Ready for the NCLEX® Examination!

Key Points

- Pain is often something we can all understand or experience.
- For many years, patients suffered with pain because there was a fear that they would become addicted to opioids. New guidelines have tried to change this.
- Morphine is the standard against which all other opioid analgesics are judged.
- There are now many new synthetic opioid analgesics available to help reduce pain.
- Nurses have a special job in learning and following the many rules for giving opioids and in preventing abuse of these drugs.

Additional Learning Resources

SG Go to your Study Guide for additional learning activities to help you master this chapter content.

evolve Go to your Evolve website (http://evolve.elsevier.com/Edmunds/LPN/) for additional online resources.

Review Questions for the NCLEX® Examination

1. The patient is being treated with an opioid medication. She has nausea when the medication dosage is slightly reduced. The patient is experiencing:
   1. addiction
   2. dependence
   3. tolerance
   4. withdrawal symptoms

2. The patient who is the best choice for treatment with an opioid medication is:
   1. a 70-year-old man with a history of hypertension
   2. a 32-year-old woman who is 6 months pregnant
   3. a 55-year-old man who has experienced two heart attacks
   4. a 42-year-old woman who has abdominal pain

3. The patient is started on an opioid medication. He complains to the nurse of having flushing. The nurse recognizes that this is:
   1. an expected side effect of the medication
   2. an anaphylactic reaction to the medication
   3. indication of a toxic dosage of the medication
   4. an unexpected side effect of the medication

4. To help patients get the best pain relief, a good schedule for oral treatment of acute pain is:
   1. 1 tablet by mouth every 12 hours
   2. 1-2 tablets by mouth every 4-6 hours
   3. 2-4 tablets by mouth every 6 hours
   4. 3-4 tablets by mouth every 8 hours

5. The physician says the patient has neuropathic pain. The nurse recognizes that this pain will most likely be described by the patient as:
   1. dull or aching
   2. throbbing or stinging
   3. shooting or stabbing
   4. pinching or burning

Get Ready for the NCLEX® Examination!—cont'd

Case Study

Mr. Rim, a hard-working Korean immigrant, works in an inner-city convenience store. He has recently hurt his back lifting heavy boxes.

1. What is the most appropriate form of initial pain control?
2. The pain continues, and now Mr. Rim experiences pain shooting from his lower back down his left leg. X-ray studies reveal a ruptured vertebral disk, and he undergoes surgery. What type of analgesia is likely to be ordered after surgery?
3. Mr. Rim does not want to take any pain medication. He believes he should only have pain medication if his pain is so bad that he cannot tolerate it. What would the nurse tell him?
4. Is there any reason why Mr. Rim is likely to become addicted to his medication?
5. What type of behavior might lead the nurse to believe that a patient has become addicted to pain medication?

Drug Calculation Review

1. Order: Morphine sulfate 5 mg IM every 4 hours as needed for pain. Supply: Morphine sulfate 10 mg/mL.
   Question: How many milliliters of morphine sulfate is needed for each dose?
2. Order: Dilaudid 0.5 mg/hr IV continuous drip. Supply: Dilaudid 20 mg in 200 mL 0.9% normal saline.
   Question: How many milliliters per hour should the IV infusion device be set for?

3. Order: Narcan 0.4 mg IV for respiratory rate (RR) less than 8 breaths/min. Supply: Narcan 0.2 mg/mL.
   Question: How many milliliters of Narcan should be given if the RR is less than 8 breaths/min?

Critical Thinking Questions

1. Why are increased caution and lower doses of opioid analgesics recommended for use in older adult patients?
2. The patient who is postoperative from abdominal surgery has been requesting increasingly frequent pain medication. Her medication has been ordered every 4 hours, but she is now requesting it every 2 to 2½ hours. What is the most appropriate nursing action for this patient?
3. A nursing entry on a patient's chart read, "Quiet evening." Also recorded was that the same nurse had administered "ASA 625 mg PO for headache" to the patient. What information is missing?
4. Mr. Taylor has just returned to the surgical unit from the postanesthesia care unit, following left total knee-replacement surgery. When is the best time to administer pain medication to Mr. Taylor?
5. Mr. Robbins was started on an opioid agonist analgesic immediately after his surgery. Several days after the surgery, he seems to be requesting medication more often than the nurse had anticipated. Mr. Robbins is not addicted to his medication, but both he and his family are concerned about that possibility. Draw up a teaching plan for a patient taking an opioid agonist analgesic.

18

Antiinflammatory, Musculoskeletal, and Antiarthritis Medications

*e*volve

http://evolve.elsevier.com/Edmunds/LPN/

Objectives

1. List medications commonly used for the treatment of minor musculoskeletal pain and inflammation.
2. Compare the actions of various antiinflammatory and muscle relaxant agents.
3. Identify the appropriate use for musculoskeletal relaxants.
4. Explain the mechanisms of action for different antiarthritis medications.
5. Describe adverse reactions frequently found in the use of antiarthritis medications.
6. Describe the clinical situations in which uricosuric therapy may be indicated.

Key Terms

arthritis (ărth-RĪ-tĭs, p. 324)
gout (gŏwt, p. 328)
nonsteroidal antiinflammatory drugs (NSAIDs) (p. 319)
osteoarthritis (ŏs-tē-ō-ărth-RĪ-tĭs, p. 324)
rheumatoid arthritis (RŪ-mă-tŏyd, p. 324)

salicylates (să-LĬS-ĭl-āts, p. 314)
skeletal muscle relaxants (SKĔL-ĭ-tăl, p. 321)
uric acid (Ū-rĭk, p. 328)
uricosuric agents (Ū-rĭ-kō-SŪR-ĭk, p. 328)

OVERVIEW

This chapter includes the medications helpful in treating problems affecting the bones, joints, muscles, and ligaments. There are many musculoskeletal disorders that cause pain, stiffness, and boney deformity. Powerful drugs are used for the more serious problems; safer over-the-counter (OTC) drugs are used for less serious conditions. Many acute problems, such as sprains, fractures, or tears, require only short-term therapy. Some disorders, such as arthritis, may require long-term therapy with simpler drugs used initially, advancing to advanced drugs as the pain and mobility problems increase. Most of these products—even the drugs sold OTC have serious adverse reactions, and patient response to therapy must be monitored closely.

This chapter is divided into four sections. The first section deals with antiinflammatory and analgesic medications such as the salicylates and nonsteroidal antiinflammatory drugs (NSAIDs), which are used to treat both minor and severe pain and common orthopedic problems. The second section presents skeletal muscle relaxants. The third section introduces a variety of medications used to treat arthritis, the disease-modifying antirheumatic medications (DMARDS) and immune modulators. Agents used to treat high uric acid levels found in gout are presented in the fourth section. These are all common conditions that licensed practical and vocational nurses see and medicines they use frequently.

MUSCULAR AND SKELETAL SYSTEMS

The muscular and skeletal systems work together to provide support and movement for the body (Figures 18-1 and 18-2). The skeletal system is made up of the bones, cartilage, ligaments, and joints, and the muscular system is those muscles attached to the skeleton.

The skeleton protects, supports, and allows body movement, produces blood cells in the long bones, and stores minerals. The muscular system helps the body parts move, holds the body upright, and produces body heat.

Disease may attack just a small part of the body or the whole muscular and skeletal system. Injuries are often due to trauma, wear over many years, or overuse. Although some traumatic skeletal injuries heal well, some injury sites may continue to have pain and deformity.

THE INFLAMMATORY RESPONSE

The inflammatory response is necessary for the body's survival when faced with stress or injury. A number of things can trigger the inflammatory response. These include infectious agents, ischemia (lack of blood

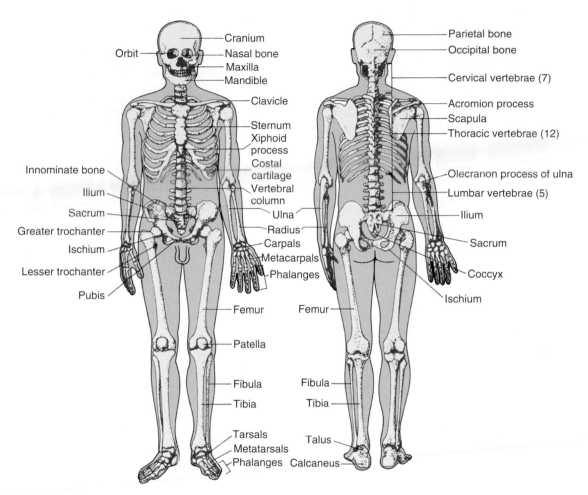

FIGURE 18-1 The skeletal system.

supply to a tissue), antigen-antibody interactions, and thermal (heat or cold) or other injury. The inflammatory response has three phases:

1. Acute, brief, local vasodilation (opening up of the blood vessels) and increased capillary permeability
2. A delayed, subacute infiltration (movement) of leukocytes and phagocytic cells into the tissue
3. Chronic proliferative tissue degeneration (breakdown) and fibrosis

The inflammatory response of the body produces the symptoms of erythema (redness or irritation), edema (fluid buildup in the body tissues), tenderness, and pain. This happens when the affected blood cells release a variety of inflammatory mediators (substances that continue the inflammatory response). The inflammatory mediators act to increase blood flow to the area and increase capillary permeability, allowing movement of large molecules across cell walls into the site. One of the most important inflammatory mediators is histamine, which causes vasodilation to increase blood flow to the area. Cytokines help control the inflammatory process. Prostaglandins also have a role in the inflammatory reaction.

Prostaglandins have several actions in the body. The useful functions of prostaglandins have to do with "housekeeping" actions in the tissues, especially in protecting the mucosa of the gastrointestinal (GI) tract. They also maintain normal renal function, platelet aggregation (clumping together), consciousness and mental functions in the brain, and temperature. Prostaglandins also cause erythema and an increase in local blood flow, and they can remove the vasoconstrictor effects of substances such as norepinephrine and angiotensin. These actions of prostaglandins are controlled by a series of reactions at sites of tissue injury and inflammation. Prostaglandins are helpful when they are kept in check, but harmful when they are not.

The housekeeping functions of prostaglandins are controlled by cyclooxygenase-1 (COX-1). Cyclooxygenase-2 (COX-2) is created where there is inflammation caused by cytokines and other inflammatory mediators. It is also found in the brain, where it plays a role in fever and perception of pain. COX-2 is an active participant in the inflammatory process and produces harmful results in the body if not controlled.

Although it is important to have medications that can block the harmful actions of prostaglandins, the important physiologic functions of prostaglandins that are helpful in the body must be preserved. Most

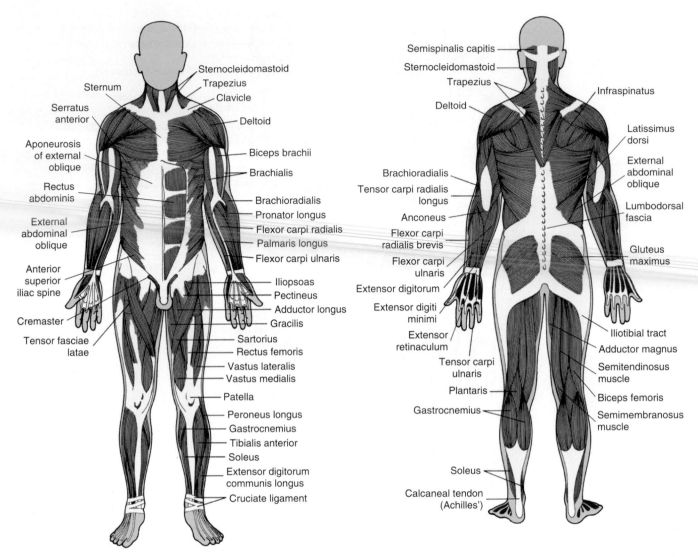

FIGURE 18-2 The muscular system.

antiinflammatory drugs block the actions of both COX-1 and COX-2. A group of drugs known as *COX-2 inhibitors* or *blockers* was developed to reduce the inflammatory response in some tissues without destroying the tissue of the GI tract (Figure 18-3). Although these drugs reduce the incidence of gastric bleeding, current research suggests that they may do so at the expense of the heart. All but one of these drugs have been removed from the market because of this problem.

ANTIINFLAMMATORY AND ANALGESIC AGENTS

OVERVIEW

Aspirin is one of the most commonly taken medications. The ease with which it can be bought and the fact that people decide when and if they need it should not decrease the importance given to this drug

in treating common and significant musculoskeletal problems. Aspirin (acetylsalicylic acid [ASA]) has greater antiinflammatory action than other salicylates and is preferred in the treatment of many problems. Acetaminophen is also used for analgesia in generalized pain and arthritis because of its safety. Acetaminohen is an analgesic but not an NSAID because it has no antiinflammatory properties. The NSAIDs are powerful agents to help decrease pain and inflammation. Prostaglandins may make peripheral pain receptors more sensitive to painful stimuli. Both salicylates and NSAIDs are thought to limit the production of prostaglandins.

SALICYLATES

ACTION

Salicylates have analgesic (pain-reducing), antipyretic (temperature-reducing), and antiinflammatory effects. It also has growing use as an emergency antiplatelet

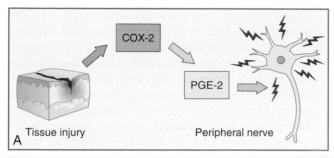

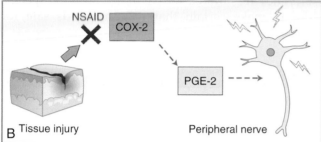

FIGURE 18-3 Model for nociceptive pain. A, Tissue injury triggers cyclooxygenase-2 (COX-2) in peripheral tissue to convert arachidonic acid to prostaglandin E2 (PGE2), resulting in stimulation of the nociceptor in peripheral nerve to send a signal for pain to the central nervous system. B, Nonsteroidal antiinflammatory drug (NSAID) interfering with COX-2–mediated prostaglandin synthesis.

drug in patients who are having a myocardial infarction (MIs) or to prevent other MIs or strokes in men. Salicylates stop the production of prostaglandins, which affects the pain and inflammatory processes through a depressant effect on the central and peripheral pain receptors. They do this by blocking the production of cyclooxygenase, an enzyme that is necessary for the production of prostaglandins.

USES

Aspirin is stronger or more potent in stopping prostaglandin synthesis than are other salicylates, and it has greater antiinflammatory effects. Aspirin is used in the treatment of mild to moderate pain. Aspirin is the only drug in this category to slow the clumping of platelets for the life of the platelet (7 to 10 days). It also interferes with factor III of the clotting mechanism. This makes it useful in reducing the risk for strokes or for treating transient ischemic attacks (TIAs) in patients who have had some types of TIAs. However, it is of no benefit for men who have already had strokes. Research shows that aspirin does not seem to prevent TIAs or strokes in women.

Small daily doses of aspirin are also used to reduce the risk of death or nonfatal MI in patients with previous infarction or unstable angina pectoris. Lower doses are just as effective and have fewer side effects than higher doses for this purpose. Unlabeled uses of aspirin in low doses also include prevention of colorectal cancer and preeclampsia.

Salicylates are used as first-line therapy to treat various forms of arthritis (rheumatoid arthritis, osteoarthritis, degenerative joint disease) through inhibition of cyclooxygenase (COS). The inflammatory and analgesic effects of aspirin are roughly equivalent to those of many other NSAIDS. Their use has declined somewhat with the option of NSAIDS. They are used to treat fever produced by bacterial illnesses and in therapy for pain from trauma to soft tissue or muscle. Pain in the muscles, nerves, and joints (myalgias, neuralgias, and arthralgias), as well as headache and dysmenorrhea, are also treated with salicylates. The antiinflammatory effects are useful in treating systemic lupus erythematosus, acute rheumatic fever, and similar conditions. An aspirin should be chewed immediately by any patient suspected of having an acute MI to help limit tissue damage.

ADVERSE REACTIONS

The greatest concern in use of aspirin for chronic disease is the production of GI distress and bleeding. Bleeding may often occur suddenly and without pain. It is estimated that a normal person taking Aspirin loses 10 mL of blood every day from minor GI irritation. Hypersensitivity (allergy) is also common and may produce anaphylaxis. In those with allergy, there may also be cross-sensitivity to other medications, including NSAIDS and acetaminophen. Other adverse reactions to antiinflammatory analgesics include tinnitus (ringing in the ears), visual disturbances, edema, urticaria (hives), rashes, anorexia (lack of appetite), epigastric discomfort, and nausea. Aspirin has been associated with the occurrence of Reye syndrome when given to children with varicella (i.e. chickenpox) or influenza. In Reye syndrome, symptoms may affect all organs of the body, but most seriously affects the brain and liver. Rapid development of severe neurological symptoms, including lethargy, confusion, seizures, and coma, make Reye syndrome a life-threatening emergency. Most authorities advise against the use of aspirin in these and other viral infections. In overdosage, symptoms may progress from mild to severe, beginning with hyperventilation, diaphoresis (sweating), thirst, headache, drowsiness, skin eruptions, and electrolyte imbalance, and progressing to central nervous system (CNS) depression, stupor, convulsions and coma, tachycardia (rapid heartbeat), and respiratory insufficiency. Respiratory and metabolic acidosis are most often seen in children.

DRUG INTERACTIONS

Alcohol taken with any of the antiinflammatory analgesics increases the chance of GI bleeding. There is an increased effect of anticoagulants, sulfonylureas, and sulfonamides if they are used at the same time as salicylates. Ascorbic acid increases the effect of salicylates by increasing renal tubular reabsorption. Salicylates interact with other NSAIDs to increase effects, side effects, and toxicities. Salicylates also increase or potentiate the effects of phenytoin (Dilantin) and inhibit hyperuricemia produced by pyrazinamide. Salicylates can affect the results of many laboratory test results.

❖ NURSING IMPLICATIONS AND PATIENT TEACHING

▪ Assessment

Learn all possible details about the patient's health history. Check for the presence of allergy to aspirin or other NSAIDs, history of asthma or nasal polyps, GI problems or ulcer disease, current use of other drugs that may cause interactions, or other hepatic or renal disease. These conditions are precautions or contraindications to the use of salicylates.

The health care provider may ask the nurse to get a stool specimen to check for occult blood before beginning the medication. This will help decide whether or not the patient had bleeding in the stool before the medication was started.

▪ Diagnosis

Careful attention should be paid to other medications and disease processes of the patient. Are there conditions that would make the use of NSAIDs or salicylates dangerous? What is the risk for GI bleeding in this patient? How much caffeine, alcohol, or tobacco does this patient use? Are there other problems related to weight, mobility, safety, or nutrition?

▪ Planning

Antiinflammatory analgesics should not be used in patients with hepatic (liver) disease. Patients on anticoagulant therapy or with blood clotting problems must be very careful when they use these products. These drugs also should not be used before surgery (because of their effect on platelet aggregation) or before labor (because bleeding may increase). They should be used with caution in patients with symptoms suggesting TIAs. In patients with musculoskeletal pain that persists for more than 10 days, further evaluation of the pain is needed.

Antiinflammatory analgesics should not be used during pregnancy, especially during the third trimester, because they may have adverse effects on the fetus. Salicylates are excreted in breast milk.

These drugs should be used carefully if the patient has gastric irritation, especially in patients with a past history of upper GI problem, blood dyscrasias, or decreased renal function.

Hydration (supply of fluids) should be monitored carefully in children, because they seem to be more likely to get salicylate intoxication or overdose.

Reye syndrome is an acute, life-threatening problem seen in children that produces vomiting and lethargy that may go on to delirium and coma with permanent brain damage and possible death. Use of aspirin after influenza, chickenpox, or other viral conditions in children seems to be closely related to the development of Reye syndrome and should be avoided.

Many salicylate products are not recommended for use in children younger than 12 years of age. When salicylates are ordered for children, check the specific drug to make certain that the product is safe for children.

 Clinical Pitfall

Reye Syndrome

Children who have repeated instances of viral upper-respiratory-tract infections within a short time or who have disorientation due to high fever should not be given salicylates. These drugs have been linked to the development of Reye syndrome post viral infection.

▪ Implementation

The administration and dosage for each of the salicylate products vary. There are tablets, capsules, drops, chewable preparations, suppositories, and injectable forms of these products. Aspirin is the most active agent and has the greatest amount of salicylate per unit. Individual products should be checked for dosing specifics by age.

Patients (particularly poorer patients or immigrants) with diabetes who are testing their urine with Benedict's Clinitest may get incorrect readings. They may need to switch to another form of urine testing while using salicylate products. Salicylates also increase the action of oral hypoglycemic agents, and patients with diabetes should be alert to signs of hypoglycemia (low blood sugar level).

A summary of dosing information for the salicylates is provided in Table 18-1.

▪ Evaluation

The patient should be monitored to see that symptoms resolve (i.e., pain is gone and temperature is reduced to 101° F or lower). The dosage should be reduced or the drug stopped if tinnitus (ringing in ears) develops. Observe for fever that does not fall or other symptoms that suggest the patient is getting worse, and notify the health care provider.

For arthritis, higher dosages are usually needed to control pain and stiffness. The dosage should be slowly increased as necessary while the patient is watched not only for pain relief, but for improvement in such things as increased strength of grip, increased mobility, and improved ability to carry on normal activities of daily living. Patients taking medication over a long time

Table 18-1 **Antiinflammatory Analgesics**

GENERIC NAME	TRADE NAME	COMMENTS
Salicylates and Acetaminophen		
acetaminophen ★	Acephen Aceta Acetaminophen Apacet FeverAll Panadol Tempra 3 Tylenol	Used as an analgesic-antipyretic in the presence of aspirin allergy and for patients with blood coagulation disorders being treated with oral anticoagulants, bleeding diatheses, upper GI disease, gastritis, hiatal hernia, and gouty arthritis. Also used for a variety of soft-tissue injuries and for acute pain relief.
acetylsalicylic acid (ASA, aspirin) ★	Aspergum Bayer Ecotrin Empirin	The most commonly used antiinflammatory agent. Standard against which all other agents are compared. Hypersensitivity often exists.
acetylsalicylic acid (ASA) buffered choline salicylate	Alka-Seltzer Ascriptin Bufferin	Aspirin-antacid combinations are used in patients who experience GI distress from plain aspirin. Dosage and administration are the same as for plain aspirin.
diflunisal	Dolobid	Salicylic acid nonsteroidal derivative.
magnesium salicylate	Doan's caplets	Sodium-free salicylate with lower incidence of GI problems than ASA.
salsalate	Amigesic Salflex	Take in divided doses.
sodium salicylate	Sodium Salicylate	Comes in an enteric-coated pill.
Nonsteroidal Antiinflammatory Drugs		
diclofenac	Cataflam Voltaren ♣	Used for chronic long-term therapy. Also comes in a delayed-release tablet.
fenoprofen	Nalfon	Administer medication 30 min before or 2 hr after meals; food interferes with absorption.
flurbiprofen	Ansaid	Used in rheumatoid arthritis and osteoarthritis.
ibuprofen ★	Advil Motrin Nuprin	Approved for use in the treatment of dysmenorrhea. Used in acute, chronic pain and for inflammatory processes.
indomethacin	Indocin	A potent prostaglandin synthesis inhibitor with significant toxic side effects; many adverse reactions (including blood dyscrasias) and drug interactions. Acute gouty arthritis. Take for 5 days, then reduce dosage. Patient should be weaned off medication as soon as possible.
ketorolac	Toradol	Given IM for short-term management of pain and orally for short duration. Do not use longer than 5 days.
meclofenamate		Has ability to block action of prostaglandins and inhibit their synthesis, whereas other NSAIDs only inhibit prostaglandin synthesis.
mefenamic acid	Ponstel	Recommended for treatment of dysmenorrhea rather than arthritis or other acute musculoskeletal problems.
meloxicam	Mobic	Take with or without food.
naproxen	Aleve Anaprox Naprosyn	Used for mild to moderate pain, rheumatoid arthritis, osteoarthritis, ankylosing spondylitis. Long-term therapy may require the higher dosage range. If no symptomatic effect in 2 wk, trial should be continued for 2 more wk before drug discontinued. Used to treat acute gout.
piroxicam	Feldene	Indicated in the treatment of acute exacerbations and long-term management of rheumatoid arthritis and osteoarthritis.
sulindac	Clinoril	Used for arthritis and ankylosing spondylitis, acute painful shoulder or gout.
Cyclooxygenase-2 Inhibitor		
celecoxib	Celebrex	Used in osteoarthritis, rheumatoid arthritis, acute pain, and dysmenorrhea. Long-term use may damage heart. Do not use in patients allergic to sulfa.

GI, Gastrointestinal; *IM*, intramuscular; *NSAID*, nonsteroidal antiinflammatory drug.
★ Indicates "Must-Know Drugs," or the 35 drugs most prescribers use.

should be monitored for signs of occult (hidden) bleeding with regular blood counts and stool checks. Check for signs of aspirin toxicity, especially tinnitus. Periodic checks of serum salicylate levels may be helpful if the dosage is reaching maximum levels or if there is a question of patient compliance.

■ Patient and Family Teaching

Tell the patient and family the following:

- These drugs may cause stomach upset because they are so strong. This symptom may be reduced by taking medicine with food, milk, or a full glass of water. Patients should never take the medication without adequate liquid, because it may lead to GI distress and pain.
- The patient should contact the health care provider right away if ringing in the ears; abnormal bleeding or bruising; or bloody or black, tarry stools are noted.
- Chronic problems may require taking the medicine for more than a week before the patient notices any decrease in symptoms.
- The medication should be taken regularly to reduce inflammation. If the medication is taken regularly, a stable serum level is kept in the blood, and symptoms can be reduced more easily.
- The patient should not take any other medications at the same time without the knowledge of the health care provider. This includes drugs the patient may purchase OTC.
- The health care provider should be contacted if the patient is taking the medicine for a fever and: (1) the fever does not come down in 24 to 48 hours, or (2) the patient becomes lethargic (sleepy) or hard to awaken.
- This medication should be kept out of the reach of children and all others for whom it is not prescribed. Even small doses may be fatal to small children.
- If the patient is unable to take the medication in the form prescribed, the health care provider should be contacted so another form may be ordered. Medication is available in chewable tablets and suppositories to make it easier for some patients to take.

ACETAMINOPHEN

OVERVIEW

Acetaminophen (Tylenol) is an OTC medication commonly used to decrease fever and mild pain. It can be used in patients who have experienced gastric irritation with aspirin or other NSAIDs. Acetaminophen is similar to aspirin in its effectiveness in treating fever and pain. It is the drug of choice for relief of minor pain in children. Acetaminophen is different from aspirin in that it does not have an antiinflammatory effect or an effect on platelet aggregation.

Acetaminophen is a metabolite of phenacetin, a product that was taken off the market because of a link with nephropathy (kidney damage). It is also linked to hepatotoxicity (liver damage) when dosage is increased. Acetaminophen may be included with other OTC drugs used to treat common illnesses.

Clinical Pitfall

Safety with Acetaminophen

Parents frequently do not realize that acetaminophen is in many products and miscalculate the dosage of acetaminophen given to young children, exceed the dosage, or give the dose too often. This may produce liver toxicity and death due to liver failure. Always remind parents to be careful in giving this drug. Drug manufacturers voluntarily removed many children's cough and cold OTC products containing acetaminophen to help avoid this problem.

ACTION AND USES

Acetaminophen works as an antipyretic by direct action on the hypothalamic heat-regulating center, lowering the temperature to a normal level. It does this by blocking the action of pyrogenic cytokines on the heat-regulating center. This helps get rid of body heat via vasodilation and sweating.

The mechanism of analgesic action is not clear. It may be due to inhibition of prostaglandin synthetase in the CNS. Acetaminophen differs from aspirin in that it does not inhibit peripheral prostaglandin synthesis. This may account for the absence of inflammatory and platelet-inhibiting effects. Acetaminophen is a very effective medication for treating chronic pain of both malignant and nonmalignant origin. Other medications are often combined with acetaminophen to enhance their effectiveness.

Acetaminophen is the initial drug of choice for treatment of osteoarthritis. It is effective in pain relief and has fewer adverse reactions than aspirin or NSAIDs.

ADVERSE REACTIONS

If used as directed, adverse reactions are rare. The symptoms of hypersensitivity are skin eruptions, urticaria, erythema, and fever. Extremely rare hematologic reactions include hemolytic anemia, leukopenia, neutropenia, and pancytopenia. Other reactions are hypoglycemia, liver toxicity, and jaundice (yellow color of skin, eyes, and mucous membranes). Overdosage is possible and may be fatal. This is particularly a problem in young children and older adults.

DRUG INTERACTIONS

Use of acetaminophen with the following drugs may increase the risk of hepatotoxicity (damage to the liver): barbiturates, hydantoins (Dilantin), carbamazepine (Tegretol), rifampin, and ethanol.

Activated charcoal reduces acetaminophen absorption. Acetylcysteine (Mucomyst) is used as an antidote in acetaminophen overdose.

❖ NURSING IMPLICATIONS AND PATIENT TEACHING

■ Assessment

Learn as much as possible about the patient's health history. Ask questions to learn about other problems the patient may have that might have produced pain. Does the patient have any risk factors for drug interactions?

■ Diagnosis

What other products does that patient take for symptoms of common colds or minor pains at the same time as using it for treatment of osteoarthritis? If so, do the products contain acetaminophenen that might place them at risk for overdose or developing toxicity.

■ Planning

Acetaminophen is available OTC, and many patients decide when and how much medicine to take. Ask specifically about acetaminophen use when taking a medication history to include all OTC medications, herbal medicine, and prescription drugs. Generic acetaminophen is equally effective and less expensive than brand-name products.

■ Implementation

Acetaminophen is the drug of choice for reduction of fever. Treatment of minor fever is not indicated unless the fever is making the patient uncomfortable. Symptomatic relief of a temperature greater than 40° C is usually required. Treatment of a temperature higher than 41° C or 105° F to 106° F is a medical emergency. Caution the patient against overdosing.

Dosing information for acetaminophen is provided in Table 21-1.

■ Evaluation

Monitor fever or pain control. Watch for symptoms of gastric distress, nausea, or bleeding.

■ Patient and Family Teaching

Tell the patient and family the following:
- The patient should not exceed the recommended dosage.
- Have the patient look at or bring in all of their medications to assess for the drugs that may have acetaminophen.
- This medication should be kept out of the reach of children.
- The patient should stop using this medication if a sensitivity reaction occurs.

- Severe pain or high fever may indicate serious illness. If symptoms persist, the patient should contact the health care provider.
- The patient should avoid consumption of excessive alcohol while taking this medication because of increased risk of liver damage.

NONSTEROIDAL ANTIINFLAMMATORY DRUGS

ACTION

Nonsteroidal antiinflammatory drugs (NSAIDs) have analgesic, antiinflammatory, and antipyretic effects and are used to treat rheumatic diseases, degenerative joint disease, osteoarthritis, and acute musculoskeletal problems. The exact mode of action of NSAIDs is not known, although it is believed that the analgesic and antiinflammatory effects of NSAIDs are largely the result of their ability to stop the production of prostaglandins. All NSAIDs inhibit cyclooxygenase, thus blocking the production of prostaglandins. One NSAID celecoxib (Celebrex) specifically works to inhibit COX-2, the chemical created at sites of inflammation by cytokines and inflammatory mediators. These agents also inhibit platelet clumping or aggregation, but this effect appears to be dose related.

USES

Use of NSAIDs may be indicated for acute or chronic musculoskeletal pain.

Most NSAIDs are used in the treatment of both rheumatoid arthritis and osteoarthritis. They are used specifically in the relief of arthritic signs and symptoms, in treatment of acute inflammatory flare-ups and worsening of symptoms, and for long-term management of arthritis. NSAIDs are also used in treatment of pain from dental extraction, minor surgery, and soft-tissue athletic injuries. Ibuprofen (Advil, Motrin) has been approved for use in dysmenorrhea because of its inhibition of prostaglandin production.

ADVERSE REACTIONS

Adverse reactions to NSAIDs include asthma, fluid retention, hypertension (high blood pressure), confusion, dizziness, blurred or decreased vision, malaise (weakness), sleepiness, tinnitus, pruritus, skin irritation or rash related to sun exposure, abdominal pain, anorexia, bloating, constipation, diarrhea, dyspepsia (stomach discomfort after eating), excessive gas in the GI tract, GI bleeding (upper or lower), heartburn, nausea, vomiting, hematuria (blood in the urine; occurs with some NSAIDs or with worsened renal failure), and many forms of blood-cell changes.

DRUG INTERACTIONS

Because the various NSAIDs are somewhat different structurally, their specific drug interactions vary. Therefore each agent should be checked for drug interactions that should be monitored. Most products have many significant drug interactions.

Lifespan Considerations
Older Adults

NSAIDS

The incidence of perforated peptic ulcers or bleeding is more common in older adult patients taking an NSAID than in younger adults. Serious consequences occur more often in this age group.

Older adult patients with renal impairment may be at higher risk for NSAID-induced hepatotoxicity or nephrotoxicity (damage to the kidney) and often require a lower dose to prevent drug levels from building up in the blood.

Clinicians have recommended that patients 70 years or older be started at half of the usual adult dose, with close monitoring and careful dosage increases. A dosage increase is based on reduction in symptoms and no signs of toxicity. Specific drug warnings include the following:

- Flurbiprofen (Ansaid) may result in increased peak serum levels in women between 74 and 94 years old. This increased serum level has not been seen in older adult men. Therefore older adult women may need a lower dose to produce a therapeutic response.
- Indomethacin (Indocin) is responsible for a higher incidence of CNS side effects, especially confusion, in older adult patients.
- Naproxen (Naprosyn) is protein bound and when given to older adults with lower protein levels, results in a higher proportion of unbound (free) naproxen, which may be reflected by the total serum level. The concentration of unbound naproxen may be nearly double that in a younger adult, which may result in an increase in side effects, adverse effects, or toxic effects, even with a normal serum level range. Be aware this might happen, because the health care provider may need to be notified about the possible need for a dosage reduction.

Modified from McKenry LM, Tessier E, Hogan MA: *Mosby's pharmacology in nursing*, ed 22, St Louis, 2006, Mosby.

❖ NURSING IMPLICATIONS AND PATIENT TEACHING

■ Assessment

Learn as much as possible about the health and drug history of the patient, including sensitivity to aspirin or any of the products within this group, GI problems, renal dysfunction, history of asthma or allergic respiratory problems, anticoagulant therapy, bleeding problems, other drugs being taken that may cause drug interactions, and the possibility of pregnancy or breastfeeding.

Low doses of ibuprofen are often the first choice for pain relief in the older adult patient. The patient may complain of musculoskeletal pain or tenderness of involved areas, inflammation, stiffness, and an alteration in the normal activities of life. The onset may be gradual—the patient may show only tiredness—or it may be sudden or may occur after a change in activity or minor trauma, depending on the type of arthritic problem. The individual history of onset, duration, and location are important factors in diagnosing the type of arthritis. Evaluate the patient for signs of inflammation: tenderness, erythema, increased warmth, and swelling. Joint stiffness, decreased range of motion, or crepitus (a peculiar crackling sound) may also be present. Distribution, location, pattern (for example, on one side of the body or on both sides), and number of involved joints must be determined.

NSAIDs are not to be used in patients with past sensitivity to the drug. They are also not to be used in patients who have allergy or hypersensitivity to aspirin, because all of the specific agents are closely related to aspirin, and there is the chance for cross-sensitivity. (That is, a patient who is sensitive to aspirin may be sensitive to NSAIDs also.) Other agents in this category should not be given to patients who have had symptoms of bronchospasm, asthma, rhinitis, urticaria, nasal polyps, or angioedema (swelling of the skin and mucous membranes) after using any agents within this group.

■ Diagnosis

What other medical problems or risk factors does the patient have that might make taking this drug a problem? Does the patient have concerns about weight, nutrition, safety, or mobility? Is the patient suffering from depression? Does the patient drink alcohol, smoke, or have high caffeine intake that may make his or her GI tract more sensitive to problems with this drug?

■ Planning

Some agents will only be prescribed for short-term therapy because of their toxic side effects. The length of therapy should be considered by the health care provider when a particular drug is selected for treating chronic arthritis.

In problems that occur in only one joint, all infectious processes should be ruled out. This is because NSAIDs may relieve symptoms but will not affect any infectious agent. That would allow greater damage to take place if the patient continues to take NSAIDs.

■ Implementation

NSAIDs are first-line drugs in the treatment and control of various forms of arthritis and in many of the single-joint inflammatory processes (for example, bursitis). If symptoms fail to improve with the use of one agent, this does not mean there will be no improvement with another. Because of the low cost, efficacy, and low toxicity of salicylates, all NSAIDs are compared with them in terms of their therapeutic benefits and side or adverse effects (see Table 18-1).

▪ Evaluation

Watch the patient for therapeutic effects: reduction of symptoms and ability of the patient to return to previous activities without pain. The patient should be evaluated 3 to 4 weeks after starting the medication for the first signs of improvement. If there is no reduction in symptoms or if side effects develop, another drug in the NSAID group can be tried.

The patient should be asked about adverse effects, particularly GI and CNS symptoms. Periodic laboratory analysis should also be carried out while the patient is taking this medication. Collect stool specimens to check for occult bleeding. Complete blood cell counts with differential for anemia or other blood dyscrasia problems, and ability to fight infection should be done at least twice a year.

Clinical Pitfall

Gastrointestinal Upset

GI upset is the most common adverse effect of NSAID use and should be reported to the health care provider. Bowel movements should also be checked for the presence of blood or tarry stools, which result from excessive irritation. This should not be confused with black stools in patients taking iron preparations.

▪ Patient and Family Teaching

Tell the patient and family the following:
- These medications should be taken only as ordered. The dosage should not be increased or decreased unless the patient is told to do so by the drug prescriber. Evaluation of the action of these drugs requires returning to the health care provider regularly for checkups.
- These medications should be taken with meals or milk to minimize gastric irritation. The patient may use an antacid with the medicine, unless told not to do so.
- Patients who have chronic arthritic problems may need to take the medication for 1 to 2 weeks before noting any improvement. The medication should be taken as ordered during this time to evaluate effectiveness.
- A certain level of medication must be maintained within the body at all times to maintain the antiinflammatory effect of the drug. If the patient does not take the medication regularly, the drug level may become too low to be effective.
- If a dose is missed, it should be taken as soon as possible. If the patient remembers the missed dose close to the time when the next dose is to be taken, only the regular dose should be taken, and the missed dose should be skipped. An increased amount of medication should not be taken to make up for a missed dose.
- Blurred vision or any other eye problems, ringing in the ears, and rashes should be reported immediately to the health care provider.
- Some patients have drowsiness, light-headedness, or less alertness when taking this medication. Patients should not drive or perform tasks requiring alertness until they know their reaction to this drug.
- The patient should not take aspirin or any other antiinflammatory drug while using this product.

MUSCLE RELAXANTS

OVERVIEW

Muscle relaxants are used to help reduce pain caused by muscular tension or tightness.

ACTION

Skeletal muscle relaxants limit the transmission or movement of impulses in the motor pathways at the level of the spinal cord and brainstem (centrally acting), or they interfere with the mechanism that shortens skeletal muscle fibers (direct myotrophic blocking), so they contract.

The main action of **skeletal muscle relaxants** is to reduce muscle tone and involuntary (uncontrolled) movement without loss of voluntary (controlled) motor function. Other actions include mild sedation, reduction of anxiety and tension, and changes in pain perception.

USES

Skeletal muscle relaxants are used to relieve pain in musculoskeletal and neurologic disorders involving peripheral injury and inflammation, such as muscle strain or sprain, arthritis, bursitis, low back syndrome, cervical syndrome, cerebral palsy, and multiple sclerosis. They are often used following trauma, such as a motor vehicle or sporting accidents, when many muscles may be tender or stiff.

ADVERSE REACTIONS

Adverse reactions to skeletal muscle relaxants include flushing (red color in the face and neck), hypotension, syncope (light-headedness and fainting), tachycardia, ataxia (poor coordination), blurred vision, confusion, drowsiness, headache, insomnia (inability to sleep), irritability, abdominal pain, anorexia, bleeding, diarrhea, hiccups, nausea, many blood cell disorders, anaphylactic (shock) reactions, asthma-like reaction, dermatoses, erythema, fever, pruritus, rash, dysuria (painful urination), incontinence, urinary retention, dyspnea (uncomfortable breathing), nasal congestion, shortness of breath, wheezing, dyspepsia, euphoria (excessive happiness), metallic taste, pain or sloughing at injection site, and tremors. Cyclobenzaprine (Flexeril) has a contraindication against using the drug in patients with cardiovascular problems and hyperthyroidism. It may also be associated with Long QT syndrome, leading to lethal arrhythmias.

DRUG INTERACTIONS

Skeletal muscle relaxants are known to increase the effect of CNS depressants, including sedatives, narcotic analgesics, antianxiety agents, hypnotics, and alcohol. They also increase the effects of general anesthetics, monoamine oxidase inhibitors, and tricyclic antidepressants. Cyclobenzaprine (Flexeril) and orphenadrine (Norflex) have the same effects as anticholinergic drugs. Cyclobenzaprine may interfere with the antihypertensive activity of the alpha-adrenergic blockers.

❖ NURSING IMPLICATIONS AND PATIENT TEACHING

■ Assessment

Learn as much as possible about the patient's health history, including the presence of hypersensitivity, use of other drugs that might produce drug interactions, and history of respiratory, renal, hepatic, or cardiac dysfunction. These drugs should not be given to women who are pregnant or breastfeeding or to persons with a history of drug dependency.

The patient may have a history of pain caused by acute muscular injury or inflammation (sprains or strains), low back pain syndrome, arthritis, multiple sclerosis, muscular tension with or without intermittent relief, headache, and muscle rigidity.

■ Diagnosis

Does this patient have other problems that the nurse should be concerned about? Is the patient able to take care of activities of daily living, including personal hygiene and eating? Is the patient able to travel or is he or she confined at home? Is depression a problem? Has the problem made a significant difference in the patient's activity level? All of these things may require nursing intervention. Is the patient upset or worried about being involved in a lawsuit or criminal inquiry as a result of the trauma? Is the patient concerned about legal or financial issues that make him or her tense or stressed?

■ Planning

Using a skeletal muscle relaxant with other CNS drugs, including alcohol, increases the sedative actions of this drug. Therefore these drugs are not recommended for persons with a history of alcoholism or alcohol abuse.

While there are pediatric doses for some of the drugs to treat spasticity, the efficacy and safe use of these drugs have not been established in children.

The nurse should be particularly careful in recording observations and patient care and be aware of the likelihood that nursing records might be examined if a law suit is involved because of the injury.

■ Implementation

Skeletal muscle relaxants are often given to hospitalized patients and available in both tablet and injectable forms. Although many muscle relaxants are given orally (PO), research suggests these drugs may not always be effective when given by this route. The oral dose must be 5 to 10 times greater than the injectable (parenteral) dose to obtain true muscle relaxation. For this reason, the parenteral form of these drugs is recommended versus the oral form. However, the parenteral form of the drug can cause local tissue irritation with injection.

In rare instances, the first dose of skeletal muscle relaxants produces an idiosyncratic (unique and unknown cause) reaction within minutes or hours. Symptoms include extreme weakness, transient quadriplegia, dizziness, ataxia (imbalance in walking), temporary loss of vision, diplopia (double vision), mydriasis, dysarthria, agitation, euphoria, confusion, and disorientation.

Table 18-2 provides a summary of skeletal muscle relaxants.

■ Evaluation

Hepatotoxicity (liver toxicity), nephrotoxicity (kidney toxicity), and abnormal blood cells have been reported with the use of skeletal muscle relaxants. Signs of hepatotoxicity include abdominal pain, high fever, nausea, and diarrhea. Signs of blood dyscrasias include fever, sore throat, mucosal irritation, malaise, and petechiae (tiny red spots on the skin). Side effects that occur most commonly include drowsiness, diplopia, dizziness, weakness, mild muscular incoordination, anorexia, nausea, vomiting, syncope, and hypotension.

The lowest dosage possible should be used, and the patient should be checked for signs and symptoms of hepatotoxicity, blood dyscrasias, dependence, and adverse drug reactions. The drug should be discontinued by the health care provider if no improvement occurs after 45 days, because the risk of hepatotoxicity increases with long-term use of these drugs.

The severity of the musculoskeletal or neurologic problem determines how long the patient should take the drug. Discontinuing the drugs suddenly may cause withdrawal symptoms after long-term use, so the dosage should be gradually reduced before being stopped.

The patient should be checked for relief of signs and symptoms, and increase in range of motion, relief from muscle spasm, pain relief, and so on.

Table 18-2   Skeletal Muscle Relaxants

GENERIC NAME	TRADE NAME	COMMENTS
Centrally Acting		
baclofen	Lioresal	Muscle relaxant, antispastic: Dosage regimen begun with 5 mg 3 times daily for 3 days. Thereafter dosage increased until desired response is obtained. Dosage adjusted according to reversal of spasticity symptoms. Maximum daily dose: 80 mg.
carisoprodol	Soma	Muscle relaxant: Take daily and at bedtime. Administration with meals will help reduce gastric distress.
chlorzoxazone	Paraflex Parafon Forte DSC Remular-S	Initial dose for painful musculoskeletal conditions: If adequate response not obtained, dosage increased, then gradually reduced to maintenance dose once therapeutic effect achieved. Administration with meals may help avoid GI irritation.
cyclobenzaprine	Flexeril	Relieves acute skeletal muscle spasm of local origin without interfering with muscle function. Not to be administered for longer than 2-3 wk.
diazepam ★	Valium	For use with geriatric or debilitated patients. This is strongly addictive and should be used for a short time.
metaxalone	Skelaxin	Used for muscle relaxation. Use for short time.
methocarbamol	Robaxin	Drug may change color of standing urine to green or black. Used for relief of muscle spasm.
orphenadrine citrate	Norflex Banflex	Used for relief of muscle spasm.
tizanidine	Zanaflex	Given as a single oral dose. Effects are dose related.
Direct Acting		
dantrolene	Dantrium	Spasticity: Each dosage level should be maintained 4-7 days to determine patient's response.
Combination Products		
carisoprodol and aspirin (also comes with codeine)	Soma Compound	Combination centrally acting skeletal muscle relaxant. Used to treat acute muscle spasms and relieve pain associated with musculoskeletal conditions. Has CNS depressant effects and physical and psychologic addictive effects; withdrawal effects occur if drug abruptly stopped.
orphenadrine citrate, aspirin, and caffeine	Norgesic	Combination centrally acting skeletal muscle relaxant indicated for relief of mild to moderate pain and muscle spasms of acute musculoskeletal conditions.

CNS, Central nervous system; *GI*, gastrointestinal.
★ Indicates "Must-Know Drugs," or the 35 drugs most prescribers use.

■ Patient And Family Teaching

Tell the patient and family the following:

- The patient should take this medication as advised and not stop taking it suddenly or increase the dosage without the knowledge of the health care provider.
- The patient should avoid driving, operating heavy machinery, or doing tasks requiring alertness while taking skeletal muscle relaxants.
- The patient should avoid taking other medications that depress CNS functions at the same time. These include antihistamines, allergy or cold medications, sedatives, tranquilizers, sleeping medications, anticonvulsants, narcotic analgesics, and tricyclic antidepressants.
- If a dose of medication is missed, it may be taken within an hour of when it was scheduled. If the patient remembers the missed dose close to the time when the next dose is to be taken, only the regular dose should be taken, and the missed dose should be skipped.
- The health care provider should be contacted immediately if any of the following adverse effects occur: dizziness or fainting, mental depression, unusually fast heartbeat, wheezing, shortness of breath, difficult breathing, abdominal pain, high fever, nausea, diarrhea, sore throat, malaise, mucosal ulceration, or petechiae.
- The patient should take the last dose at bedtime so that drowsiness will help them go to sleep.

- This medication must be kept out of the reach of children and all others for whom it is not prescribed.

ANTIARTHRITIS MEDICATIONS

OVERVIEW

The term **arthritis** covers more than 100 different types of joint disease in which inflammation or destruction is present. The most common types are rheumatoid arthritis and osteoarthritis. **Rheumatoid arthritis** is a systemic disease that involves an autoimmune response caused by failure of the body to recognize its own tissue; this results in the body destroying its own joints. **Osteoarthritis** is a more localized form of joint destruction, particularly in joints that carry weight like hips and knees or have a lot of stress like hands and feet. This type of arthritis progresses gradually over time from overuse and increasing age.

Symptoms of arthritis depend upon the type of arthritis but almost all include swelling, pain, and

Complementary and Alternative Therapies

Arthritis

PRODUCTS	COMMENTS
OSTEOARTHRITIS	
Grape seed	Potential interaction with anticoagulants, aspirin, NSAIDs, antiplatelet agents, methotrexate
Ginger	Potential interaction with anticoagulants, aspirin, NSAIDs, antiplatelet agents, cardiac glycosides
Cat's claw	Potential interaction with anticoagulants, aspirin, NSAIDs, antiplatelet agents
Turmeric	Potential interaction with anticoagulants, aspirin, NSAIDs, antiplatelet agents
Boswellia	No reported interactions
Chondroitin sulfate	No reported interactions
Glucosamine sulfate	No reported interactions
RHEUMATOID ARTHRITIS	
Cat's claw	Potential interaction with anticoagulants, aspirin, NSAIDs, antiplatelet agents
Boswellia	No reported interactions
Devil's claw	No reported interactions
Evening primrose	Potential interaction with anticoagulants, aspirin, NSAIDs, antiplatelet agents
Tumeric	Potential interaction with anticoagulants, aspirin, NSAIDs, antiplatelet agents
Bromelain	Potential interaction with anticoagulants, aspirin, NSAIDs, antiplatelet agents
Chondroitin sulfate	No reported interactions
Glucosamine sulfate	No reported interactions

Modified from Krinsky DL, LaValle JB, Hawkins EB et al: *Natural therapeutics pocket guide*, ed 2, Hudson, Ohio, 2003, Lexi-Comp, Inc.

stiffness in one or more joints. In rheumatoid arthritis, as the disease progresses, there is degeneration and destruction of the joint with permanent changes that produce deformities and immobility.

Arthritis is one of the most common disorders. Patients often do not get much relief from any of the medications they try, so they may turn to alternative medicine and herbal products to reduce arthritic symptoms and reduce pain. These herbal products have many possible interactions with other medications (see the Complementary and Alternative Therapies box).

✤ DISEASE-MODIFYING ANTIRHEUMATIC MEDICATIONS AND IMMUNE MODULATORS

Salicylates and NSAIDs are first-line drugs for the treatment of arthritis. Steroids may also be used for antiinflammatory antirheumatic purposes and these will be discussed in Chapter 21. DMARD medications are prescribed primarily by specialists and used only in diagnosed cases of rheumatoid arthritis that have been getting worse despite other types of treatment, including high doses of NSAIDs. Nurses should know something about these drugs because none of these agents is without significant risk and toxic effects. Patients taking these drugs need constant follow-up and regular evaluation and may be admitted to the hospital or seen in offices for other problems.

The DMARDs or **conventional drugs** are useful in treating significant cases of rheumatoid arthritis and include hydroxychloroquine sulfate (Plaquenil), a drug typically used for malaria, a sulfonamide (sulfasalazine), and methotrexate (Rheumatrex, Folex). Most of these medications are designed to reduce pain, swelling, and inflammation; these drugs cannot stop the arthritic process. Gold compounds and penicillamine were once prescribed but have fallen into disuse because of severe allergic reactions and will not be discussed here.

The specialty drugs most commonly used now are the immunomodulators. These include the cytokine-blockers Tumor Necrosis Factor (TNF)-α inhibitors, cytokine blockers, IL-1 receptor antagonists, and T-cell modulators. These drugs do have the ability to reduce pain and halt the destructive inflammatory processes that deform the joints.

Each of these two categories are briefly described below and summarized in Table 18-3.

✤ DMARDS OR CONVENTIONAL ANTIRHEUMATIC DRUGS

HYDROXYCHLOROQUINE SULFATE

ACTION

The mechanism of action of hydroxychloroquine sulfate (Plaquenil) is not understood. This is an antimalarial drug that in some way stops the formation of

Table 18-3 | **Antiarthritic Medications**

GENERIC NAME	TRADE NAME	COMMENTS
Conventional or DMARDs Antirheumatic Drugs		
hydroxychloroquine	Plaquenil	Rheumatoid arthritis: Take with meals or food to prevent GI upset. Maintenance dose: Take daily for 4-12 wk until patient has symptomatic improvements; dose then reduced and maintained.
methotrexate	Trexall Rheumatrex ♦	To detect any extreme sensitivity reactions, initial test dose usually given before beginning regular dosage schedule. See package insert for specific guidelines. Therapeutic response generally seen in 3-6 wk; patient may continue to improve for another 12 wk. Optimal duration of therapy unknown. Arthritis may worsen within 3-5 wk of ending therapy.
sulfasalazine	Azulfidine	Give in divided doses; use in patients that have not responded to other drugs.
Immumomodulators		
Cytokine Blockers TNF-α Inhibitors		
adalimumab	Humira	Has many drug interactions. Use with care.
etanercept	Enbrel	Has many drug interactions. May not be used in immunocompromised patients.
Cytokine Blockers, IL-1 Receptor Antagonists		
anakinra	Kineret	Use with care in immunocompromised patients.
infliximab	Remicade	Adults: Begin as an IV infusion, followed with similar doses at 2 and 6 wk after first infusion, then every 8 wk. Dose may be adjusted as often as every 4 wk. Watch for postinfusion reactions within 1-2 hr after infusion is finished.
T-Cell Modulators		
Abatacept	Orenca	
leflunomide	Arava	Check liver enzymes prior to beginning therapy.

GI, Gastrointestinal; *IV,* intravenous; *PO,* by mouth.

antigens in the body. These antigens produce the hypersensitivity reactions leading to the physiologic changes of rheumatoid arthritis and systemic lupus erythematosus.

Clinical Pitfall

Hydroxychloroquine Sulfate

The most serious side effect of hydroxychloroquine sulfate (Plaquenil) is damage to the eyes, which usually appears in two forms: (1) retinopathy with irreversible visual loss, and (2) corneal infiltration that may be somewhat reversible when the medication is stopped.

USES

Hydroxychloroquine sulfate (Plaquenil) is used in diagnosed cases of rheumatoid arthritis that have been getting worse despite other methods of therapy, including high doses of NSAIDs. This agent is not without significant risk and toxic effects. Patients taking this drug need constant follow-up and regular evaluation. This drug may also be used in confirmed diagnosis of systemic or discoid lupus erythematosus.

ADVERSE REACTIONS

Hydroxychloroquine requires 4 to 12 weeks of therapy before improvement is seen. If there is no improvement after 6 months, the drug should be stopped.

If the drug is stopped because the patient is feeling relief from the symptoms, the agent can be reintroduced if the disease flares up again. Corticosteroids or NSAIDs may be used with this drug until the effects of this slow-acting drug become apparent.

Retinopathy is a serious adverse effect. The retinopathy does appear to be dose related, so patients should have an expert ophthalmologic evaluation before beginning the drug and periodic checkups every 3 to 6 months throughout therapy. The drug should be stopped if there are any visual complaints or symptoms, such as seeing flashes or streaks of light, because the retinal damage may progress even after the drug is stopped.

This product must not be used with other conventional antirheumatics because combined use will greatly increase the chance of dermatologic reactions.

DRUG INTERACTIONS

Antacids and kaolin have been reported to reduce absorption of hydroxychloroquine. Use with digoxin can increase the serum digoxin levels. Hydroxychloroquine inhibits CYP2D6 in the liver and may increase anticholinergic side effects if these drugs are given at the same time. The drug may also reduce the renal clearance of methotrexate, another antiarthritic drugs. Close monitoring to detect methotrexate toxicity should be done, especially in patients with reduced renal function.

SULFASALAZINE

ACTION AND USES

Sulfasalazine (Azulfidine) is a sulfonamide used in the treatment of rheumatoid arthritis and ulcerative colitis. Sulfasalazine is metabolized to its active components by bacteria in the colon into chemicals that have inflammatory actions.

ADVERSE REACTIONS

The most common (up to 33% of patients) adverse reactions occurring during sulfasalazine therapy I include anorexia, diarrhea, GI distress, headache, and nausea/vomiting. Agranulocytosis, aplastic anemia, and many other blood dyscrasias occur infrequently but can be fatal. These blood dyscrasias present as fever, pale skin, sore throat, fatigue, and unusual bleeding and bruising and require immediate discontinuation of the drug. Skin reactions such as rash, urticaria, and pruritus are also relatively frequent. Consult product information for other adverse reactions.

DRUG INTERACTIONS

Sulfasalazine interacts with a wide variety of other drugs. It can inhibit the absorption and reduce the bioavailability of cardiac glycosides; has antifolate activity; potentiates the effects of warfarin and coumarin; and may be associated with methotrexate-induced pulmonary toxicity. It may reduce the action of Dilantin and diabetic drugs. It has many other drug interactions.

METHOTREXATE

ACTION AND USES

Methotrexate (Rheumatrex, Trexall) is an antineoplastic medication that has been used for years to treat various cancerous and psoriatic conditions. The mechanism of action in rheumatoid arthritis is unknown. It may affect immune function. It reduces joint swelling and tenderness in 3 to 6 weeks, but there is no evidence that it causes remission of the disease or limits bone erosions.

Methotrexate is used in cases of severe rheumatoid arthritis that are unresponsive to other treatment. This product has a high possibility of severe adverse reactions, including death. It is most toxic to the bone marrow, liver, kidney, and lungs. It has many contraindications to use, drug interactions, and dosage precautions. Consult the package insert for specific information.

ADVERSE EFFECTS

In general, the incidence and severity of acute adverse reactions are related to the dose and frequency of administration. The most common adverse reactions are stomatitis, esophagitis, oral ulceration, nausea/ vomiting, and abdominal distress. Drug-induced bone marrow suppression occurs rapidly and may cause numerous blood dyscrasias, acute and chronic hepatotoxicity, severe opportunistic infections, a transient acute neurologic syndrome with a stroke-like encephalopathy, and renal toxicity. Methotrexate is a category X drug.

DRUG INTERACTIONS

Methotrexate interacts with a wide variety of drugs and only a few of the most important are listed here. Concurrent NSAID use reduces the clearance of methotrexate, resulting in elevated and prolonged serum methotrexate levels. Caution should be used in giving salicylates with methotrexate. The drug is partially bound to plasma proteins and drugs that can displace methotrexate from these proteins, such as oral sulfonylureas, phenylbutazone, hydantin anticonvulsants, or sulfonamides could cause methotrexate-induced toxicity. Oral antibiotics may decrease intestinal absorption of methotrexate or interfere with liver circulation.

✤ IMMUNOMODULATORS

Three different subclasses of immunomodulators are in current use. They are the cytokine blockers TNF-α inhibitors, the cytokine blocker IL-1 antagonists, and the T-cell modulators.

CYTOKINE BLOCKERS TNF-α INHIBITORS

ACTION AND USES

These drugs are monoclonal antibodies specific for tumor necrosis factor-alpha and are approved as sole therapy in the treatment of rheumatoid arthritis (RA), and are administered subcutaneously. In addition to reducing the signs and symptoms of RA and ankylosing spondylitis, and several other arthritic-type diseases. The drugs reduce disease progression, and significantly improve pain and inflammation.

The cytokine blockers TNF-α inhibitors such as adalimumab (Humira), and etanercept (Enbrel) act to neutralize the biological activity of tumor necrosis factor-alpha by binding to it and blocking its interactions with TNF receptors.

ADVERSE EFFECTS

Adalimumab may cause myositis. The most common adverse events are rash, headache, and pruritus. Cutaneous vasculitis and erythema multiforme have also been reported. Rare cases of blood dyscrasias are also reported.

One of the most common adverse reactions reported with etanercept is an injection site reaction lasting 3-5 days. The drug may worsen psoriasis. Infections including active tuberculosis, invasive fungal infections, and other opportunistic bacterial and viral infections have been reported. Pancytopenia and other blood dyscrasias are common. Diarrhea and inflammatory bowel disease have been noted. It may also increase the risk of secondary malignancy.

DRUG INTERACTION

These drugs should not be used with other TNF-alpha blockers. The immune response to vaccines or toxoids may be decreased. Safety for use immunocompromised patients is unknown. Do not give abatacept with adalimumab.

Concurrent use of etanercept and cyclophosphamide or sulfasalazine is not recommended. There is only limited data examining the safety and efficacy of vaccine or toxoids given with this drug. Serious infections may develop if given with anakinra.

CYTOKINE BLOCKERS, IL-1 RECEPTOR ANTAGONISTS

ACTION AND USES

These cytokine blockers IL-1 receptor antagonist drugs, such as infliximab (Remicade) and anakinra (KIineret), are used in combination with methotrexate to reduce the signs and symptoms of rheumatoid arthritis and limit the worsening of damage to joints. This leads to improved physical function in patients with moderate to severe active rheumatoid arthritis who have had an inadequate response to methotrexate alone. It is also used in Crohn disease (inflammatory bowel disease) and some orthopedic inflammatory or destructive processes.

ADVERSE REACTIONS

This drug may activate tuberculosis, invasive fungal infections, and other opportunistic infections. (A test for tuberculosis should be given and any latent tuberculosis treated prior to beginning the patient on this therapy.) There is a high mortality rate in patients who have preexisting congestive heart failure. Watch for hypersensitivity and infusion-related reactions (for example, dyspnea, flushing, headache, and rash that may occur within 1 to 2 hours of the infusion).

DRUG INTERACTIONS

Infliximab shuld not be given with abatacept, anakinra, rilonacept, and tocilizumab as the incidence of serious infections increases. Anakinra should not be given with rilanacept or any TNF modifiers because of the increased risk of serious infections.

For both drugs, the immune response to vaccines or toxoids may be decreased. Safety for use immunocompromised patients is unknown.

T-CELL MODULATORS

ACTION AND USES

T-cell modulators such as abatacept (Orencia) and leflunomide (Arava) are pyrimidine synthesis inhibitors that have an antiinflammatory effect. They are used in treatment of active rheumatoid arthritis in adults to reduce signs and symptoms and to slow structural damage in joints.

ADVERSE REACTIONS

The Federal Drug Administration requires a warning label that pregnancy must be ruled out and avoided in all women who are of childbearing age while they are taking this drug. This is a category X drug that is contraindicated during pregnancy.

Leflunomide may produce hepatotoxicity, and there is some evidence of increased risk of cancer of the lymph system. In patients taking abatacept, common reactions were headache, dizziness, hypertension, and dyspepsia and these may start within 1 hour of taking the medicine. Hypersensitive reactions may also develop. As T cells mediate cellular responses, these drugs may affect host defenses against infections and malignancies.

DRUG INTERACTIONS

Use of abatacept and anakinra together is not recommended. Do not give with TNF modifiers. Abatacept may increase the onset of respiratory infections and should not obe used with drugs that decrease mucus production and clearance such as general anesthetics or atropine and scopolamine. Live viruses should not be given concurrently with abatacept or within 3 months of its discontinuation.

Leflunomide should not be given with other hepatotoxic drugs as it increases the risk of hepatotoxicity. It inhibits the cytochrome P45 2C9 system. Increased International Normalized Ratio when this drug and warfarin are coadministered is possible. It also appears to interact with rifampin.

❖ NURSING IMPLICATIONS AND PATIENT TEACHING

■ Assessment

After reading specific information from the package insert about the medication, learn as much as possible about the patient's health history, including the treatment history of the patient's arthritis; presence of drug sensitivities; underlying diseases such as renal, liver, cardiovascular, or hematopoietic diseases that contraindicate any of these products; the possibility of pregnancy; and other drugs taken at the same time that might cause drug interactions.

■ Diagnosis

What is the patient's general level of mobility? Do pain and joint deformity interfere with the ability to perform activities of daily living or required tasks on the job? Is the patient able to comply with the treatment regimen? Does the patient experience side effects from antiarthritis medication? What effect has chronic rheumatoid disease had on emotions and the ability to cope? Does the patient have other kidney disease?

■ Planning

These drugs are not without significant adverse reactions. The benefits of the medication must be weighed against the risks and serious adverse reactions.

■ Implementation

These drugs will be given by rheumatologists. Nurses do not often administer these drugs. A summary of dosage information concerning antiarthritis medications is provided in Table 18-3.

■ Evaluation

The nurse should observe for the therapeutic effect and monitor closely for the numerous and serious adverse effects that may develop.

■ Patient and Family Teaching

Tell the patient and family the following:

- These drugs are very potent and slow acting. They may be helpful in some patients in reducing symptoms or actually halting joint destruction caused by arthritis. They do not help all patients, and a thorough trial will sometimes take weeks before full response to the drug can be determined.
- There are serious toxic effects that can occur with these drugs. These toxic effects may last for a long time even after the drug is stopped. The patient must work closely with the health care provider, keep appointments, and have laboratory work performed as requested in order for greatest safety.
- The patient and the health care provider should be alert for problems that may develop in the kidneys, lungs, liver, skin, or blood.
- These medications may require frequent response and dosage monitoring.
- The health care provider should be contacted as soon as possible if the patient notes any unusual or new symptoms.

ANTIGOUT MEDICATIONS

OVERVIEW

Uric acid comes from the metabolism of protein and is present in the blood within a very specific range. Several pathologic processes, metabolic changes, or drug interactions may be responsible for increasing the uric acid level of the blood above an acceptable amount. High uric acid levels cause the excess uric acid to form crystals, usually in the kidneys and in joint spaces. These crystals have very long, sharp, and jagged edges. These crystals tear and bruise the tissues with which they come in contact. The result is swelling or increased tissue edema, heat, inflammation, and severe pain—the syndrome called gout. Gout is a form of arthritis caused when the body makes too much (overproduction) or does not get rid of (underexcretion) uric acid, and may manifest in any joint.

The drugs used to treat gout vary in their method of action. Those used to treat acute attacks act to relieve pain and inflammation. Other drugs called *uricosurics* alter the body's response to, production of, or distribution of uric acid to prevent gout attacks.

ACTION

The management of gout involves three different steps: reducing the inflammatory response (colchicine, glucocorticoids and ACTH, and NSAIDS), decreasing uric acid production allopuruinol (Zyloprim), and increasing uric acid clearance (probenecid and sulfinpyrazone). The glucocorticoids and ACTH are reserved for acute attacks when the patient is resistant to therapy or if there is a contraindication to use of colchicine or NSAIDS. Chronic gout is usually treated with uricosuric agents, allopurinol, or daily colchicine given in low doses.

Uricosuric agents increase the excretion of urate salts in the urine by blocking tubular reabsorption of these salts in the kidney. They also decrease the amount of circulating urate and the deposition of urate and promote reabsorption of urate deposits. Sulfinpyrazone also has platelet inhibitory and antithrombotic effects. Uricosuric agents do not have significant antiinflammatory or analgesic properties and therefore are of little help during an acute episode of gout.

Colchicine is a special drug used to treat acute gouty attacks. It is not an antiinflammatory, analgesic, or uricosuric agent. The mechanism of action of colchicine in relieving gouty attacks is not completely known. It is believed to be involved in the inhibition of leukocyte migration and phagocytosis that causes the inflammatory response in gout. It also decreases uric acid deposits in the tissues. In addition to use in the acute stage, it may also be used with allopurinol or other uricosuric agents to prevent an acute attack.

Probenecid inhibits tubular reabsorption of urate, increasing uric acid excretion.

Allopurinol inhibits the production of uric acid by decreasing the production of xanthine oxidase, an enzyme that metabolizes purine hypoxanthine to xanthine and xanthine to uric acid. This drug has no analgesic or antiinflammatory properties and therefore is not beneficial in the treatment of acute gout. Instead, it is used in prophylactic (preventive) therapy for repeated or chronic gout. It is also used in patients with renal failure severe enough to increase their uric acid levels to a point at which they may develop gouty attacks.

Corticosteroids and ACTH decrease inflammation in gout. They do this by inhibiting the release of leukocyte adhesion to the capillary wall, inhibiting histamine release, and interfering with the formation of scar tissue, as well as other processes.

USES

Usually the patient comes in with an acute attack and the diagnosis of gout is made. The joint with acute gout is very painful, red, and swollen. Even a sheet on a toe might not be tolerated. Oral colchicine and/or NSAIDS are first-line agents for systemic treatment of acute attacks. Colchicine is used to treat gouty attacks when the diagnosis of gout is either confirmed or suspected by the patient's history and physical examination and when examination of joint fluid is not possible. Colchicine relieves the pain of acute attacks but it does not decrease the levels of uric acid. Intraarticular aspiration and injection of a long-acting steroid is safe and effective for acute gout attacks.

For those patients with recurrent acute attacks, arthropathy, tophi, or x-ray changes, urate-lowering therapy, usually with allopurinol, is used long term to maintain the serum uric acid level below 6.8 mg/dL and to dissolve urate crystals. Uricosuric agents such as probenecid are an alternative to allopurinol. Colchicine may also used along with allopurinol or uricosuric agents to prevent a gouty attack until the serum uric acid level is reduced to normal and stabilized. It has no effect on uric acid levels itself. It may be used prophylactically along with NSAIDs (such as indomethacin, naproxen, and sulindac) to prevent recurrent attacks, but only in combination with a uricosuric agent.

Uricosuric agents are primarily used to reduce uric acid levels in patients who do not excrete enough uric acid. The diagnosis of gout is confirmed by serum uric acid levels greater than 7 mg/100 mL and a 24-hour urine test for uric acid of less than 800 mg/day. The patient has usually had more than one acute episode before being started on these agents.

Sulfinpyrazone (Anturane) is used only in patients who do not respond to all other drugs. It is the preferred drug for patients with gout secondary to hypertensive diuretic therapy and may have other risk factors for coronary artery disease.

Allopurinol (Zyloprim) generally is used when objective findings show any of the following conditions:

- Overproduction of uric acid on a general diet (24-hour urine test shows uric acid excretion greater than 700 mg/day)
- Uric acid nephropathy with impaired renal function (creatinine clearance less than 80 mL/min)

- Tophi, or small masses of crystals, on bony prominences (often the elbow or ankle)
- When kidney stones are seen by flat plate x-ray study of the abdomen
- Primary or secondary hyperuricemia associated with blood dyscrasias and their treatment
- When gout is not controlled by uricosuric drugs alone, or is caused by the patient's intolerance of the drug or when the drug is not effective
- A need for prophylactic therapy in patients with lymphomas, leukemias, or other malignancies requiring chemotherapy or radiation therapy that results in an increase in the serum uric acid level as tissue is broken down
- Febuxostat (Uloric) is a new selective xanthine oxidase inhibitor that is used as an alternative to allopurinol. It is particularly useful in patients who have renal insufficiency and who cannot tolerate allopurinol.

Probenecid is also often used with penicillin preparations to treat venereal diseases because of its ability to increase the plasma level of penicillin. Levels may increase two to four times normal, regardless of the route of penicillin administration.

Corticosteroids (such as methylprednisolone) are often injected into the joints if 1 or 2 accessible joints are involved. Where systemic steroids are required, doses of oral prednisone are given for several days and then gradually the dose tapered over 10-14 days.

ADVERSE REACTIONS

Uricosuric agents may produce drug fever, dizziness, pruritus, rashes, anorexia, constipation, diarrhea, nausea, vomiting, and exacerbation of acute attacks of gout. Rarely, anaphylaxis, nephrotic syndrome, hepatic necrosis, and aplastic anemia are seen.

Colchicine may cause abdominal pain, hemorrhagic gastroenteritis, severe diarrhea, nausea, and vomiting. Chronic use may cause bone marrow depression, agranylocytosis, aplastic anemia, alopecia (hair loss), peripheral neuritis, purpura (bruising), and myopathy. There is usually a delay between overdosage and onset of symptoms. Deaths have been reported with as little as 7 mg. Risk of colchicine-related deaths increases when it is given with cyclosporine, erythromycin, calcium channel antagonists (verapamil and diltiazem), tellithromycin, ketoconazole, HIV protease inhibitors, or nefazodone.

The most common adverse effect with use of a allopurinol (Zyloprim) is skin rash that may develop up to 2 years after the beginning of treatment. It may also produce drowsiness, alopecia, purpura, diarrhea, abdominal pain, nausea, vomiting, and blood dyscrasias. It may produce idiosyncratic potential fatal toxicity syndrome shown by fever, chills, arthralgias (joint pain), skin rash, pruritus, nausea, vomiting, interstitial nephritis, occasional development of cataracts, and vasculitis that may lead to hepatotoxicity and death.

Febuxostat (Uloric) has a higher rate of risk of cardiovascular thromboembolic events compared to allopurinol.

All of the NSAIDs produce similar adverse effects, the most common being nausea, anorexia, abdominal pain, and ulceration. (See Chapter 17 for a discussion of these drugs.)

All glucocorticoids, by stimulating negative feedback, can suppress the HPA axis. These drugs are also discussed in greater detail in Chapter 21.

DRUG INTERACTIONS

Salicylates antagonize (interfere with) the uricosuric action of these drugs. Uricosurics increase the effects of the following drugs by decreasing renal tubular excretion: sulfonamides, sulfonylureas, naproxen, indomethacin, rifampin, dapsone, pantothenic acid, aminosalicylic acid, and methotrexate. Additionally, sulfinpyrazone affects anticoagulants by increasing their platelet aggregation effects.

The effects of colchicine are blocked by acidifying agents and increased by alkalinizing agents. Patients taking this drug may have an increased sensitivity to CNS depressants. Colchicine also decreases gut absorption of vitamin B_{12}. The effects of sympathomimetics are increased by colchicine.

Hypersensitivity may occur in patients with renal compromise who are taking thiazides and allopurinol at the same time. Use at the same time as ampicillin may increase the chance for skin rashes. Allopurinol increases the half-life of anticoagulants and many other drugs.

Febuxostat (Uloric) is contraindicated in patients treated with azathioprine, mercaptopurine, or theophylline.

❖ NURSING IMPLICATIONS AND PATIENT TEACHING

■ Assessment

Learn as much as possible about the patient's health history, including the presence of hypersensitivity, other drugs being taken that could cause drug interactions, history of other disease, or the possibility of pregnancy. These conditions are precautions or contraindications to the use of antigout medications. The frequency and severity of the attacks should be recorded to help determine whether therapy with colchicine is indicated.

The patient may complain of an initial or recurrent attack of inflammation, erythema, swelling, extreme tenderness, and pain, usually in a single joint. At least 50% of initial attacks occur in the great toe at the metatarsal-phalangeal joint (podagra). This disease usually develops in the lower extremities. Joints affected may be in the instep, ankles, heels, or knees, although some patients are also bothered in wrists, fingers, and elbows. In patients with a severe or worsening form of the disease, additional joints may be involved. These symptoms are sudden in onset, and the patient may complain of being unable to tolerate clothing, shoes, or even bed coverings touching the site of inflammation. In some cases, there is a history of minor trauma to the involved joint, obesity, alcohol intake, use of a new drug such as hydrochlorothiazide, or low-dose aspirin consumption.

■ Diagnosis

In addition to the medical diagnosis, what other problems exist for the patient? Are there general concerns about weight, diet, stress, or conditions that would limit the use of medication? How can the nurse help the patient prevent future attacks? What does the patient need to learn about gout and its treatment?

■ Planning

The nurse can assist in collecting a 24-hour urine test for uric acid level and creatinine clearance and baseline laboratory tests as ordered by the health care provider.

Uricosuric agents are to be started only after the acute attack has resolved. Prophylactic therapy is recommended in patients having more than one acute attack per year. If affected less often, the patient should try to control attacks by having colchicine on hand and beginning treatment as soon as symptoms develop.

Initiation of therapy with uricosuric agents may cause an acute attack of gout, so colchicine is often given to prevent such an attack.

The use of salicylates in small or large doses is contraindicated in patients taking probenecid, because salicylates antagonize the uricosuric action of this drug. Patients needing mild pain relief for other conditions should be told to use only acetaminophen products.

Allopurinol (Zyloprim) may also cause a gouty attack during the initial treatment phase. This is easily prevented by prophylactic use of colchicine 0.5 mg twice daily PO for 2 weeks to 1 month. Good fluid intake and neutral or alkaline pH of the urine are important to prevent the possibility of xanthine stone or calculi forming. Patients with poor renal function require smaller doses, and renal function should be carefully watched.

When patients switch from uricosuric agents to allopurinol, a gradual increase of allopurinol with a gradual decrease of the other agent should be made over a period of several weeks. The patient should be watched for complications, and blood work will likely be ordered to monitor serum uric acid levels.

■ Implementation

The patient's urine should be alkalinized to prevent hematuria or formation of urate stones, especially during the initial stages of therapy. Injectable doses of colchicine are not to be given intramuscularly or subcutaneously, but must be given only intravenously.

With an acute attack, colchicine should be given immediately, and then a dose should be given every hour until either symptoms go away or the patient develops signs of toxicity.

Table 18-4 provides a summary of dosage information concerning some common antigout medications.

■ Evaluation

Colchicine must be started as soon as the patient has gout pain. Observe for therapeutic effects and adverse reactions. The patient being treated for acute attacks with a loading dose can usually reach a maximum dose level before the onset of GI side effects. The patient should be checked frequently for weakness, anorexia, nausea, vomiting, or diarrhea, because these are the first indications of toxicity. If these symptoms appear, the dosage should be reduced. If the patient has taken colchicine for a long time, vitamin B_{12} deficiency may develop.

If the nurse is seeing the patient over several months, watch for the therapeutic effects (decrease in frequency and severity of gouty attacks) of these drugs and watch for symptoms of the arthritis process (joint deformity, destruction, or formation of tophi).

The effect of allopurinol is seen 5 to 10 days after therapy is started. The dosage should be adjusted to maintain a serum uric acid level of less than 7 mg/100 mL. Uric acid levels as low as 2 to 3 mg/100 mL are not harmful. Adverse reactions such as rash, appearance of tophi, and change in joint deformities should be monitored.

If a maculopapular rash develops in the patient taking allopurinol at any time during therapy, the drug should be stopped immediately and it should not be restarted.

Table 18-4   Antigout Medications

GENERIC NAME	TRADE NAME	COMMENTS
Antigout Analgesic Preparations for Acute Gouty Attacks—First Line Drugs to Reduce Inflammation		
colchicine	Colchicine	Acute attack of gout: Therapy should be started at first warning of an acute attack. Delay of even a few hours greatly reduces therapeutic effectiveness. PO: Follow directions closely. Give medication every hour or two until pain is relieved or nausea, vomiting, or diarrhea develops. Pain usually relieved in 12 hr and gone in 24-48 hr. IV: Give until pain is relieved. Prophylactic therapy: Give daily in single or divided doses, usually in combination with a uricosuric agent.
NSAIDS		
naproxyn	Aleve	Used in reducing inflammation and swelling in acute gouty attacks.
indomethacin	Indocin	Used in reducing inflammation and swelling in acute gouty attacks.
sulindac	Clinoril	Used in reducing inflammation and swelling in acute gouty attacks.
Corticosteroids		
Methylprednisolone		For injection into painful joints.
prednisone ★		For systemic steroid use
Uricosuric Agents—Decrease Uric Acid Production		
allopurinol	Zyloprim	Effective in reducing uric acid levels in blood
febuxostat	Ulonic	New product used primarily when patient unable to tolerate allopurinol.
Uricosuric Agents—Increase Uric Acid Clearance		
probenecid		Increases urate excretion. Often used with penicillin to treat venereal disease. Cross-sensitivity to phenylbutazone and other pyrazoles.
sulfinpyrazone	Anturane	Drug reserved for patients refractory to all other modalities of therapy. Initial dose: Should be taken with meals. Maintenance dose: Therapy should be continued even during acute episodes. Patient may be switched from other uricosuric agents to this drug at full maintenance dose.

★ Indicates "Must-Know Drugs," or the 35 drugs most prescribers use.
IV, intravenous; *PO*, by mouth.

■ Patient and Family Teaching

Tell the patient and family the following:
- Things the patient may do to help prevent or control gouty attacks include:
  - Control weight with daily exercise
  - Limit the amount of red meat eaten
  - Replace eating fish with omega-3 fatty acids supplements
  - Stop eating foods and drinks containing high fructose
  - Eat 1-2 servings of dairy or calcium supplements daily
  - Eat nuts and vegetables daily
  - Take a vitamin C supplement
- The uricosuric drugs do not have an effect on acute gouty attacks, but they help prevent attacks if they are taken regularly. After the initial dose, an acute attack may be precipitated, but the medicine will decrease future chances of severe attacks. Uricosuric medication should be taken as outlined by the health care provider. They should be taken with meals to help decrease GI upset. This is particularly helpful with colchicine.
- The patient should drink at least 8 glasses of fluid (especially water or citrus juices) every day while taking uricosuric medication to prevent kidney stones from developing. The patient should observe stools and urine for blood.
- The health care provider should be contacted immediately if any rash, stomach problems, any skin rash, fever, sore throat, unusual bleeding, bruising, or new or troublesome symptoms develop.
- The medication must be kept in a locked cabinet out of the reach of children and all others for whom it is not prescribed.
- Colchicine should be kept on hand in case the patient develops an attack of gout. At the first sign of gout, the patient should take two tablets, and then one tablet every hour or every 2 hours until the symptoms are relieved or until he or she develops nausea, diarrhea, or vomiting. The patient should not take more than 12 tablets.
- If the patient is taking colchicine regularly with other drugs, it should be taken with meals to reduce GI upset.
- While the patient is taking colchicine on a daily basis, the drug should be stopped if the patient notices symptoms of nausea, vomiting, or diarrhea. In this situation, the patient should contact the health care provider. The patient should not take any other medications without the knowledge of the health care provider. Some drugs interact adversely with allopurinol because it can block the action of the P-450 enzyme system.

Get Ready for the NCLEX® Examination!

Key Points

- This chapter discusses musculoskeletal and antiarthritis medications, which are used to treat problems affecting bones, joints, muscles, and ligaments.
- The specific drug used to treat the disorder is selected based on the severity of the problem and the mechanism causing the problem.
- Many acute problems require only short-term therapy. Some disorders, such as arthritis, may require long-term therapy with a variety of medications, including more powerful medications as the disease gets worse.
- Many of these products have significant side effects and therefore require close monitoring.

Additional Learning Resources

SG Go to your Study Guide for additional learning activities to help you master this chapter content.

℮volve Go to your Evolve website (http://evolve.elsevier.com/Edmunds/LPN/) for additional online resources.

Review Questions for the NCLEX® Examination

1. The patient is admitted to the emergency department and suspected of having an MI. The first medicine the patient will probably be given is:
   1. morphine
   2. nitroglycerin
   3. an aspirin
   4. acetaminophen (Tylenol)

2. The patient tells the nurse they have had musculoskeletal-type pain for the past 2 weeks. The highest priority action on the part of the nurse should be:
   1. document the patient's complaints of persistent pain
   2. assess the symptoms that the patient experiences in addition to pain
   3. ask the physician to order a different medication for pain relief
   4. notify the physician that the patient's pain has been persisting for this long

Get Ready for the NCLEX® Examination!—cont'd

3. The patient has been started on colchicine for an acute gouty attack. What will the nurse tell the patient about why this medicine is given?

1. It reduces pain
2. It reduces the level of uric acid in the blood
3. It increases the level of uric acid in the blood
4. It increases the level of uric acid in the urine

4. The patient recovers from their acute gouty attack. What drug are they most likely to take next?

1. febuxostat (Uloric)
2. ACTH injections into joints
3. allopurinol (Zyloprim)
4. naproxyn (Aleve)

5. The patient has severe buttocks and back pain from a ruptured disk but refuses to have surgery. Which type of NSAID might be useful for long term analgesia?

1. Aspirin
2. acetaminophen (Tylenol)
3. indomethacin (Indocin)
4. celecoxib (Celebrex)

Case Study

Larry Stephenson is a 43-year-old Air Force colonel. He comes into the medical clinic with severe back pain from a herniated vertebral disc. The pain starts in his left buttock and travels down his left leg. He is sent home with the following medications:

- Ibuprofen (Motrin) 800 mg q8h PO
- Medrol Dose Pack as ordered for 7 days
- Hydrocodone 5 mg q6h prn

1. Describe why each of these medications is ordered for this problem.

2. The dose of ibuprofen is very high. Why is this dose ordered? Colonel Stephenson returns to the clinic in 1 week. He is not feeling any better. He continues to have severe buttock pain and has trouble sleeping. He also complains of severe itching.

3. The health care provider discontinues the hydrocodone and orders acetaminophen #2 with codeine. Why did she did this?

4. The health care provider also started the patient on orphenadrine (Norflex). Why was this medication ordered?

5. Does this patient have any contraindications to the use of this product?

6. Col. Stephenson develops slight tachycardia, headache, dizziness, and blurred vision. Under questioning, he also reports increasing problems with constipation. Are these serious problems related to any of his medications?

7. Col. Stephenson also reports that he has been having a lot of gastric burning. What is happening, and what can be done about it?

8. After a month, Col. Stephenson still reports a little pain, particularly at night. He is feeling a little discouraged that he has not made a complete recovery. The health care provider starts him on amitriptyline (Elavil). Why is this medication ordered?

Drug Calculation Review

1. Order: Acetaminophen (Tylenol) 280 mg oral every 4 hours prn T >100.6. Supply: Acetaminophen 80 mg/0.8 mL.
Question: How many milliliters of acetaminophen should be given with each dose?

2. Order: Toradol 15 mg IV every 6 hours (maximum of 6 doses). Supply: Toradol 30 mg/mL.
Question: How many milliliters of Toradol will be given with each dose?

3. Order: Aspirin 650 mg by mouth daily. Supply: Aspirin 325 mg/tablet.
Question: How many aspirin tablets should be given with each dose?

Critical Thinking Questions

1. Mr. Lionhart has started taking aspirin for treatment of arthritis. He says he has a sister with lupus who is also takes aspirin. Mr. Lionhart wonders about the difference in their dosages, because that he and his sister are similar in body weight and size. Explain the importance of different dosages, depending on the problem.

2. In assessing Mr. Lionhart, his health care provider asks the nurse to test for "occult blood." What is occult blood, and how does nurse test for this?

3. Mr. Franklin is being checked for worsening of his gout, which was diagnosed 3 years ago. He tells the nurse he "doesn't think the doctor knows what he's doing, because the pills he told me to take don't help the pain at all." How would the nurse address this with Mr. Franklin?

4. Ms. French is receiving an NSAID for her rheumatoid arthritis. Why might this drug be preferred over aspirin or salicylate therapy? What adverse reactions should Ms. French be told to watch out for?

5. Mr. Henson has been prescribed an oral skeletal muscle relaxant. Mr. Henson asks, "Wouldn't an injection or something be more helpful?" What is a possible reason for the oral form?

6. Because oral skeletal muscle relaxants pose serious risks to patients, carefully prepare a teaching plan that includes a discussion of the high incidence of serious and potentially fatal adverse effects. This plan should stress the importance of good patient compliance.

7. Discuss the two causes of high uric acid levels, comparing the signs and symptoms of each.

8. When managing pain associated with orthopedic injuries, what nursing interventions can be implemented for increasing patient comfort from analgesics?

Gastrointestinal Medications

Objectives

1. Identify common uses for antacids and histamine H2-receptor antagonists.
2. Compare and contrast the actions of anticholinergic and antispasmodic medications on the gastrointestinal tract.
3. Compare the actions and adverse reactions of the five major classifications of laxatives.
4. Identify indications for the use of at least two common antidiarrheals, antiflatulents, digestive enzymes, and emetics.
5. Describe indications for disulfiram use and what is meant by "disulfiram reaction."

Key Terms

antacids (ănt-ĂS-ĭdz, p. 336)
antidiarrheals (ăn-tĭ-dĭ-ă-RĒ-ălz, p. 340)
antiflatulents (ăn-tĭ-FLĂ-tū-lĕnts, p. 347)
digestive enzymes (dī-JĔS-tĭvĔN-zīmz, p. 349)
disulfiram reaction (dī-SŬL-fĭ-răm, p. 350)

emetics (ĕm-ĔT-ĭks, p. 347)
histamine H2-receptor antagonists
(HĬS-tă-mēn, ăn-TĂG-ō-nĭsts, p. 336)
laxatives (LĂK-să-tĭvz, p. 341)
motility (mō-TĬL-ĭ-tē, p. 340)

OVERVIEW

This chapter discusses medications used to treat the many diseases and disorders that affect the gastrointestinal (GI) tract. Many of these drugs are available over the counter (OTC); many others are used, often in combination, to relieve the symptoms of common GI tract problems.

There are three major types of GI medications. The first type includes products designed to help restore or maintain the lining that protects the GI tract. These drugs include antacids, which act to neutralize or reduce the acidity of the gastric contents; histamine H_2-receptor antagonists, which reduce gastric acid secretion by limiting the action of histamine at the H_2 receptors in the stomach; and proton pump inhibitors, which reduce gastric acid by blocking the proton pump. These medications are described in the first section.

A second type of GI medication affects the general motility, or movement, of the GI tract. These medications include the anticholinergics and antispasmodics, which not only reduce gastric motility but also decrease the amount of acid secreted by the stomach, and the antidiarrheals, which reduce diarrhea by slowing the intestinal peristalsis. These drugs are discussed in the second section.

The third type of GI drugs also affect motility, but their action is primarily in the colon. These are the laxative agents. These preparations promote bowel emptying in a variety of ways. They may increase intestinal bulk, lubricate the intestinal walls, soften the fecal mass by retaining water, or produce increased peristalsis through local tissue irritation or by direct action on the intestine. These drugs are discussed in the third section.

The fourth section presents miscellaneous medications. These preparations include antiflatulents, which are used to reduce gas and bloating; and digestive enzymes, which are used in deficiency states to break down fats, starches, and proteins in the digestive process. (Antiemetic preparations are discussed in Chapter 16, along with antivertigo agents.)

DIGESTIVE SYSTEM

The digestive system is composed of the mouth, esophagus, stomach, intestines, and accessory structures (Figure 19-1). This system performs the mechanical and chemical process of digestion, absorbs nutrients, and eliminates waste.

Digestion begins in the mouth with chewing and mixing of food with enzyme-rich saliva secreted by salivary glands. The passages and spaces from the mouth to the anus are called the *alimentary canal*. Here is where the complex compounds created in the mouth are reduced to soluble substances that can be absorbed; the usable food substances are absorbed; and the

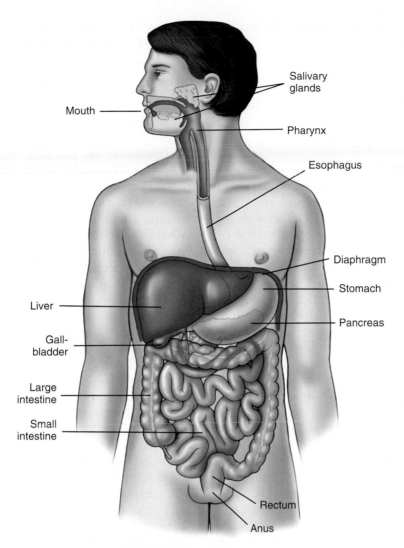

FIGURE 19-1 The digestive system.

indigestible and waste material is eliminated. The digestive glands secrete enzymes and other chemicals essential to the breakdown of food substances and their absorption into the bloodstream. The salivary glands, gallbladder, liver, and pancreas are included as accessory glands.

Almost all oral medications use the digestive system as a means to reach target organs or tissues. Many of the side effects, such as diarrhea, nausea, or constipation, are results of the direct action of medications on the alimentary tract itself. Medications, as well as all swallowed materials, are acted on by the digestive tract and are metabolized and excreted.

The digestive tract must work without being destroyed by the strong acid it makes to digest food. Several factors work together to protect the GI tract mucosa from injury. The gastric mucosal barrier resists backward diffusion of hydrogen and thus has the ability to have a high concentration of hydrochloric acid (HCl) within the gastric lumen unless something breaks this barrier. Endogenous prostaglandins (those

produced in the GI tract) are thought to protect the cells against agents that would be harmful. Prostaglandins are produced in great numbers in the mucosa of the stomach and duodenum. They are known to produce both mucus and bicarbonate and to maintain mucosal blood flow. Mucus helps protect the mucosa. It is secreted by surface epithelial cells and forms a gel that covers the mucosal surface and physically protects the mucosa from abrasion. It also resists the passage of large molecules such as pepsin. Bicarbonate is produced in small amounts by surface epithelial cells and moves up from the mucosa to create a thin layer of alkalinity between the mucus and the epithelial surface. Other protective factors include mucosal blood flow, epithelial healing or renewal, and epidermal growth factor that is secreted in saliva and by the duodenal mucosa.

There is a lot of variability in the body's ability to absorb medications from the GI tract over the course of a lifetime. Changes in GI blood flow, amount of surface available, and motility are found in very young and older adult patients. Thus dosages of some medications may need to be changed when the patient is very young or very old.

ANTACIDS, H₂-RECEPTOR ANTAGONISTS, PROTON PUMP INHIBITORS

OVERVIEW

The lining of the stomach is usually strong enough to resist the powerful digestive juices and acids that bathe it. When stress or disease produce excess secretion of gastric acids, or when there is destruction of the protective mucosal lining because of alcohol, chemicals, or disease, gastric distress is produced. If the protective lining is not repaired or the gastric acid level reduced, duodenal, gastric, or peptic ulcers are produced, leading to increased pain and bleeding. Antacid therapy, histamine H₂-receptor antagonists, and proton pump inhibitors reduce gastric acidity and promote healing. More than one medication may be used at the same time to help in healing. Two unique medications, sucralfate and misoprostol, are designed to assist in the protection of GI mucosa from the effects of nonsteroidal antiinflammatory drugs (NSAIDs).

ACTION

Antacids are OTC agents that neutralize HCl and increase gastric pH, thus inhibiting pepsin (a gastric enzyme). Antacids work in a variety of ways. Some antacids cause hydrogen ion absorption (buffering the acid), tightening of the gastric mucosa, and increased tone of the cardiac sphincter. Formation of gas that may be released by burping is another way in which antacids work.

Histamine H₂-receptor antagonists are unique, because they promote healing of ulcers and act with antacids to produce more alkaline conditions in the GI tract. Histamine H₂-receptor antagonist drugs can bind to the H₂ receptor, thereby displacing histamine from receptor binding sites and preventing stimulation of the secretory cells. Thus they block histamine, inhibit the secretion of gastric acid, and are rapidly absorbed; they reach their peak of effectiveness in 45 to 90 minutes.

Another class of drugs that works to heal gastric ulcers is proton pump inhibitors. These drugs irreversibly stop the acid secretory pump embedded within the gastric parietal cell membrane by altering the activity of H⁺, K⁺-ATPase, the enzyme inhibiting hydrogen ion transport into the gastric lumen, and thus decrease acid secretion. Because proton pump inhibitors act on the basolateral membrane of the parietal cells, they do not affect gastric emptying, basal or stimulated pepsin output, or secretion of intrinsic factor. These drugs do not seem to affect the level of adenosine triphosphatase (ATPase) of other organ systems.

USES

Antacids are used with other drugs to treat peptic ulcer disease, gastritis, gastric ulcer, peptic esophagitis, hiatal hernia, gastric hyperacidity, and esophageal reflux.

Histamine H₂ blockers are generally considered first-line therapy to relieve symptoms and prevent complications of peptic ulcer disease when used for 6 to 8 weeks. (It is common for the patient to have a relapse after the medication is stopped.) They are also used in the prophylaxis and treatment of peptic esophagitis, benign gastric ulcers, duodenal ulcers, stress ulcers, and Zollinger-Ellison syndrome. The H₂ blockers are similar in effectiveness and side effects.

Many peptic ulcers may be caused by *Helicobacter pylori*. This organism may be controlled and the ulcer healed by use of antibiotics plus products such as ranitidine.

Proton pump inhibitors are used in the short-term treatment of active duodenal ulcers, usually after adequate courses of H₂-receptor antagonists have not been successful. Longer therapy is not indicated. Severe erosive esophagitis and poorly responsive gastroesophageal reflux disease (GERD) are indications for these types of medications as well. Long-term treatment with proton pump inhibitors is needed for pathologic hypersecretory conditions.

There are other important drugs that do not fit into these three categories but also assist in the healing of ulcers. Sucralfate is an aluminum salt of sulfated sucrose and a polysaccharide with antipeptic activity. It aids in the healing of ulcers by forming a protective layer at the ulcer site, providing a barrier to hydrogen ion diffusion, but does not alter gastric pH. It also works to stop pepsin's action and adsorbs bile salts. Misoprostol is a synthetic prostaglandin analogue with both an antisecretory and a mucosal protective action. It is indicated for use in patients who have gastric distress or ulceration secondary to the use of NSAIDs.

ADVERSE REACTIONS

Some adverse reactions occur only with a certain category of antacids; others are common to most. Antacids may produce malaise (weakness), anorexia (lack of appetite), bowel obstruction, constipation, diarrhea, frequent burping, thirst, and muscle weakness. In cases of extreme hypermagnesemia, cardiotoxicity with bradyarrhythmia (slow heart beat), asystole (no heart beat), and hypotension may be seen. The most severe reactions include coma, decreased reflexes, and respiratory depression.

With histamine H₂-receptor antagonists, side effects are unusual, but the patient may have mild and self-limiting problems such as dizziness, headaches, somnolence, mild and brief diarrhea, some hematologic changes, rash, impotence, mild gynecomastia (enlargement of the breasts in men), muscle pain, and fever. With proton pump inhibitors, reactions include headache, diarrhea, abdominal pain, and nausea. Rare reactions include rash, vomiting, and dizziness.

DRUG INTERACTIONS

Antacids prevent the absorption of the antibiotic tetracycline. Enteric coatings of various medications dissolve more quickly in the presence of antacids, leaving the upper GI tract more sensitive to irritation. Some antacids have been known to either bind with or alter the absorption rate of digitalis products, anticoagulants, iron, phenothiazines, antiinflammatory agents, antihypertensives, antiarthritic agents, hydantoin, and possibly propranolol. Aluminum-magnesium hydroxide gel may increase absorption of aspirin.

 Clinical Pitfall

Cimetidine

Cimetidine inhibits the cytochrome P-450 system and interacts with many other medications. Care should be used when any other medications are taken at the same time as cimetidine.

Antacids may increase the absorption of cimetidine, a histamine antagonist agent. Cimetidine may increase the effects of anticoagulants, hydantoin, beta-adrenergic blocking agents, lidocaine, benzodiazepine derivatives, and theophylline. Decreased white blood cell counts have been reported in cimetidine-treated patients who also received other drugs and treatments known to produce neutropenia. Apnea, confusion, and muscle twitching may be produced when cimetidine is administered with morphine. Serum digoxin levels may be reduced when digoxin and cimetidine are administered together. Cigarette smoking may neutralize the action of cimetidine. Ranitidine does not appear to interact with warfarin-type anticoagulants, theophylline, or diazepam, although it does produce false-positive urine protein tests.

Proton pump inhibitors also inhibit the cytochrome P-450 system and may interfere with the metabolism of other drugs using the P-450 system. They may also increase concentration of oral anticoagulants, diazepam, and phenytoin, making overdosage a possibility.

❖ NURSING IMPLICATIONS AND PATIENT TEACHING

▪ Assessment

Learn everything possible about the patient's health history, including GI symptoms, the presence of disease (especially renal failure), the presence of allergy, and whether any medications that might cause drug interactions are currently being taken by the patient.

▪ Diagnosis

In addition to the medical diagnosis, what is the source of the patient's problem? Does the patient drink too much coffee or alcohol or use cigarettes extensively—all of which are harmful to the gastric mucosa? Is the patient under stress from financial, family, or job-related difficulties? Does the patient experience gastric distress because of other medications (such as NSAIDs) or disease processes? Look beyond the symptoms to find the cause of increased gastric acid production. This may assist the patient in focusing on the true source of the problem.

▪ Planning

The patient's fluid intake should be increased, and the patient who is taking antacids that cause constipation, such as those containing calcium or aluminum, should be carefully monitored. These drugs may be alternated with antacids that have cathartic-like actions, such as those containing magnesium.

▪ Implementation

Antacids are available in several different forms. Liquids or solutions are the preferred choice whenever possible, because they neutralize acid more rapidly. Suspensions, gels, chewable tablets, effervescent tablets, and powders are also available. Tablets should be considered the last alternative, even though they may be the patient's first choice. The gastric emptying time of the peptic ulcer patient may vary, so it is wise to individualize the antacid schedule. The neutralizing abilities of antacids vary, requiring different quantities of medication, depending on the product. Discuss flavor preferences with the patient. Many patients discontinue antacid therapy because they dislike the flavor. Products come in many flavors, and various drugs may be tried if compliance becomes a problem.

Antacids with a laxative effect should be taken at bedtime to allow adequate rest before the bowel is stimulated.

The sodium content of various antacids must be carefully assessed before giving them to patients who are on restricted sodium intake. These patients include pregnant women and patients with congestive heart failure (CHF) or other cardiac conditions, hypertension (high blood pressure), edema (fluid buildup in the body tissues), or renal failure.

Histamine H$_2$-receptor antagonists may be given via intravenous (IV) or oral (PO) medications. Preparations given PO should be given with meals and at bedtime. IV injections should be diluted and injected over 1 to 2 minutes or given by infusion, and are usually given to patients with hypersecretion of gastric acid or intractable pain from ulcers. These medications should be given for 2 to 6 weeks, until endoscopy tests reveal healing. This drug may mask underlying malignancy.

 Lifespan Considerations
Older Adults

ANTIULCER THERAPIES

- GI problems are very common in older adult patients. Every concern should be evaluated before starting drug therapy.
- In older adults, melena (a black stool that contains digested blood) is more common than pain as an indication of ulcer disease.
- Acid secretion reaches its peak during sleep between the hours of 10 PM and 2 AM. Therefore H$_2$-receptor antagonists given once a day should be taken at bedtime.
- Cigarette smoking, which increases the amount of acid produced in the stomach, may decrease the effect of H$_2$ blockers. Patients should be advised to stop smoking, if possible, or at least to not smoke after the last dose of medication is taken.
- Confusion and dizziness with the use of H$_2$ blockers are more commonly reported by older adults than by younger adults. Mental status changes have been seen with cimetidine (Tagamet), especially in older adults who have damaged liver or renal function or who are severely ill. Acute mental changes in older adult patients may show a need to lower the drug dose or to stop the medication.
- Antacids neutralize gastric acid; food also serves as a buffer for gastric acid. Thus antacids are most beneficial if given between meals and at bedtime.
- When H$_2$-receptor antagonists are ordered with antacids, the medications should be scheduled at least 1 hour apart, with the antacid taken first.

Modified from McKenry LM, Tessier E, Hogan MA: *Mosby's pharmacology in nursing*, ed 22, St Louis, 2006, Mosby.

Table 19-1 presents a summary of antacids and histamine H$_2$-receptor antagonists.

■ Evaluation

Watch to see if the patient seems to have less GI distress or develops any adverse reactions.

■ Patient and Family Teaching

Tell the patient and family the following:

- The patient should take the medication exactly as ordered. Antacids are generally taken 1 hour after meals. If the patient is being treated for peptic ulcer, the gastric emptying time (usually between 1 and 3 hours) will determine when the antacid should be taken. The patient should not switch to another antacid or take new drugs without telling the health care provider.
- Antacids may cause diarrhea or constipation. The patient should report any major problems with

these symptoms to the health care provider. A good fluid intake should be maintained, and the amount of fluids and fiber in the diet should be increased if constipation becomes a problem.

- The chewable tablets should be chewed thoroughly before swallowing and followed with a full glass of water.
- Liquid preparations should be shaken well before taking them, to ensure accurate dosage.
- The health care provider should be asked about whether the antacids will affect any other medications the patient may need to take. Spacing of other medication at different times may limit drug interactions.
- Liquid medications should be stored in a cool place but not allowed to freeze; refrigeration makes them taste better.
- Antacids lose their effectiveness over time; the patient should not use old medication.
- If the physician or nurse practitioner prescribes an aluminum-containing antacid, the patient's diet must contain adequate amounts of dietary phosphorus (up to 1.5 g/day). Phosphorus is found in the protein of meat, almonds, beans, barley, bran, cheese, cocoa, chocolate, eggs, lentils, liver, milk, oatmeal, peanuts, peas, walnuts, whole wheat, rye, asparagus, beef, carrots, cabbage, celery, cauliflower, chard, chicken, clams, corn, cream, cucumbers, eggplant, fish, figs, prunes, pineapples, pumpkins, raisins, and string beans.
- The patient with a peptic ulcer will need to make several follow-up visits to the health care provider for examination and laboratory tests; this is done to assess the healing process.
- Peptic and duodenal ulcers tend to recur, so it is important to determine what causes the problem and to try to correct it. The medication is only part of the therapy. Controlling stress, avoiding irregular eating and stressful living habits, and eliminating other diseases and infections are also important.
- Antacids are often taken with histamine H$_2$-receptor antagonists. The patient should keep medications at home, at school, or at the office so they can be used as soon as there is any gastric distress.
- Antacids dissolve the enteric coating on tablets. Thus antacids should not be taken within 1 hour of a medication with an enteric coating.
- Patients taking proton pump inhibitors must swallow the tablets whole. The patient must not crush or chew tablets.
- Proton pump inhibitors should be taken before meals.
- Proton pump inhibitors and H$_2$ blockers should not be used at the same time. Now that H$_2$ blockers may be purchased OTC in half-strength doses, patients should be reminded of this each time proton pump inhibitors are prescribed.

Table 19-1 Antacids, Histamine H$_2$-Receptor Antagonists, and Proton Pump Inhibitors

GENERIC NAME	TRADE NAME	COMMENTS
Antacids		
aluminum carbonate gel	Basaljel	Take between meals and at bedtime, followed by a sip of water if desired.
aluminum hydroxide gel	Dialume	Helps delay stomach emptying and binds bile salts. Drug of choice in peptic ulcer disease. Take between meals and at bedtime, followed by a sip of water if desired.
calcium carbonate	Tums	Very effective; promotes prolonged and powerful neutralizing effect greater than aluminum hydroxide. Primarily suited for short-term therapy; given in small doses. Constipating effects may be minimized by alternating with doses of a magnesium-containing antacid such as magnesium carbonate.
magaldrate	Losopan Riopan	Combination of magnesium and aluminum hydroxide. Effectiveness depends on GI pH. Give between meals and at bedtime; not to be taken for more than 2 wk.
magnesium hydroxide	Milk of Magnesia	Helpful because cathartic effect counteracts constipation of aluminum hydroxide. Osmotic diarrhea may occur when given alone. Take with water up to 4 times daily.
magnesium oxide	Mag-Ox Maox Uro-Mag	Acts more slowly than sodium bicarbonate but has a more prolonged action and increased neutralizing ability. As with other magnesium antacids, osmotic diarrhea may develop, but it may be alleviated if alternated with aluminum or calcium salts.
sodium bicarbonate	Bell/ans	Take 1 to 4 times/day.
sodium citrate	Citra pH	Take daily.
Antacid Combinations		
aluminum hydroxide and magnesium hydroxide	Maalox	Combined to provide a nonconstipating, noncathartic antacid for relief of hyperactivity of peptic ulcer. Suspension may be followed by a sip of water.
aluminum hydroxide, magnesium hydroxide, and simethicone	Gelusil	Products use simethicone to reduce gas formation; come in many flavors and a variety of combinations.
calcium carbonate	Titralac	Form an insoluble antacid-protective compound for the relief of hyperacidity. Take after meals; tablets can be chewed, swallowed, or allowed to dissolve slowly in the mouth.
Histamine H$_2$-Receptor Antagonists		
cimetidine	Tagamet	Widely used in prophylaxis and treatment of ulcers. Has more drug interactions than other preparations and a much wider range of actions than other preparations. Should be taken with antacids.
famotidine	Pepcid	Reduce dose in those with decreased renal function.
nizatidine	Axid	Give reduced dose for those with decreased renal function.
ranitidine	Zantac	Similar in action to cimetidine, but has fewer drug interactions. Headaches are frequent; extrapyramidal symptoms may be noted. Dose should not exceed 150 mg/24 hr if creatinine clearance is below 50 mL/min.
Agents to Treat *Helicobacter pylori*		
bismuth subsalicylate, metronidazole, and tetracycline	Helidac Pylera	Each dose includes 4 pills: 2 pink chewable 262.4-mg tablets (bismuth subsalicylate); 1 white 250-mg tablet (metronidazole); and 1 pale orange and white 500-mg capsule (tetracycline). Patient should take each dose 4 times daily, with meals and at bedtime, chew and swallow pink tablets, swallow others whole, and drink plenty of water with medication, especially at night.
Miscellaneous Products		
misoprostol	Cytotec	Take daily with meals and at bedtime; reduce dose if higher dose cannot be tolerated. Patient should use throughout the course of NSAID therapy.

Continued

Table 19-1 Antacids, Histamine H₂-Receptor Antagonists, and Proton Pump Inhibitors—cont'd

GENERIC NAME	TRADE NAME	COMMENTS
sucralfate	Carafate	Antacids may be prescribed as needed for pain relief, but patient should not take within ½ hr before or after this medication.
Proton Pump Inhibitors		
esomeprazole	Nexium	Take delayed-release capsule 1 hr before eating.
lansoprazole	Prevacid ♦	Adults: 15 mg once daily before meals for 4 wk. May also use 30 mg with 500 mg clarithromycin and 1 g amoxicillin twice daily for 14 days; or 30 mg with 1 g amoxicillin 3 times daily for 14 days for those intolerant to clarithromycin.
omeprazole	Losec ♦	Adults: 20 mg daily before eating for 4-8 wk. Most ulcers heal within 4 wk, but some require an additional 4 wk. Do not open, chew, or crush capsule.
	Prilosec	
pantoprazole	Protonix	Use delayed-release capsule once daily for 8 wk; also available as an IV infusion.
rabeprazole	Aciphex	Use delayed-release tablet every morning for 4-8 wk.

GI, Gastrointestinal; *IV*, intravenous; *NSAID*, nonsteroidal antiinflammatory drug.

ANTICHOLINERGICS, ANTISPASMODICS, AND ANTIDIARRHEALS

OVERVIEW

Motility is the spontaneous but unconscious or involuntary movement of food through the GI tract. Much of the discomfort of GI disease is caused by increased intestinal peristalsis (muscle contraction). Abdominal cramping, bloating, and pain may be related either to acute minor illnesses associated with diarrhea and increased gas, or to chronic diseases such as ulcers or colitis. Also, many drugs have both diarrhea and increased bowel motility as common adverse reactions.

The medications used to treat these problems are classified as anticholinergics, antispasmodics, or antidiarrheals. Their actions are somewhat different, although they are often used interchangeably.

ACTION

The anticholinergic-antispasmodic agents are parasympatholytic drugs (natural and synthetic) that act with antacids in prolonging or continuing the therapeutic benefits of both drug categories. Anticholinergics reduce GI tract spasm and intestinal motility, acid production, and gastric motility and thus reduce the associated pain. Gastric emptying time is slowed, and neutralization is increased. Pancreatic secretions of fluid, electrolytes, and enzymes are also stopped. However, the adverse reactions resulting from the high dosages necessary to obtain these effects make the use of such dosages questionable. GI motility stimulants are also available and are particularly helpful in the elderly patient with GERD because they do not have cholinergic activity.

Antidiarrheals reduce the fluid content of the stool and decrease peristalsis and motility of the intestinal tract. They increase smooth muscle tone and diminish digestive secretions. The bismuth salts absorb toxins and provide a protective coating for the intestinal mucosa.

USES

Anticholinergic-antispasmodic agents are used primarily to treat peptic ulcer, pylorospasm, biliary colic, hypermotility, hyperacidity, irritable colon, and acute pancreatitis.

Antidiarrheals are used to treat nonspecific diarrhea or diarrhea caused by antibiotics.

ADVERSE REACTIONS

Adverse reactions are common in anticholinergic therapy because high dosages are usually required. The most common adverse reactions include rapid, weak pulse; blurring of vision; dysphagia (difficulty swallowing); difficulty talking; dilation of pupils; drowsiness; excitation; photophobia (sensitivity to light); confusion; restlessness; staggering; talkativeness; rash primarily over the face, neck, and upper trunk (especially in children); flushing of skin; constipation; dry mouth; great thirst; urinary urgency; and difficulty emptying the bladder. Anticholinergics containing phenobarbital may produce convulsions, delirium, excitement, musculoskeletal pain, and various dermatologic and allergic responses. Antidiarrheals may cause tachycardia (rapid heartbeat), dizziness, drowsiness, fatigue, headache, sedation, pruritus (itching), urticaria (hives), abdominal distention, constipation, dry mouth, nausea, vomiting, urinary retention, and physical dependence.

DRUG INTERACTIONS

Anticholinergics containing phenobarbital may decrease the effects of anticoagulants, requiring higher doses of the anticoagulant. Anticholinergics have many drug interactions (see Chapter 16 for a more specific discussion). The newer GI stimulants may cause serious dysrhythmias (irregular heartbeats) when given with other drugs that inhibit the cytochrome P-450 3A4 system and must be used with caution.

❖ NURSING IMPLICATIONS AND PATIENT TEACHING

■ Assessment

Learn everything possible about the patient's health history, including the presence of allergy, underlying diseases, current use of medications, previous GI history, and history of bowel function (regularity, consistency, and frequency). The patient with diarrhea may have frequent loose, watery stools, often with mild, cramping abdominal pain before bowel movements.

■ Diagnosis

Determine if the patient has other problems relating to hydration or nutrition. Is the patient eating enough fiber? Are other medications or foods producing constipation? Does the patient need education to help in managing GI symptoms?

■ Planning

Preparations with phenobarbital may be habit forming, so they should not be given to patients with a history of addiction. Initial doses should be small. These drugs should be used with caution in patients who have hepatic dysfunction or prostatic hypertrophy or who are at risk for glaucoma.

Opiates, loperamide, and diphenoxylate may cause psychologic or physical dependence if used in high dosages or for long periods. The nonspecific antidiarrheal agents provide symptomatic relief until the cause of the diarrhea can be determined and specific therapy can be instituted. These agents should not be used in patients with diarrhea caused by poisoning until the toxin has been removed from the GI tract.

■ Implementation

Anticholinergics may be given orally or parenterally (when oral dosages cannot be retained or when immediate relief is needed). It is usually better to begin the oral dosage as soon as possible. All of the antidiarrheal agents are given orally; individual dosages are determined by need. Dietary changes are usually part of the treatment plan. The patient's diet is restricted to clear liquids for 24 hours, and then foods are gradually added as tolerated.

Table 19-2 gives a summary of anticholinergic, antispasmodic, and antidiarrheal medications. Synthetic forms of these anticholinergic drugs are more expensive than the natural forms (belladonna, atropine, and scopolamine).

■ Evaluation

Long periods of diarrhea can cause dehydration and electrolyte imbalance. Encourage the patient to increase fluid intake to replace the fluid lost in the stool.

Patients who are also taking diphenoxylate and atropine sulfate (Lomotil) or laxatives and narcotics should be watched for signs of central nervous system (CNS) depression. CNS side effects are rare with synthetic anticholinergic therapy, which is one of the advantages of the synthetic products.

Antidiarrheals should not be used on a long-term basis. Watch for diarrhea to decrease and to see if any adverse effects develop.

Long-term anticholinergic therapy may mask or alter the symptoms of GI disease, so it may be difficult to tell if GI disease has occurred again.

■ Patient and Family Teaching

Tell the patient and family the following:
- The patient should take this medication exactly as ordered by the health care provider.
- This medication should be kept out of the reach of children and all others for whom it has not been prescribed.
- Many people experience mild side effects with these medications. The patient should alert the health care provider if any new or troublesome problems occur, especially diarrhea, so that the problems may be evaluated.
- High environmental temperatures may make the patient feel unusually hot and fatigued. The patient should avoid becoming overheated while taking this drug.
- The antidiarrheal agents are used to relieve symptoms and to prevent dehydration until the underlying cause can be found and treated.
- The patient with diarrhea should be restricted to clear liquids (tea, gelatin, broth, carbonated beverages) for 24 hours; the patient can then begin adding bland foods and continue to add more solid foods if diarrhea does not reappear.
- Diarrhea that persists for more than 48 hours should not be self-treated. The patient should return to the health care provider for further evaluation and diagnosis.
- Some antidiarrheal medications contain habit-forming drugs; therefore they should be used only at the dosage recommended and for the length of time prescribed.

LAXATIVES

OVERVIEW

Laxatives are drugs that help draw fluid into the intestine to promote fecal softening, speed the passage of feces through the colon, and aid in the elimination of

Table 19-2 | Anticholinergic, Antispasmodic, and Antidiarrheal Medications

GENERIC NAME	TRADE NAME	COMMENTS
Anticholinergics		
Belladonna Alkaloids		
atropine sulfate ★	Sal-Tropine	Among the most effective of the anticholinergic drugs; minimal side effects.
belladonna tincture	Cystospaz	Used in adults and children.
l-hyoscyamine	Levsin	Reduces hypermotility and hyperacidity; several contraindications for use. Children: Dosage calculated based on weight.
scopolamine	Scopace	Similar to atropine in peripheral action, but parenteral dosages cause CNS depression, resulting in drowsiness, euphoria (excessive happiness), relief of fear, sleep, relaxation, and amnesia. May be given subcutaneously, IM, or through transdermal system, as well as PO.
Quaternary Anticholinergics		
clidinium	Librax	Give daily before meals and at bedtime.
glycopyrrolate	Robinul	Used orally as adjunctive treatment in peptic ulcer disease.
mepenzolate	Cantil	Decreases gastric acid and pepsin secretion while slowing contractions of the colon. Give PO with meals and at bedtime.
methscopolamine	Pamine	Synthetic substitute for atropine as an antispasmodic. Give 30 min before eating and at bedtime.
propantheline	Pro-Banthine	Analogue to methantheline; more effective than methantheline in reduction of volume and acidity of stomach's secretions. Give with meals and at bedtime; dosage adjusted according to therapeutic response.
Antispasmodics		
dicyclomine	Antispas Bentyl Di-Spaz	Synthetic antispasmodic controls spasms of the GI tract; also used in irritable bowel syndrome. Give PO or IM.
Anticholinergic Combination Drug		
Hyoscyamine atropine scopolamine phenobarbital ★	Donnatal	One of many combination products combining anticholinergic and sedative drugs. Because of the phenobarbital, these products may be habit forming. Individualize dose as needed and tolerated. Also comes as an Extentab.
Gastrointestinal Stimulant		
metoclopramide	Reglan	Nocturnal heartburn related to GERD. Adults: Give 30 min before each meal and at bedtime for 2-8 wk; increase dosage if needed.
Antidiarrheals		
bismuth subsalicylate	Bismatrol Pepto-Bismol	Contains salicylates; ask patient about aspirin sensitivity. Has risk of producing Reye syndrome in children. May cause temporary darkening of the stool and tongue. Give PO every 30 min to 1 hr until symptoms are relieved or until a maximum of 8 doses have been given. Children: Dosage calculated by weight. Give with oral rehydration solution in children with severe diarrhea.
difenoxin with atropine	Motofen	Adults: 2 tablets, then 1 after each loose stool to a maximum of 8 tablets in 24 hr.
diphenoxylate and atropine sulfate	Lomotil Logen	These are Schedule V controlled substances. Addition of atropine sulfate helps prevent abuse. Adults: 2 tablets or 2 teaspoonfuls 4 times daily until diarrhea is controlled. Children: Dosage calculated by weight.

Table 19-2 Anticholinergic, Antispasmodic, and Antidiarrheal Medications—cont'd

GENERIC NAME	TRADE NAME	COMMENTS
kaolin and pectin	Kaopectate Parepectolin	Nonprescription products widely used in self-treatment of diarrhea; clinical effectiveness has not been established. Adults: Take 2 tablespoonfuls at once and 1 or 2 tablespoonfuls after each bowel movement. Children: Dosage calculated by weight.
lactobacillus	Bacid Lactinex	Nonprescription product specifically used to treat diarrhea caused by antibiotics. Reestablishes normal intestinal flora and may be used prophylactically in patients with a history of antibiotic-induced diarrhea. Adults: Take 2 capsules or 4 tablets of Bacid; or use 1 packet of granules of Lactinex, 2 to 4 times daily, preferably with milk.
loperamide	Imodium	More potent drug with a longer duration of action with less CNS depression than diphenoxylate; now available OTC. Adults: Initial dose 4 mg PO, then 2 mg after each unformed stool; maximum of 16 mg PO daily.
mesalamine	Asacol Rowasa	Used daily for 6 wk in ulcerative colitis.
olsalazine	Dipentum	Give PO in 2 divided doses for ulcerative colitis.
opium tincture (tincture of opium, paregoric)		Opium tincture contains 25 times the amount of morphine than Paregoric. Schedule III controlled substance. Given orally mixed with water. A white, milky fluid forms when they are mixed together. *Tincture of opium* Adults: Take 0.6 mL PO 4 times daily. *Camphorated opium tincture (paregoric)* Adults: Take 5-10 mL PO 4 times daily until diarrhea subsides. Children: Take 0.25-0.5 mL/kg PO 4 times daily until diarrhea subsides.
sulfasalazine	Azulfidine	Used for mild to moderate ulcerative colitis. Give in evenly divided doses.

CNS, Central nervous system; *IM*, intramuscular; *OTC*, over the counter; *PO*, by mouth.
★ Indicates "Must-Know Drugs," or the 35 drugs most prescribers use.

stool from the rectum. They are classified in five major categories, based on their mechanism of action. These categories are bulk-forming agents, fecal softeners, hyperosmolar or saline solutions, lubricants, and stimulant or irritant laxatives.

Laxatives are one of the major groups of drugs used by patients as self-treatment for constipation, with use increasing as patients age. Laxatives have a high rate of overuse, and they destroy the body's natural emptying rhythm when they are used excessively. Laxatives are used in bowel training of individuals who have lost neurogenic control of the bowel, and are commonly used in preparing patients for x-ray, obstetric, or surgical procedures.

ACTION

Bulk-forming laxatives absorb water and expand, increasing both the bulk and the moisture content of the stool. The increased bulk stimulates peristalsis, and the absorbed water softens the stool. These agents do not have systemic effects.

Fecal softeners soften stool by lowering the surface tension, which allows the fecal mass to be softened by intestinal fluids. They also inhibit fluid and electrolyte reabsorption by the intestine.

Hyperosmolar laxatives such as lactulose and glycerin produce an osmotic effect in the colon by distending the bowel with fluid accumulation and promoting peristalsis and bowel movement. Saline laxatives also produce an osmotic effect by drawing water into the intestinal lumen of the small intestine and colon.

Lubricant laxatives create a barrier between the feces and the colon wall that prevents the colon from reabsorbing fecal fluid, thus softening the stool. The lubricant effect also eases the passage of feces through the intestine.

Stimulant or *irritant laxatives* increase peristalsis by several mechanisms, depending on the agent. These mechanisms include primary stimulation of colon nerves (senna preparations), stimulation of sensory nerves in the intestinal mucosa (bisacodyl), or direct stimulation of smooth muscle and inhibition of water and electrolyte reabsorption from the intestinal lumen (castor oil).

USES

Bulk-forming laxatives are used in simple constipation and in atonic constipation, when the colon loses muscle tone as a result of overuse of other cathartics. Bulk-forming laxatives are also very useful in postpartum, older adult, and weakened patients. They have been used to treat diverticulosis and irritable bowel syndrome.

Fecal softeners help relieve constipation produced by a delay in rectal emptying. They are also useful when it is important to reduce straining at stool, such as in patients with hernia or cardiovascular disease, postpartum patients, or patients after rectal surgery.

Saline laxatives are used to cleanse the bowel in preparation for endoscopic or colonoscopic examination, x-ray studies, or surgery. They are used to hasten evacuation of worms after the administration of anthelmintics, and after the ingestion of poisons to help get rid of toxic material quickly. Lactulose and glycerin are most commonly used to treat simple constipation.

Lubricant laxatives are used to soften stool in conditions in which straining at stool should be avoided, such as in patients with myocardial infarction, aneurysm, stroke, or hernia or after abdominal or rectal surgery. They are also used to prevent discomfort and tearing or laceration of hemorrhoids or fissures.

Stimulant or irritant laxatives are used to treat constipation resulting from prolonged bed rest or poor dietary habits or constipation induced by other drugs. They are also used to cleanse the bowel in preparation for endoscopic or colonoscopic examination, x-ray studies, or surgery.

ADVERSE REACTIONS

Bulk-forming laxatives may produce abdominal cramps, diarrhea, strictures (narrowing), and obstructions (blockages) when taken without sufficient liquid. Nausea and vomiting are also common. Hypersensitivity may be demonstrated by development of asthma, dermatitis, rhinitis, and urticaria.

Fecal softeners may cause mild cramping or diarrhea.

Hyperosmolar or saline laxatives may produce abdominal cramping, nausea, and fluid and electrolyte disturbance if used daily or in patients with renal impairment. Hypermagnesemia may occur in patients with chronic renal insufficiency and is aggravated by increased intake of magnesium in hyperosmolar laxatives. In patients with cardiac disease or CHF, the increased sodium intake in the sodium-containing saline cathartics can start or worsen the condition.

Lubricant laxatives may produce abdominal cramps, vomiting, decreased absorption of nutrients and fat-soluble vitamins, diarrhea, and nausea. Lipid pneumonia caused by aspiration and deficiency syndromes resulting from low absorption of the fat-soluble vitamins may occur with long-term or excessive use.

Stimulant or irritant laxatives may produce muscle weakness (following excessive use of laxatives), dermatitis, pruritus, abdominal cramps, diarrhea, nausea, vomiting, alkalosis, and electrolyte imbalance (with excessive use).

Some patients believe they should have a bowel movement every day and may rely on laxatives to achieve this. Long-term or excessive use of stimulant laxatives may result in irritable bowel syndrome or a severe, prolonged diarrhea. These conditions may lead to hyponatremia and hypokalemia (decreased sodium and potassium in the blood) and dehydration. Cathartic colon, a syndrome resembling ulcerative colitis both radiologically and pathologically, may develop after chronic misuse.

DRUG INTERACTIONS

Antibiotics, anticoagulants, digitalis preparations, and salicylates may have reduced effectiveness if used at the same time as bulk-forming agents because of binding and hindrance of absorption. A 2-hour interval between doses of these medications is required.

Fecal softeners should never be used along with mineral oil or other laxatives. The systemic absorption of other agents is enhanced, causing an increased laxative effect and greater risk of toxic effects, especially to the liver. Hyperosmolar saline laxatives should not be taken within 1 to 3 hours of tetracyclines, because they may form nonabsorbable complexes. Lubricant laxatives may reduce the effectiveness of anticoagulants, contraceptives, digitalis, and fat-soluble vitamins if taken together.

Antacids or milk should not be taken with bisacodyl tablets because together they cause the enteric coating to dissolve too rapidly, resulting in gastric irritation. Some laxatives cause rapid transit through the bowel, and so current use of many medications that require time to dissolve may be adversely affected.

❖ NURSING IMPLICATIONS AND PATIENT TEACHING

■ Assessment

Learn everything possible about the patient's health history, including underlying disease, allergies, edema, or CHF; use of a sodium-restricted diet; and other drugs being taken. The patient should be evaluated for potential abuse. Constipation that persists should always be evaluated for serious organic causes. Changes in bowel habits, especially waking up at night to defecate, should always be investigated.

The patient may complain of increased hardness of stool or of difficulty in passing stool. Decreased frequency of stools, mild abdominal discomfort and distention, and occasionally mild anorexia may be present. Confused geriatric patients may show only increased restlessness when they are constipated.

Laxatives should not be given to patients with abdominal pain, nausea, vomiting, other signs of appendicitis, or acute surgical abdominal conditions. Other contraindications include fecal impaction, intestinal ulcerations, stenosis or obstruction, disabling adhesions, or dysphagia.

Lifespan Considerations
Older Adults

LAXATIVES

Older adult patients often use and abuse laxatives, even though studies have indicated that 80% to 90% of people older than 60 years have at least one bowel movement daily.

To reduce the potential for chronic laxative use and dependency, the older adult patient should be taught nondrug measures to prevent constipation, such as increasing fluid intake to 6 to 8 glasses of water each day if permitted and tolerated. Also recommended is a regular exercise routine, such as a daily walk or active and passive exercise for bedridden patients.

Get a dietary and laxative history from the patient. Consistent intake of a low-fiber diet or a regular intake of foods that tend to harden stools (cheese, hard-boiled eggs, liver, cottage cheese, high-sugar-content foods, rice) may result in constipation.

High-fiber or high-residue diets, along with adequate fluid intake, serve to speed up food travel time in the GI tract and have a mild laxative effect.

High-fiber foods include orange juice with pulp or a fresh orange, bran or whole-grain cereals, whole-grain or bran breads, leafy vegetables, and fresh fruits. Although prunes, bananas, figs, and dates are high in dietary fiber, prunes also contain a laxative substance that stimulates intestinal motility.

Modified from McKenry LM, Tessier E, Hogan MA: *Mosby's pharmacology in nursing,* ed 22, St Louis, 2006, Mosby.

▪ Diagnosis

What are the factors that have caused constipation? Does the patient have other problems in terms of hydration, lack of nutritional fiber, or eating disorders that underlie the development of constipation? Is the patient taking codeine, morphine, or other opioids that may cause constipation?

▪ Planning

Many bulk-forming products contain significant amounts of dextrose, galactose, and sucrose and should be avoided in patients with diabetes mellitus. Allergic reactions (urticaria, rhinitis, and asthma) may occur as a result of the plant gums present in these agents. This should be considered in patients with a history of allergic reactions, especially to plants.

Bulk-forming agents may become dry, thick, and hardened in the throat or within the intestine if they are swallowed without sufficient water. They can cause esophageal or intestinal obstruction or impaction if this occurs. The drugs should never be chewed or swallowed without one or more full glasses of water. Before giving medication for constipation, ensure that the patient is well hydrated (has enough fluids).

Products with sodium salt should be avoided in patients with edema, pregnancy, CHF, and sodium-restricted diets. Potassium salt should be avoided in patients with renal impairment. Because laxatives are available without prescription, it is especially important to teach the patient about these serious side effects.

Begin educating the patient by explaining the usefulness of exercise, diet, and liquids to reduce constipation. The patient should be taught to eat bulk-forming foods, fruits, vegetables, and whole-grain cereals and encouraged to perform more physical activities if able to do so. Proper bowel habits should be discussed and encouraged, and increased fluid intake should be stressed.

Overdosage or overuse of stimulant laxatives may cause excessive fluid loss and electrolyte imbalance, particularly hypokalemia. Overuse of any laxative can lead to atonic constipation and create dependence on the laxative.

If the patient does not really need a laxative, or must use a laxative because of constipation resulting from pain medication, the bowel must be retrained to function without laxative use. Good hydration, high fiber intake, and exercise all help patients make this change.

▪ Implementation

All bulk-forming and stimulant laxatives are given orally with one or more glasses of liquid. Most other laxatives are available for oral administration or as enemas.

Plan medication administration to allow the drug's effects to occur at a time that will not interfere with the patient's rest or digestion. Administration of lubricant laxatives should be timed so that they are not given within 2 hours of meals or medication.

Bisacodyl enteric-coated tablets must be swallowed whole, never chewed or crushed, and never taken with milk or antacids.

A summary of laxative products is given in Table 19-3. The need for mixtures of laxatives has not been documented. The actions of various laxatives show that combinations are unnecessary and may produce harmful or undesirable effects. They also tend to be more expensive than drugs sold individually. A partial listing of some of the available drug mixtures that patients may ask the nurse about is provided in Table 19-4, but it is not recommended that combination drugs be used.

▪ Evaluation

Laxatives should be used only for short periods and should not require any patient monitoring. If for any reason they are used on a long-term basis, ask the patient about bowel habits, diet, and exercise, and monitor for adverse reactions. Many of the stimulant laxatives discolor alkaline urine reddish pink and acidic urine yellow brown. They may give a reddish color to feces.

Table 19-3 Laxatives

GENERIC NAME	TRADE NAME	COMMENTS
Bulk-Forming Laxatives		
methylcellulose	Citrucel Unifiber	Produces a laxative effect in 12-72 hr. All doses should be taken with a full glass or more of liquid. Adults: Give PO 3 times daily with a full glass of water; or may be taken PO 4 times daily with meals and at bedtime.
psyllium seed	Fiberall Metamucil	This product is indigestible and not absorbed; does not interfere with absorption of nutrients. These laxatives are least likely to cause laxative abuse. Adults: Give PO in full glass of water 1 to 3 times daily; follow with second glass of water.
Fecal Softeners or Wetting Agents		
docusate	Colace Modane	Give once daily.
Hyperosmolar or Saline Laxatives or Enemas		
glycerin	Sani-Supp	Suppository: Use 1 and retain for 15 min before expelling.
lactulose	Cephulac Cholac	Available by prescription only. Usually taken as needed.
magnesium (magnesium citrate, milk of magnesia)	Philips Milk of Magnesia	Usually products are taken at bedtime and produce results overnight.
sodium salts	Fleet Enema Phospho-Soda	Approximately 10% of the sodium in these products may be absorbed. Oral: Give PO mixed with half a glass of water; follow with another full glass of water; should be taken as soon as patient gets up in the morning. Enema: Take 4 oz PR for adults; 2 ½ oz for children older than 2 yr.
Lubricant Laxatives		
castor oil	Purge Emulsoil	Used orally and also given rectally as an enema for retention and softening. Should be given at least 2 hr after meals. Children over 6 yr: Give PO; or 4 oz PR as enema.
Stimulant or Irritant Laxatives		
bisacodyl	Dulcolax Correctol Feen-a-Mint	Enteric-coated tablets must be swallowed whole; do not chew or crush. Do not take within 1 hr of antacids or milk. Drink at least 1 full glass of water with each dose. Suppository should be inserted at time bowel movement is desired; acts within 15-60 min. Enema is administered rectally at time evacuation is desired. Adults: Give PO in evening or before breakfast. Approximately 30 mg PO may be safely used in preparation for special procedures.
Cascara sagrada	Cascara, Aromatic	Fluid extract contains 18% alcohol. Sold under various brand names; some tablets are sugar coated, others are uncoated. May discolor alkaline urine reddish pink and acidic urine yellow brown. Adults: Comes as aromatic liquid or PO.
senna	Senokot Ex-Lax Agoral	May cause yellow or yellow green cast to feces; reddish pink discoloration of alkaline urine, yellow brown color in acid urine.

PO, By mouth; *PR*, per rectum.

Table 19-4   Laxative Combination Products

TRADE NAME	CHEMICAL COMBINATION
Peri-Colace	casanthranol, docusate sodium
Senokot-S	senna, docusate sodium

■ Patient and Family Teaching

Tell the patient and family the following:

- Bulk-forming laxatives require large amounts of fluid to work properly; they should never be chewed or swallowed without water. The patient must take at least one full glass of liquid with each dose.
- Laxatives should be taken exactly as specified by the health care provider and are indicated for short-term use only. Overuse of laxatives robs the bowel of its ability to perform on its own.
- Some agents are high in sodium or glucose. The content should be checked if the patient is on a restricted diet or has diabetes.
- Laxatives should be used only as additional therapy when regular bowel habits, daily exercise, and the use of high-bulk foods and fruits in the diet fail to maintain regularity.
- Bulk-forming laxatives should not be taken within 2 hours of any other medications.
- Allergic reactions may occur in response to any of these products. If rash, itching, nasal congestion, or wheezing occurs, the patient should stop taking the medication immediately and contact the health care provider.
- The laxative effect of bulk-forming laxatives may occur within 12 hours or may take up to 3 days to appear. Fecal softeners act within 24 to 48 hours. Lactulose may require 24 to 48 hours to produce a normal bowel movement. Saline laxatives produce results within 2 to 8 hours and should not be taken at bedtime. The fastest effect of hyperosmolar products is obtained when the drug is taken on an empty stomach with a full glass of water. Mineral oil should not be taken within 2 hours of taking food or other medication. The stimulant laxatives act within 6 to 10 hours, except castor oil, which acts within 1 to 3 hours. The stimulant laxatives include many of the chewing gum and chocolate types and are the kind most often abused.
- Fecal softeners should be used only in addition to good, regular bowel habits, daily exercise, and the use of high bulk or fiber in the diet to help maintain regularity. They do not treat preexisting constipation, but do prevent constipation from developing.
- The patient should take milk or fruit juice with fecal softeners to mask the bitter taste. The flavor of the hyperosmolar laxatives may be improved by taking the medication with fruit juice or a citrus-flavored carbonated beverage. Fruit juices or carbonated drinks may help disguise the oily taste of lubricant laxatives.
- The health care provider should give the patient a list of foods high in bulk or fiber that can assist in maintaining bowel regularity.
- Saline laxatives should not be taken daily on a prolonged basis or used in children younger than 6 years of age.
- Large doses of lubricant laxatives may cause a leakage of oil from the rectum. The use of pads to protect clothing may be necessary if tight sphincter control is not present.

MISCELLANEOUS GASTROINTESTINAL DRUGS

OVERVIEW

Many diseases and symptoms affect the GI tract; there are also many drugs used in their treatment. Antiflatulents, such as simethicone, break up GI gas bubbles through a defoaming action so they may be more easily expelled by belching or as flatus. Pancreatic digestive enzymes are used as replacement therapy for individuals with pancreatic enzyme insufficiency. **Emetics** are used mostly in emergency situations to produce vomiting by direct action on the vomiting center. Chenodiol acts on the liver to increase breakdown of radiolucent cholesterol gallstones. Disulfiram is used in alcoholic patients to produce a severe sensitivity to alcohol. Each of these drugs is briefly described.

Table 19-5 summarizes the important miscellaneous GI medications.

ANTIFLATULENTS

ACTION

Simethicone is an **antiflatulent** that breaks up and prevents mucus-surrounded pockets of gas from forming in the intestine. Mucus surrounding the gas bubbles is broken down, and the gas bubbles all come together, freeing the gas. Gastric pain is then reduced. Charcoal is occasionally used as an antiflatulent but is used primarily in the treatment of drug overdosage to absorb chemicals.

USES

Antiflatulents are used to treat problems that produce bloating, flatulence, or postoperative gas pains. They may also be used for chronic air swallowing, functional dyspepsia (stomach discomfort after eating), peptic ulcer, spastic or irritable colon, and diverticulitis. The patient may complain of being bloated or distended, of feeling "full" or gaseous, or of frequent belching. Gas pains may also be noted, especially after surgery. Determine if the flatulence is caused by food and whether changing the diet may decrease the

Table 19-5   Miscellaneous Gastrointestinal Medications

GENERIC NAME	TRADE NAME	COMMENTS
Antiflatulents		
activated charcoal	CharcoCaps	Adults: Take after meals or at first sign of discomfort; repeat PRN.
simethicone	Mylanta Gas Relief Mylicon	Available in both drops and tablet form. Chew tablets thoroughly before swallowing. Shake drops well before using.
Gallstone Dissolution		
ursodiol	Actigall	Adults: Take daily in 2 or 3 divided doses.
Digestive Enzymes		
pancreatin	Creon	Product tends to be cheaper than pancrelipase, although not as effective. Take with meals.
pancrelipase	Ku-Zyme HP Pancrease Viokase	Pancrelipase is a prescription drug combination of the pancreatic enzymes used in replacement therapy. Works more effectively than pancreatin. Provides a catalyst effect in the hydrolyzation of fats, proteins, and starch. Amount of dietary fat is the key to dosage: for every 17 g of fat, 300 mg of pancrelipase should be taken. Adults: Take capsules or tablets (or 1-2 packets) just before each meal or snack.
Antialcoholic Product		
disulfiram	Antabuse	Take specific dosage daily for 1-2 wk, followed by a daily maintenance dose. May take up to 3 wk for drug to reach full effectiveness; drug remains effective for approximately 2 wk after therapy is discontinued. Average maintenance dosage is 250 mg daily. Maintenance therapy is needed until the patient is fully recovered socially, and a basis for permanent self-control has been established. May take months or even years.

PRN, As needed.

symptoms. Antiflatulents are often used together with antacid therapy. This medication is intended for short-term use only. More rigorous evaluation should be undertaken if symptoms do not disappear with therapy.

GALLSTONE-SOLUBILIZING AGENTS

ACTION

Gallstone-solubilizing agents act on the liver to suppress cholesterol and cholic acid synthesis. Biliary cholesterol desaturation is enhanced, and breakup or dissolution of radiolucent cholesterol gallstones (those that allow x-rays to pass through and thus show up as dark images) eventually occurs. There is no effect on calcified or radiopaque gallstones (those that absorb x-rays and thus show up as white images) or radiolucent bile pigment stones.

USES

Gallstone-solubilizing agents are useful in selected patients with radiolucent stones in gallbladders that opacify well (show up when dye is used). These patients are poor surgical risks because of disease or advanced age. Success is likely to be higher with small stones that float.

ADVERSE REACTIONS

Adverse reactions to gallstone-solubilizing agents may include dose-related diarrhea, anorexia, constipation, cramps, dyspepsia, epigastric distress, flatulence, heartburn, nausea, nonspecific abdominal pain, and vomiting. Laboratory test results may be altered; nonspecific decreases in white cell count may also develop.

DRUG INTERACTIONS

Biliary cholesterol secretion and gallstones may be increased by estrogens, clofibrate, and oral contraceptives. Therefore these drugs may counteract the effectiveness of gallstone-solubilizing agents. Bile acid–sequestering agents such as cholestyramine and colestipol may reduce the absorption of gallstone-solubilizing agents. Aluminum-based antacids may absorb bile acids and also reduce the absorption of gallstone-solubilizing agents.

These medications should not be used in patients with known liver or other gallbladder disease. If the gallbladder fails to show up after two consecutive single doses of dye, or if radiopaque or radiolucent bile pigment stones are seen, these medications will likely not be used. These products may produce hepatotoxicity (damage to the liver), ranging from mild toxicity to fatal hepatic failure. They should be used only in patients without previous hepatic problems, and careful monitoring of the patient's liver function is required. There is also the chance that chenodiol therapy might contribute to the development of colon cancers in individuals who are predisposed to develop them.

If diarrhea develops, reducing the dosage usually eliminates the symptoms. The patient is often able to resume higher dosages without diarrhea occurring again.

Evaluation of patient compliance is important. The patient must be reliable in keeping appointments, reporting problems, and having periodic health evaluations.

 Memory Jogger

Gallstone Recurrence

Stone recurrence can be expected within 5 years in 50% of all patients using gallstone-solubilizing agents. Low-cholesterol, low-carbohydrate diets with increased dietary bran may help reduce biliary cholesterol. Weight reduction may help postpone stone recurrence.

DIGESTIVE ENZYMES

ACTION

Pancreatic **digestive enzymes** promote digestion by acting as replacement therapy when the body's natural pancreatic enzymes are lacking, not secreted, or not properly absorbed. They are made from pork pancreas. Healthy patients may find intestinal gas is decreased when they take the medication.

USES

Digestive enzymes are often indicated for individuals with poor digestion, for predigestive purposes, and as replacement therapy. They may be used to relieve the symptoms of cystic fibrosis, cancer of the pancreas, or chronic inflammation of the pancreas causing malabsorption syndromes. Patients who have had GI bypass surgery may also be helped. Obstruction of the pancreatic or common bile duct by a tumor may produce a need for these enzymes.

ADVERSE REACTIONS

If a proper dietary balance of fat, protein, and starch is not maintained, temporary indigestion may develop. Nausea, abdominal cramps, and diarrhea have been reported in patients taking high doses. Inhalation of the powder may provoke asthma.

DRUG INTERACTIONS

Antacids containing calcium carbonate or magnesium hydroxide may cancel out the therapeutic effect of digestive enzymes. In addition, serum iron levels produced by iron supplements may be decreased by these enzymes.

❖ NURSING IMPLICATIONS AND PATIENT TEACHING

The patient may complain of sudden, intense pain in the gastric region; hiccups; belching of gas; vomiting; constipation; pain radiating to the back; weakness; diarrhea; indigestion; ravenous appetite without weight gain; and chronic cough and infections.

Patients who are hypersensitive to pork protein should avoid this therapy. The patient should avoid breathing the powdered form of the enzymes or allowing it to come into contact with the skin, because it may produce irritation.

Digestive enzymes are given with meals or snacks. They are available in tablet or capsule form, which is swallowed, not chewed. They also come in a powder, or the capsules may be opened and sprinkled on food for those who have difficulty swallowing tablets. Medication granules are not to be taken without food, because this will destroy the enzymes.

The correct dosage can be determined after several weeks of therapy. Different flavors are available for this medication.

Monitor the patient for the therapeutic effect and the absence of adverse reactions. Question the patient about the appearance of stools, because this may help evaluate the degree of malabsorption present.

■ Patient and Family Teaching

Tell the patient and family the following:

- The patient should take this medication exactly as ordered. The capsules or tablets should be swallowed at mealtime, or the capsules of powder can be opened and sprinkled on food if the patient has difficulty swallowing pills.
- The granules should always be taken with meals or snacks. The body will destroy the granules and not receive any benefit from them if the patient does not take them with food.
- The patient must be careful not to breathe in the powder or touch it with the hands when opening the powder and pouring it. Direct exposure to the powder produces a strong irritation.
- The patient should eat a well-balanced diet with adequate amounts of fat, starch, and protein and develop and maintain a normal eating routine; this will help prevent indigestion.
- The patient can try the various flavors of medication until a preferred flavor is found.
- The patient should report any discomfort or troublesome symptoms to the health care provider.

DISULFIRAM

ACTION

Disulfiram (Antabuse) produces a severe sensitivity to alcohol that results in a very unpleasant reaction. This **disulfiram reaction** includes severe nausea, vomiting, and diarrhea, as well as many other adverse reactions, when even small amounts of alcohol are swallowed. This drug causes excessive amounts of acetaldehyde to develop by stopping the normal liver enzyme activity after the conversion of alcohol to acetaldehyde. Increased levels of acetaldehyde produce the disulfiram reaction. The reaction is present until the alcohol is completely metabolized. The intensity of the reaction is variable, but it is usually related to the amount of disulfiram and alcohol swallowed.

 Clinical Pitfall

Disulfiram Reaction

A disulfiram (or Antabuse) reaction may include the following symptoms: flushing and warming of the face, severe throbbing headache, shortness of breath, chest pain, nausea, vomiting, sweating, weakness, hyperventilation, tachycardia, syncope (light-headedness and fainting), and confusion. Severe reactions could include dysrhythmias, respiratory distress, cardiovascular collapse, myocardial infarction, acute CHF, convulsions, and death.

USES

Disulfiram (Antabuse) is used only for the management of alcoholism. It is used to discourage alcohol intake, which in turn forces the patient to be sober. This drug is used in addition to psychiatric therapy or alcohol counseling and in patients who are motivated and fully cooperative.

ADVERSE REACTIONS

Disulfiram may produce drowsiness, fatigue, headache, optic neuritis (with impaired vision, decreased color perception, and blindness), psychotic reactions, restlessness, acneiform eruptions, dry mouth, elevation of serum liver enzyme levels, hepatotoxicity, metallic or garlic-like aftertaste, and impotence.

DRUG INTERACTIONS

Use of disulfiram with even small amounts of alcohol produces a severe reaction. When used together, disulfiram increases the effects of anticoagulants, phenytoins, and barbiturates, and may increase the side effects of isoniazid. Use with metronidazole and marijuana has an additive effect and may produce psychotic episodes. Exaggerated clinical effects of diazepam and chlordiazepoxide are produced when these drugs are taken at the same time as disulfiram. Use with paraldehyde may produce the disulfiram-alcohol reaction.

Some medications, such as metronidazole, produce a similar reaction when taken with alcohol. Patients must be warned of these disulfiram-like reactions.

❖ NURSING IMPLICATIONS AND PATIENT TEACHING

Disulfiram should not be used if the patient has consumed alcohol in any form within the last 12 hours. This includes the use of cough mixtures, tonics, vanilla, vinegar, some sauces, aftershave lotions, back-rubbing solutions, some creams, or other products containing alcohol. Do not use disulfiram if there has been recent ingestion of paraldehyde or metronidazole. Do not use in the presence of severe myocardial disease or coronary occlusion, psychoses, or hypersensitivity (allergy) to disulfiram. Do not use disulfiram in pediatric patients.

Disulfiram should be used with extreme caution in patients with any of the following conditions: diabetes mellitus, epilepsy, cerebral damage, hypothyroidism, chronic and acute nephritis, hepatic cirrhosis or insufficiency, conditions requiring multiple drug usage, coronary artery disease, and hypertension. In these patients, there is the possibility of an accidental disulfiram reaction.

The patient should give permission for disulfiram therapy. The patient and a responsible family member need to understand the consequences of this therapy. Disulfiram reactions may occur for up to 2 weeks after a single dose of disulfiram. The longer patients take this drug, the more sensitive they will become to alcohol. The disulfiram reaction may be provoked by even small amounts of alcohol. The patient should be cautioned against hidden forms of alcohol (tonics, cough syrups, aftershave lotions).

Disulfiram users should wear a MedicAlert bracelet or necklace or carry a medical identification card indicating that they use this drug and describing the symptoms most likely to occur in the disulfiram reaction. Cards to give to patients taking this drug may be obtained from the drug company.

The patient should be actively involved in support and counseling to reduce psychologic dependence and should be monitored for compliance and development of adverse effects.

COMPLEMENTARY AND ALTERNATIVE THERAPIES

The Complementary and Alternative Therapies box describes herbal preparations commonly used by patients and potential drug interactions with other medications.

Complementary and Alternative Therapies

Gastrointestinal Problems

CONDITION	PRODUCT	COMMENTS
Constipation	Cascara Senna Milk thistle Psyllium	Use may decrease absorption of oral medications; potential interaction with antiarrhythmics, digoxin, phenytoin, laxatives, lithium, and theophylline. No toxicity or serious side effects noted.
Diarrhea	Grapefruit seed extract Olive leaf Green tea Bilberry	Avoid concurrent administration of terfenadine, astemizole, and cisapride; use other medications metabolized by the cytochrome P-450 (CYP) 3A4 subsystem with caution. No reported toxicities. Potential interaction with anticoagulants, aspirin, NSAIDs, and antiplatelet agents.
Gallbladder and gallstones	Milk thistle Artichoke Goldenseal	No reported toxicities with any of these products.
Indigestion and heartburn	Bromelain Ginger Cayenne Artichoke Chamomile Peppermint	Potential interactions with anticoagulants, aspirin, NSAIDs, and antiplatelet agents. Potential interactions with anticoagulants, aspirin, NSAIDs, antiplatelet agents, and cardiac glycosides. Potential interaction with anticoagulants, aspirin, NSAIDs, and antiplatelet agents; potential interference with monoamine oxidase inhibitors and antihypertensives. No known interactions with the rest of these products.
Irritable bowel	Cat's claw Grapefruit seed extract Evening primrose Peppermint	Potential interaction with anticoagulants, aspirin, NSAIDs, and antiplatelet agents. Avoid concurrent administration of terfenadine, astemizole, and cisapride; use other medications metabolized by the CYP 3A4 subsystem with caution. Potential interaction with anticoagulants, aspirin, NSAIDs, and antiplatelet agents. No known interactions.
Nausea/ vomiting	Chamomile Ginger	No known interactions. Potential interactions with anticoagulants, aspirin, NSAIDs, antiplatelet agents, and cardiac glycosides.
Ulcer	Licorice Mastic Marshmallow	Potential interaction with nitrofurantoin. No known interactions. Potential interactions with insulin and oral hypoglycemic agents.

Modified from Krinsky DL, LaValle JB, Hawkins EB, et al: *Natural therapeutics pocket guide*, ed 2, Hudson, Ohio, 2003, Lexi-Comp, Inc.

Get Ready for the NCLEX® Examination!

Key Points

- Many medications are used to treat the variety of diseases or disorders affecting the GI tract.
- The major medications covered in this chapter are antacids, which neutralize or reduce stomach acidity; histamine H$_2$-receptor antagonists, which stop the action of histamine at receptor cells in the stomach; anticholinergics and antispasmodics, which reduce gastric motility and decrease acid secretions; antidiarrheals, which reduce diarrhea; laxatives, which promote emptying of the bowel; antiflatulents, which reduce gas and bloating; digestive enzymes, which break down fats, starches, and proteins; and emetics, which produce vomiting.
- Many of these medications are self-administered by patients. Therefore it is important that the nurse teach the patient or family about serious adverse reactions to watch for and any special administration considerations, such as fluid intake or foods to avoid.

Additional Learning Resources

SG Go to your Study Guide for additional learning activities to help you master this chapter content.

evolve Go to your Evolve website (http://evolve.elsevier.com/Edmunds/LPN/) for additional online resources.

Review Questions for the NCLEX® Examination

1. The nurse is taking care of a patient being treated with disulfiram (Antabuse). The patient complains to the nurse of not having the full effects of the medication after taking the drug for 10 days. The most appropriate response from the nurse is:
   1. "The effects of this medicine are seen mainly when you drink alcohol."
   2. "You may need a larger dose of the medication."
   3. "It may take 3 weeks for the drug to reach its full effectiveness."
   4. "This is evidence that the medication is not effective for you."

Get Ready for the NCLEX® Examination!—cont'd

2. The patient has been placed on simethicone (Mylicon). The highest priority instruction that the nurse should give the patient is:

   1. swallow tablets whole; do not chew
   2. chew tablets thoroughly before swallowing
   3. swallow tablets with at least 8 ounces of water
   4. take tablets with food or milk

3. The patient has been started on senna (Senokot). The patient tells the nurse she has a reddish-pink color to her urine. The most appropriate response from the nurse should be:

   1. "This is an expected response to the medication."
   2. "This is evidence of a toxic dose of the medication."
   3. "This is an allergic response to the medication."
   4. "This is an unexpected response to the medication."

4. The patient begins to take famotidine (Pepcid). The patient has a history of decreased renal function. The nurse recognizes that:

   1. the patient will need an increased dosage of the medication
   2. the patient must be placed on a different drug
   3. the patient is at high risk of an allergic reaction
   4. the patient will need a decreased dosage of the medication

5. The patient tells the nurse that she has started taking the herbal preparation cat's claw to treat irritable bowel syndrome. The patient also is being treated with an anticoagulant medication. The most important thing that the nurse should tell the patient is:

   1. "Cat's claw is known to be a safe herbal medication with few side effects."
   2. "Cat's claw is known to interact with anticoagulants. You should talk with your doctor."
   3. "Cat's claw may decrease the effectiveness of the anticoagulant. Talk with your doctor."
   4. "Cat's claw may increase the effectiveness of the anticoagulant, so you may need less of it."

Case Study

Mr. Frost is a 73-year-old patient, who is being treated for CHF that developed after an acute myocardial infarction. His stay in the hospital has been upsetting for him, and both his eating and bowel habits have changed. He usually reports a bowel movement every morning but has been unable to pass stool for the last 3 days. He is currently sitting on a commode and straining. The doctor orders:

- Metamucil: 1 rounded tsp 1 to 2 times/day
- Lanoxin: 0.25 mg PO daily
- Hydrochlorothiazide: 50 mg daily

   1. Why is the Metamucil ordered?
   2. If the Metamucil does not work, what type of laxative might be effective?
   3. What type of laxative would not be indicated for this patient?

4. Why is the Lanoxin ordered?
5. What is the purpose of the hydrochlorothiazide?
6. Are there any things to be concerned about in a patient taking hydrochlorothiazide?
7. What dietary modifications might assist Mr. Frost in returning to normal bowel activity?

Drug Calculation Review

1. Order: Famotidine (Pepcid) 20 mg by gastrostomy tube (per GT) twice a day. Supply: Pepcid 40 mg/5 mL.
   Question: How many milliliters of Pepcid are needed with each dose?

2. Order: Dolasetron (Anzemet) 1.8 mg/kg 30 min before chemotherapy. Supply: Anzemet 20 mg/mL.
   Question: How many milligrams of Anzemet should be given to a patient weighing 143 lb?

3. Order: Sucralfate (Carafate) 1.5 g per GT 4 times per day. Supply: Sucralfate 1 g/10 mL.
   Question: How many milliliters of sucralfate are needed with each dose?

Critical Thinking Questions

1. Ms. McKelvey has been taking OTC antacids for her stomach ulcer. Now, however, the health care provider has added a histamine H_2-receptor antagonist. When the health care provider leaves the room, Ms. McKelvey tells the nurse she is unhappy about this, because she has prided herself on keeping her "medical costs" down by using only home remedies and OTC drugs. "If they're both for ulcers," she says, "then what's the difference? Why can't I just double my dose of the antacid?" Describe the differences between these two drugs in their actions and uses in a way that makes it easy for Ms. McKelvey to understand.

2. Explain why adverse reactions are more frequent with anticholinergics than with antidiarrheals.

3. Mrs. Harris, age 82, has been admitted to the hospital for treatment of severe diarrhea. She is placed on antidiarrheal therapy and is under observation. Identify signs of dehydration and electrolyte imbalance, as well as any adverse reactions that might be associated with antidiarrheal therapy, particularly in the older adult patient.

4. On the second day of treatment, Mrs. Harris does show signs of both dehydration and electrolyte imbalance, as the nurse had anticipated. Draw up a treatment plan for this patient.

5. Mr. Weigand has been using fecal softeners on an almost daily basis "for quite a while," he says, but is still having constipation. The health care provider has examined Mr. Weigand and tells him that he needs to be switched to a lubricant type of laxative instead of the softeners. Mr. Weigand is uncomfortable with this and asks the nurse why he cannot use his "old stand-by."

Get Ready for the NCLEX® Examination!—cont'd

6. A digestive enzyme has been ordered for Mrs. Magid. What are the possible indications for this drug? What kind of patient teaching should the nurse give Mrs. Magid about this drug? How can she minimize adverse reactions?

7. Why would digestive enzymes be prescribed for a child with cystic fibrosis?

8. What is a "disulfiram reaction?" Why is disulfiram prescribed? Explain why patient compliance is so important with this drug.

Hematologic Products

Objectives

1. Describe the influence of anticoagulants on blood clotting.
2. Develop a teaching plan for patients taking anticoagulants on a long-term basis.
3. Identify at least three adverse reactions associated with hematologic products.
4. Identify drugs that act in the formation, repair, or function of red blood cells.

Key Terms

anticoagulants (ăn-tĭ-kō-ĂG-ū-lĕnts, p. 354)
fibrin (FĪ-brĭn, p. 354)
fibrinogen (fĭ-BRĬN-ō-jĕn, p. 354)

thrombi (THRŎM-bī, p. 354)
thromboplastin (thrŏm-bō-PLĂS-tĭn, p. 354)

OVERVIEW

Hematologic products act in the formation, repair, or function of red blood cells. There are four major groups of medications that have hematologic effects. They include the anticoagulants (heparin and warfarin [Coumadin]) and the heparin antagonist protamine sulfate. Thrombolytic agents and antiplatelet factors also have a major influence on blood clotting. Related vitamins and minerals needed for red blood cell development are iron, vitamin K, vitamin B_{12}, and folic acid; these are presented in Chapter 24.

ANTICOAGULANTS

One of the body's protective functions is to clot blood in response to tissue injury. Any damage to the cells starts a series of chemical reactions to protect the body (Figure 20-1). Cellular damage results in the formation of **thromboplastin**, which then acts on prothrombin to form thrombin. Calcium must be present for this reaction to occur. Thrombin then acts on **fibrinogen** (a protein found in the blood plasma) to produce **fibrin**, a netlike substance in the blood that traps red and white blood cells and platelets and forms the matrix, or skeleton, of the clot. Vitamin K must be present to produce prothrombin and other clotting factors that are made in the liver. All **anticoagulants** prevent the formation of blood clots, or thrombi, by interfering with this complex clotting mechanism of blood and increasing the time it takes for blood to clot. In cases

of overdose, protamine sulfate is given to counteract the effect of heparin. In response to some bleeding disorders, vitamin K may be given either orally or parenterally to manufacture prothrombin and serve as an anticoagulant antagonist (see Chapter 24).

ACTION

There are two major categories of anticoagulants. The first category, the coumarin and indanedione derivatives, limits formation of blood coagulation factors II, VII, IX, and X in the liver by interfering with vitamin K. These drugs do not destroy existing blood clots; however, they may limit the extension of existing blood clots or thrombi.

The second category, heparin sodium, acts at multiple sites in the normal coagulation system to stop reactions that lead to the clotting of blood and the formation of fibrin clots. It increases the action of antithrombin III (heparin cofactor) on several other coagulation factors, primarily activated factor X (Xa), to slow new clot development. Heparin does not dissolve existing clots either, although thrombolytic agents do. Low-molecular-weight heparin is a special formulation used in special circumstances, such as to prevent deep vein thrombosis (DVT) after surgery.

USES

As part of the circulatory system, the arterial vessels carry oxygenated blood throughout the body. If these small arteries become plugged with **thrombi** (clots

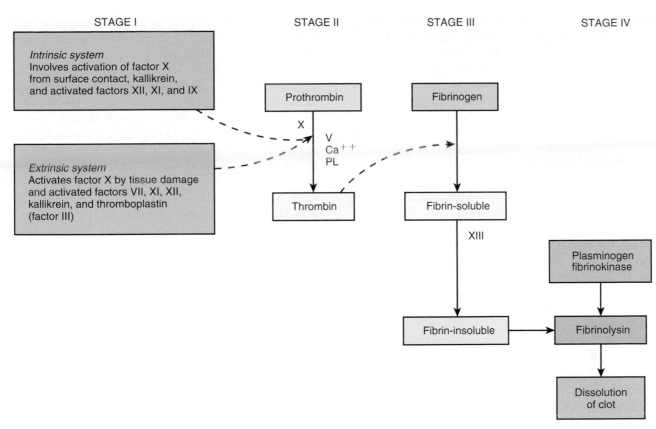

FIGURE 20-1 Blood coagulation and clot resolution. *PL*, Phospholipid.

made of fibrin, platelets, and cholesterol), oxygen cannot get to the tissues, and death may result. Abnormal blood clotting may produce a thrombus in the coronary artery, which nourishes the heart muscle. Emboli (small pieces of a blood clot) may break off from a site of thrombophlebitis (inflammation and blood clot in a vein) in the lower extremities and travel through the bloodstream to block vessels in areas of the heart, brain, or lung. (See Chapter 15, Figure 15-7.) This blockage can cause stroke or death. Drugs that can slow or reduce clotting, then, are very helpful.

Anticoagulant therapy is used to prevent new clot formation or to stop existing clots from growing in size. Anticoagulant therapy is used prophylactically during and after many types of surgery, especially surgery involving the heart or circulation. It is also used in patients with heart valve disease, in patients with some dysrhythmias (irregular heartbeats), and in patients receiving hemodialysis. Any patient on bed rest for a long time is at risk for development of blood clots, especially patients with a history of clotting problems or recent orthopedic, thoracic, or abdominal surgery.

Heparin is the anticoagulant of choice when an immediate effect is needed. For long-term therapy, a coumarin or indanedione derivative is used. The U.S.

Food and Drug Administration has classified coumarin preparations as "possibly" effective as part of the therapy for treatment of transient cerebral ischemic attacks. Indanedione derivatives (phenindione) are used to treat pulmonary emboli and as prophylaxis to treat DVT, myocardial infarction, rheumatic heart disease with valve damage, and atrial dysrhythmias. Low-intensity warfarin therapy (prothrombin time [PT] ratio between 1.2 and 1.5) greatly decreases the risk of stroke from nonrheumatic atrial fibrillation and has few side effects.

ADVERSE REACTIONS

By far, the most common adverse reactions from heparin and warfarin are excessive bleeding and thrombocytopenia. Early signs of overdose or internal bleeding include bleeding from gums while brushing teeth, excessive bleeding or oozing from cuts, unexplained bruising or nosebleeds, and unusually heavy or unexpected menses in women. These are the "must know" symptoms that suggest the patient needs prompt attention.

There are a number of other adverse reactions that may occasionally be seen. Warfarin may produce alopecia (hair loss), rash, urticaria (hives), cramping, diarrhea, intestinal obstruction, nausea, paralytic ileus, vomiting, excessive uterine bleeding, hemorrhage with excessive dosage, leukopenia, and fever. Heparin sodium may produce hypertension (high blood pressure); headache; hematoma, irritation, and pain at the injection site; conjunctivitis; tearing of eyes; rhinitis; frequent or persistent erection; hemorrhage; thrombocytopenia; shortness of breath; wheezing; chills; fever; alopecia; and hypersensitivity (allergic) reaction.

DRUG INTERACTIONS

Other anticoagulants (coumarin or indanedione derivatives), methimazole, and propylthiouracil increase the anticoagulant effect of heparin.

Antihistamines, digitalis, nicotine, and tetracycline decrease the anticoagulant effect of heparin.

Acetylsalicylic acid (ASA), coumarin-derivative anticoagulants, dextran, nonsteroidal antiinflammatory drugs (NSAIDs), and other selected drugs increase the risk of bleeding and hemorrhage in a patient receiving heparin.

ASA, corticotropin, ethacrynic acid, glucocorticoids, and NSAIDs increase the risk of gastrointestinal (GI) bleeding and hemorrhage in a patient receiving heparin.

Allopurinol, ASA, anabolic steroids, antibiotics, androgens, many sedatives, some antacids, dextran, disulfiram, drugs affecting blood elements, glucagon, heparin, narcotics (with prolonged use), phenylbutazone, propylthiouracil, quinidine, quinine, salicylates, thyroid drugs, and vitamin E increase the PT response of patients receiving warfarin.

Adrenocorticosteroids, antacids, antihistamines, barbiturates, contraceptives (oral), estrogens, griseofulvin, haloperidol, meprobamate, primidone, rifampin, thiazide diuretics, and vitamin K decrease the PT/International Normalized Ratio (INR) response of a patient on warfarin.

Anticoagulant effects may be increased with acute alcohol intoxication and decreased with chronic alcohol abuse. Oral hypoglycemics taken with anticoagulants may increase the effect of either the hypoglycemic or anticoagulant.

Alkylating agents, antimetabolites, corticosteroids, ethacrynic acid, indomethacin, quinidine, and salicylates increase the risk of bleeding in a patient taking warfarin.

❖ NURSING IMPLICATIONS AND PATIENT TEACHING

Patients requiring rapid anticoagulation are commonly hospitalized. Coagulation and PT/INR tests are ordered when the patient is started on anticoagulants. Heparin is usually started for an immediate effect and gradually replaced by oral anticoagulants. Thereafter, the physician or other health care provider orders coagulation and PT/INR tests at regular intervals. When the oral anticoagulant shows proper effect, and the prothrombin activity is in the therapeutic range, heparin therapy may be stopped and the oral anticoagulant therapy continued.

Standard heparin dosing protocols have been controversial for many years. Weight-based dosing is now the standard of care for determining the dosing of heparin. Weight-based dosing uses the patient's body weight in kilograms, infusing 80 units/kg as an intravenous (IV) bolus. The maintenance infusion is 18 units/kg/hr through an infusion pump. There are indications that weight-based dosing is safer, achieves therapeutic levels in less time than with standard dosing, and results in fewer bleeding complications and a lower rate of thromboembolic recurrences.

The standard tests for determining the general effect of heparin on clotting are the Lee-White coagulation time, the whole-blood activated partial thromboplastin time, and the activated partial thromboplastin time (aPTT). The most commonly used test is the aPTT. The dosage of heparin is considered adequate when the whole blood clotting time is approximately 1.5 to 2.5 times the control value. The recommended method for establishing the unfractionated therapeutic range is by the anti-Xa method. This method is the most specific and is least affected by the variables inherent to the in vitro technique. Samples are collected from patients on unfractionated heparin. The samples are tested with aPTT and anti-Xa assays. The range of aPTT values correlate to anti-Xa levels in a range of 0.3-0.7 U/mL of heparin.

PTs are used to determine the dosage for coumarin preparations. These PT tests are done daily until the results stabilize in the therapeutic range ($1\frac{1}{2}$ to $2\frac{1}{2}$ times the normal control value). After stabilization, tests are performed at 1-week to 4-week intervals, depending on patient status. Unfortunately, these test results vary from laboratory to laboratory and from day to day because of variations in the reagent chemical used to perform the test. However, this test is still used in many countries.

To avoid test variation, a system called the International Normalized Ratio (INR) is used to standardize PT reporting so that all laboratory reports are the same. The INR is based on the PT ratio supplied by the drugmaker that would be obtained if a standard reference testing chemical was used. PT numbers are changed to INR measurements by a standard math equation. Laboratories commonly report both numbers (PT/INR) when a PT is ordered.

The goal of prolonging the PT to 1.5 to 2.5 times the normal has largely been replaced in the United States and some other countries by specific INR goal recommendations for each clinical indication. The typical INR goal is 2 to 3, except in mechanical cardiac valve replacement, in which a higher INR is necessary to prevent clot formation.

Assessment

Learn as much as possible about the patient's health history, including the presence of hypersensitivity, underlying systemic disease, the current nature of the problem, and use of other medications. Inquire about conditions that contraindicate use of some anticoagulants, such as alcoholism; blood dyscrasias; bleeding tendencies of the GI, genitourinary, or respiratory tracts; or malignant hypertension. Patients with congestive heart failure may be more sensitive to coumarin anticoagulants and indanedione derivatives.

Heparin is derived from animal tissue and should be used with caution in any patient with a history of allergy. This drug should be used cautiously in patients with hepatic or renal disease or hypertension, during menses, after delivery, or in patients with indwelling catheters. A higher incidence of bleeding may be seen in women older than the age of 60. Make absolutely sure that female patients taking a coumarin or indanedione derivative are not pregnant or breastfeeding. These drugs are usually not given to children.

Diagnosis

There are many medical and surgical contraindications to the use of anticoagulant drugs, particularly in patients who have recently had surgery, trauma, or obstetric complications. Review the patient's problems and make certain that none of these contraindications exist.

Planning

The dosages listed for heparin are given in United States Pharmacopeia heparin units. Heparin is not effective if given orally and should be given by IV injection, IV infusion, or deep subcutaneous (intrafat) injection. Heparin should not be given via intramuscular (IM) injection because these injections produce hematomas, irritation, and pain at the injection site. Use a small (25-gauge) needle and a tuberculin syringe for the subcutaneous intrafat injection.

 Clinical Pitfall

Planning for Safety

Patients who are anticoagulated and require dental or surgical procedures may need to discontinue the medication before surgery to avoid problems with bleeding. Patients should be encouraged to tell the dentist, physician, or surgeon they are taking anticoagulants. Surgical procedures may be a particular risk if patients have a traumatic injury or require emergency surgery.

Implementation

Anticoagulant drugs should not be used if good laboratory facilities are not available, or if the patient is not compliant in taking medications or keeping appointments for laboratory and health assessment. Coumarin derivatives should not be used in a patient undergoing diagnostic or therapeutic procedures with risk for uncontrolled bleeding.

The sites of intrafat injections of heparin should be rotated to avoid formation of hematomas. (See Chapter 10, Figure 10-16, for rotation site suggestions.) Because of the adverse effects if inaccurate doses are given, once the heparin is drawn into the syringe, double check the dose with another nurse. There are several

 Lifespan Considerations

Older Adults

ANTICOAGULANTS

Older adults may be more sensitive to the effects of anticoagulants, and a lower maintenance dose is usually recommended for the geriatric patient, along with very close supervision and monitoring. This is particularly true for clients who receive warfarin and may be Vitamin-K deficient because of low intake of green leafy vegetables.

The primary adverse effects of excessive drug dosages are prolonged bleeding from the gums from small shaving cuts or when brushing teeth, excessive or easy skin bruising, blood in urine or stools, and unexplained nosebleeds. There may be early signs of overdose that indicate the need for medical intervention.

Caution patients to wear a MedicAlert bracelet or carry an identification card indicating the use of an anticoagulant. Also, remind patients to always consult the prescriber before starting any new drug (including over-the-counter [OTC] medications and vitamins), if changing a medication dose, or when any drug product is discontinued. Many medications can change the effects of an anticoagulant in the body.

Be aware that when drugs that may cause gastric irritation are given to clients on anticoagulant therapy, the risk for GI bleeding is increased. Drugs such as NSAIDs (e.g., ibuprofen, indomethacin) that are commonly prescribed for the older adult patient often cause GI effects.

Alcohol consumption can alter the effect of anticoagulants in the body. Patients should be instructed to avoid alcohol or at the least limit their alcohol intake to one alcoholic drink a day. Alcohol may cause liver damage and minor GI bleeding, both of which increase the individual's sensitivity to anticoagulants.

The nurse should be aware that diet can interfere with the anticoagulant effect. In a previously stabilized person, vitamin C deficiency, chronic malnutrition, diarrhea, or other illness may result in an increased anticoagulant effect. Increased intake of green leafy vegetables (e.g., broccoli, cabbage, collard greens, lettuce, spinach) or consumption of a nutritional supplement or multivitamin containing vitamin K can result in decreased anticoagulant effectiveness.

Modified from McKenry LM, Tessier E, Hogan MA: *Mosby's pharmacology in nursing*, ed 22, St Louis, 2006, Mosby.

things to remember about heparin injection that make the process unique. First, do not attempt to pull back on the plunger or aspirate blood before injection. Second, the nurse must be extra careful to not move the needle while the heparin is being injected. Third, injection sites should not be massaged before or after injection. Patients receiving heparin are not good candidates for IM injections of other medications, because hematomas and bleeding into nearby areas may occur.

If the heparin solution is discolored or contains a precipitate (solid at the bottom), it must not be used. Heparin is strongly acidic and is chemically incompatible with many other medications in solution, so it must not be piggybacked with other drugs into an infusion line. Never mix any drug with heparin in a syringe when bolus therapy is given.

If intermittent IV therapy is being given, blood for partial thromboplastin time determination should be drawn ½ hour before the next scheduled heparin dose. Blood for partial thromboplastin times can be drawn anytime after 8 hours of continuous IV heparin therapy. However, blood should not be drawn from the tubing of the heparin infusion line or from the vein being used for infusion. Blood should always be drawn from the arm not being used for heparin infusion.

If heparin is being given at the same time as a coumarin or an indanedione derivative, blood should not be drawn for PTs within 5 hours of IV heparin administration or 24 hours if heparin is given subcutaneously. IV heparin infusions should be checked frequently, even if pumps are in good working order, to make sure the proper dose is being given.

If anticoagulant therapy is started with heparin and continued with a coumarin or indanedione derivative, it is recommended that both drugs be given until the PT or INR results indicate an adequate response to the coumarin or indanedione derivative.

A summary of anticoagulants is provided in Table 20-1.

 Clinical Pitfall

Internal Bleeding

Signs suggesting internal bleeding include abdominal pain or swelling, back pain, bloody or tarry stools, bloody or cloudy urine, constipation (resulting from paralytic ileus or intestinal obstruction), coughing up blood, dizziness, severe or continuous headaches, and vomiting blood or "coffee-ground" substance.

■ Evaluation

If heparin is given by continuous IV infusion, the coagulation time should usually be determined every 4 hours in the early stages of treatment. Many medical centers have adopted evidenced-based protocols that indicate heparin dosing based on previous aPTT results and when the next aPTT should be drawn.

Watch for signs of overdose of anticoagulants and internal bleeding as therapy progresses. This might include bleeding gums when brushing teeth, blood in the urine, or coughing up blood.

Determine whether the patient understands why he or she is taking the medicine and the symptoms of overdose. Have the patient explain to the nurse if he or she notices signs of bruising or easy bleeding. More accurate patient monitoring of anticoagulant response is a Joint Commission National Patient Safety Goal, and many hospitals are adopting new protocols for required patient teaching and clinical monitoring.

■ Patient and Family Teaching

Tell the patient and family the following:
- The patient should take the oral medication only as directed. If a dose is missed, it should be taken as soon as possible, but not if it is almost time for the next dose. The doses should not be doubled. The patient should keep a record of all missed doses.
- The patient will need regular PT/INR time or coagulation blood tests, and regular visits to the physician to ensure that blood clotting stays within the narrow therapeutic range. The dosage may require changes from time to time, based on results of laboratory tests.
- The patient should not take other medications without checking with the health care provider; this includes aspirin or any OTC medicines.
- The patient should wear a MedicAlert bracelet or necklace, or carry a medical information card stating the name of the anticoagulant.
- The patient should inform all nurses, physicians, dentists, podiatrists, and other health care providers about being on anticoagulant therapy.
- The patient should use caution in brushing teeth, trimming nails, and shaving. (An electric razor should be used when possible.)
- Pressure should be used to stop bleeding from accidental cuts or scrapes; if bleeding persists after 10 minutes, the health care provider should be contacted.
- The patient should not engage in contact sports or other activities that could lead to injuries.
- The patient should eat a normal, balanced diet, but should avoid eating excessive amounts of foods high in vitamin K (tomatoes, onions, dark leafy greens, bananas, or fish).
- The patient should avoid alcohol.
- The patient should know the possible side effects of anticoagulants: active bleeding or signs of bleeding such as tarry stools, blood in the urine, bleeding gums, nosebleeds, dizziness, coughing up blood, abdominal or joint pains, unexplained bruising, or unusually heavy or unexpected menstrual periods in women.

Table 20-1   Anticoagulants and Other Drugs Affecting the Blood

GENERIC NAME	TRADE NAME	COMMENTS
Anticoagulants		
Coumarin and Indanedione Derivatives		
warfarin (sodium) ★	Coumadin	Dosage individualized for patient and problem. Usual initiation dose is 2-5 mg/day, with dosage adjustments based on the results of INR and/or PT ratio determinations. Store tablets at 59° F to 86° F, and protect from air and light.
Heparin		
heparin ★	Heparin	Dosage is adjusted according to patient's coagulation time. q4h
Low-Molecular-Weight Heparins		
dalteparin sodium	Fragmin	Given SQ for DVT prophylaxis and treatment for DVT/PE, MI.
enoxaparin	Lovenox ♦	Given SQ for DVT prophylaxis and treatment for DVT/PE, MI.
tinzaparin	Innohep	Given for DVT/PE treatment.
Heparin Antagonist		
protamine sulfate	Protamine Sulfate	The onset of action for protamine sulfate is 0.5-1 min. The duration of action is 2 hr. Adults and children: 1 mg of protamine sulfate for every 90 USP units of beef lung heparin or for every 115 USP units of porcine intestinal mucosa heparin to be neutralized. Administer IV at a slow rate over 1-3 min (limit is 50 mg given in 10 min). Additional doses may be given if need is indicated by coagulation studies.
Thrombolytic Agents		
Tissue Plasmogen Activators		
alteplase, recombinant	Activase	For lysis of coronary artery thrombi (accelerated infusion): Best results if given IV within 6 hr of onset of symptoms of MI. Dosage is determined by patient weight. An IV bolus is given first followed by IV infusion over 60 min. May be slightly more effective but costs 10 times more than other products. Pulmonary embolism or acute ischemic stroke: Must administer within 3 hr after onset of symptoms. 10% of the total dose is given as an IV bolus over 1 min then the remaining dose is administered over 60 min.
reteplase	Retavase	Given as a double bolus with first bolus IV over 2 min then another IV bolus 30 min later.
tenecteplase	TNKase	Dose is weight based. Do not give more than 50 mg; by IV administration only. Do not exceed recommended volume per 5 sec when giving as IV bolus.
Antiplatelet Agents		
abciximab	ReoPro	Give IV bolus administered 10-60 min before the start of PTCA, followed by a continuous IV infusion for 12 hr.
acetylsalicylic acid ★	ASA	Give 325-650 mg PO (chewed) stat with first indication of MI. Do not give ASA in addition to coumarin anticoagulants.
anagrelide	Agrylin	Used in treating essential thrombocythemia to reduce elevated platelet count and the risk of thrombosis. Give daily for about 1 wk and then adjust to lowest effective dosage required to reduce and maintain platelet count, 600,000/mL.
cilostazol	Pletal	For intermittent claudication, give daily approximately 30 min before or 2 hr after breakfast and dinner. May need a smaller dose if concurrent administration of some CYP3A4 drugs.
clopidogrel	Plavix	Give with or without food. No adjustment necessary for older adult patients or those with renal disease.
dipyridamole	Persantine	Give daily as adjunct to warfarin therapy.
ticlopidine	Ticlid	Give with food.

Continued

Table 20-1	Anticoagulants and Other Drugs Affecting the Blood—cont'd	
GENERIC NAME	**TRADE NAME**	**COMMENTS**
Other Miscellaneous Products		
antihemophilic factor	Hemofil M/E Koate- HPMonoclate P	Used in treating patients with hemophilia A. Individualize dosage based on needs of patient.
antiinhibitor coagulant complex	Autoplex T/E Feiba VH	Individualize dosage based on needs of patient.
antithrombin III	Thrombate III	Used in treating patients with hereditary antithrombin III deficiency. Individualize dosage based on needs of patient.
eptifibatide	Integrilin	Give IV bolus as soon as possible after diagnosis of acute coronary syndrome, followed by continuous infusion of 2 mcg/kg/min until hospital discharge or CABG surgery.
hydroxyurea	Droxia	Antisickling agent. The patient's CBC count must be monitored every 2 wk.
pentoxifylline	Trental	Used in intermittent claudication from chronic occlusive arterial disease and in cerebrovascular insufficiency. Give with meals. Decrease dosage if GI side effects develop.
tirofiban	Aggrastat	Used with heparin in the treatment of acute coronary syndrome, including patients who are to be managed medically and those with PTCA. Can be administered in the same IV catheter as heparin. Give for 48-108 hr, including during surgical procedure and after. Medication must be diluted and administered according to the patient's weight.

ASA, Acetylsalicylic acid; *CABG*, coronary artery bypass grafting; *CBC*, complete blood cell; *DVT*, deep vein thrombosis; *INR*, international normalized ratio; *IV*, intravenous; *MI*, myocardial infarction; *PE*, pulmonary embolism; *PO*, by mouth; *PT*, prothrombin time; *PTCA*, percutaneous transluminal coronary angioplasty; *SQ*, subcutaneous.
★ Indicates "Must-Know Drugs," or the 35 drugs most prescribers use.

- After anticoagulation therapy has been stopped, the patient should use caution until the body recovers its blood-clotting abilities.

PROTAMINE SULFATE

ACTION

Protamine sulfate is a strongly basic (alkaline) protein that acts as a heparin antagonist to neutralize (reverse) the actions of heparin. However, it may also serve as an anticoagulant when used as the sole medication. In the presence of heparin, it forms a stable salt, which is strongly acidic. This cancels out the anticoagulant activity of both drugs. When protamine sulfate is used with heparin, these results occur almost immediately and may persist for 2 hours or more.

USES

Protamine sulfate is used to treat heparin overdose. It may also be used after surgical procedures to neutralize the effects of heparin given during extracorporeal circulation on a heart-lung machine.

ADVERSE REACTIONS

Adverse reactions to protamine sulfate include bradycardia (slow heartbeat), dyspnea (uncomfortable breathing), lassitude (weariness), sudden drop in blood pressure, transitory flushing (red color in the face and neck), and a feeling of warmth. Overdose may produce anticoagulant effects.

❖ NURSING IMPLICATIONS AND PATIENT TEACHING

■ Assessment

Because of the anticoagulant activity of protamine sulfate, overdoses of this drug when used as a heparin antagonist may produce additional anticoagulation.

■ Diagnosis

Does the patient have any other problems that might result from excessive anticoagulation? Is the patient taking other medications or using a diet that would interfere with anticoagulation?

■ Planning

Protamine sulfate may be inactivated by blood. Thus there may be a rebound effect when a large dose is used to neutralize heparin. This requires an increased dose of protamine sulfate. Hyperheparinemia or bleeding may be seen in some patients 30 minutes to 18 hours after open-heart surgery, even when adequate amounts of protamine sulfate have been given.

■ Implementation

Protamine sulfate should be given only by a physician. The nurse would usually assemble the medications but allow the physician to draw up the dose. It should be given slowly by IV injection over 1 to 3 minutes in doses not exceeding 50 mg of protamine sulfate activity (5 mL) during any 10-minute period. It is rare that more than 100 mg is given at a time.

Severe hypotension and anaphylactic-like reactions may be provoked if it is given too rapidly. This drug contains no preservatives, so the unused portion of the medication in the ampule should be discarded.

▪ Evaluation

Closely monitor the patient for signs of further anticoagulant activity, and have equipment readily available to treat shock.

▪ Patient and Family Teaching

The family and patient should know that this is a standard drug used to neutralize heparin. See Table 20-1 for information on protamine sulfate and other hematologic products.

THROMBOLYTIC AGENTS

ACTION

Thrombolytics convert plasminogen to the enzyme plasmin, which degrades or breaks down fibrin clots, fibrinogen, and other plasma proteins. These products are used for lysis (dissolving) of thrombi.

USES

Thrombolytic agents are used in acute myocardial infarction for lysis of thrombi blocking coronary arteries, in acute pulmonary emboli for clot lysis when the patient is hemodynamically unstable, and in acute ischemic stroke and acute arterial occlusion. Use of thrombolytics reduces the extent of cellular damage from blockage.

ADVERSE REACTIONS

Bleeding is the most obvious adverse effect. Dysrhythmias, hypotension (low blood pressure), polyneuropathy, cholesterol embolism, pulmonary embolism, and hypersensitivity are all possible effects.

DRUG INTERACTIONS

Administering these products together with other anticoagulants may increase the potential for bleeding.

❖ NURSING IMPLICATIONS AND PATIENT TEACHING

▪ Assessment

These medications are given by the physician in life-threatening situations of vascular block caused by thrombosis. They are most helpful if administered within the first hour after the thrombosis.

Learn as much as possible about the health history of the patient. Through talking to the patient or other primary witnesses, attempt to determine the exact time sequence of events and what happened before the patient was seen. Determine whether any other medications have been taken. For example, because aspirin helps reduce platelet adhesion, patients who are suspected of having a myocardial infarction are urged to chew a 325-mg aspirin (ASA) tablet. Obtain the history of any recent surgery.

▪ Diagnosis

What other factors in addition to the medical diagnosis are important? Does this patient have risk factors for bleeding, myocardial infarction, stroke, or pulmonary emboli? This patient is probably very frightened and anxious, as well as seriously ill. Accompanying worries about finances, career, and family may arise.

▪ Planning

These medications come as a powder that requires reconstitution. Are all the equipment and materials the physician will require for infusion present?

▪ Implementation

Carefully monitor the vital signs of the patient receiving thrombolytic therapy. Report these findings frequently to the physician or other health care provider.

▪ Evaluation

Observe the patient carefully for bleeding. Bleeding may be superficial, coming from the infusion site. Other more significant bleeding indicates overdose and is shown by hematuria (blood in the urine), hematemesis (blood in the vomitus), signs of abdominal tension, and internal bleeding.

▪ Patient and Family Teaching

Explain the basis of thrombolytic therapy to the patient and family as necessary. Make sure the physician speaks with them about what is being done.

ANTIPLATELET AGENTS

ACTION

Through a variety of mechanisms, these products act to limit or inhibit platelet aggregation (clumping) and thus reduce thrombus formation.

USES

ASA reduces the incidence of myocardial infarction–related deaths in men older than 50 years of age. ASA is the drug of choice in ischemic stroke; it plays no role in hemorrhagic stroke.

Clopidogrel (Plavix) is used for myocardial infarction prophylaxis for men and as additional or adjunct therapy with thrombolytics in preventing infarction or stroke. Abciximab (ReoPro), eptifibatide (Integrilin), bivalirudin (Angiomax), and a variety of other specialty products may be used during cardiac catheterization or other cardiovascular procedures.

ADVERSE REACTIONS

Bleeding is the most frequently seen adverse event. Diarrhea, nausea, dyspepsia (stomach discomfort after eating), rash, GI pain, neutropenia, purpura (bruising), vomiting, flatulence, pruritus (itching), dizziness, and anorexia (lack of appetite) are also seen.

DRUG INTERACTIONS

Variable interactions with antacids, cimetidine, digoxin, and theophylline are possible.

❖ NURSING IMPLICATIONS AND PATIENT TEACHING

■ Assessment

These drugs are used in critically ill patients to help limit damage from thrombosis or occlusion. The nurse will be involved in monitoring vital signs and assisting with monitoring the patient's cardiovascular status.

 Clinical Goldmine

Myocardial Infarction

ASA is often given as soon as it is suspected that the patient may be having a myocardial infarction.

■ Diagnosis

Evaluate for changes in level of consciousness, renal function, and respiration. Be alert for any signs of bleeding.

■ Planning

Have all materials available for monitoring the patient's vital signs and for giving medications.

■ Implementation

Assist in recording the medications given and the patient's response. Assist in the ordering and collection of any blood work required to monitor therapy.

■ Evaluation

Changes in vital signs and levels of consciousness provide important feedback about the status of blood circulation.

■ Patient and Family Teaching

Assist in calming the patient, explaining the situation to the family, and providing information. Some of these medications may be given orally over time to help maintain a good circulation.

Get Ready for the NCLEX® Examination!

Key Points

- Hematologic products act in the formation, repair, or function of red blood cells.
- There are four major groups of hematologic products. They are the anticoagulants, the heparin antagonist protamine sulfate, thrombolytics and antiplatelet factors, and the vitamins and minerals needed for red blood cell development (discussed in Chapter 24).
- Patient and family teaching is especially important for the patient undergoing long-term therapy.

Additional Learning Resources

SG   Go to your Study Guide for additional learning activities to help you master this chapter content.

⊝volve   Go to your Evolve website (http://evolve.elsevier.com/Edmunds/LPN/) for additional online resources.

Review Questions for the NCLEX® Examination

1. The nurse is caring for a patient who is being treated with heparin. The patient complains to the nurse of experiencing unusually heavy periods. The most appropriate response from the nurse should be:

   1. "Have you noticed any other changes in your menstrual cycle?"
   2. "Let me know if you notice any other unusual symptoms."
   3. "Please keep a chart of your periods so that we can note any unusual trends developing."
   4. "I will notify the physician right away of your symptom."

2. The nurse is caring for a patient who is taking tetracycline and has also been ordered to be treated with heparin. Based on this combination of medications, the nurse anticipates that the patient will experience:

   1. decreased effect of the heparin
   2. increased effect of the heparin
   3. decreased effect of the tetracycline
   4. increased effect of the tetracycline

3. An appropriate menu selection for a patient who is being treated with an anticoagulant is:

   1. bacon, lettuce, and tomato sandwich and iced tea
   2. chef salad, whole grain crackers, and orange juice
   3. baked chicken, macaroni and cheese, and low-fat milk
   4. pork chops, broccoli and cheese, and iced tea

Get Ready for the NCLEX® Examination!—cont'd

4. The nurse is preparing a heparin injection. An important principle to remember when administering such an injection is:
   1. always pull back on the plunger before giving the injection
   2. do not move the needle while injecting the medication
   3. massage the injection site after giving the injection
   4. heparin mixes well with other medications during injection

5. The nurse is caring for a patient who is ordered to be treated with cilostazol (Pletal). The nurse anticipates that the most appropriate dosage schedule for this patient will be:
   1. give 1 hour before or 1 hour after breakfast and dinner
   2. give 2 hours before or 2 hours after breakfast and dinner
   3. give 30 minutes after or 1 hour before breakfast and dinner
   4. give 30 minutes before or 2 hours after breakfast and dinner

Case Study

Mrs. Lily, 34 years old, arrives at the office late for her appointment. She is limping and says her right calf is very sore. It is swollen, red, and very painful to touch. Mrs. Lily is a heavy smoker, takes oral birth control pills, and was recently involved in a car accident in which her right leg was badly bruised. The physician admits her to the hospital with the following orders:

* Bed rest.
* Right leg elevated and wrapped with warm, moist compresses.
* Begin heparin therapy after admission blood work drawn.

1. If Mrs. Lily has thrombophlebitis, what is the probable cause?
2. What risk factors does she have now for other adverse reactions?
3. What blood test is useful in determining how much heparin should be given?
4. The dosage of heparin is considered adequate when the whole blood clotting time is approximately ____ the control value.
5. Low-intensity coumarin-derivative therapy (PT ratio between 1.2 and 1.5) greatly decreases the risk of stroke from what condition?
6. The nurse is talking to Mrs. Lily about her warfarin. What is important to teach her regarding signs of warfarin overdose?

Drug Calculation Review

1. Order: Heparin 7500 units subcutaneously twice a day.
   Supply: Heparin 20,000 units/mL.
   Question: How many milliliters of heparin should be given with each dose? (Round to the nearest hundredth.)

2. Order: Give 500 mL of dextran 40 over 24 hr.
   Question: How many milliliters per hour should the IV infusion device be set for? (Round to the nearest whole number.)

3. The physician orders enoxaparin (Lovenox) 30 mg subcutaneously twice daily for 7 to 10 days for prevention of DVT after hip replacement surgery. Available are prefilled syringes of 150 mg/1 mL concentration. How many milliliters will the nurse expect to administer to this patient with each dose?

Critical Thinking Questions

1. Briefly point out the major differences in the three major groups of hematologic agents with regard to actions and uses.
2. Mrs. Gardner is being treated for a DVT. She is concerned about her treatment regimen, pointing out differences in the treatment her sister received for the same thing. As the nurse listens to Mrs. Gardner's worries, she realizes she keeps referring to her "embolism." Explain to Mrs. Gardner the difference between a thrombus and an embolism and why this difference may affect methods of treatment.
3. Mr. Pierce is brought to the unit and placed on anticoagulant therapy. Explain the rationale for needing to know why this patient is being put on anticoagulation therapy. Why are laboratory values used to validate accurate dosage?
4. Describe the possible problems that can arise if anticoagulants are used in conjunction with some other specific drugs.
5. In the emergency department, Ms. Zukerman needs an immediate anticoagulant effect. Which is the drug of choice? Why?
6. Ms. Zukerman receives the appropriate medication, as indicated by Question 5, but now she exhibits signs of overdose. What are the signs and symptoms of overdose with this drug? Describe the needed interventions, both nursing and pharmacologic.
7. Which coagulation value is most accurate in monitoring the effect of Ms. Zukerman's therapy and why?
8. Ms. Zukerman's condition is stabilized now, but she is experiencing pain at injection sites. How can the nurse respond?
9. Mrs. Martinez has just started taking warfarin 2.5 mg every day. She is also "cutting down" on her caloric intake, at her doctor's recommendation, to help control her type 2 diabetes. She seems confused at her follow-up visit, however, and asks the nurse, "If I'm supposed to lose weight, why can't I have salads? I thought they were low in sugar and calories, and I should eat a lot of vegetables on a diet." What does Mrs. Martinez need to know about warfarin therapy?
10. Mr. Harris wants to know if his "Coumadin is working. I had some blood taken yesterday, and my doctor told me my platelets were OK. I thought the Coumadin was supposed to make me take longer to clot. Does this mean I need to take more?" What would the nurse explain to Mr. Harris?

Objectives

1. Describe the use of antidiabetic medications.
2. Identify preparations that act on the uterus.
3. Compare and contrast the action of adrenal and pituitary hormones.
4. Describe at least five adverse reactions that may result from the use of glucocorticoids and mineralocorticoids.
5. Compare the actions of various male and female hormones.
6. List the indications for the use of thyroid preparations.

Key Terms

abortifacients (ă-BŎR-tĭ-FĀ-shĕnts, p. 375)
androgens (ĂN-drō-jĕnz, p. 383)
corticosteroids (KŎR-tĭ-kōSTĔR-ŏydz, p. 378)
diabetes mellitus (dī-ă-BĒ-tēz mĕ-LĪ-tĭs, p. 366)
estrogen (ĔS-trō-jĕn, p. 383)
glucometer (GLŪ-kŏ-mēt-ĕr, p. 369)
hormones (HŎR-mōnz, p. 364)
hyperglycemia (hī-pĕr-glī-SĒ-mē-ă, p. 368)
hyperthyroidism (hī-pōr-THĪ-rŏyd-ĭzm, p. 393)
hypoglycemia (hī-pō-glī-SĒ-mē-ă, p. 368)
hypothyroidism (hī-pō-THĪ-rŏyd-ĭzm, p. 393)
incretins (ĭn-krētĭns, p. 367)
insulin (ĬN-sū-lĭn, p. 366)
insulin-dependent diabetes mellitus (IDDM) (dī-ă-BĒ-tēz mĕl-Ī-tĭs, p. 366)

lipodystrophy (lĭp-ō-DĬS-trō-fē, p. 367)
myxedema (mĭk-sĕ-DĒ-mă, p. 394)
non–insulin-dependent diabetes mellitus (NIDDM) (dī-ă-BĒ-tēz mĕl-Ī-tĭs, p.367)
oral hypoglycemic (hī-pō-glī-SĒM-ĭks, p. 373)
oxytocic agents (ŏk-sē-TŌ-sĭk, p. 375)
progesterone (prō-JĔS-tĕr-ōn, p. 383)
sex hormones (HŎR-mōnz, p. 378)
Somogyi effect (SŎM-ō-jē, p. 372)
steroids (STĔR-ŏydz, p. 364)
systemic acidosis (sĭs-TĔM-ĭk ăs-ĭ-DŌ-sĭs, p. 368)
tocolytics (tō-kō-LĬT-ĭks, p. 375)
type 1 diabetes (dī-ă-BĒ-tēz, p. 366)
type 2 diabetes (dī-ă-BĒ-tēz, p. 366)
uterine relaxants (Ū-tĕr-ĭn rē-LĂK-sănts, p. 375)

OVERVIEW

This chapter discusses the different hormones and steroids used in medical therapy. Unlike many other categories of medications, many of these are natural or synthetic preparations that replace, increase, or decrease natural chemicals already present within the patient. At times, the body may produce too much of a hormone (for example, in hyperthyroidism), and medication is given to reduce the hormone (such as methimazole, which limits the production of thyroid hormones). In diabetes mellitus, medication is given to replace the hormone insulin when not enough is produced by the pancreas.

Hormones are chemicals that are made in an organ or gland and carried through the bloodstream to another part of the body. Once it arrives, the hormone stimulates that part of the body to increase its activity or secretion. **Steroids** are a specific chemical group of hormones that have powerful effects on cell sensitization, healing, and development. They are all part of a complex message system of the body, linking together various organs and systems. Lack of one basic hormone stimulates, or signals, the glands to produce more hormone. When the right amount of the hormone is reached, the signal is turned off, and the gland slows production of the hormone. This is called a *feedback mechanism* and is important in creating stability of the body. If some part of the system does not work properly, failure in one organ system may then cause changes in other hormonal systems.

This chapter is divided into five basic sections. The first section describes insulin and the oral hypoglycemic agents used to treat diabetes mellitus. The various drugs that act on the uterus are presented in the second section. The third section describes the pituitary and adrenocortical hormones, the major steroids that act throughout the body. The fourth section presents the male and female hormones and the different hormones in oral contraceptives. The fifth section describes various drugs used to treat the overproduction and underproduction of thyroid hormones.

ENDOCRINE SYSTEM

The regulation and coordination of body activities happens in two ways: (1) through nerve impulses carried by the nervous system; and (2) through chemical substances or hormones carried by the blood and lymph. The organs that secrete hormones are called *endocrine glands,* or glands of internal secretion. All together, these glands make up the endocrine system (Figure 21-1). This system includes the pituitary gland, thyroid gland, parathyroid glands, adrenal glands, pancreas, duodenum, testes, ovaries, and placenta.

Sometimes the thymus gland and the pineal body are listed as part of the endocrine system. Endocrine glands are ductless; their secretions go directly into the blood or lymph and are then carried to all parts of the body. In this respect, they are different from exocrine glands (glands of external secretion) such as salivary or sweat glands, whose products go through ducts that open onto a surface.

Of special importance are the hormones that affect the reproductive system. The gonads, accessory structures, and genitals of males and females are involved in reproduction and control sexual function and behavior (Figures 21-2 and 21-3). How these reproductive organs develop and function is under the control of hormones.

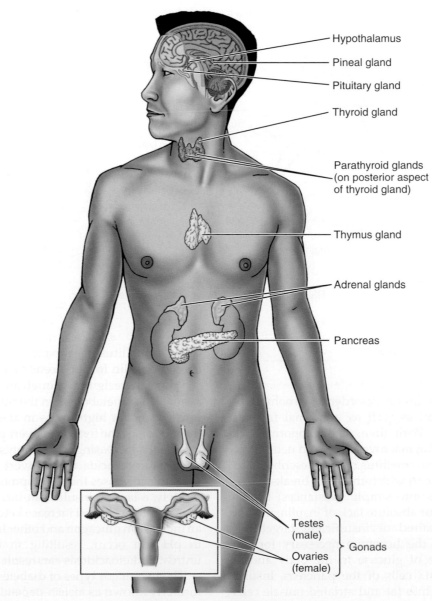

FIGURE 21-1 The endocrine system.

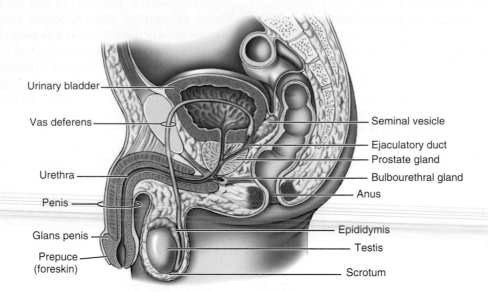

Urinary bladder

Vas deferens

Urethra

Penis

Glans penis

Prepuce
(foreskin)

Seminal vesicle

Ejaculatory duct

Prostate gland

Bulbourethral gland

Anus

Epididymis

Testis

Scrotum

FIGURE 21-2   The male reproductive system.

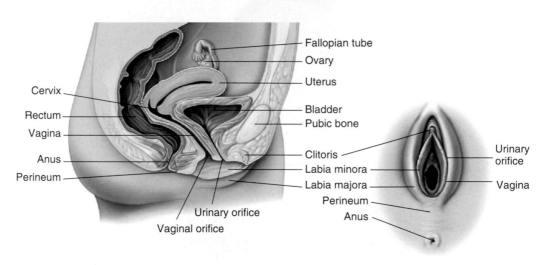

Cervix

Rectum

Vagina

Anus

Perineum

Urinary orifice

Vaginal orifice

Fallopian tube

Ovary

Uterus

Bladder

Pubic bone

Clitoris

Labia minora

Labia majora

Perineum

Anus

Urinary
orifice

Vagina

FIGURE 21-3   The female reproductive system.

ANTIDIABETIC DRUGS

 ## OVERVIEW

Diabetes mellitus is a chronic disorder of carbohydrate (glucose) metabolism, as well as abnormal fat and protein metabolism. With time, these abnormalities result in microvascular, macrovascular, and neurologic complications. Diabetes mellitus can be described as a catabolic state (a state in which the body breaks down complex compounds into simple substances) that is caused by a relative or absolute lack of insulin, insulin resistance, and impaired or insufficient target cell receptors. **Insulin** is the hormone necessary for the metabolism and use of glucose in the body and is produced by the beta cells of the pancreas. Insulin helps glucose move into fat and striated muscle cells by turning on a carrier system. The patient with

diabetes mellitus has a pancreas that fails to produce enough insulin for the needs of the body.

When there is not enough insulin, glucose is not available for metabolism in the cell, and so it circulates unused and at high levels in the blood. The lack of insulin forces the liver to convert protein and fat to use for energy, increasing the amounts of fatty acids. Some of these fatty acids will convert to cholesterol; over time, this increases the development of atherosclerosis. Acutely, a lack of insulin can increase the production of free fatty acids and increase ketogenesis. Along with an increase in glucagon and other hormones, a decrease in pH can occur, resulting in ketoacidosis. If left untreated, ketoacidosis can result in death.

The two major types of diabetes are **type 1 diabetes**, formerly known as **insulin-dependent diabetes mellitus (IDDM)** or juvenile diabetes, and **type 2 diabetes**, formerly known as **non–insulin-dependent diabetes mellitus (NIDDM)** or latent-onset diabetes. Patients with type 2 diabetes usually have a pancreas that functions a little and can be encouraged by medication to produce more insulin. Patients with type 1 diabetes usually have little or no production of insulin by the pancreas. These patients must take insulin to control the symptoms of diabetes mellitus. Insulin may also be necessary for some cases of type 2 diabetes, although diet, weight reduction, and oral hypoglycemic agents are usually effective in controlling symptoms.

Insulin replacement and antidiabetic agents are used along with diet, exercise, and lifestyle changes to control blood glucose levels. These agents include insulin and a variety of oral agents from different drug classes.

☀ INSULIN

ACTION

Insulin's primary effect is to lower blood glucose levels by helping glucose move into target tissues. Once insulin binds to and stimulates an insulin receptor, a series of reactions take place in the cell, making it easier for glucose to pass into the cell. In addition to its role in glucose control, insulin is also very important in fat metabolism. Adequate amounts of insulin inhibit lipoprotein lipase, thereby preventing the release of fatty acids into the blood. Insulin also promotes glucose transport and storage of glucose as triglycerides in fat cells. Thus *insulin is an anabolic hormone* (one that converts simple substances into more complex compounds) that helps maintain stores of fatty acids, glycogen, and protein.

USES

Patients with type 1 diabetes do not produce enough insulin and must receive insulin to survive and prevent ketosis. This disorder is thought to be caused by an autoimmune T-lymphocyte attack on the beta cells of the pancreas, leading to destruction of the insulin-producing cells in the individual who has a genetic risk of diabetes.

In type 2 diabetes, tissues are insensitive to insulin, and beta-cell response to glucose is altered. This results in a lack of the circulating insulin that is needed by the body. Unlike type 1 diabetes, ketosis is not likely to occur, because some insulin is present. A nonketotic state with high osmotic pressure may occur in patients with infection or other underlying disease. Lack of tissue sensitivity to insulin, particularly in the muscles and liver, leads to hyperglycemia and insulin resistance. Therefore, higher levels of insulin are necessary to overcome the resistance.

The Diabetes Control and Complications Trial and the Kumamoto Study clearly showed that intensively treated type 1 and 2 patients with diabetes had a delay in the onset and the progress of diabetic complications. The American Diabetes Association consensus statement recommends treatment to produce glucose levels as close to normal as possible.

The best glucose control in type 1 diabetes can be reached with multiple insulin injections. Multiple injection insulin pumps, or continuous subcutaneous insulin delivery devices now allow insulin to be delivered in much the same way as it would be normally in the nondiabetic patient and have made dramatic changes in how insulin is given to patients. Over the last several years, various devices have also been developed to simplify insulin injection. However, the standard insulin syringe and vial of insulin are still used by most patients.

Patients with type 2 diabetes may require insulin because of oral antidiabetic agent failure or to provide an additional glucose-lowering effect when oral agents alone are not adequate. Insulin is also used in patients with type 2 diabetes if the patient has oral agent allergies, liver or renal dysfunction, or is pregnant or contemplating pregnancy. Most patients with type 2 diabetes can be successfully treated with oral antidiabetic medications for years.

Insulin has been produced from various animal sources and by recombinant technology. Animal-source insulins are produced from the pancreas glands of cows and pigs. Synthetic human insulin is prepared using a nonpathogenic strain of *Escherichia coli* bacteria or *Saccharomyces cerevisiae* fungus. Since 1999, only pure pork insulin and synthetic insulin have been produced. The advantage of using synthetic human insulin or purified pork insulin is a decrease in the production of antibodies in the diabetic patient. In addition, there is a lower risk of developing **lipodystrophy**, or shrinkage and loss of the fatty tissue, when insulin is given in the same spot too frequently. Human insulin is also now less expensive than animal-source insulin. However, substituting human insulin is not required when successful treatment has already been achieved with pork insulin.

Insulin lispro, a rapid onset, short-duration insulin, was introduced in the 1990s. This *insulin analogue* offers quick absorption, an earlier insulin peak, and a faster postpeak decline than regular insulin; its action is more like the body's natural insulin response.

Use of new drugs known as *incretin mimetic agents* has also made great changes in how diabetics are treated. **Incretins** are hormones that are released from the gut postprandially (after eating) and are often in low concentrations in persons with type 2 diabetes. The incretin that has received the most attention is glucagon-like peptide (GLP-1). Incretins stimulate insulin secretion in pancreatic beta cells and have been shown to restore both phases of insulin release. GLP-1 regulates glucose homeostasis. Incretins are also known to:

- Stimulate glucose-dependent endogenous insulin secretion (and perhaps insulin sensitivity).
- Inhibit endogenous glucagon secretion.
- Suppress appetite and induce satiety.
- Reduce the speed of gastric emptying.
- Possibly stimulate islet growth.
- Protect beta cells from cytokine and free fatty acid–mediated injury.

Another drug, exenatide (Byetta), is made from part of the saliva of the Gila monster lizard. It is approved as adjunctive therapy for type 2 diabetes. Exenatide binds to GLP-1 receptors and stimulates insulin secretion when blood sugar is high. It is the first drug that has been shown to restore first-phase insulin secretion, which is missing in persons with type 2 diabetes. It is given as an injection before the morning and evening meals. Adverse effects of exenatide include nausea, vomiting, diarrhea, and upper respiratory symptoms. Many patients lose weight when taking this drug.

ADVERSE REACTIONS

Adverse reactions to insulin include local itching, swelling, or erythema (redness or irritation) at the injection site, lipodystrophy, and symptoms of insulin allergy or resistance. The most important adverse reaction is **hypoglycemia** (serum glucose levels <60 mg/dL), which is caused by taking too much insulin. Symptoms of hypoglycemia include sudden onset of nervousness; hunger; malaise (weakness); cold, clammy skin; lethargy (sleepiness); no urine glucose or acetone; pallor (paleness); diaphoresis (sweating); change in level of consciousness (awareness and ability to respond); and shallow respirations.

 Memory Jogger

Hypoglycemia

Hypoglycemia may develop, especially with insulin overdosage, increased work or exercise, skipping a meal or eating the meal later than usual, or an illness associated with vomiting, diarrhea, or delayed digestion. Meals must be timed with respect to the activity of the insulin (i.e., onset, peak, and duration).

If the patient does not take enough insulin or does not take it on a regular schedule, **hyperglycemia** (fasting blood glucose levels >50 mg/dL) may develop. Signs of hyperglycemia include glycosuria and ketonuria (abnormal amounts of glucose and ketone bodies in the urine), Kussmaul respirations (deep, rapid, sighing breaths), tachycardia (rapid heartbeat), and acetone breath (fruity odor to the breath).

DRUG INTERACTIONS

Insulin needs may be increased by insulin antagonists such as oral contraceptives, corticosteroids, epinephrine, and preparations used for thyroid hormone replacement therapy. Thiazide diuretics may elevate glucose levels. A variety of other drugs, alcohol, and anabolic steroids may increase the hypoglycemic effects of insulin. Insulin promotes the movement of potassium into cells and lowers the serum potassium levels. Propranolol and other beta blockers can mask the signs and symptoms of hypoglycemia.

❖ NURSING IMPLICATIONS AND PATIENT TEACHING

■ Assessment

A patient whose diabetes mellitus was not previously diagnosed or is poorly controlled or out of control may have a history of polyuria (excretion of a large amount of urine), polydipsia (excessive thirst), polyphagia (excessive uncontrolled eating), weight loss, blurred vision, and fatigue. In severe cases of hyperglycemia, the patient may develop **systemic acidosis**, a condition in which the basic fluid and electrolyte balance of the body is disturbed, and the blood pH is decreased. Symptoms of systemic acidosis include nausea, vomiting, and changes in level of consciousness.

Ask the patient about signs of pregnancy, infection, and kidney, liver, or thyroid disease, because these conditions alter the requirement for insulin. Find out about any earlier sensitization (allergy to a foreign protein) to beef or pork and whether the patient is taking other drugs that may interact with insulin.

 Clinical Goldmine

Patients Taking Insulin

In patients taking insulin, look for a history of hypoglycemia. Symptoms include cold, clammy sweats; sudden onset of nervousness; hunger; malaise; lethargy; serum glucose levels less than 60 mg/dL; no urine glucose or acetone; pallor; diaphoresis; change in level of consciousness; and shallow respirations. These symptoms are relieved by having the patient eat or drink a source of fast-acting sugar. The nurse may also see signs of hyperglycemia: elevated fasting blood glucose levels (greater than 150 mg/dL), glycosuria, ketonuria, Kussmaul respirations, tachycardia, and acetone breath.

■ Diagnosis

What other needs does the patient have? Does the patient need information on weight loss, nutrition, or other knowledge? What other diseases does this patient have that might influence the therapy for diabetes?

■ Planning

Successful management of diabetes mellitus depends on the patient understanding the disease. Control and maintenance require that the patient know about the nature of the disease, proper diet and the need for weight control, and the importance of hygiene and exercise. The patient must understand how to do blood and urine testing and how to correctly draw up and inject insulin. A diabetic must know the signs and symptoms of hypoglycemia and hyperglycemia and the appropriate actions to take for each, as well as procedures to follow during illness.

The patient should be shown the proper injection technique, including drawing up, injection, and storage of insulin. Ask the patient to demonstrate how to give the injection.

The patient should be taught about rotation of injection sites to prevent lipodystrophy. Although use of human insulin has reduced the incidence of lipodystrophy, all patients should be encouraged to rotate injection sites regularly to help with absorption. (See Chapter 10, Figure 10-15.)

It may be preferable to have patients use prefilled insulin cartridges and syringes that automatically dispense standard dosages if their vision is bad or they have difficulty understanding. Routine follow-up and evaluation of injection technique is important. The patient should be asked periodically to give a demonstration of the technique on return visits to the clinic or office.

 Clinical Pitfall

Errors in Insulin Administration

Errors in insulin administration by diabetic patients are among the most common drug errors. Errors in the amount of medication, coupled with reduced vision or difficulty drawing up or injecting insulin, contribute to the potential for problems. Review the patient's technique regularly.

Patients must also be taught how to test the blood glucose level using a **glucometer** (hand-held testing machine). Have the patient practice using the machine and accurately interpreting the results; the requirements of the specific equipment being used will vary. Provide a booklet or chart in which the patient can record findings. Information on times when the blood should be tested for glucose should be given to the patient as part of written instructions. Times to test blood glucose may vary, based on the type of medication taken and the degree of control required.

Individuals with cerebral vascular disease, coronary disease, or advanced complications may be at higher risk of hypoglycemia and may not benefit from tight glucose control. In general, the goal for the fasting blood sugar (FBS) is less than 120 mg/dL.

The goal for the average preprandial glucose level should be between 80 and 120 mg/dL. The goal for the bedtime glucose level is 110 to 140 mg/dL. Treatment adjustment should occur if the glucose is less than 100 mg/dL or greater than 160 mg/dL.

 Clinical Pitfall

Insulin Dosage Adjustment

Dosage adjustment should occur if the FBS is less than 80 mg/dL or greater than 140 mg/dL. The goal is to keep the hemoglobin (Hb)A_{1c} level less than 7%, which is equivalent to a blood glucose level of 150 mg/dL.

Insulin allergy (transient local itching, swelling, and erythema at the injection site) commonly develops when therapy is started, particularly with pork insulin. Use of produced by recombinant deoxyribonucleic acid technology has decreased this problem. Insulin resistance (requirements of more than 200 units of insulin per day) is rare and may be caused by infection, inflammatory diseases, obesity, or stress. To make sure that hypoglycemia is avoided, closely monitor the patient with insulin resistance who is being treated with a concentrated insulin injection. Long-acting insulins are not adequate in the treatment and management of acidosis and emergencies.

Administration of insulin by an aerosol inhaler allows some diabetic patients to give up injections. Not all persons with diabetes can use this format.

▪ Implementation

Techniques for calculation of insulin dosage, preparation of injection, mixing of insulin types, injection sites, and injection technique are all presented in Chapter 10. Refer to this material to review this information.

Insulin is a protein and therefore is inactivated by gastrointestinal (GI) enzymes. Thus insulin is generally given subcutaneously and timed so that it is available in the body when the glucose level rises after eating. The time of administration also depends on the type of insulin preparation. Only regular insulin can be administered intravenously, as is done during ketoacidosis or diabetic coma.

Various substances such as protamine or zinc may be added to delay insulin absorption or turn it into a suspension. Different insulin preparations with different onsets, peaks, and durations of action are required so that patients can individualize their treatment. Premixed insulin products are also available as combinations of neutral protamine Hagedorn (NPH) and regular insulin in ratios of 70/30, 30/70, and 50/50. Information about these products is summarized in Tables 21-1 and 21-2.

Insulin dose depends on the patient's response. The dosage will be gradually increased or decreased (titrated) to get the best response with the lowest dosage. Generally, the minimal goal of therapy is to avoid extremes of ketoacidosis and hypoglycemia.

The individual presenting with ketones in the blood is usually started on insulin. The goal of therapy is to maintain blood glucose levels as follows: fasting,

Table 21-1 Insulin Characteristics and Duration of Action

INSULIN	COLOR	ONSET	PEAK	DURATION
Rapid Acting				
lispro (Humalog) ★	Clear	5-15 min	30-90 min	3-4 hr
aspart (NovoLog)	Clear	5-15 min	1-3 hr	3-5 hr
glulisine (Apidra)	Clear	5-15 min	30-90 min	3-4 hr
Short Acting				
Regular (R)	Clear	30-60 min	2-4 hr	6-8 hr
Intermediate Acting				
NPH (N)	Cloudy	2-4 hr	6-10 hr	10-16 hr
Long Acting				
glargine (Lantus)	Clear	2 hr	No peak	20-24 hr
detemir (Levemir)	Clear	1 hr	No peak	6-24 hr
Mixtures				
70/30	Cloudy	15 min	30 min-12 hr	10-16 hr
50/50	Cloudy	30 min	3-5 hr	10-16 hr
Humalog 75/25	Cloudy	15 min	30-90 min	10-16 hr
NovoLog 70/30	Cloudy	5-15 min	1-3 hr	10-16 hr

NPH, Neutral protamine Hagedorn.
★ Indicates "Must-Know Drugs," or the 35 drugs most prescribers use.

90-110 mg/dL; 1 hour after eating (postprandial), less than 180 mg/dL; and 2 hours postprandial, less than 150 mg/dL. There are a variety of recommendations for how insulin might be given daily to achieve these goals:

1. Basal insulin therapy in combination with oral agents
   - Start with glargine (Lantus) or detemir (Levemir) insulin 10 units or 0.3 unit/kg at bedtime. Increase dosage by 2 to 4 units every 3 to 5 days to achieve FBS goal.
   - Start with NPH insulin 10 units at suppertime or bedtime. Increase dose by 1 to 2 units every 3 to 5 days to achieve FBS goal.
2. Premixed insulin regimens
   - Start with 70/30 insulin at suppertime or NPH/regular insulin at suppertime. This is a good combination if bedtime and fasting blood glucose levels are elevated. Increase dose by 10% to 20% every 3 to 5 days to achieve blood sugar goals.
   - Start 70/30 at breakfast and at suppertime. This is a good combination if glucoses are elevated throughout the day and if the patient is not a candidate for additional oral therapy.
3. NPH/regular insulin before breakfast and before dinner
   - Use 0.5 to 1 unit per kilogram of patient's weight as total daily insulin dose.
   - Divide dose so that two-thirds of total dose is given in the morning and one-third of the total dose is given before dinner.
   - Divide each morning and dinner dose so that two-thirds of the dose is NPH and one-third is regular.
4. Basal-bolus regimens (long-acting insulin in combination with premeal rapid insulin injection)

After the patient is started on a basal dose of long-acting insulin (glargine or detemir), rapid- or short-acting insulin is added before meals. This requires that blood glucose levels be monitored frequently. One option is to add premeal rapid- or short-acting insulin to the largest meal. Then prandial boluses of rapid-acting insulin can be added at other meal times. Rapid- and short-acting insulin can be added as standing doses or on a sliding scale based on blood sugar readings.

This is the most physiologic approach to insulin therapy; however, this regimen can be daunting for many diabetic patients. Consequently, twice-daily premixed insulin (given before breakfast and before dinner) is an acceptable alternative for the patient who is not willing or able to take multiple daily injections.

The insulin vial in use may be stored outside of the refrigerator for 1 month, provided it does not get extremely hot or cold. An extra supply of insulin should be stored in the refrigerator. Insulin should be warmed to room temperature for use, because the injection of cold insulin may irritate the tissues. The expiration date on the bottle should be checked regularly to make sure the insulin is not too old to use safely.

Table 21-2 Oral Treatment of Type 2 Diabetes

GENERIC NAME	TRADE NAME	COMMON INSTRUCTIONS
Second Generation Sulfonylureas		
glimepiride	Amaryl 1-, 2-, 4-mg tablets	After reaching 2 mg/day, dose often increased by no more than 2 mg at 1- to 2-wk intervals.
glipizide extended release	Glucotrol XL 5-, 10-mg tablets	Premeal dosing not necessary.
glipizide	Glucotrol 5-, 10-mg tablets	Divide daily doses >15 mg; take 30 min before meals.
glyburide	DiaBeta Micronase 1.25-, 2.5-, 5-mg tablets	Can divide daily doses >10 mg; doses >10 mg may not further lower glucose levels.
micronized glyburide	Glynase PresTabs 1.5-, 3-, 6-mg tablets	Small particle size facilitates rapid absorption; can divide doses >6 mg.
Biguanides		
metformin	Glucophage 500-, 850-mg tablets	Take with meals to decrease GI symptoms; avoid in liver and kidney disease; hold dose for contrast studies; lactic acidosis potential; called an *insulin sensitizer*.
Thiazolidinediones		
rosiglitazone	Avandia	Usual dosage up to 8 mg daily. May be used as monotherapy or with existing dosages of sulfonylurea or metformin. Only available to select patients because of safety concerns.
pioglitazone	Actos	Taken once daily without regard to meals. May be used with sulfonylurea, metformin, or insulin.
α-Glucosidase inhibitors		
acarbose	Precose 25-, 50-, 100-mg tablets	Take with the first bite of the meal; adjust dose at 4- to 8-wk intervals based on glucose level 1 hr after meal; increase to 100 mg 3 times daily only if weight >60 kg; avoid in liver and intestinal disorders; treat hypoglycemia with glucose or lactose.
miglitol	Glyset	Take medication with first bite of each meal. May be used as monotherapy or in combination therapy with a sulfonylurea.
Non-sulfonylurea Secretagogues (Meglitinides)		
repaglinide	Prandin 0.05-, 1-, 2-mg tablets	Dosing: up to 30 min before a meal; if meal is added or skipped, add or skip dose; if not previously treated or if hemoglobin A1c <8%, will usually start with 0.5 mg; if previously treated or A1c 8%, may begin at 1-2 mg before meals; the dose should be doubled, up to 4 mg before meals, until glucose goal is achieved.
nateglinide	Starlix	May be used as monotherapy or with metformin.
Icretin Agents		
exenatide	Byetta	Usual dose is 10 mcg SQ bid but may go up to 20 mcg.
pramlintide	Symlin	May increase by 15 mcg SQ every 3 days if tolerated.
Dipeptidyl-Peptidase-IV Inhibitors (DPP-IV)		
sitagliptin	Januvia, Onglyza	DPP-IV Inhibitor drug used in adjunctive therapy. Adjust dose based on creatinine clearance. Does not promote weight loss.

GI, Gastrointestinal; *SQ*, subcutaneous.

Rapid-acting insulin is used during treatment of ketoacidosis and in other acute situations (infection, surgery) when the patient's food intake is variable. It is also used in combination with longer-acting insulins to achieve greater control. Regular insulin may be used in divided dose therapy. The dosage is determined by the level of blood glucose. Long-acting insulin is used primarily for patients whose blood sugar level is constantly high at night.

For insulin suspensions, the vial is gently rolled and tipped from end to end before the insulin is drawn up, so that any particles that may have settled out are returned to suspension. Vigorous shaking may result in air bubbles that can make it difficult to accurately draw the insulin. Shaking also breaks down protein molecules in the insulin.

Most patients with diabetes can control their symptoms with 40 to 60 units of insulin per day. Occasionally a patient develops resistance to the insulin or becomes so unresponsive to insulin that several hundred or even thousands of units of insulin may be necessary. Patients who require dosages in excess of 300 to 500 units often have impaired insulin receptors. Concentrated insulin injection allows a larger dose to be given in a smaller amount of fluid. Each milliliter of the concentrated insulin contains 500 units of purified pork, rather than the 100 units in the normal products. Glargine is an insulin product that provides a basal level of insulin for 24 hours.

■ Evaluation

The patient's response to the insulin dose is seen by testing the blood. The nurse, physician, or other health care provider should inform the patient about how frequently to return for checkups, what blood levels are being found at these visits, and what the desired levels should be. The patient must be encouraged to take responsibility for managing his or her own disease.

Patients with type 2 diabetes are frequently overweight. As the patient's blood sugar level is under control and they begin to lose weight, the dosage of insulin they require is less. The clinician will often reduce the dosages of medications prescribed when weight loss has taken place.

The plan of insulin therapy is to keep blood glucose levels within specific limits and to prevent symptoms of hyperglycemia and hypoglycemia. Patients with home glucometers should be told when to check their blood glucose level, depending on the type of insulin they are taking. Urine ketones should be measured during acute illness or periods of increased glycosuria and in ketosis-prone diabetic patients. The records the patient keeps will provide information regarding control between office visits and should be taken to each visit with the health care provider.

If hypoglycemia occurs, the patient should be taught to eat some form of carbohydrate immediately. The family should also be involved in patient teaching about therapy for hypoglycemia. If the patient is unconscious, honey or corn syrup may be put under the tongue or on the buccal mucosa in the mouth. Additional carbohydrates, such as bread, crackers, or milk, should be provided for the next 2 hours; a sandwich should be eaten if a snack or meal would not be regularly eaten within an hour. Glucagon, a glucose-rich liquid, may be administered by a family member or a care provider to quickly raise blood glucose levels if the patient has accidentally taken too much insulin.

The Somogyi effect (rebound elevation of glucose levels brought on by hypoglycemia) can lead to overtreatment of the patient with insulin when less insulin is actually needed. Patients older than 60 years of age are often sensitive to hypoglycemia. They should be observed for confusion and abnormal behavior, because repeated episodes of hypoglycemia may cause brain damage.

Regular appointments with the clinician will be timed with laboratory blood work to measure blood sugar control. The hemoglobin (Hb) A1c blood test reflects the state of glycemia the patient has experienced for the last 90 days, which is the lifetime of the red blood cell. The goal is to keep the HbA1c level less than 7%, which is equivalent to a blood glucose level of 150 mg/dL. The blood glucose level goes up by approximately 30 points for every 1% increase of the HbA1c (e.g., 8% = 180 mg/dL; 9% = 210 mg/dL). Evaluation of this blood level will tell the clinician about general blood sugar levels, not just the blood sugar level on the day of the appointment.

■ Patient and Family Teaching

Tell the patient and family the following:
- The patient should maintain a specific diet (regular meals, snacks, and caloric requirements) and maintain an ideal body weight to promote glycemic control and prevent hypoglycemia.
- The patient must know the signs and symptoms of hypoglycemia (too little sugar) and hyperglycemia (too much sugar), their causes, prevention, and treatment. The patient should notify the nurse, physician, or other health care provider if any of the symptoms occur.
- Pork insulin can cause an increase (hypertrophy) or a decrease (atrophy) in the size of fatty tissue when injected into the same site frequently. A plan for rotation of insulin injection sites should be developed, followed, and recorded.
- The patient must use the proper syringe and the correct type, strength, and dose of insulin to avoid dosage errors.
- The patient should avoid drinking alcohol because it can intensify the hypoglycemia produced by insulin, causing blood glucose levels to fall too low.

- The patient's blood glucose levels can be measured by daily blood testing. The patient should be taught the proper technique for testing, recording, and interpreting the results. This will help the patient and the nurse, physician, or other health care provider manage the disease successfully.
- Insulin requirements increase when the patient is under stress or becomes ill, especially with an infection. The patient must faithfully test the urine or blood when ill and must not stop taking insulin. A liquid nutritional supplement can substitute for a meal if the patient has an upset stomach, nausea, or vomiting. The nurse, physician, or other health care provider should be contacted for information on how to adjust the insulin dosage.
- The patient must be prepared for emergency situations by:
  - Carrying a medical identification card.
  - Wearing a MedicAlert bracelet or necklace.
  - Carrying a readily available source of sugar at all times.
- When traveling, patients should carry an extra supply of insulin, syringes, and needles in a separate container kept with them in case they cannot get to their luggage. Patients will need to make adjustments for time zone changes to avoid hypoglycemia.
- The patient should be alert for hypoglycemia when driving, operating machinery, or engaging in activities that require alertness.

☀ ORAL HYPOGLYCEMICS

ACTION

The primary action of the oral hypoglycemics is to stimulate insulin release by the beta cells of the pancreas. Therefore the patient must have some functioning beta cells if these drugs are to work. These products also increase the peripheral use of insulin and influence other fat and carbohydrate processes.

USES

The number of classes of oral antidiabetic agents has dramatically increased since the 1980s. They can be used in monotherapy (therapy with one drug) or combined oral agent therapy, or can be combined with insulin to achieve the optimal (best) glucose control in patients with type 2 diabetes. The first available class of oral agents was the sulfonylureas. Sulfonylureas lower serum glucose levels by increasing beta cell insulin production and, to a lesser extent, by decreasing insulin resistance. In the early 1980s, a second generation of sulfonylureas became available, and over time these have replaced the first-generation sulfonylureas. Second-generation sulfonylureas are approximately 1000 times more potent than first-generation

agents. Unlike first-generation oral agents, which bind to ionic and nonionic sites, second-generation agents bind only to nonionic sites. This type of binding usually results in fewer interactions with other medications. The major side effect of sulfonylureas is hypoglycemia. These drugs can be used as monotherapy or in combination with insulin, acarbose, or metformin.

The second class of oral agents that became available was the biguanides. The only drug in this class that is still available in the United States is metformin. Metformin use is associated with a very small risk for lactic acidosis, usually in patients who may also have some renal dysfunction. This class of medication lowers glucose levels by decreasing glucose production in the liver, decreasing insulin resistance, and slowing the absorption of glucose from the intestines. As monotherapy, metformin generally does not cause hypoglycemia. Metformin can be used in combination with insulin, and all of the other oral agents.

Alpha-glucosidase inhibitors became available in the 1990s. Acarbose and miglitol are the drugs available in this class. They lower glucose by slowing the breakdown of polysaccharides into simple sugars. As monotherapy, they cannot cause hypoglycemia. Alpha-glucosidase inhibitors can be used with sulfonylureas, insulin, or metformin.

Another class of oral antidiabetic agents, the meglitinides, was released in 1998. The drugs repaglinide and nateglinide, although chemically unrelated to the sulfonylureas, work by stimulating the release of insulin from the beta cells of the pancreas. Their use can result in hypoglycemia. Meglitinides can be used as monotherapy or in combination with metformin.

The thiazolidinedione class of drugs has introduced many new options for treatment of patients with diabetes. These agents increase the body's response to insulin without increasing insulin secretion. The drugs rosiglitazone (Avandia) and pioglitazone (Actos) have revolutionized the way patients can be treated. Thiazolidinediones have been associated with severe cardiovascular side effects, however, and must be used with care. Currently rosiglitazone is a drug only available to selected patients but pioglitazone is still generally available, although closely monitored.

A whole new class of drugs, the incretins, have also provided new treatment options. The amylin analog drug pramlintide (Symlin), the GLP-1, exenatide, and the DPP-4 inhibitor sitagliptin phosphate (Januvia) are included in this class. Incretins are hormones that are released from the gut postprandially; they often are found in low concentrations in persons with type 2 diabetes. The incretin that has received the most attention is GLP-1. Incretins stimulate insulin secretion in pancreatic β-cells and have been shown to restore both phases of insulin release. GLP-1 regulates glucose homeostasis via multiple complementary actions and along with other incretins is known to:

- Stimulate glucose-dependent endogenous insulin secretion (and perhaps insulin sensitivity).
- Inhibit endogenous glucagon secretion.
- Suppress appetite and induce satiety.
- Reduce the speed of gastric emptying.
- Possibly stimulate islet-cell growth.
- Protect β-cells from cytokine and free fatty acid–mediated injury.

New drugs as well as new treatment delivery systems such as the pump have changed how diabetes is treated.

ADVERSE REACTIONS

Hypoglycemia is the most common adverse reaction. Allergic reactions, manifested by urticaria (hives), rash, pruritus (itching), and erythema, may occur at the beginning of therapy, generally temporarily. More common reactions to sulfonylureas include heartburn, nausea, vomiting, abdominal pain, and diarrhea caused by increased gastric acid secretion. Occasionally, sulfonylureas cause hepatotoxicity (damage to the liver) and cholestatic jaundice, with symptoms of jaundice (yellow color of skin, eyes, and mucous membranes), dark urine, and light-colored stools. Leukopenia, agranulocytosis, thrombocytopenia, hemolytic anemia, aplastic anemia, and pancytopenia have also been reported. There are rare reports of disulfiram-like reactions when alcohol is taken with tolbutamide. Lactic acidosis may rarely occur with metformin, and the risk is increased with the use of alcohol. Nausea, vomiting, diarrhea, flatulence, and anorexia are the most common adverse reactions with metformin; these problems tend to improve over time.

 Clinical Pitfall

Alcohol Consumption

Alcohol consumption with some oral hypoglycemics may result in a violent disulfiram-like reaction.

DRUG INTERACTIONS

The hyperglycemic effects of the sulfonylureas and metformin are potentiated (made worse) by oral anticoagulants and various other drugs. Sulfonamide-type antibacterial agents and salicylates displace the sulfonylureas from protein-binding sites, and this leads to high blood levels of the active drug. Barbiturates, sedatives, and hypnotics may have a prolonged effect when taken at the same time as the sulfonylureas because of a decreased rate of elimination from the body. Thiazide diuretics oppose the secretion of insulin from the beta cells and decrease the effectiveness of sulfonylureas. Many of these drugs, when used along with oral contraceptives that contain ethinyl estradiol and norethindrone, may decrease contraceptive effectiveness.

❖ NURSING IMPLICATIONS AND PATIENT TEACHING

■ Assessment

Try to learn as much as possible about the patient's health history, including what other drugs the patient is taking that may interact with the oral products, and if the patient is pregnant or has renal insufficiency, impaired liver function, or a history of ketoacidosis. Ask if the patient has any sensitivity (allergy) to sulfa drugs, because he or she may have cross-sensitivity to sulfonylureas (a patient who is sensitive to one type of sulfa drug may be sensitive to all types).

■ Diagnosis

Does the patient have any other problems that would interfere with drug therapy? Are there problems with weight, nutrition, vision, or finances? Does the patient have past history or behavior that might cause the nurse to suspect this patient might not be compliant with diet, exercise, medication, and testing requirements?

■ Planning

No transition period is necessary when a patient is switched from one oral hypoglycemic to another. Plan the teaching that will be necessary as the nurse works with this patient.

■ Implementation

These products are administered orally. The duration of the hypoglycemic effect is the main difference between the various products. The duration of action, dosage range, and approximate doses per day are given in Tables 21-1 and 21-2.

■ Evaluation

The patient's blood glucose levels should be monitored, and the patient should be watched for signs and symptoms of hypoglycemia.

Rashes may develop when sulfonylurea therapy begins, but they generally last only a short time. If they persist, the medication should be stopped. Cholestatic jaundice has been reported in a small number of patients on oral hypoglycemic therapy. Any liver damage that has developed generally goes away when the drug is stopped. Watch for any signs of blood dyscrasias, GI intolerance, or allergic reactions.

■ Patient and Family Teaching

Teach the patient and family about diabetes, diet, and exercise, just as the patient is taught about starting to take insulin. Teach patients specifically about nutrition, blood testing, and general precautions to follow. In addition, tell the patient and family the following:

- The patient taking oral hypoglycemic agents should report jaundice, dark urine, light-colored stools,

- fever, sore throat, fatigue, or any unusual bleeding or bruising to the nurse, physician, or other health care provider.
- Allergic skin reactions may develop when oral hypoglycemic therapy begins. Red, raised rashes are generally brief and will disappear with continued drug therapy.
- The patient should avoid drinking alcohol when taking these products because lactic acidosis or a disulfiram-like reaction, with severe nausea and vomiting, dizziness, headache, diaphoresis, and flushing (red color in the face and neck), may develop.

SELECTED DRUGS USED WITH PREGNANCY AND DELIVERY

OVERVIEW

Medications used throughout the end of pregnancy and during delivery are a special category of drugs beyond the scope of this text. However, any drug used for the mother also affects the fetus, so paying special attention to drug use is required during the immediate delivery period. Therefore a few of these products are selected for discussion. Excluding anesthetics, most drugs used during the antepartum (before), intrapartum (during), and postpartum (after birth) periods are given primarily for their effect on the uterus. These include tocolytics, oxytocics, uterine relaxants, and abortifacients. These products are used primarily to slow labor at the time of delivery or to help expel the fetus from the uterus to terminate pregnancy.

ACTION

Abortifacients stimulate or increase uterine contractions and cause the uterus to empty. **Oxytocic agents** and ergot preparations cause the uterus to contract, helping labor move on to delivery. Oxytocin acts directly on the smooth muscles of the uterus, especially when the mother is at or near full term, to produce firm, regular contractions. They also act on the blood vessels to produce vasoconstriction (narrowing) and on the mammary gland cells in the postpartum phase to stimulate the flow of milk. Because these drugs are given so frequently, most of the information presented here is about oxytocics.

In contrast to abortifacients, oxytocin, and the ergots, the **uterine relaxants** act on the beta-adrenergic receptors to stop uterine smooth muscle contractions. **Tocolytics** are agents used to stop preterm labor. They generally act through uterine relaxation.

USES

Abortifacients are used early in pregnancy to end pregnancy by emptying the uterus. Oxytocics are used for a number of purposes:

- To stimulate or induce labor at term when there are medical problems threatening the life of the mother or fetus
- To assist in the delivery of the shoulder of the infant
- To assist in the release of the placenta
- To control postpartum bleeding or lack of muscle tone in the uterus
- To relieve breast swelling or engorgement caused by lack of lactation
- To stimulate uterine contraction after a cesarean section birth or other uterine surgery
- To treat incomplete abortion

The ergots are used to prevent or control hemorrhage after the delivery of the placenta and in the postpartum period.

Uterine relaxants and tocolytics are used when a mother goes into preterm labor and the goal is to delay delivery. Women who show signs of preterm delivery may be treated with a subcutaneous injection and then sent home on an oral maintenance dose. Magnesium sulfate, a common anticonvulsant, has some success as a tocolytic; however, it is not a first-line agent. It has also been used with ritodrine therapy, although with questionable efficacy and an increase in adverse reactions. Hydroxyprogesterone caproate (Makena) is a drug to help reduce the risk of preterm delivery before 37 weeks of pregnancy. This indication is for pregnant women with a history of at least one spontaneous preterm birth, but not for use in women with a twin pregnancy or other risk factors for preterm birth. The Food and Drug Administration has warned that injectable or oral terbutaline, a drug long used off-label to prevent premature birth, should not be used beyond 48-72 hours of preterm labor because of the potential for serious maternal cardiovascular events and death.

ADVERSE REACTIONS

Abortifacients may produce severe cramping and pain. Tocolytics often produce visual disturbances, malaise, nausea, and confusion. Oxytocin may produce dysrhythmias (irregular heartbeats), edema (fluid buildup in the body tissues), fetal and neonatal bradycardia (slow heartbeat), anxiety, redness of skin during administration, nausea and vomiting, anaphylaxis (shock), postpartum hemorrhage, cyanosis (blue color to the skin), and dyspnea (uncomfortable breathing).

In the appropriate dosage and in the absence of contraindications, the ergots are fairly safe. The most common adverse reactions are nausea and vomiting. More unusual reactions include allergic reactions, bradycardia, hypotension (low blood pressure), hypertension (high blood pressure), or cerebral-spinal symptoms and spasms. The most common side effects reported with hydroxyprogesterone caproate include pain, swelling, or itching at the injection site; hives; nausea; and diarrhea. Serious adverse reactions are rare.

Excessive doses of oxytocics during labor can produce uterine hypertonicity (extreme muscle tension), spasm, and tetanic contractions and ruptures of the uterus. Smaller overdoses in labor yield a sustained, forceful contraction without rest. Overdose with ergots during labor yields a similar reaction, with cardiovascular and GI symptoms progressing to more dangerous problems.

DRUG INTERACTIONS

Vasoconstrictors and local anesthetics increase the effects of oxytocics.

❖ NURSING IMPLICATIONS AND PATIENT TEACHING

■ Assessment

It is important to determine the exact due date for delivery. The patient may be past the anticipated due date for the baby or have a history of engorged breasts. A history of incomplete abortion, cesarean section births, or excessive postpartum bleeding may require use of oxytocics or ergots. Finally, a patient may also want to terminate an unwanted pregnancy early in gestation.

■ Diagnosis

What additional problems might this patient have? Is there unreasonable anxiety or fear associated with the delivery? Does the mother have concerns about the health of the child? Have previous experiences been positive? What other medical conditions might make this delivery more risky?

■ Planning

The uterine contractions produced by oxytocics should be about the same as those of spontaneous, normal labor.

There are numerous precautions or contraindications to the use of oxytocics. These medications must be given by qualified nurses under the direct supervision of physicians or other health care providers. Inappropriate use of either oxytocic or ergot preparations has caused fetal and maternal death or injury, subarachnoid hemorrhage, and uterine rupture.

■ Implementation

Oxytocin is the drug of choice to cause or induce labor in many areas of the country. However, prostaglandins are now preferred in some regions. These are usually given by intravenous (IV) infusion pump.

Ergonovine is now the drug of choice to control postpartum bleeding. It can be given sublingually, intramuscularly, or intravenously in emergency situations. Methylergonovine is the synthetic homologue of ergonovine and has been found to produce fewer vasoconstrictive or hypertensive side effects than ergonovine. It is noted that IV administration of either of these ergot preparations increases the danger of side effects.

A summary of drugs acting on the uterus is provided in Table 21-3.

■ Evaluation

If oxytocin is used during induction of labor, the patient should be monitored for degree of contractions and the development of adverse reactions. The blood pressure and pulse should be checked frequently, and there should be continuous monitoring of the fetal heart rate. Monitor the dilation of the cervix and the progression of contractions. Drastic increases in the frequency, force, and duration of contractions and in resting uterine tone may require the drug to be stopped. The contractions should not be more than 50 mm Hg, the frequency should be no longer than every 2 minutes, and the duration should be no longer than 90 seconds. Both the mother and fetus should be monitored with internal monitoring equipment (fetal scalp electrode and intrauterine pressure catheter).

Watch out for the symptoms of ergotism: vomiting; diarrhea; unquenchable thirst; tingling, itching, and coldness of the skin; a rapid, weak pulse; confusion; and unconsciousness.

Ergonovine might stimulate cramping. If this becomes too uncomfortable, the physician may either decrease the dosage or treat the symptoms.

The most common side effects of ergonovine are nausea and vomiting. These symptoms can sometimes be stopped if the patient is given a phenothiazine antiemetic.

If overdosage of an oxytocic occurs, producing a continuous contraction, the drug must be stopped immediately. It may be necessary to give a general anesthetic to relax the uterus, particularly if the fetus is threatened.

■ Patient and Family Teaching

Tell the patient and family the following:
* Oxytocics or ergots are given to augment the body's natural action during and after labor and delivery.
* The patient will be watched continually throughout this treatment.
* Contractions should not be more intense than normal contractions.
* Ergonovine might stimulate cramping; if this becomes intense, the patient should inform the nurse or physician.

Table 21-3   Drugs Acting on the Uterus

GENERIC NAME	TRADE NAME	COMMENTS
Oxytocics		
ergonovine	Ergotrate	Used to prevent or control postpartum hemorrhage secondary to uterine atony or subinvolution. Note similarity in names between ergotamine (used for migraines) and ergonovine; they are not the same, although they may be listed the same in some books. Sublingual (appropriate in nonemergency situations and for prophylaxis after leaving the labor and delivery suite): Give daily for 48 hr postpartum.
methylergonovine	Methergine	Synthetic ergonovine produces stronger and more prolonged contractions. Protect vials from heat and light, and discard colored vials. Onset of action from IV is immediate; after IM, it is 2-5 min, and with PO it is 5-10 min. Give IV, IM, or PO.
oxytocin	Pitocin	Used to induce or stimulate labor at term and secondarily in the stimulation of milk flow. Drug of choice in many areas of the country for medical induction of labor. Never administer intravenously in undiluted form or in high concentrations. To induce labor: Give medication 1 L D_5W or isotonic saline as an IV infusion. If no response within 15 min, dose gradually increased to a maximum of 20 milliunits/min. The total induction dose ranges from 600 to 12,000 milliunits, with the average being 4000 milliunits. For postpartum bleeding: Given IM after delivery of the placenta; or in 1 L isotonic saline IV at a rate to control the bleeding.
Abortifacients		
carboprost	Hemabate	Give IM.
dinoprostone	Prostin E_2	1 suppository high into vagina; repeated PRN.
mifepristone	Mifeprex	Patient takes tablets after reading and signing consent form. If abortion does not occur within 3 days, the patient is seen and must take misoprostol. Patient returns for examination 14 days later.
Tocolytics		
magnesium sulfate	Magnesium Sulfate	Drug has a narrow therapeutic range of 4-7 mEq/L. Also used for treatment of preeclampsia and eclampsia conditions. Dosage must be accurate.
terbutaline sulfate	Brethine I	Initiate IV administration; titrate dosage upward. Maintain IV dosage at the minimum effective dose for 4 hr. Oral doses q4-6h have been used as maintenance therapy until term. This use has been off-label and is now discouraged by FDA because of potential for serious maternal CV events and death. Inhalation products no longer on market.
Agents for Cervical Ripening		
dinoprostone	Cervidil Prepidil	Used in pregnant women at or near term with a medical or obstetric need for labor induction 10-mg gel insert: Physician should use aseptic technique to insert endocervical catheter and introduce gel into cervical canal. Bring to room temperature just before administration. Wash hands after handling product. Patient should remain in supine position for 15-30 min to help retain fluid. May be repeated after 6 hr if no response. IV oxytocin given 6-12 hr after gel insertion as needed

CV, Cardiovascular; *D_5W*, 5% dextrose in water; *FDA*, Food and Drug Administration; *IM*, intramuscular; *IV*, intravenous; *PO*, by mouth; *PRN*, as needed.

PITUITARY AND ADRENOCORTICAL HORMONES

OVERVIEW

The pituitary, or "master" gland, lies in the sella turcica in the sphenoid bone in the skull and is connected to the brain by a slender stalk. This area is almost directly between the eyes in the middle of the brain. The anterior (front) portion of the pituitary, or the *adenohypophysis*, and the posterior (back) portion of the pituitary, or the *neurohypophysis*, produce hormones that control growth, metabolism, electrolyte balance, water retention or loss, and the reproductive cycle.

The adrenal cortex manufactures the **corticosteroids** and a small amount of the **sex hormones**. These hormones are substances that influence many organs, structures, and life processes of the body. The corticosteroids are composed of the glucocorticoids and the mineralocorticoids, and the sex hormones include the androgens and estrogens.

✤ PITUITARY HORMONES
ANTERIOR PITUITARY HORMONES

ACTION AND USES

The major anterior pituitary hormones include two gonadotropins: follicle-stimulating hormone (FSH) and luteinizing hormone (LH). They are called *gonadotropins* because they influence the gonads, which are the organs of reproduction. They influence the production of sex hormones, the development of secondary sex characteristics, and the pattern and regularity of the reproductive cycle. An additional anterior pituitary hormone, prolactin, stimulates the production of breast milk after childbirth.

There are a number of sources for gonadotropins that are used clinically. Human chorionic gonadotropin is taken from human placentas and contains FSH and LH. A purified form of FSH and LH, known as *menotropins,* is taken from the urine of postmenopausal women. These hormones may be given to produce ovulation in women with ovulatory failure, to stimulate production of sperm in men, or to assist in treatment when the testes have failed to descend into the scrotum. Clomiphene is a synthetic nonsteroidal compound that is also used to promote ovulation.

Somatotropic hormone (somatotropin) and adrenocorticotropic hormone (ACTH, or corticotropin) are also produced by the anterior pituitary. Somatotropin comes from human pituitary glands removed at autopsy. This hormone regulates growth during childhood and is given to children who have failed to grow because of a growth hormone deficiency. ACTH stimulates the adrenal cortex to produce and secrete hormones, primarily glucocorticoids. ACTH is used in diagnostic testing and in the treatment of some acute neurologic problems.

Adverse Reactions

Because all of these medications are hormones, their primary adverse reactions include systemic or local hormonal reactions. Menotropins may produce ovarian enlargement, blood inside the peritoneal cavity, and febrile reactions; when it is used to increase fertility, multiple births may be produced. Clomiphene may produce abdominal discomfort, ovarian enlargement, blurred vision, nervousness, and nausea and vomiting. Vasomotor flushes (hot flashes), much like those seen in menopause, may also occur. Chorionic gonadotropin may cause headache, irritability, restlessness, fatigue, and edema. Precocious puberty (onset of sexual development at an early age) may result from its use in treatment for undescended testes.

Somatotropin may provoke antibody stimulation in some individuals, resulting in failure of the drug to produce any growth. ACTH is involved with numerous adverse reactions because it stimulates the adrenal gland. A summary of the most commonly used types of ACTH is provided in Table 21-4.

POSTERIOR PITUITARY HORMONES

ACTION AND USES

The posterior pituitary gland produces the antidiuretic hormone (ADH) vasopressin, as well as oxytocin, a hormone that stimulates the uterus. Vasopressin regulates the reabsorption of water by the kidneys. This hormone is specifically released whenever the brain senses that the urine is becoming concentrated because the patient has had severe diarrhea or vomiting or has become dehydrated through some other condition.

Vasopressin may be given when the body loses water when it should not do so, as in diabetes insipidus, or when the pituitary fails to secrete vasopressin because of disease or surgical removal. Vasopressin is also used in some GI problems and in the treatment of nighttime bedwetting. Pituitary extract is also given to increase smooth muscle contraction of the digestive tract and blood vessels. Information on vasopressin and desmopressin (DDAVP, the synthetic form) is provided in Table 21-5.

Table 21-4	Common Anterior Pituitary Hormones	
GENERIC NAME	**TRADE NAME**	**COMMENTS**
corticotropin (ACTH)	Acthar	Very rapid absorption and use necessitates administration q6h to maintain desired production; give IM or SC.
corticotropin repository	HP Acthar Gel	Slowly absorbed and can be administered in a single daily IM dose.
cosyntropin	Cortrosyn	Synthetic subunit of ACTH but exhibits all the pharmacologic properties of natural ACTH. Cosyntropin 0.25 mg is equivalent in action to 25 units natural ACTH and is less likely to produce allergies. Adrenocortical insufficiency testing: Give IM or IV.

ACTH, Adrenocorticotropic hormone; *IM,* intramuscular; *IV,* intravenous; *SQ,* subcutaneous.

Table 21-5   Posterior Pituitary Hormones

GENERIC NAME	TRADE NAME	COMMENTS
desmopressin	DDAVP Stimate	Synthetic antidiuretic inhalant; drug of choice in patients with mild to moderate diabetes insipidus. Offers prolonged antidiuretic activity without vasopressor or oxytocic side effects. Adults: Give in the evening. Effect noted and increased nightly by 2.5 mcg until satisfactory sleep duration attained.
vasopressin	Pitressin Vasopressin tannate	Water-insoluble derivative of vasopressin with longer duration of action; of use in long-term treatment of diabetes insipidus in children and some adults. Adults: Give IM or SQ, 2 to 4 times daily.

IM, Intramuscular; *SQ*, Subcutaneous.

Oxytocin acts directly on the smooth musculature of the uterus to produce firm, regular contractions, as described in the second section of this chapter.

ACTH usually is reserved for testing and replacement therapy. ACTH stimulates the adrenal cortex to secrete cortisol, corticosterone, aldosterone, and several other weaker substances.

ADVERSE REACTIONS

Adverse reactions to small doses of vasopressin include abdominal cramps, anaphylaxis, bronchial constriction, circumoral (around the mouth) pallor, diarrhea, flatus (gas in the intestine), intestinal hyperactivity, nausea, "pounding" headaches, sweating, tremors, urticaria, uterine cramps, vertigo (feeling of dizziness and spinning), and vomiting. Vasopressin given in larger doses may produce death.

ACTH use, particularly over a sustained period, is associated with substantial adverse effects of the cardiovascular, endocrine, GI, musculoskeletal, and ophthalmic systems. The patient must be monitored closely while using these products. Suddenly stopping the medication may worsen symptoms.

DRUG INTERACTIONS

Oral antidiabetic agents, urea, and fludrocortisone increase the effects of vasopressin, and large doses of epinephrine, heparin, and alcohol decrease the effect. The antidiuretic effect of desmopressin is decreased by lithium, large doses of epinephrine, demeclocycline, heparin, and alcohol. The antidiuretic effect of desmopressin may be increased by chlorpropamide, urea, and fludrocortisone.

ACTH interacts with aspirin, anticholinesterases, diuretics, barbiturates, and hydantoins.

❖ NURSING IMPLICATIONS AND PATIENT TEACHING

▪ Assessment

Learn everything possible about the patient's health history to determine medication use and the presence of other diseases or conditions that would influence whether it is safe to use pituitary hormones.

▪ Diagnosis

Patients needing anterior pituitary hormones often have many symptoms that must be dealt with while the primary problems are resolved. These patients often have emotional, financial, and physical problems. Diagnosing problems that bother the patient and helping take care of them will be important in meeting the long-term treatment goals for each individual.

▪ Planning

There are no oral forms of pituitary hormones. They are given intramuscularly, subcutaneously, intravenously, or intranasally. Patients taking posterior pituitary products must be monitored closely. Additional doses may be required in times of stress.

▪ Implementation

The dosages of desmopressin are individualized so that the patient has an adequate daily rhythm of water metabolism and adequate duration of sleep. Generally the administration should be at the same time as polyuria or polydipsia and before sleep.

Even though vasopressin is given in an injection, the patient should drink one to two glasses of water at the time of administration to reduce the incidence of adverse effects.

▪ Evaluation

Monitor the patient taking ADH for a decrease in the frequency and the amount of urination, monitor the specific gravity of the urine, and watch for water intoxication or signs of dehydration.

▪ Patient and Family Teaching

Tell the patient and family the following:
• The patient and family should meet regularly with the nurse, physician, or other health care provider. No medications should be stopped, or the dosage altered, without the prescriber's knowledge and approval.
• Patients taking ADH should measure fluid intake and the amount and specific gravity of their urine. They should keep accurate records that should be

reviewed by the nurse, physician, or other health care provider.

- The patient should be aware of the symptoms of water intoxication: drowsiness, listlessness, headache, and convulsions. The drug should be stopped and the nurse, physician, or other health care provider should be contacted at once if any of these symptoms develop. Signs of dehydration—failure to urinate, dry skin and mouth, complaint of thirst, and furrowed tongue—should also be reported.

ADRENOCORTICAL HORMONES

ACTION

The adrenal cortex manufactures glucocorticoids, mineralocorticoids, and small amounts of sex hormones. Hydrocortisone and cortisone are two of the many glucocorticoids produced by the adrenal glands. These hormones regulate glucose, fat, and protein metabolism and control the antiinflammatory response and the immune response system. The mineralocorticoids consist of aldosterone and desoxycorticosterone. These hormones work with others to maintain the fluid and electrolyte balance in the body. They conserve sodium and increase the elimination of potassium. They are used in replacement therapy for adrenal insufficiency.

USES

Glucocorticoids may be given in normal or physiologic doses for replacement of missing hormones in adrenal insufficiency (Addison disease). They are more commonly given in pharmacologic doses to reduce inflammatory, allergic, or immunologic responses and with antineoplastics to treat hematologic and malignant diseases. Examples of when glucocorticoids might be used are acute emergencies, allergic states, collagen diseases, connective tissue disease, diagnostic testing of adrenocortical hyperfunction, edematous states, hematologic and neoplastic diseases, ophthalmologic diseases, respiratory diseases, and miscellaneous conditions such as acute Bell palsy, chronic kidney disease, ulcerative colitis, and thromboembolic disease.

Local steroids might be used for intraarticular (into joints), soft tissue, or intrabursal (into bursae) problems, or for intralesional (into lesions) or subcutaneous dermatologic problems. Steroids might also be used topically for acute and chronic dermatoses, rectal problems, and some eye or ear problems.

ADVERSE REACTIONS

The side effects of systemic corticosteroids in pharmacologic doses are predictable exaggerations of the actions of the corticosteroids that are normally produced by the adrenal glands, or the results of reduced function of the hypothalamic-pituitary-adrenal axis. These are not benign drugs. Some adverse reactions are quite common; others are more unusual. Adverse reactions that might develop are listed in Table 21-6.

DRUG INTERACTIONS

Corticosteroids increase the effects of barbiturates, sedatives, narcotics, and anticoagulants. They decrease the effects of insulin and oral hypoglycemics, coumarin anticoagulants, isoniazid, aspirin, and broad-spectrum antibiotics. Drugs that increase the effects of steroids are indomethacin, aspirin, and oral contraceptives, especially estrogen. Drugs that decrease the effects of steroids include ephedrine, barbiturates, phenytoin, antihistamines, chloral hydrate, rifampin, and propranolol. Some drugs produce exaggerated side effects when given with steroids. These include alcohol, aspirin and antiinflammatory drugs, amphotericin B, thiazides and other potassium-wasting diuretics, anticholinergics, cardiac glycosides, and stimulants such as adrenalin, amphetamines, and ephedrine. Steroids also interfere with numerous laboratory tests.

❖ NURSING IMPLICATIONS AND PATIENT TEACHING

■ Assessment

There are many contraindications and precautions to the use of these drugs. Learn everything possible about the patient's health history, including other diseases, other medications that might interact with corticosteroids, and whether the patient might have an infection or be pregnant.

■ Diagnosis

Once a patient has started glucocorticoids, there is a constant need to look for adverse effects, both physical and psychologic. The nurse must be constantly aware of new symptoms that may represent pathologic conditions or disease.

■ Planning

Steroids come in many forms. Corticosteroids may be administered by the following routes: oral, inhalation, intranasal, IV, intramuscular, subcutaneous, intrabursal, intradermal, intrasynovial, intralesional, soft tissue injection, topical, and per rectum. Only corticosteroid preparations with specific labels should be used for ophthalmologic or otic administration.

Steroids that are used topically affect only a small part of the body. Steroids that are injected or taken by mouth affect the whole body—they have effects throughout the body's systems. Although glucocorticoids are highly potent drugs, short-term use of even very large doses is not likely to cause long-term problems. However, intermediate and long-term administration (longer than 6 days of systemic treatment)

| Table **21-6** | Adverse Reactions Associated with Corticosteroids |

BIOLOGIC SYSTEM	POTENTIAL ADVERSE REACTIONS
Endocrine	Atrophy of adrenal cortex* (can occur after 10 days); anterior pituitary suppression; diabetes* (catabolism of fat, protein, glycogen, resulting in hyperglycemia); fluid/electrolyte imbalance* (from overlapping mineralocorticoid effect); hypokalemia; muscle cramps; irregular heart rate; redeposition of lipids* (moon face, buffalo hump, truncal obesity, striae, hirsutism, acne); and androgenic effects from sex hormones
Gastrointestinal	Gastritis,* peptic ulcer* (unrelated to local irritation of oral tablets); esophagitis; and pancreatitis
Immune	Absence of signs of infection*; uninhibited invasion and proliferation of virus, bacteria, fungus; and inhibition of fibroplasia with delayed wound healing
Musculoskeletal	Muscle wasting* (catabolism of protein) and osteoporosis
Neurologic	Mood changes (euphoria, insomnia, nervousness, irritability); mood swings (psychotic episodes, depression, exaggerated sense of well-being); and EEG changes
Ophthalmologic	Induces or aggravates glaucoma by decreasing aqueous outflow; cataracts; optic nerve damage; increased susceptibility to viral or fungal infection; and corneal perforation (when used in conditions that cause cornea to thin)
Vascular	Thrombosis, thromboembolism, thrombophlebitis, hypercholesterolemia, and atherosclerosis; these problems are especially prominent with cortisone
Miscellaneous	Hypertension; collagen tissue breakdown can activate latent TB by liberating organisms from deposits in pulmonary tissue; hypersensitivity reactions

EEG, Electroencephalogram; *TB*, tuberculosis.
*Most common potential adverse effects.

places the patient at high risk for a large number of serious adverse effects. How much risk is involved and how much benefit the patient will receive must be carefully considered. These medications stop production of steroids by the body, so if the medication is suddenly stopped, the body may be unable to function. The immediate and long-term effects of these drugs vary greatly and depend on the disease, the route of administration, dosage, duration, and frequency and time of administration.

Generic forms of the drugs are much less expensive than brand-name drugs. Generally, prednisone is considered the drug of choice to reduce inflammation and depress the immune system. It is recommended that antacids be taken with or between doses to help reduce the chance of peptic ulcer. Systemic corticosteroids are given orally, except in emergency circumstances or when the patient is unable to take oral medication. The onset of action is 2 to 8 hours, and the effects last for 24 hours. Oral corticosteroids are almost completely absorbed in the GI tract.

When corticosteroids are given orally to patients with functioning adrenal glands, the total dose should be taken first thing in the morning. This is the time when the adrenal glands are normally secreting the most hormones, so the corticosteroid dose will not cause problems with the body's feedback loop.

For conditions requiring a local injection, a single injection yields sufficient antiinflammatory effects to reduce symptoms in many cases. The slowly absorbed forms (acetate, diacetate, tebutate) of corticosteroids generally give relief for 1 to 2 weeks.

■ **Implementation**

Dosages vary a lot; the dose will be determined for each patient and each problem, based on the diagnosis, severity, prognosis, and estimated length of the disease. Patient response and tolerance will also be considered when deciding on dosage. Individuals may respond better to one form than another, but this is unpredictable. The general rule the physician follows, regardless of route of administration, is to prescribe as high a dose as necessary initially to get a favorable response, then decrease the amount gradually to the lowest level that will maintain the therapeutic effect but not produce complications.

In systemic administration, dosage regimens are of two types: (1) physiologic, for replacement of glucocorticoids in adrenal insufficiency; and (2) pharmacologic, to reduce symptoms.

Corticosteroids cannot be stopped without tapering (slowly reducing) the dose over time. Stopping the drug suddenly leads to steroid withdrawal syndrome, with symptoms of anorexia, nausea and vomiting, lethargy, headache, fever, joint pain, skin peeling, myalgia (widespread muscle pain), weight loss, and hypotension. Abruptly stopping the drug may also result in a rebound of symptoms of the condition being treated.

When corticosteroids are administered for longer than 1 to 2 weeks at pharmacologic doses, pituitary release of ACTH is stopped, and this causes secondary adrenocortical insufficiency. Patients undergoing physiologic, emotional, or psychologic stress may need additional support through larger amounts of steroids. This suppression of ACTH may last up to 2 years after the patient stops taking the drug.

During tapering to maintenance doses or to stop the drug, the patient must be watched carefully and taught the signs of adrenal insufficiency (malaise, hypotension, and anorexia [lack of appetite] are common, but many other symptoms may also occur). If these symptoms occur, or if the patient's disease flares up, the steroid dose is increased until symptoms go away. Tapering then begins again on a more gradual plan. After shorter steroid courses (1 to 2 weeks), the dosage is reduced by 50% each day. The same scheduled dose intervals are kept.

Table 21-7 provides a summary of adrenocortical hormones.

▪ Evaluation

All patients receiving systemic corticosteroids should be watched carefully, and the dosage should be adjusted to reflect reduced or increased symptoms, the patient's response, and any periods of stress in the patient's life (injury, infection, surgery, and emotional crisis). Patients should be monitored for 1 or 2 years after high-dosage or long-term treatment. To prevent unmonitored steroid use while patients are receiving steroids, they are usually given prescriptions that cannot be refilled.

Corticosteroids hide infection and increase the patient's risk for infection. Corneal fungal infections are particularly likely to develop with extensive ophthalmologic corticosteroid use. Corticosteroids are particularly dangerous to use in patients with a history of tuberculosis, because the disease can be reactivated. With long-term use, active psychologic disorders may be made worse or hidden disorders made active because steroids affect mood. Long-term use may also produce osteoporosis, leading to vertebral collapse.

Although steroids are often used illegally in sports because they affect muscle size and strength, it is dangerous to take steroids for a long time because of all the damage they can do to the body.

▪ Patient and Family Teaching

Tell the patient and family the following:
- The patient will need to visit the nurse, physician, or other health care provider frequently to monitor progress during and after steroid therapy.
- Nicotine raises the blood level of naturally produced cortisone; therefore heavy smoking may add to the expected action.
- Alcohol may enhance the tendency of steroids to cause ulcers. The patient should avoid alcohol during the course of therapy.

Table 21-7 Adrenocortical Hormones

GENERIC NAME	TRADE NAME	COMMENTS
Glucocorticoids		
Short-Acting		
cortisone	Cortone	Initially: Give PO or IM.
hydrocortisone ★	Cortef	Initially: Dosage may be as low as 0.1 mg 3 times/wk.
hydrocortisone acetate	Hydrocortisone Acetate	For intralesional, intraarticular, or soft tissue injection only. Do not give IV. Adults: Dosage depends on site.
hydrocortisone sodium succinate	Solu-Cortef	Adults: Give IV or IM and repeat at 2-, 4-, or 6-hour intervals, depending on patient response.
Intermediate-Acting		
methylprednisolone	Depo-Medrol	Give IM.
prednisolone	Delta-Cortef	Give PO.
prednisone ★	Meticorten	Give PO.
triamcinolone	Aristocort	Give PO.
triamcinolone diacetate	Aristocort Forte	Give IM, intraarticular, or intrasynovial.
Long-Acting		
betamethasone	Celestone	Give PO, IM, or IV.
dexamethasone	Decadron	Give PO.
Mineralocorticoids		
fludrocortisone acetate	Florinef Acetate	Adults: Give IV or IM, repeated at 2-, 4-, or 6-hour intervals, depending on patient response.

IM, Intramuscular; *IV,* intravenous; *PO,* by mouth.
★ Indicates "Must-Know Drugs," or the 35 drugs most prescribers use.

- Steroids may decrease resistance to infection and the ability to tolerate stress, injury, or surgery (including dental surgery). The patient should inform the nurse, physician, or other health care provider or dentist or surgeon that a steroid is being taken.
- The patient may need an increased dosage of steroids during times of injury, illness, or emotional or psychologic stress for up to 2 years after long-term treatment with steroids.
- The patient and family should know the signs and symptoms of adrenal insufficiency. Malaise, weakness, hypotension, anorexia, nausea and vomiting, aching of bones and muscles, headache, increased temperature, and diarrhea are common, but many other symptoms may also develop. The nurse, physician, or other health care provider should be contacted immediately if any of these problems develop.
- The patient must not stop taking the steroids suddenly. The body will slowly grow to depend on them and will not be able to survive well without them.
- During and after corticosteroid treatment, the patient should wear a MedicAlert bracelet or necklace or carry a medical identification card with the name of the drug.
- The patient should not receive any immunizations without consulting the nurse, physician, or other health care provider first.
- The patient should take oral medication with food to minimize stomach upset.
- The patient may need to eat a diet rich in potassium and low in sodium. The nurse, physician, or other health care provider should give the patient a list of foods to eat and foods to avoid.
- The patient should keep the tablets in tightly sealed, brown bottles away from heat.
- The female patient should tell the nurse, physician, or other health care provider if she becomes pregnant or begins to take medications from another health care provider, especially aspirin, diuretics, digitalis preparations, insulin, oral hypoglycemics, phenobarbital, rifampin, phenytoin, and somatotropin.
- If the patient misses a dose:
  - If the patient is on an alternate-day schedule, the dose should be taken as soon as possible, and the regular schedule should be followed. If the patient does not remember until the evening, the missed dose should be taken the next morning, the day after that should be skipped, and a new schedule should be started.
  - If the patient is on a daily-dose schedule, the dose should be taken as soon as possible. If the patient does not remember until the next day, only the normal dose should be taken, and the normal schedule should be followed.
  - If the patient is on divided doses (taking medication more than once a day), the dose should be taken as soon as possible, and the normal schedule should be followed. If the patient forgets to take the medication until it is time for the next dose, that dose should be doubled, and then the patient should go back on the regular schedule.
- Patients should call the nurse, physician, or other health care provider if they have rapid weight gain; black or tarry stools; unusual bleeding or bruising; or signs of hypokalemia (decreased potassium in the blood), including anorexia, lethargy, confusion, nausea, and muscle weakness.
- It is important to have frequent appointments to monitor therapy while the patient is taking this drug.

SEX HORMONES

OVERVIEW

The sex hormones are produced under the influence of the anterior pituitary gland. The male hormone testosterone and its related hormones are called *androgens*; the female hormones are *estrogen* and *progesterone*. **Androgens** help to develop and maintain the male sex organs at puberty and develop secondary sex characteristics in men (facial hair, deep voice, body hair, body fat distribution, and muscle development). They promote the anabolic or tissue-building processes in the body. Anabolic steroids are synthetic drugs with the same use and actions as androgens. These medications may be given as replacement therapy for testosterone deficiency. Androgen therapy may also be given to women as part of the treatment for estrogen-dependent inoperative metastatic breast carcinoma in patients who are past menopause. Androgens are also used to reduce postpartum breast pain and engorgement. Some postmenopausal women also use low-dose androgen therapy to treat a relative androgen deficiency. This helps reverse some of the masculinizing symptoms of menopause.

In addition to the two naturally occurring female hormones estrogen and progesterone, there are also a number of synthetic estrogen and progesterone preparations. **Estrogen** is secreted by the ovarian follicle and the adrenal cortex. Estrogens help develop and maintain the female reproductive system and the primary and secondary sex characteristics in women. They also are part of the feedback system to the pituitary, providing signals for the release of the gonadotropins. Estrogens play a role in the fluid and electrolyte balance in the tissues, especially in relation to calcium. They are active in most of the tissue and muscular processes involved in pregnancy and labor.

Progesterone is produced by the corpus luteum in the ovary, by the placenta, and in small amounts by the adrenal cortex. Progesterone is essential for the development of the placenta and helps maintain pregnancy once it occurs. Progesterone also helps prevent pregnancy by inhibiting the pituitary gonadotropins that cause the ovarian follicle to mature and produce ovulation.

Estrogen, progesterone, and combinations of the two hormones are very effective as oral contraceptives. They prevent ovulation and cause a state that mimics pregnancy in the female.

✤ MALE SEX HORMONES

ANDROGENS

ACTION

The main action of androgens is to develop secondary male sex characteristics. Androgens are anabolic, increasing the building of tissue. Androgens are also antineoplastic when used to treat certain breast cancers in women. Erythropoiesis, or an increase in red blood cell formation, occurs with the administration of androgens.

USES

Androgens are used in hypogonadism, hypopituitarism, dwarfism, eunuchism, cryptorchidism, oligospermia, and general androgen deficiency in males. They are used to restore a positive nitrogen balance in patients with chronic, debilitating illness or trauma; in treatment of anemia secondary to renal failure and in other blood dyscrasias in which increased erythropoiesis is needed; for palliative therapy (therapy to treat symptoms in terminal cases) for advanced breast cancer in postmenopausal women; and for treatment of endometriosis in younger women. Androgens are also used to suppress milk production. They are commonly misused by body builders and athletes who wish to have bigger and stronger muscles.

ADVERSE REACTIONS

Adverse reactions to androgens include edema caused by sodium retention (usually only with large doses), acne, hirsutism (excessive body hair), male pattern baldness, cholestatic hepatitis with jaundice, buccal irritation, diarrhea, nausea, and vomiting. In women, androgens may produce clitoral enlargement and masculinization. In men, androgens may cause a decrease in sperm count, excessive sexual stimulation, gynecomastia (enlargement of the breasts), impotence, and urinary retention. In children, use of androgens may produce precocious puberty. Children may also develop short stature because of premature bone epiphyseal closure.

DRUG INTERACTIONS

Anabolic steroids may increase the effects of anticoagulants, antidiabetic agents, and other drugs. Corticosteroids given at the same time as androgens increase the possibility of edema. Barbiturates decrease the therapeutic effects of androgens because of increased breakdown in the liver. Androgens may affect the results of many laboratory tests.

❖ NURSING IMPLICATIONS AND PATIENT TEACHING

■ Assessment

Learn as much as possible about the health history of the patient, including the presence of carcinoma; cardiac, renal, or liver dysfunction; other drugs the patient may be taking; and the possibility of pregnancy.

The male patient may have a history of impotence, reduced libido (sex drive), weight loss, male climacteric, or castration. There may be a history of traumatic castration or failure to develop secondary sex characteristics by 15 to 17 years of age.

■ Diagnosis

These patients often have other problems that need to be diagnosed and addressed. In addition to their medical problems, they often have great concern about their sexuality, body image, and self-esteem.

■ Planning

When androgens are given for hypogonadism, careful descriptions of secondary sex characteristics and measurements should be recorded for a baseline to monitor the therapeutic effects.

If cholestatic jaundice develops or liver function decreases, the drug should be stopped. Stomatitis (inflammation of the mouth) may result from buccal administration.

■ Implementation

Androgens can be taken buccally, sublingually, and through the skin as a patch, depending on the specific drug and the reason for therapy. Dosages vary from 2 to 10 mg daily for replacement therapy. Higher divided doses are given for antineoplastic therapy.

Patients must be taught not to swallow the pill and not to eat, drink, or smoke or chew tobacco until the buccal tablet is absorbed.

Table 21-8 provides a summary of androgen products.

■ Evaluation

The therapeutic response may be slow, requiring 3 or more months to affect symptoms. Monitor for the development of secondary sex characteristics and improvement in sexual functioning.

Table 21-8 Androgens

GENERIC NAME	TRADE NAME	COMMENTS
danazol	Androxy	Synthetic androgen is used to treat endometriosis, fibrocystic breast disease, and hereditary angioedema through suppression of pituitary gonadotropins and subsequent reduction in menstruation. Endometriosis: Give twice daily for 3-6 mo; may be continued for 9 mo. Used only for those who cannot tolerate other drugs or who fail to respond; therapy begun during menstruation to rule out pregnancy. Fibrocystic breast disease: Give PO twice daily for 4-6 mo; begun during menstruation; used only when pain is severe.
fluoxymesterone	Androxy, Halotestin	GI disturbances are more frequent with this product than with other oral androgens. Oral medication used for hypogonadism or breast cancer treatment.
methyltestosterone	Android Testred Virilon	Patient should not drink, eat, or smoke or chew tobacco until tablet is absorbed buccally. Check mouth each visit for signs of local irritation. Used for male eunuchism, androgen deficiency, undescended testicle after puberty, and female breast cancer.
testosterone gel	AndroGel Testin	Primary hypogonadism: 1% gel (5 g tube contains 50 mg testosterone) applied in the morning to clean, dry, intact skin of shoulders, upper arms. AndroGel may be applied to abdomen, Testin is not used on abdomen. Application adjusted based on blood levels of testosterone.
Testosterone cypionate (in oil)	Depo-Testosterone	Give injection every 2-4 wk.
testosterone pellets	Testopel	Use pellets given SQ every 3-6 mo. Each pellet contains 75 mg of testosterone. Number of pellets to be implanted gradually increases as parenteral injection dosage decreases.
Testosterone transdermal system	Androderm	5 mg/day or two systems initially. System applied at night to a clean, dry area of skin on the back, abdomen, upper arms, or thighs. Should *not* be applied to scrotum. Patches worn for 24 hours. Blood levels tested and drug titrated up or down through use of additional patch.
	Testoderm	Primary or secondary hypogonadism: Therapy started with a 6-mg/day system applied daily. Patch placed on a clean, dry scrotal area and worn 22-23 hr daily. After 3-4 wk of use, blood levels checked 2-4 hr after applying patch. Patient should achieve adequate blood levels in 6-8 wk or shift to another form of therapy.
testosterone buccal	Striant	Mucoadhesive tablets for replacement therapy: 1 tablet taken morning and night; rounded side placed against gum and held firmly in place for 30 seconds to ensure adhesion. Tablet remains in position until the next tablet is applied. Protect tablet from heat and moisture.
Androgen Hormone Inhibitors		
finasteride	Propecia Proscar	Used in benign prostatic hyperplasia and prostatic carcinoma; 5 mg once daily. May require 6 mo of therapy or more. Also used in treating male pattern alopecia

GI, Gastrointestinal; *PO,* by mouth; *SQ,* subcutaneous.

■ Patient and Family Teaching

Tell the patient and family the following:

- The patient should take this medication as instructed by the prescribing health care provider.
- Response to the drug may take several weeks or months.
- The patient should eat a diet high in calories, protein, vitamins, and minerals unless otherwise instructed by the nurse, physician, or other health care provider.

- The patient should report any new or troublesome symptoms that may develop. Men should report fluid retention, especially in the feet and hands; enlargement of breasts; shortness of breath; excessive physical or sexual stimulation; prolonged or painful erection of the penis; impotence; urinary retention; and jaundice. Women should report jaundice; fluid retention, especially in the feet and hands; shortness of breath; changes in vaginal bleeding; increased sex drive; and masculinization of appearance. (Signs of masculinization in women usually are reversed when the drug is discontinued.)

- If medicine is taken under the tongue (sublingually) or buccally (putting medicine in cheek), the patient should rinse the mouth and brush the teeth after taking medicine.

✣ FEMALE SEX HORMONES

ESTROGENS

ACTION

Exogenous estrogens (those produced outside the body) aid in the development of both primary and secondary sex characteristics, including growth and development of the uterine musculature and endothelium, vaginal epithelium, and fallopian tubes; development of breasts; increased cervical mucus and decreased vaginal pH; increased uterine motility; growth of axillary and pubic hair; decreased long bone growth in prepubertal and pubertal girls; and decreased calcium loss from bones. Estrogens suppress the release of gonadotropins (FSH and LH) from the pituitary or hypothalamus through a feedback mechanism. Estrogens are anabolic and cause retention of salt, water, and nitrogen, an increase in serum lipoproteins and triglycerides, and a decrease in cholesterol. They suppress ovulation when given in adequate doses.

USES

Estrogens are used for hormone replacement therapy in menopause or other conditions in which the natural estrogens are decreased, such as ovarian failure, primary amenorrhea, and oophorectomy. They are used in infertility work-ups, for palliative therapy in prostatic cancer, and in breast cancer that occurs at least 5 years after menopause. After many years of controversy, it has now been demonstrated conclusively that estrogens are effective for prevention of postmenopausal osteoporosis when used with other measures, but they do increase the risk for stroke, heart attack, and breast cancer. Estrogen-progestin combinations also seem to provide a decreased incidence of uterine cancer. Use of these drugs should be determined for each patient after a careful weighing of the risks and benefits.

ADVERSE REACTIONS

Adverse reactions to estrogens include edema, hypertension, thrombophlebitis, depression, migraine headaches, skin rash, decreased glucose tolerance, intolerance to contact lenses, abdominal cramps, diarrhea, nausea, vomiting, breast tenderness and enlargement, changes in vaginal bleeding, worsening of estrogen-dependent malignancies, increase in size of uterine fibroids, vaginal candidiasis, and changes in weight and libido.

DRUG INTERACTIONS

Rifampin and barbiturates may reduce the effects of estrogen. Estrogens may reduce the effects of oral anticoagulants, tricyclic antidepressants, anticonvulsants, and antidiabetic agents. They may potentiate anti-inflammatory or glycosuric effects of hydrocortisone and the effect of meperidine. Estrogens alter the results of many diagnostic tests.

PROGESTINS

ACTION

Progestins cause the uterine endometrium to shed during menses after tissue growth stimulated by estrogen. They maintain the endometrium and vaginal epithelium and decrease uterine motility during pregnancy. Acting with estrogen, they cause the breasts to secrete milk and become more vascular. Some progestins have estrogenic or androgenic effects. Progestins suppress pituitary gonadotropins through a feedback mechanism. They can suppress ovulation, control uterine bleeding caused by hormonal imbalance, increase sodium excretion, and cause a negative nitrogen balance.

USES

Progestins are used for contraception, control of excessive uterine bleeding caused by hormonal imbalance, treatment of secondary amenorrhea, dysmenorrhea, and premenstrual tension, and control of pain in endometriosis. They may be used in the diagnosis and treatment of infertility. They are also used as palliative therapy for endometrial cancer. When used for contraception, progestin-only preparations are known as "mini-pills."

ADVERSE REACTIONS

Adverse reactions to progestins include fluid retention, thromboembolic events (including pulmonary embolism), dizziness, headache, mental depression, rashes, decrease in glucose tolerance, weight gain or loss, cholestatic jaundice, diarrhea, nausea, vomiting, amenorrhea, breast tenderness or enlargement, decreased libido, galactorrhea, increased vaginal discharge, spotting, and withdrawal bleeding (bleeding that occurs when the drug is stopped). Overdosage produces changes in menses, nausea, vomiting, and withdrawal bleeding.

DRUG INTERACTIONS

Progestins alter the results of several laboratory tests.

❖ NURSING IMPLICATIONS AND PATIENT TEACHING

■ Assessment

For patients who have not had menses, ask about primary amenorrhea and sexual infantilism. For women of childbearing age, ask about the possibility of pregnancy, history of ovarian failure, need for contraception, and dysmenorrhea. For patients near the age of menopause, see if they have a history of hot flashes, menstrual irregularities, dyspareunia (pain during intercourse), vaginal discharge, vulvar pruritus, urinary frequency, and history of oophorectomy or hysterectomy.

There is an increased dose-related risk of thromboembolic disease, especially in premenopausal women. Progestins should not be used during pregnancy, especially the first 3 months, because of the risk of congenital anomalies and of vaginal adenosis or vaginal or cervical cancer in female offspring when they reach childbearing age. There is an increased risk of gallbladder disease with long-term use. Postmenopausal estrogen therapy is associated with an increase in the risk of endometrial cancer of 5 to 15 times the normal risk; the level of risk is related to the length of treatment. Administration of estrogen may result in hypercalcemia in patients with breast or bone cancer.

■ Diagnosis

Based on the assessment, the nurse should be prepared to recognize and deal with other emotional or physical problems arising from estrogen or progestin use. As women go through their reproductive years, they have different concerns and physical problems. Determine age-related factors that may be of concern to the patient. Individualize therapy as much as possible.

■ Planning

Estrogen therapy affects many body systems. When estrogens are used before puberty, short stature and decreased growth can result. Use in adult women can increase the risk for migraine headaches, hypertension, diabetes, and certain benign and malignant tumors. Because estrogens are metabolized in the liver and excreted through the kidneys, renal or hepatic dysfunction can alter their actions. Fibroid tumors of the uterus may increase in size. Because fluid is retained, symptoms of hypertension, asthma, epilepsy, migraine, and heart or kidney dysfunction may be increased. Topical estrogens are readily absorbed and may have systemic effects.

Progestins are especially valuable in women who cannot take estrogen. Progestins often cause menstrual cycle changes, and patients must understand this before taking these drugs if they are to have a successful experience. These medications can be used for contraception in women who are breastfeeding.

■ Implementation

Estrogens can be given orally, intramuscularly, or topically. For control of menopausal symptoms, ovarian failure, or postoophorectomy symptoms, they are usually given in cycles of one tablet daily for 3 weeks, followed by 1 week off the drug. Usually, the lowest effective dose is given for the shortest period. High doses or long-term therapy should be tapered gradually.

Natural progestins are poorly absorbed orally; therefore oral progestins are synthetic products. Tablets are given daily. Progestins are quickly metabolized in the liver, but daily doses are effective.

Table 21-9 presents a summary of estrogens and progestins.

■ Evaluation

Patients on female hormone therapy should be monitored regularly, and the nurse should watch for adverse effects. Problems that should raise concern are thrombophlebitis and edema in women and feminizing changes or impotence in men.

Timing and description of any vaginal bleeding should be noted to determine if response is therapeutic or adverse.

■ Patient and Family Teaching

Tell the patient and family the following:
- Estrogenic drugs, by law, must be dispensed with a patient package insert titled "What You Should Know About Estrogens." The patient should look for this package insert and read it thoroughly.
- Some patients experience side effects when taking this medication. If any of the following symptoms develop, the patient should stop taking the medication and contact the nurse, physician, or other health care provider immediately: chest pain, abdominal or leg pain or swelling, sudden severe headaches, visual changes, sudden loss of coordination, sudden shortness of breath, or slurred speech.
- The patient should discontinue the drug immediately if she believes she is pregnant.
- Less dangerous symptoms that require care or consultation with a health care provider include changes in vaginal bleeding or discharge, skin rash, breast lumps, jaundice, hypertension, abdominal pain, and mental depression.
- Nausea and breast tenderness may occur early in therapy but should lessen after 1 to 3 weeks; taking oral medicines with food may reduce nausea.
- Less common side effects are changes in libido, photosensitivity, chloasma (facial skin changes often seen in pregnancy), and vomiting.
- Use of estrogens for replacement is associated with an increased risk of developing endometrial cancer. The patient should report any vaginal bleeding after

Table 21-9   Estrogens and Progestins

GENERIC NAME	TRADE NAME	COMMENTS
Estrogens		
conjugated estrogens	Premarin	Contain 50%-65% sodium estrone sulfate and 20%-35% sodium equilin sulfate; these are naturally occurring and extracted from the urine of pregnant mares. Store in closed containers. Medication should be given for 3 wk on a daily basis, with 1 wk off the medication. Used for shortest time possible due to long-term adverse effects on heart.
esterified estrogens	Menest	Contain 75%-85% sodium estrone sulfate and 6%-15% sodium equilin sulfate. Store medication in a tightly closed container. Vasomotor menopausal (natural or surgical) symptoms: Adjusted to lowest dose that controls symptoms.
estradiol	Climara Delestrogen Estrace Estraderm	Vasomotor menopausal symptoms, senile vaginitis, kraurosis vulvae, or replacement therapy in hypogonadism or female castration, ovarian failure. Give PO daily, cycled 3 wk on and 1 wk off. Lowest therapeutic dosage should be used. Transdermal system: Use patch 2 times/wk, increasing dose until symptoms resolve. May use 3-wk cycle on patch, 1 wk off.
estrogen vaginal creams	Estrace Estring Premarin	Preparations used vaginally and on vulva to treat atrophic epithelial changes related to low estrogen levels. Can be absorbed systemically and produce side effects. Most effective when used at bedtime. Contain various synthetic estrogens. Usual dose: Use applicator included or rub on topically; lowest dose for shortest time that will control symptoms.
estropipate or piperazine estrone	Ogen	Composed of crystalline estrone and piperazine for stability. Prevention of postmenopausal osteoporosis, senile vaginitis, or vasomotor menopausal symptoms: Cycled 3 wk on, 1 wk off; lowest dose that controls symptoms should be used.
Estrogen and Progestin Combination		
conjugated estrogens; medroxyprogesterone	Prempro Premphase	Moderate to severe vasomotor symptoms associated with menopause, prevention of osteoporosis: Give tablet once daily. Atrophic vaginitis: Vaginal cream daily for 1-2 wk then reduced dose 1-3 times/wk.
Estrogen Agonist/Antagonists		
raloxifene	Evista	Use for osteoporosis prevention.
Progestins		
medroxyprogesterone acetate	Provera	Duration of action is long and somewhat variable. Secondary amenorrhea, abnormal uterine bleeding caused by hormonal imbalance: Give daily for 5-10 days, beginning on 16th or 21st day of menstrual cycle. Maximum therapeutic effect will be noted with 10 mg/day for 10 days beginning on 16th day of cycle. Withdrawal bleeding should occur 3-7 days after last dose.
megestrol acetate	Megace	Used for appetite enhancement in AIDS and cancer patients and for palliative treatment of advanced carcinoma of the breast or endometrium.
norethindrone	Micronor Nor-QD Ovrette	This medication represents the only ingredient in some "mini-pill" contraceptives. Should be taken with meals to reduce nausea and stored in a closed container. Amenorrhea or uterine bleeding caused by hormonal imbalance: Give daily on 5th to 25th day of the menstrual cycle. Endometriosis: Give daily for 2 wk, increasing at 2-wk intervals until a target dose is reached. Continued 6-9 mo or until breakthrough bleeding occurs. Then it can be stopped temporarily.

GENERIC NAME	TRADE NAME	COMMENTS
Table 21-9		**Estrogens and Progestins—cont'd**
norethindrone acetate	Aygestin	This medication is twice as strong as norethindrone. It is mildly androgenic. Should be taken with meals to reduce nausea and stored in a closed container. Uterine bleeding caused by hormonal imbalance: Give daily on 5th to 25th day of the menstrual cycle. Endometriosis: Give daily for 2-wk, increasing at 2-wk intervals until a target dose is reached. Continued 6-9 mo or until breakthrough bleeding occurs. Then it can be stopped temporarily. The object of therapy is to prevent menstruation
progesterone	Crinone	For amenorrhea, abnormal uterine bleeding, AIDS wasting: Give daily for 6-8 days by IM injection.

AIDS, Acquired immunodeficiency syndrome; *IM*, intramuscular; *PO*, by mouth.

menopause to the nurse, physician, or other health care provider.

- If surgery is anticipated, the surgeon should be notified so that doses may be changed or briefly stopped.
- Patients of all ages should be monitored regularly while on any estrogen preparation.
- The patient should take the pills exactly as directed and keep them out of the reach of children or anyone for whom they are not prescribed.
- When used for a short period to treat dysfunctional bleeding, progestins should first stop the bleeding and then cause the endometrial lining to shed when the drug is stopped (withdrawal bleeding). Improvement of heavy bleeding should occur in 24 to 48 hours.
- Breakthrough or withdrawal bleeding can occur, especially in long-term use for contraception. The patient should report abnormal or unexplained vaginal bleeding to the nurse, physician, or other health care provider.
- The patient should not take progestins if there is a history of breast or genital cancer, except as palliative treatment in advanced disease.
- Diabetic patients should tell the health care provider if they begin developing positive urine tests so that antidiabetic medication can be adjusted.
- Many herbal products are marketed to provide hormone replacement therapy. These products are not regulated, standardized, or tested, and caution should be used in their use.

ORAL CONTRACEPTIVES

ACTION

Most oral contraceptives are combination drugs that contain both an estrogen and a progestin. The principal action is to prevent ovulation by inhibiting FSH and LH. The progestin-only "mini-pill" prevents ovulation by the same mechanism but is more variable in suppressing the gonadotropins. The progestins in both types of oral contraceptive pills have several other contraceptive effects: creating thick cervical mucus hostile to sperm, slowing ovum transport by decreasing motility of the fallopian tubes, and blocking implantation. Oral contraceptive pills come in a variety of combinations, including those like Yasmin with very low estrogen content.

USES

Oral contraceptives are used to prevent pregnancy when a highly effective method is needed and heterosexual activity is regular.

ADVERSE REACTIONS

Information on adverse reactions to oral contraceptives is provided in the previous sections on estrogen and progestin. Most adverse reactions are caused by hormonal imbalance. The types of hormonal imbalance and the symptoms they cause include the following:

- Estrogen excess may produce nausea, dizziness, edema, cyclic weight gain, bloating, increase in fibroid size, uterine cramps, irritability, increased fat deposition, poor contact lens fit, vascular-type headache, hypertension, suppression of lactation, cystic breast changes, breast tenderness, thrombophlebitis, cerebrovascular infarction, myocardial infarction, and hepatic adenoma.
- Progestin excess may cause increased appetite and weight gain (noncyclic), tiredness, malaise, depression and decrease in libido, acne, alopecia (hair loss), cholestatic jaundice, decreased length of menstrual flow, hypertension, headaches during the "resting" phase of the cycle (the time that the patient is off the drug), breast tenderness, decreased carbohydrate tolerance, dilated leg veins, and pelvic congestion syndrome.
- Androgen excess may produce increased appetite and weight gain, hirsutism, acne, oily skin, rash, increased libido, cholestatic jaundice, and pruritus.

- Estrogen deficiency may cause irritability, nervousness, hot flashes, vasomotor symptoms, uterine prolapse, pelvic relaxation symptoms, early and midcycle spotting, decreased amount of menstrual flow, no withdrawal bleeding, decreased libido, dry vaginal mucosa, atrophic vaginitis and dyspareunia, headaches, and depression.
- Progestin deficiency may produce late breakthrough bleeding and spotting, heavy menstrual flow and clots, delayed onset of menses, dysmenorrhea, and weight loss.

Emergency Contraception

Any time a woman has unprotected intercourse and does not want to become pregnant, she may use an emergency contraception kit containing two tablets (or take two multiple-tablet doses) of selected combined oral contraceptive pills. Treatment must be started within 72 hours of intercourse, with two doses taken 12 hours apart. Emergency contraceptive pills work primarily by blocking or delaying ovulation or by changing the way sperm or ova are transported, thereby preventing conception. The risk of pregnancy is decreased by 75%. The pills often produce nausea and irregular menstrual bleeding.

DRUG INTERACTIONS

There may be an increase in breakthrough bleeding and a decrease in contraceptive effectiveness in patients taking antitubercular medication, many antibiotics, barbiturates, and anticonvulsants.

Oral contraceptives may decrease the effectiveness of anticoagulants, antihypertensives, anticonvulsants, tricyclic antidepressants, oral hypoglycemics, and vitamins. When oral contraceptives are given with troleandomycin, the effect may be additive in causing jaundice. Oral contraceptives may alter many laboratory test results.

 Clinical Goldmine

Obtaining a History

Ask the patient for a detailed menstrual history and history of any thromboembolic events, migraine headaches, and liver or kidney problems.

❖ NURSING IMPLICATIONS AND PATIENT TEACHING

■ Assessment

To determine the most appropriate type of contraception for a patient, learn as much about the patient's history as possible, including a thorough menstrual, contraceptive, and reproductive history. This must include any current diseases, the patient's drug history, and whether the patient smokes. The nurse should

make certain the patient is not breastfeeding or pregnant, assess the patient's sexual activity and knowledge of contraceptive methods, and discover whether there are any contraindications for drug use (Box 21-1).

■ Diagnosis

Does the patient have other knowledge deficits or financial, nutritional, or social problems that would interfere with her taking this medication? For example, women who smoke and use oral contraceptives are at

---

Box 21-1	Contraindications for Oral Contraceptives

ABSOLUTE CONTRAINDICATIONS

History or presence of thromboembolic disorders, cerebrovascular accident, coronary artery disease, hepatic adenoma, malignancy of breast or reproductive system, known impairment of liver function, and pregnancy.

STRONG RELATIVE CONTRAINDICATIONS

Severe headaches (particularly vascular or migraine)*; hypertension (with resting diastolic blood pressure of 90 mm Hg or greater on three or more separate visits or an accurate measurement of 110 mm Hg or more on a single visit)*; diabetes*; prediabetes or a strong family history of diabetes; gallbladder disease, including cholecystectomy*; previous cholestasis during pregnancy; congenital hyperbilirubinemia (Gilbert disease); mononucleosis (acute phase); sickle cell disease or sickle C disease*; undiagnosed, abnormal vaginal bleeding†; elective surgery (planned in next 4 weeks or major surgery requiring immobilization)*; long leg casts or major injury to lower leg; patient older than 40 years of age*; patient older than 35 years of age with a history of heavy smoking*; and impaired liver function within the past year.

OTHER RELATIVE CONTRAINDICATIONS

Termination of term pregnancy within past 10 to 14 days,* weight gain of 10 pounds or more while on the pill,* failure to have established regular menstrual cycles,* profile suggestive of anovulation and infertility problems (late onset of menses and very irregular, painless menses),* presence of or history of cardiac or renal disease,* conditions likely to make patient unreliable at following dosage instructions (mental retardation, major psychiatric problems, alcoholism, history of repeatedly taking pills incorrectly),* lactation (oral contraceptives may be started as weaning begins and may be an aid in decreasing the flow of milk).*

Women with the following problems may begin taking oral contraceptives but should be observed carefully for worsening or improvement of the problem: depression,* hypertension (with resting diastolic blood pressure of 90 to 99 mm Hg at a single visit),* presence of or history of chloasma or alopecia related to pregnancy,* asthma,* epilepsy,* uterine fibromyoma,* acne, varicose veins,* history of hepatitis (but liver function tests are normal now and have been for at least 1 year).

*These are contraindications to estrogen-containing pills. They may not be contraindications to progestin-only pills or may be less of a contraindication to progestin-only pills than to combined pills.
†Some believe this to be an absolute contraindication.

much greater risk for venospasm and thromboembolic events. These women should either not be placed on oral birth control (OBC) if they are older than 35 years or should be helped to discontinue smoking.

 Clinical Pitfall

Adverse Effects of Smoking

Patients should be questioned about smoking while taking the pill. Patients who smoke while taking oral contraceptives, especially if they are older then 35 years, are at increased risk of adverse effects.

For women using emergency contraception, do they understand other more effective ways to prevent pregnancy?

■ Planning

Although breakthrough bleeding may be a side effect, nonfunctional causes should be investigated. Bleeding irregularities are more common with progestin-only pills.

There is some risk of infertility after oral contraceptives are stopped, especially in women who have had irregular or scanty periods before taking pills.

Research suggests that many women forget to take pills, resulting in many unintentional pregnancies. Discuss with the patient how the pill will fit into her lifestyle in such a way that she will remember to take it.

■ Implementation

To be effective, oral contraceptives must be taken at about the same time each day. This is particularly true with progestin-only pills. Taking medication with meals will reduce the nausea common in the first cycles.

All oral combination contraceptives are to be taken for 21 days. Usually, therapy is started either the fifth day after or the Sunday after menstruation starts. Another method of contraception should be used for the first 7 to 10 days of the first cycle. Pills are packaged in a 1-month packet with the days named or numbered. Some preparations contain 28 pills to be taken daily, 7 of which contain an inert substance or iron. Others require the patient to go 7 days without pills before starting another 28-day cycle. During the "resting" phase of the cycle, vaginal bleeding should occur.

Combination pills vary in the type and amount of estrogen and progestin they contain (Box 21-2). All have at least one estrogen and one progestin. Two estrogens, ethinyl estradiol and mestranol, may be used in the different pills. Mestranol is half as strong as ethinyl estradiol. Several progestins are

---

Box 21-2   Content of Oral Combination (Estrogen and Progestin) Contraceptive Pills

MESTRANOL AND NORETHINDRONE
- Norinyl 1+50
- Ortho-Novum 1/50

ESTRADIOL AND NORETHINDRONE
- Brevicon
- Modicon
- Norinyl 1+35
- Ortho-Novum 1/35
- Ovcon-50; Ovcon-35

ESTRADIOL AND NORETHINDRONE BIPHASIC OR TRIPHASIC PILLS
- Ortho-Novum 10/11 (Norethindrone dose increases in phase 2)
- Ortho-Novum 7/7/7 (Norethindrone dose increases in phases 2 and 3)
- Tri-Levlen (Norethindrone dose increases in phases 2 and 3)
- Tri-Norinyl (Norethindrone dose increases in phases 2 and 3)
- Triphasil (Norethindrone dose increases in phases 2 and 3)

ESTRADIOL AND NORETHINDRONE ACETATE
- Loestrin 21 1.5/30; Fe 1.5/30; 21 1/20; Fe 1/20

ESTRADIOL AND ETHYNODIOL DIACETATE
- Demulen 1/35; 1/50

ESTRADIOL AND LEVONORGESTREL
- Levlen
- Nordette

ESTRADIOL AND NORGESTREL
- Lo/Ovral
- Ovral

ESTRADIOL AND DESOGESTREL
- Ortho-Cept

ETHINYL ESTRADIOL AND DROSPIRENONE
- Yasmin
- YAS

---

used in combination with them. Some progestins are estrogenic, antiestrogenic, or androgenic in effect. A dose of 50 mcg or less of estrogen is used to start therapy. Less than this dose may cause breakthrough bleeding, but doses of less than 50 mcg are increasingly being prescribed. Yasmin and YAS are low-estrogen formulations containing drospirenone and ethinyl estradiol. YAS may also be effective in preventing mild premenstrual syndrome. New combinations are introduced frequently. For the progestin-only pills, the medication is taken daily on a continuous basis.

Table 21-10 provides a summary of oral contraceptives.

Table 21-10 Oral Contraceptives

GENERIC NAME	TRADE NAME	COMMENTS AND DOSAGE
estrogen and progestin combinations	**Monophasic:** Demulen Loestrin Lo/Ovral Lunelle Modicon Nordette Norinyl Ortho-Cept Ortho-Novum Ovcon Ovral **Biphasic:** Mircette Necon Ortho-Novum 10/11 **Triphasic:** Estro Step Fe Estro Step 21 Ortho Novum 7/7/7 Ortho-Tri-Cyclin Tri-Levlen Tri-Norinyl Triphasil Trivora-28	The patient should take 1 pill each day for 21 days, beginning with the regimen the prescribing health care provider suggests, either starting the Sunday after a period begins or 5 days after the onset of the period. If there are 7 inert pills, they should be taken after the 21-day cycle. If not, the patient should start a new pack 7 days after finishing the 21-day cycle. If 1 pill is missed, the forgotten one should be taken and a backup contraceptive method used. If 2 pills are missed, 2 should be taken for 2 consecutive days and another method used until the end of the cycle. If 3 are missed, a new pack should be started on the 8th day or the first Sunday after the last pill was taken. Another birth control method must be used for 7-14 days, depending on the dosage.
progestin only (mini-pills)	Micronor Nor-QD Ovrette	Pills must be taken at the same time each day to be most effective. Only the most reliable patients should use these pills. These pills are slightly less effective than combination products in preventing pregnancy. Incidence of pregnancy highest in first 6 mo of use. Breakthrough bleeding more common than with combination pills; therefore undiagnosed genital bleeding is an important contraindication, especially in older women. Patient should take 1 pill at the same time every day continually and not stop during menses.

Other Contraceptive Forms

GENERIC NAME	TRADE NAME	COMMENTS AND DOSAGE
emergency contraception	Plan B Preven Emergency Contraceptive Kit	Initiate treatment within 72 hr of intercourse, with 2 doses taken 12 hr apart. (Patients may also use 2 multiple-tablet doses of combined oral contraceptive medications such as Ovral, Lo/Ovral, Levlen, Nordette, Tri-Levlen, and Triphasil according to the instructions given in the package insert.)
levonorgestrel intrauterine system	Mirena	For women who have had at least one child, this system is implanted in the uterus. It provides contraception for up to 5 yr.
medroxyprogesterone acetate	Depo-Provera	Long-term injectable contraceptive. Patient given 150 mg every 3 mo after onset of normal menses. Injected in gluteal or deltoid muscle. Make certain patient is not pregnant.
progesterone intrauterine insert	Progestasert	A T-shaped unit containing a reservoir of 38 mg progesterone with barium sulfate dispersed in a silicone fluid is inserted into the uterine cavity. Contraceptive effectiveness is maintained for 1 yr, and then the unit must be replaced. Bleeding and cramps may occur during the first few weeks after insertion, sometimes requiring removal.

■ Evaluation

Monitor for adverse effects, which may vary in severity. They may be a result of the different strengths of estrogen and progestin. Side effects may be avoided by changing to a different combination of estrogen and progestin pill. Some spotting can be tolerated in younger women.

Evaluate the patient's compliance in taking medications. Patients who have trouble remembering to take other medications are not good candidates for oral contraceptives.

■ Patient and Family Teaching

Tell the patient and family the following:

- The patient must take the pills exactly as prescribed. If a pill is missed, the patient should follow the directions given by the nurse, physician, or other health care provider. Usually the patient takes two pills the next day or discards one tablet and takes one tablet the next day. The risk for bleeding or conception increases with two or more pills missed. The patient may need to use a backup method of contraception for a period of time. Another method should also be used in the first 3 weeks of the first cycle and if vomiting for several days occur because of illness.
- Certain side effects should be reported to the nurse, physician, or other health care provider immediately: pain in the chest, groin, or legs; sudden, severe headaches; sudden slurring of speech; sudden loss of coordination; sudden visual changes; and sudden shortness of breath. Other symptoms may require attention but are not emergencies: changes in vaginal bleeding, hypertension, breast lumps, jaundice, vaginal discharge, stomach or side pains, and mental depression. Other side effects may be present but are not serious: nausea, anorexia, acne, stomach cramps, edema of ankles and feet, breast swelling and tenderness, tiredness, brown spots on the skin, changes in libido, changes in weight, hirsutism, some hair loss on the scalp, and sensitivity to the sun.
- The patient must return for scheduled checkups.
- The patient should immediately stop taking the pill if she thinks she is pregnant or if she misses two periods. The patient must not take oral contraceptives while breastfeeding.
- The patient should keep one extra month's supply of pills on hand so there is no chance of running out and breaking the cycle.
- The patient should not smoke while taking the pill.
- All other medications the patient is taking should be reported to the nurse, physician, or other health care provider because of possible drug interactions. This is particularly true for antibiotics, which may make the pill less effective and thus allow the woman to get pregnant.

- For women younger than 40 years of age, the risk of death from complications from the pill is less than the risk of death from complications of pregnancy. (Patients should not be so frightened of taking the pill that they fail to recognize that it is safer statistically to take the pill than to be pregnant.)
- For patients using the Progestasert system, special instructions are needed. Patient should watch for signs of infection or excessive bleeding after insertion. Difficulties should be reported to the nurse, physician, or other health care provider immediately.

Each visit to the health care provider should include a history of possible side effects or adverse reactions since the previous visit, a review of whether the patient is taking the pill correctly, and a reminder of signs and symptoms to report.

THYROID HORMONES

OVERVIEW

The thyroid gland, located in the neck in front of the trachea, produces the hormones thyroxine (T_4) and triiodothyronine (T_3), which influence almost every organ and tissue of the body. Although their exact mechanism of action is unknown, their primary action is to control the metabolic rate of the tissues.

The anterior pituitary gland secretes thyroid-stimulating hormone (TSH), which tells the thyroid gland to release the hormones it has stored. When the level of circulating thyroid hormones is high, TSH from the anterior pituitary gland is withheld; when the circulating level falls, this information is also signaled, and TSH is once again released. This type of arrangement is called a *feedback mechanism*, because physiologic action influences the organ sending the signals.

Two general types of diseases can influence the hormone-producing activity of the thyroid gland. A decrease in the amount of thyroid hormones manufactured or secreted is called **hypothyroidism**. Symptoms include fatigue, malaise, lethargy, moderate weight gain (around 10 pounds) with minimal appetite, cold intolerance, menorrhagia, dry skin, coarse hair, hoarseness, impaired memory, and constipation. An increase in the amount of thyroid hormones manufactured and secreted is called **hyperthyroidism**. Symptoms include weight loss, decreased or absent menstruation, rapid or pounding heart, heat intolerance, nervousness, irritability, diarrhea, sweaty skin, insomnia (inability to sleep), fever, or chest pain.

Synthetic hormones, natural hormones, or a combination product may be given to increase the level of thyroid hormone in hypothyroid conditions or given as replacement therapy when the thyroid gland has been surgically removed. In hyperthyroid conditions, other preparations are given that slow the rate of thyroid production. Both thyroid supplements and antithyroid medications are described.

THYROID SUPPLEMENTS OR REPLACEMENTS

ACTION

The main action of the thyroid hormones is to increase metabolic rate. This results in an increase in tissue oxygen consumption, body temperature, heart and respiratory rate, cardiac output, and carbohydrate, lipid, and protein metabolism. In addition, thyroid hormones influence growth and development of the skeletal system, especially ossification in the epiphyses of long bones (the growth center).

USES

Thyroid hormones are used in replacement therapy to manage hypothyroidism, myxedema, cretinism, or nontoxic goiter caused by deficiency of thyroid hormones, atrophy, congenital defects, and the effects of surgery, antithyroid products, or radiation. They are also used to treat chronic thyroid infections and tumors that depend on thyrotropic hormone.

ADVERSE REACTIONS

Adverse reactions to thyroid replacements include dysrhythmias, hypertension, tachycardia, hand tremors, headache, insomnia, nervousness, diarrhea, vomiting, weight loss, menstrual irregularities, rash, glycosuria, hyperglycemia, increased prothrombin time, and increased serum cholesterol levels. Overdosage produces signs of hyperthyroidism.

 Lifespan Considerations
Older Adults

THYROID HORMONES

Because older adult patients are usually more sensitive to thyroid hormones and have more adverse reactions than patients in other age groups, it is recommended that thyroid replacement doses be individualized. In some patients, the dose should be 25% lower than the usual adult dose.

Hypothyroidism, the second most common endocrine disease in the older adult population, is often misdiagnosed. Only one third of geriatric patients exhibit the typical signs and symptoms of cold intolerance and weight gain. Most often the symptoms are nonspecific, such as failing to thrive, stumbling and falling episodes, weight loss, and incontinence. If neurologic change has occurred, the patient may be misdiagnosed as having dementia, depression, or a psychotic episode.

Laboratory tests for serum T_4 and TSH are used to confirm hypothyroidism.

Levothyroxine (Synthroid, others) is usually the drug of choice for thyroid replacement.

Modified from McKenry LM, Tessier E, Hogan MA: *Mosby's pharmacology in nursing*, ed 22, St Louis, 2006, Mosby.

DRUG INTERACTIONS

Thyroid preparations may increase the patient's need for antidiabetic agents. Anticoagulant effects may be exaggerated by thyroid replacement because of increased hypoprothrombinemia. Corticosteroid needs are increased for patients taking thyroid preparations because of increased tissue demands. Effects of tricyclic antidepressants are increased by thyroid hormones. Many other isolated medications may be affected.

❖ NURSING IMPLICATIONS AND PATIENT TEACHING

■ Assessment

Try to learn as much as possible about the patient's health history, including other drugs being taken that may produce drug interactions. Does the patient have diabetes mellitus, cardiovascular disease, adrenocortical insufficiency, or pregnancy? These conditions are precautions to the use of thyroid supplements. The patient may also have a history of hypothyroidism.

On examination, the nurse may find skin changes associated with **myxedema**, the most severe form of hypothyroidism. These changes include nonpitting edema; doughy skin; puffy face; large tongue; decreased body hair; and cool, dry skin. The thyroid gland may be normal in size, enlarged, or not palpable, depending on the cause of hypothyroidism. Neurologic signs include slow thinking, muscle weakness, slowed relaxation phase of the deep tendon reflexes, dull facial expression, and carpal tunnel syndrome. Cardiac signs include bradycardia and decreased blood pressure.

Laboratory findings in thyroid disease may include reduced free T_4 index and elevated serum TSH; other tests may be abnormal.

■ Diagnosis

Because thyroid disease may be insidious (hard to notice because of small changes) in onset, the patient may have many symptoms that require therapy at the time of diagnosis. Patients may have become depressed, have gained weight, or have problems with body image and self-esteem that should be addressed. Patients may find it hard to wait for the length of time it takes for thyroid medications to return them to normal functioning and resolve some of these problems.

■ Planning

Patients older than 50 years of age are often very sensitive to thyroid hormones, so it is important for them to begin on a small dose. They should be observed for signs and symptoms of cardiovascular disease before the dosage is increased.

Implementation

All treatment should begin with small doses and be increased gradually by the drug prescriber. A cut in dosage followed by a slower increase in the dose may be necessary when side effects occur. Therapy will often be withdrawn for 2 to 6 days and then restarted at a lower dosage if this happens.

The patient's age, the presence of cardiac disease, and the severity of symptoms should be considered when thyroid hormone replacement therapy is begun. Titration of dosage (gradual adjustment of dose up or down) to gain the best response with the lowest dosage is the goal of therapy. The usual maintenance dosage in the treatment of hypothyroidism is 0.5 to 2 g as a single daily dose before breakfast.

T_4 is the treatment of choice for hypothyroidism because of its purity and long duration of action. Because T_4 has a slow onset of action, therapeutic effects may not occur for 3 to 4 weeks. T_3, which has a rapid onset, may be given if rapid correction of hypothyroidism is necessary. The equivalent strengths of the various thyroid products vary, and care must be used in changing from one product to another. Patients should take the medication at the same time every day, preferably before breakfast. If medication is taken late in the day, insomnia may result.

Table 21-11 presents a summary of thyroid supplements or replacements.

Evaluation

Response to therapy is not immediate. Most patients begin to feel better within 2 weeks, and the therapeutic results are often seen in 3 months.

Teach patients the signs and symptoms of hypothyroidism and hyperthyroidism so they can determine if they are receiving too much or too little medicine.

If symptoms of overdosage occur, the prescribing health care provider should be consulted promptly. The medication will likely be stopped for several days, and therapy may be started again at a lower dosage.

Periodic blood tests should be done before thyroid hormone therapy is started and periodically once the patient is on a maintenance dose.

Patient and Family Teaching

Tell the patient and family the following:

- The patient should take the medication exactly as directed by the nurse, physician, or other health care provider. The medication should be taken at the same time every day, preferably before breakfast. If it is taken too late in the day, the patient may have difficulty going to sleep.
- Response to this medication is not immediate; symptoms should improve within 2 weeks. The patient should not increase the dosage unless instructed to do so by the nurse, physician, or other health care provider. Taking the medication regularly as ordered is very important.
- If the patient is also being treated for diabetes mellitus, any changes in blood or urine sugar and acetone test results should be reported to the health care provider.
- If the patient is receiving anticoagulant therapy, bleeding or excessive bruising should be reported to the health care provider.

Table 21-11 Thyroid Supplements or Replacements

GENERIC NAME	TRADE NAME	COMMENTS
levothyroxine	Levothroid Synthroid Unithroid	Synthetic preparation; drug of choice because effect is predictable. Increase dosage at 2-wk intervals until therapeutic effect is achieved.
liothyronine (T_3)	Cytomel Triostat	Synthetic hormone; has rapid effect and short duration of action, which allow fast dosage adjustment and quick reversibility of overdosage. Therapeutic effects achieved in 24-72 hr and persist up to 72 hr after withdrawal of drug. Mild hypothyroidism: Therapy initiated then dosage increased every 1-2 wk until effects achieved.
liotrix	Thyrolar	Liotrix is a combination of synthetic levothyroxine sodium (T_4) and liothyronine sodium (T_3) in a 4:1 ratio. Predictable therapeutic effect is an advantage. Therapy start and then increase at 1- to 2-wk intervals as needed.
thyroid, desiccated	Armour Thyroid	Desiccated thyroid contains T_4 and T_3 thyroid hormones in their natural state. Because these drugs are composed of desiccated animal thyroid glands, the hormonal content is variable, and T_3 and T_4 levels fluctuate; therefore avoid varying brands. Myxedema without hypothyroidism: Initiate therapy with increases until therapeutic effects are achieved.

T_3, Triiodothyronine; T_4, thyroxine.

- The patient should check with the health care provider before taking any other medications; this will decrease the chance of drugs interacting.
- The patient should report signs and symptoms of overdosage (hyperthyroidism) or underdosage (hypothyroidism) to the health care provider promptly (these signs and symptoms are summarized earlier).

ANTITHYROID PRODUCTS

ACTION

Antithyroid products are the main drugs used to treat hyperthyroidism or Graves disease. The principal action of antithyroid products is to stop the new production of thyroid hormones. These agents do not inactivate or inhibit thyroid hormones (T_3 and T_4) already stored or circulating in the blood.

USES

Antithyroid products are used to treat hyperthyroidism or to improve hyperthyroidism in preparation for surgery or radioactive iodine therapy.

ADVERSE REACTIONS

Adverse reactions to antithyroid products include drowsiness, headaches, neuritis, paresthesias (numbness and tingling), vertigo, epigastric distress, jaundice, nausea, vomiting, skin rash, urticaria, myalgia, edema, alopecia, and lymphadenopathy. Hypothyroidism may occur as a result of prolonged therapy. Agranulocytosis (very low number of white blood cells [WBCs]) is a rare but serious occurrence. In addition, other more serious problems may develop. Propylthiouracil now carries a safety alert for serious liver damage, including liver failure or death in some patients.

DRUG INTERACTIONS

The effects of anticoagulants are increased or potentiated by propylthiouracil. Caution should be taken when antithyroid drugs are given to patients who are receiving additional drugs known to cause agranulocytosis (e.g., hydantoin).

❖ NURSING IMPLICATIONS AND PATIENT TEACHING

▪ Assessment

Try to learn as much as possible about the patient's health history, including hypersensitivity (allergy) to antithyroid drugs, other medications being taken

that could cause drug interactions, and pregnancy or breastfeeding.

The patient may have a history of hyperthyroidism, including nervousness or tremor, weight loss with increased appetite, heat intolerance and excessive sweating, mood swings, and muscle weakness. On physical examination, the nurse may find exophthalmos (bulging eyes); thyroid enlargement; tachycardia; increased blood pressure; tremor; proximal muscle weakness; and warm, moist, smooth skin. Weight loss and the signs of chronic heart failure may be the most obvious signs of hyperthyroidism in older adults.

Laboratory findings may show elevated free T_4 index, increased T_3, or decreased TSH.

▪ Diagnosis

Because thyroid disease may be slow in onset, the patient may have many symptoms that require therapy at the time of diagnosis. Patients may be restless or anxious, have eating and sleeping problems, or have problems with concentration and memory that must be addressed. Patients may find it hard to wait for the length of time it takes for thyroid medications to return them to normal functioning and resolve some of these problems.

▪ Planning

Antithyroid drugs usually remove symptoms of hyperthyroidism if taken correctly for 1 to 2 years. Patient compliance with therapy should be encouraged to help them return to normal thyroid levels.

▪ Implementation

The therapeutic objective is to correct the hypermetabolic state with a minimum of side effects and without producing hypothyroidism. Clinical response to the antithyroid drugs usually takes 1 to 2 weeks because the drugs do not affect the release of thyroid hormone. Response depends on stopping the production of thyroid hormone in the thyroid gland. This in turn depends on the amount of hormone production materials present in the gland, and the rate of conversion of these materials into the thyroid hormones. Generally, therapy is maintained for 12 to 24 months and then reduced to see if the hyperthyroidism starts again. Titration to gain the best therapeutic response with the lowest dosage is the objective. Table 21-12 provides a summary of antithyroid products.

▪ Evaluation

Laboratory blood tests should be completed before beginning antithyroid therapy and periodically once the patient is on a regular maintenance dosage. Before

GENERIC NAME	TRADE NAME	COMMENTS
iodine products	Lugol's Iodine Thyro-Block	May have daily dose and dose before surgery.
methimazole	Tapazole Northyx	Does not inhibit peripheral conversion of thyroxine to T_3. More potent than PTU, and doses are one tenth those of PTU. Acts more rapidly but less consistently than PTU.
propylthiouracil	Propylthiouracil	PTU interferes with synthesis of thyroxine and blocks peripheral conversion of thyroxine to T_3. May cause hypoprothrombinemia and bleeding. Adults: Give initial dose at 8-hr intervals, with adjustments in dosage made after 2 wk, depending on free T_4 levels and symptoms. Therapy continued 6-18 mo before tapering. Watch for signs of liver damage.

Table 21-12 Antithyroid Products

PTU, Propylthiouracil; T_3, triiodothyronine; T_4, thyroxine.

therapy is started, a WBC count with differential is done; this should be repeated if there is any sign of infection. Serum T_4 and TSH levels are monitored initially and after every 2 weeks of therapy until a euthyroid state (normal function of the thyroid gland) is achieved, usually in 3 to 5 months. Once the patient has been euthyroid for 6 to 12 months, a decision may be made to reduce the dosage and see whether the hyperthyroidism is under control. If hyperthyroidism seems to be absent, therapy is stopped.

■ **Patient and Family Teaching**

Tell the patient and family the following:
- The patient should take this medication exactly as directed by the nurse, physician, or other health care provider.
- Because clinical response usually takes from 1 to 2 weeks to achieve, the dosage should not be increased

until the results at the present dosage level can be evaluated.
- Some patients experience side effects from this drug, such as fever, sore throat, malaise, unusual bleeding or bruising, headache, skin rash, and enlargement of cervical lymph nodes; these symptoms should be reported to the nurse, physician, or other health care provider.
- Bed rest, adequate diet, and avoidance of occupational and domestic stress are also useful modalities of therapy.

COMPLEMENTARY AND ALTERNATIVE THERAPIES

Some herbal preparations may be used by patients for the treatment of hyperglycemia, hyperthyroidism, or hypothyroidism. These products may interact with other medications, as indicated in the Complementary and Alternative Therapies box.

Complementary and Alternative Therapies

Hyperglycemia, Hyperthyroidism, or Hypothyroidism

CONDITION	PRODUCT	COMMENTS
Hyperglycemia/diabetes	Gymnema	Potential interactions with insulin, oral hypoglycemics
	Bitter melon	Potential interaction with anticoagulants, aspirin, NSAIDs, antiplatelet agents
	Evening primrose	
Hyperthyroidism	Milk thistle	No known interactions
	Passion flower	Potential interactions with antianxiety agents, antidepressants, hexobarbital, hypnotics, sedatives
	Valerian	Potential interactions with CNS depressants, sedative-hypnotics (barbiturates), antidepressants, anxiolytics, antihistamines
Hypothyroidism	Bitter melon	Potential interactions with insulin, oral hypoglycemics
	Garcinia	

Modified from Krinsky DL, LaValle JB, Hawkins EB, et al: *Natural therapeutics pocket guide*, ed 2, Hudson, Ohio, 2003, Lexi-Comp, Inc. *CNS*, Central nervous system; *NSAIDs*, nonsteroidal antiinflammatory drugs.

Get Ready for the NCLEX® Examination!

Key Points

- A variety of hormones and steroids are used in medical therapy.
- Unlike many other medications, hormones and steroids are natural or manufactured preparations that replace, increase, or decrease the effects of substances already produced in the body.
- Hormones and steroids are part of a complex message system linking together various organs and biologic systems. Increases or decreases of hormones send signals to other organ systems about whether to increase or decrease production of other substances.
- Important hormones or steroids covered in this chapter are insulin and oral hypoglycemics, agents that act on the uterus, pituitary and adrenocortical hormones, sex hormones, oral contraceptives, and thyroid preparations.
- It is important for the nurse to have a basic understanding of how these preparations work in the body, a familiarity with the major adverse effects that can occur, and a lesson plan with the important points to cover when teaching the patient and family.

Additional Learning Resources

SG Go to your Study Guide for additional learning activities to help you master this chapter content.

evolve Go to your Evolve website (http://evolve.elsevier.com/Edmunds/LPN/) for additional online resources.

Review Questions for the NCLEX® Examination

1. The nurse is scheduled to administer NovoLog 70/30 and notes that it appears cloudy. The highest priority action on the part of the nurse should be to:
   1. notify the pharmacy of the cloudy appearance
   2. administer rapid-acting insulin instead of NovoLog 70/30
   3. administer the insulin to the patient as scheduled
   4. notify the physician of the cloudy appearance

2. The patient is scheduled to be treated with metformin (Glucophage). The most appropriate dosage schedule for the patient will be:
   1. take in between meals
   2. take it with meals
   3. take with 8 oz of water
   4. take on an empty stomach

3. The nurse notes that the patient is scheduled to be treated with pioglitazone (Actos) and is already being treated with metformin. The most appropriate action on the part of the nurse should be to:
   1. administer the medication as ordered
   2. withhold the medication for this dose
   3. notify pharmacy of the medications ordered
   4. notify the physician of treatment with metformin

4. The patient is scheduled to be treated with mifepristone (Mifeprex). The nurse's highest priority action before the patient takes the medication is:
   1. verify that the patient has read and signed the consent form
   2. verify that the patient knows symptoms of an adverse reaction
   3. verify that the patient recognizes signs of an anaphylactic reaction
   4. verify that the patient has taken the medication previously

5. The patient is scheduled to be treated with vasopressin (Pitressin). The nurse anticipates that the route for the medication will be:
   1. intramuscular
   2. orally in tablets
   3. intradermal
   4. orally in a liquid

Case Study

Lucy Bradford is a 33-year-old female patient with type 2 diabetes. She developed diabetes after a pregnancy 3 years ago, and she has been able to keep her blood glucose level under control with diet until recently. Her blood sugar has been around 136 mg/dL. Over the past few months, the glucose level has begun to vary a great deal, sometimes reaching as high as 180 mg/dL. She has no other health problems or previous surgeries but has smoked a pack of cigarettes a day for 12 years. She takes oral contraceptives. She reports developing a red, itchy rash after taking sulfa as a child. Today, the physician decided she needed to start on some oral antidiabetic medication and ordered glyburide 5 mg/day PO.

1. What would the nurse tell Lucy about the medication she is going to start taking?
2. Is this a low, medium, or high dose of glyburide?
3. What blood sugar level would be an appropriate goal for Lucy?
4. What blood test monitors the effectiveness of blood sugar control over a 6- to 8-week period?
5. From this information about Lucy's condition and what is known about glyburide, how might Lucy respond to the glyburide?
6. Second-generation sulfonylureas are approximately _____ more powerful than first-generation sulfonylureas.
7. The physician decides to switch Lucy to _____, which has a mechanism of action similar to the sulfonylureas. Why is this drug a good substitute?
8. Lucy comes back several months later. Her glycohemoglobin A1c is less than 7%. Is this a problem?

Get Ready for the NCLEX® Examination!—cont'd

9. Diet and exercise are the foundation of any diabetes-management plan. Develop a teaching plan for communicating these important things to Lucy:
   a. A more ideal body weight reduces insulin resistance and can significantly affect glucose control.
   b. The total number of calories that are adequate to promote a reasonable weight and good nutrition should be established.
   c. Generally, dividing the total number of calories into three smaller meals and two to three snacks minimizes postprandial glucose spikes. Spreading out calories may also control increased hunger associated with skipped meals.
   d. Ideally, 10% to 20% of the total daily calories are from protein, 20% of calories are from saturated and polyunsaturated fat, and 60% to 70% of calories are from monounsaturated fats and carbohydrates.
   e. Exercise helps achieve and maintain an ideal body weight, resulting in decreased insulin resistance. Exercise also improves insulin sensitivity. For reasons not well understood, the exercising muscle requires little insulin but can mobilize moderate amounts of glucose.
10. Lucy's potential for hyperglycemia is increased because _____.
11. Lucy does not want to have another child. She has been taking a biphasic oral contraceptive pill. Are there any contraindications to diabetics taking oral contraceptive pills?
12. Does Lucy have any other risk factors that would limit oral contraceptive use?

Drug Calculation Review

1. The physician orders an injection of dexamethasone (Decadron) 6 mg IM for a patient with bronchial asthma. In stock is dexamethasone 4 mg/1 mL in a 5-mL multidose vial. How many milliliters of this medication will the nurse prepare?

2. Order: Synthroid 125 mcg by mouth (PO) daily. Supply: Synthroid 0.25 mcg per tablet.
   Question: How many tablets of Synthroid should be given?
3. Order: Solu-Medrol 60 mg IV push stat. Supply: Solu-Medrol 125 mg/mL.
   Question: How many milliliters of Solu-Medrol should be given? (Round to the nearest tenth.)

Critical Thinking Questions

1. Identify the major similarities in the treatment of type 1 and type 2 diabetes.
2. Seven-year-old Jessica has recently been diagnosed with type 1 diabetes. Which insulin preparation(s) is Jessica most likely to receive? Why?
3. What would indicate that a patient understands his androgen therapy regimen?
4. Ms. Marra, who is 26, has begun an initial course of oral contraceptives. What indicates that she understands and is likely to comply with her OBC regimen?
5. Mr. Moore is starting a thyroid replacement regimen. As the nurse prepares to give instruction about his medication regimen, he makes the comment, "Sounds to me like these pills will have me feeling fine in no time." How would the nurse address this?
6. What information would the nurse want to include in the education of a patient who takes oral contraceptives and has been prescribed furosemide?
7. Immunosuppression is one of the serious effects of steroid therapy. If the patient with chronic obstructive pulmonary disease (COPD) has been maintained on prednisone 40 mg PO daily for 6 months, how would the nurse instruct her to monitor herself for signs and symptoms of infection?
8. Why should the patient taking oral steroids also be receiving a histamine H_2-receptor antagonist such as ranitidine or cimetidine?

Immunologic Medications

Objectives

1. Define common terms used in immunology.
2. Explain the differences between the three different types of immunity.
3. Outline typical immunization plans for children and adults.
4. List the major adverse reactions of common immunologic drugs.
5. Identify at least three drugs used for in vivo testing.

Key Terms

antigen-antibody response (ĂN-tĭ-jĕn-ĂN-tĭ-bŏ-dē, p. 400)
antiserums (ĂN-tĭ-sĭ-rŭmz, p. 404)
artificially acquired active immunity (ĭ-MŪ-nĭ-tē, p. 400)
immunity (ĭ-MŪ-nĭ-tē, p. 400)

naturally acquired active immunity (ĭ-MŪ-nĭ-tē, p. 400)
passive immunity (PĂ-sĭv ĭ-MŪ-nĭ-tē, p. 404)
toxoid (TŎKS-ŏyd, p. 404)
vaccines (văk-SĔNZ, p. 400)

OVERVIEW

Immunologic agents are biologic preparations such as vaccines, toxoids, and other serologic agents used primarily to prevent or modify disease in an otherwise healthy person. Depending on the formulation of the biologic agents, they provide active or passive immunity to specific diseases. These different mechanisms are discussed in general, with specific product information presented later in Table 22-1.

IMMUNE SYSTEM

The immune system is part of the lymphatic system, which is made up of the lymph vessels, lymph nodes, and other lymph organs (Figure 22-1). This system removes foreign substances from the blood and lymph, combats disease, maintains tissue fluid balance, and absorbs fats. It moves lymph from its source, the body tissues, to the point where it reenters the bloodstream. The structures of the lymphatic system are of two kinds: those concerned with the transport of lymph (lymph capillaries, lymph vessels, and lymph ducts) and those composed mostly of lymphatic tissue but serving other specific functions (lymph nodes, spleen, tonsils, and thymus—together these structures are called *lymph organs*).

The lymphatic system produces the T cells that help provide immunity and moves them throughout the lymphatic system.

ACTION

A bacterium, virus, or foreign protein that invades the body is called an *antigen*. The body senses the foreign antigen and responds by making antibodies. *Antibodies* are special proteins made by the lymphatic tissue and the reticuloendothelial system; they are designed to help neutralize or resist the effects of invading foreign proteins. In this **antigen-antibody response**, a specific antigen causes the body to produce an antibody that reacts specifically with that antigen. Some antibodies keep circulating for the life of the person, providing constant active immunity to certain antigens. Other antibodies are active for only a short period, providing passive immunity.

The antigen-antibody response results in **immunity**, or resistance to invading proteins and diseases. One way a person can develop immunity is by having a disease and recovering from it. An example is when a child develops chickenpox, and the body develops antibodies to the chickenpox virus. These antibodies travel around in the bloodstream for the rest of the person's lifetime, providing **naturally acquired active immunity**.

The lymphoid tissue and the reticuloendothelial system tissues will also produce antibodies to a live but weakened antigen (known as a *live, attenuated antigen*) or an antigen that has been killed. Laboratories can produce **vaccines** that contain either attenuated or killed antigens, and people can be immunized to prevent them from getting some diseases. This is called **artificially acquired active immunity**. Whether a weak or

Table 22-1 **Agents for Immunity**

PRODUCT	COMMENTS
Agents for Active Immunity	
Toxoids	
Diphtheria and tetanus toxoids and pertussis vaccine, adsorbed Diphtheria and tetanus toxoids, combined Diphtheria, tetanus toxoid, and acellular pertussis	See CDC immunization schedules (see Figure 22-2). The FDA suggests all health care workers should have these immunizations.
Tetanus toxoid	Immunization in adults and children. May produce local reactions, fever, chills, malaise, and myalgia (widespread muscle pain). Tetanus toxoid, adsorbed: 2 doses IM at 2, 4, and 6 mo, again at 12 mo, and no later than 11-12 yr. Booster: Every 10 yr. Tetanus toxoid, fluid: 3 doses IM or SQ at 4- to 8-wk intervals and fourth dose 6-12 mo after third dose. Booster: Every 5-10 yr, depending on risk of wound.
Bacterial Vaccines	
Bacille Calmette-Guérin (BCG) vaccine	Tuberculosis protection for international travelers to high-risk areas and high-risk infants and children; use multiple-puncture disk.
Cholera vaccine	Required for travel to certain areas. May produce brief local reactions, fever, headache, and malaise. Vaccine: 2 doses SQ or IM 1 wk to 1 mo apart.
Haemophilus influenzae type b (Hib) conjugate vaccine	Routine immunization. Number of doses and amount injected vary by patient age.
Meningococcal polysaccharide vaccine Group A, Group C Groups A and C Groups A, C, Y, and W-135	Induces formation of antibodies, leading to immunity to specific organisms. Does not provide immunity against all varieties. Vaccine: SQ only. Revaccination may be required in some individuals at high risk, but standards are not specific.
Plague vaccine	Reduces incidence and severity of disease. Vaccine: 2 doses 1 mo apart, followed with third dose 1-3 mo later. Always consult dosage schedule in package insert before administering.
Pneumococcal vaccine, polyvalent	Produces immunity against a variety of pneumococcal infections. Vaccine: IM or SQ; revaccinations necessary in 3 or more yr.
Pneumococcal 7-valent conjugate vaccine (Prevnar)	Provides active immunization for infants and children against *Streptococcus pneumoniae*. Vaccine: 3 doses administered as IM injection at 2-mo intervals, followed by a fourth dose at 12-15 mo of age. Shake suspension vigorously immediately before use.
Typhoid vaccine	Given when there has been exposure to a known carrier or foreign travel to area where typhoid is endemic. May produce local reactions, fever, chills, malaise, and myalgia. Primary immunization: 2 doses SQ 4 or more wk apart. Booster every 3 yr for children younger than age 10.
Lyme disease vaccine	Given to patients at high risk who live or work in *Borrelia burgdorferi*–infested grassy or wooded areas. Primary immunization: Give initial dose, repeated in 1 and 12 mo. Vaccination with all three doses is required to achieve optimal protection. Shake container well before drawing dose. Vaccine is a turbid white suspension. Note: administer by IM injection only in the deltoid region.

Continued

Table 22-1 **Agents for Immunity—cont'd**

PRODUCT	COMMENTS
Viral Vaccines	
Hepatitis A vaccine (Havrix)	Given as primary dose and then booster 6-12 mo later. Give in deltoid muscle only. Number of doses and amount injected vary by patient age.
Hepatitis B vaccine (Heptavax-B)	For immunization against all known subtypes of hepatitis B virus. May produce local reactions, malaise, fatigue, nausea, myalgia, and headache. Adults: Give IM, repeated in 1 and 6 mo. Children younger than 10 yr: Give IM, repeated in 1, 6 mo.
Influenza virus vaccine	Annual vaccination of high-risk persons. May produce localized reactions, fever, malaise, and myalgia. Dosage schedule varies from year to year.
Measles, mumps, and rubella virus vaccine, live	Same as measles virus vaccine, live attenuated.
Measles, rubeola, and rubella virus vaccine, live	See CDC immunization schedules.
Mumps virus vaccine, live	See CDC immunization schedules.
Pertussis vaccine (in combination)	See CDC immunization schedules.
Poliomyelitis vaccine, inactivated (IPV), Salk	See CDC immunization schedules.
Poliovirus vaccine, live, oral, trivalent (TOPV), Sabin	See CDC immunization schedules.
Rotavirus	See CDC immunization schedules.
Rubella and mumps virus vaccine, live	See CDC immunization schedules.
Rubella virus vaccine, live	See CDC immunization schedules.
Varicella (Varivax)	See CDC immunization schedules.
Yellow fever vaccine	Given only at approved World Health Organization centers for people traveling abroad. Vaccine: Give SQ with revaccination in 10 yr as needed.
Agents for Passive Immunity	
Antitoxins and Antivenins	
Black widow spider species antivenin	Adults and children: Inject 1 vial IM, preferably in the region of the anterolateral thigh so that a tourniquet may be applied in the event of a systemic reaction. Symptoms usually subside in 1-3 hr.
Diphtheria antitoxin	For prevention and treatment of diphtheria. Vaccine: 20,000-120,000 units IM, IV as therapy; 10,000 units IM for prophylaxis.
Immune Serums	
Cytomegalovirus immune globulin (CMV-IGIV)	For attenuation of primary CMV disease associated with kidney transplantation. Give IV.
Hepatitis B immune globulin (HBIG; human)	For postexposure or high-risk patient prophylaxis. Produces local reactions, urticaria, and fever. HBIG: Give IM as soon as possible and repeat 28-30 days after exposure.
Immune globulin IV (IGIV)	For maintenance treatment of patients unable to produce sufficient amounts of immunoglobulin G antibodies. Used in patients with immunodeficiency syndrome, idiopathic thrombocytopenic purpura, and beta-cell chronic lymphocytic leukemia. Give IV once a month.
Immune serum globulin, human (HISG)	For hepatitis A, rubeola prophylaxis; immunoglobulin deficiency; passive immunization for varicella in immunosuppressed patients. Give IM.

Table 22-1   Agents for Immunity—cont'd

PRODUCT	COMMENTS
Lymphocyte immune globulin, antithymocyte globulin	Used in management of allograft rejection in patients who have undergone renal transplant.
Human papilloma virus (HPV) recombinant vaccine	Quadrivalent vaccine with protection against 4 HPV subtypes (6, 11, 16, 18). Trials show 100% efficacy in preventing cervical precancers and nearly 100% efficacy in preventing vulvar and vaginal precancers and genital warts caused by the targeted HPV types. Vaccine: Give IM dose of HPV vaccine in a 3-dose schedule, with initial dose followed by doses 2 mo and 6 mo later. Routine vaccination recommended for girls aged 11-12 years; vaccination series can be started in girls as young as age 9 years; catch-up vaccination recommended for females aged 13-26 years who have not been vaccinated previously or who have not completed the full vaccine series. Ideally, vaccination should begin prior to onset of sexual activity. This is a new recommendation by CDC suggested for boys.
Rh$_O$(D) immune globulin	Effectively suppresses immune response of nonsensitized Rh-negative mothers after delivery of an Rh-positive infant. Passive immunity: 1 vial IM.
Respiratory syncytial virus (RSV) immune globulin (RespiGam)	Used in prevention of serious lower respiratory tract infection caused by RSV in children less than 24 mo of age with bronchopulmonary dysplasia or a history of premature birth. Given by IV infusion, based on body mass.
Tetanus immune globulin, human (HTIG)	For temporary postexposure prophylaxis: 4 units/kg IM.
Varicella-zoster immune globulin, human (VZIG)	Provides temporary passive immunity to varicella. Given deep IM, according to dosage schedule on package insert.
Rabies Prophylaxis Products	
Rabies immune globulin, human (RIG)	Immunization for those thought to be exposed to rabies. May produce fever and soreness at injection site. Usual dose: 20 International Units/kg IM; half the dose may be used to infiltrate the wound.
Rabies vaccine, human diploid cell cultures (HDCV)	For prophylaxis and postexposure treatment. May produce nausea, headache, muscle aches, abdominal pain, and local reactions. See package insert for dosage schedule.
In Vivo Diagnostic Biologic Agents	
Coccidioidin	Used to identify people with exposure to the fungus *Coccidioides* or with active disease (coccidioidomycosis); lowest possible dose given by intradermal injection and response evaluated 24-48 hr later. Positive reaction: Area of erythema (redness) and induration (hardening) 5 mm or greater.
Histoplasmin	Used to identify people with exposure to the fungus. Histoplasma or with active disease (histoplasmosis); 0.1 mL given by intradermal injection and response evaluated 24-48 hr later. Positive reaction: Area of erythema and induration 5 mm or greater.
Mumps skin test antigen	Demonstrates cutaneous hypersensitivity to mumps virus; 0.1 mL antigen given by intradermal injection and evaluated 24-48 hr later. Positive reaction: Area of erythema and induration 5 mm or greater.
Tuberculin PPD multiple-puncture device	Used to identify persons with active tuberculosis, exposure to tuberculosis, or needing further testing.
Tuberculin Old, multiple-puncture device	Same as tuberculin PPD multiple-puncture device.
Tuberculin purified protein derivative (Mantoux)	Designed to identify persons with active tuberculosis, exposure to tuberculosis, or needing further testing; 0.1 mL of intermediate-strength PPD given by intradermal injection and evaluated in 24-48 hrs. Positive reaction: Area of erythema and induration 9 mm or more; areas 5 to 9 mm considered questionable; areas under 5 mm are negative.

CDC, Center for Disease Control and Prevention; *CMV,* cytomegalovirus; *FDA,* Food and Drug Administration; *HBIG,* hepatitis B immune globulin; *HPV,* human papilloma virus; *IM,* intramuscular; *IV,* intravenous; *PPD,* purified protein derivative; *RSV,* respiratory syncytial virus; *SQ,* Subcutaneous.

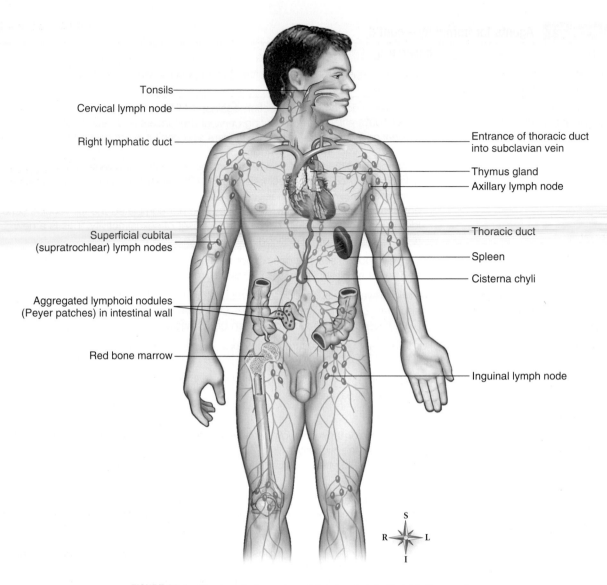

Tonsils

Cervical lymph node

Right lymphatic duct

Superficial cubital
(supratrochlear) lymph nodes

Aggregated lymphoid nodules
(Peyer patches) in intestinal wall

Red bone marrow

Entrance of thoracic duct
into subclavian vein

Thymus gland
Axillary lymph node

Thoracic duct

Spleen

Cisterna chyli

Inguinal lymph node

S
R — L
I

FIGURE 22-1   The lymphatic system. *I*, Inferior; *L*, left; *R*, right; *S*, superior.

dead antigen is given depends on the disease and on what the research has shown is the best way to protect patients. Rubeola (measles) vaccine is an example of a vaccine made from live, attenuated measles antigen. A person who is vaccinated against measles develops a very mild case of measles. The immune system then produces antibodies that protect the person from getting a full infection with measles. Some diseases may require periodic booster injections of vaccine to keep the antibody level high enough to protect the patient from disease.

Some disease-causing proteins that come from invading bacteria are called *toxins.* Toxins act like antigens to stimulate the immune system to produce antitoxins, which act to neutralize the toxins in the same way antibodies neutralize antigens. When a toxin is attenuated, or weakened, it is called a **toxoid.** A toxoid can be used to produce immunity because the body cannot distinguish between the toxin and the toxoid.

The most common example is the use of tetanus toxoid to protect patients from *Clostridium tetani.*

Once a person has had an antigen-antibody response, the antibodies are stored in the body. Immune globulins are specific types of protein antibodies that are stored in blood serum and plasma. Concentrated immune globulins are also called **antiserums;** they may be collected from human or animal sources. A common example is the hepatitis B immune globulin. These antibodies can be injected into a person who does not have immunity to the antigen. The antibodies then circulate to immediately protect this person, but the protection lasts for only a short time. This form of protection is called *artificially acquired* **passive immunity.** A type of temporary immunity can also occur when antibodies pass from the mother to the fetus through the placenta or to the nursing infant through breast milk. This is known as *naturally acquired passive immunity.*

Recommended Immunization Schedule for Persons Aged 0 Through 6 Years—United States • 2011
For those who fall behind or start late, see the catch-up schedule

Vaccine ▼ Age ►	Birth	1 month	2 months	4 months	6 months	12 months	15 months	18 months	19–23 months	2–3 years	4–6 years	
Hepatitis B[1]	HepB	HepB				HepB						
Rotavirus[2]			RV	RV	RV[2]							
Diphtheria, Tetanus, Pertussis[3]			DTaP	DTaP	DTaP	see footnote[3]	DTaP				DTaP	
Haemophilus influenzae type b[4]			Hib	Hib	Hib[4]	Hib						
Pneumococcal[5]			PCV	PCV	PCV	PCV					PPSV	
Inactivated Poliovirus[6]			IPV	IPV		IPV					IPV	
Influenza[7]						Influenza (Yearly)						
Measles, Mumps, Rubella[8]						MMR		see footnote[8]			MMR	
Varicella[9]						Varicella		see footnote[9]			Varicella	
Hepatitis A[10]						HepA (2 doses)				HepA Series		
Meningococcal[11]										MCV4		

Range of recommended ages for all children

Range of recommended ages for certain high-risk groups

This schedule includes recommendations in effect as of December 21, 2010. Any dose not administered at the recommended age should be administered at a subsequent visit, when indicated and feasible. The use of a combination vaccine generally is preferred over separate injections of its equivalent component vaccines. Considerations should include provider assessment, patient preference, and the potential for adverse events. Providers should consult the relevant Advisory Committee on Immunization Practices statement for detailed recommendations: **http://www.cdc.gov/vaccines/pubs/acip-list.htm**. Clinically significant adverse events that follow immunization should be reported to the Vaccine Adverse Event Reporting System (VAERS) at **http://www.vaers.hhs.gov** or by telephone, **800-822-7967**. Use of trade names and commercial sources is for identification only and does not imply endorsement by the U.S. Department of Health and Human Services.

1. **Hepatitis B vaccine (HepB).** (Minimum age: birth)
   At birth:
   • Administer monovalent HepB to all newborns before hospital discharge.
   • If mother is hepatitis B surface antigen (HBsAg)-positive, administer HepB and 0.5 mL of hepatitis B immune globulin (HBIG) within 12 hours of birth.
   • If mother's HBsAg status is unknown, administer HepB within 12 hours of birth. Determine mother's HBsAg status as soon as possible and, if HBsAg-positive, administer HBIG (no later than age 1 week).
   Doses following the birth dose:
   • The second dose should be administered at age 1 or 2 months. Monovalent HepB should be used for doses administered before age 6 weeks.
   • Infants born to HBsAg-positive mothers should be tested for HBsAg and antibody to HBsAg 1 to 2 months after completion of at least 3 doses of the HepB series, at age 9 through 18 months (generally at the next well-child visit).
   • Administration of 4 doses of HepB to infants is permissible when a combination vaccine containing HepB is administered after the birth dose.
   • Infants who did not receive a birth dose should receive 3 doses of HepB on a schedule of 0, 1, and 6 months.
   • The final (3rd or 4th) dose in the HepB series should be administered no earlier than age 24 weeks.
2. **Rotavirus vaccine (RV).** (Minimum age: 6 weeks)
   • Administer the first dose at age 6 through 14 weeks (maximum age: 14 weeks 6 days). Vaccination should not be initiated for infants aged 15 weeks 0 days or older.
   • The maximum age for the final dose in the series is 8 months 0 days
   • If Rotarix is administered at ages 2 and 4 months, a dose at 6 months is not indicated.
3. **Diphtheria and tetanus toxoids and acellular pertussis vaccine (DTaP).** (Minimum age: 6 weeks)
   • The fourth dose may be administered as early as age 12 months, provided at least 6 months have elapsed since the third dose.
4. ***Haemophilus influenzae* type b conjugate vaccine (Hib).** (Minimum age: 6 weeks)
   • If PRP-OMP (PedvaxHIB or Comvax [HepB-Hib]) is administered at ages 2 and 4 months, a dose at age 6 months is not indicated.
   • Hiberix should not be used for doses at ages 2, 4, or 6 months for the primary series but can be used as the final dose in children aged 12 months through 4 years.
5. **Pneumococcal vaccine.** (Minimum age: 6 weeks for pneumococcal conjugate vaccine [PCV]; 2 years for pneumococcal polysaccharide vaccine [PPSV])
   • PCV is recommended for all children aged younger than 5 years. Administer 1 dose of PCV to all healthy children aged 24 through 59 months who are not completely vaccinated for their age.
   • A PCV series begun with 7-valent PCV (PCV7) should be completed with 13-valent PCV (PCV13).
   • A single supplemental dose of PCV13 is recommended for all children aged 14 through 59 months who have received an age-appropriate series of PCV7.
   • A single supplemental dose of PCV13 is recommended for all children aged 60 through 71 months with underlying medical conditions who have received an age-appropriate series of PCV7.

• The supplemental dose of PCV13 should be administered at least 8 weeks after the previous dose of PCV7. See *MMWR* 2010:59(No. RR-11).
• Administer PPSV at least 8 weeks after last dose of PCV to children aged 2 years or older with certain underlying medical conditions, including a cochlear implant.
6. **Inactivated poliovirus vaccine (IPV).** (Minimum age: 6 weeks)
   • If 4 or more doses are administered prior to age 4 years an additional dose should be administered at age 4 through 6 years.
   • The final dose in the series should be administered on or after the fourth birthday and at least 6 months following the previous dose.
7. **Influenza vaccine (seasonal).** (Minimum age: 6 months for trivalent inactivated influenza vaccine [TIV]; 2 years for live, attenuated influenza vaccine [LAIV])
   • For healthy children aged 2 years and older (i.e., those who do not have underlying medical conditions that predispose them to influenza complications), either LAIV or TIV may be used, except LAIV should not be given to children aged 2 through 4 years who have had wheezing in the past 12 months.
   • Administer 2 doses (separated by at least 4 weeks) to children aged 6 months through 8 years who are receiving seasonal influenza vaccine for the first time or who were vaccinated for the first time during the previous influenza season but only received 1 dose.
   • Children aged 6 months through 8 years who received no doses of monovalent 2009 H1N1 vaccine should receive 2 doses of 2010–2011 seasonal influenza vaccine. See *MMWR* 2010;59(No. RR-8):33–34.
8. **Measles, mumps, and rubella vaccine (MMR).** (Minimum age: 12 months)
   • The second dose may be administered before age 4 years, provided at least 4 weeks have elapsed since the first dose.
9. **Varicella vaccine.** (Minimum age: 12 months)
   • The second dose may be administered before age 4 years, provided at least 3 months have elapsed since the first dose.
   • For children aged 12 months through 12 years the recommended minimum interval between doses is 3 months. However, if the second dose was administered at least 4 weeks after the first dose, it can be accepted as valid.
10. **Hepatitis A vaccine (HepA).** (Minimum age: 12 months)
    • Administer 2 doses at least 6 months apart.
    • HepA is recommended for children aged older than 23 months who live in areas where vaccination programs target older children, who are at increased risk for infection, or for whom immunity against hepatitis A is desired.
11. **Meningococcal conjugate vaccine, quadrivalent (MCV4).** (Minimum age: 2 years)
    • Administer 2 doses of MCV4 at least 8 weeks apart to children aged 2 through 10 years with persistent complement component deficiency and anatomic or functional asplenia, and 1 dose every 5 years thereafter.
    • Persons with human immunodeficiency virus (HIV) infection who are vaccinated with MCV4 should receive 2 doses at least 8 weeks apart.
    • Administer 1 dose of MCV4 to children aged 2 through 10 years who travel to countries with highly endemic or epidemic disease and during outbreaks caused by a vaccine serogroup.
    • Administer MCV4 to children at continued risk for meningococcal disease who were previously vaccinated with MCV4 or meningococcal polysaccharide vaccine after 3 years if the first dose was administered at age 2 through 6 years.

The Recommended Immunization Schedules for Persons Aged 0 Through 18 Years are approved by the Advisory Committee on Immunization Practices (**http://www.cdc.gov/vaccines/recs/acip**), the American Academy of Pediatrics (**http://www.aap.org**), and the American Academy of Family Physicians (**http://www.aafp.org**). Department of Health and Human Services • Centers for Disease Control and Prevention

FIGURE 22-2 Recommended immunization schedules for children and adolescents.   *Continued*

Recommended Immunization Schedule for Persons Aged 7 Through 18 Years—United States • 2011

For those who fall behind or start late, see the schedule below and the catch-up schedule

Vaccine ▼ Age ►	7–10 years	11–12 years	13–18 years	
Tetanus, Diphtheria, Pertussis[1]		Tdap	Tdap	Range of recommended ages for all children
Human Papillomavirus[2]	see footnote[2]	HPV (3 doses)(females)	HPV Series	
Meningococcal[3]	MCV4	MCV4	MCV4	
Influenza[4]	Influenza (Yearly)			
Pneumococcal[5]	Pneumococcal			Range of recommended ages for catch-up immunization
Hepatitis A[6]	HepA Series			
Hepatitis B[7]	Hep B Series			
Inactivated Poliovirus[8]	IPV Series			
Measles, Mumps, Rubella[9]	MMR Series			Range of recommended ages for certain high-risk groups
Varicella[10]	Varicella Series			

This schedule includes recommendations in effect as of December 21, 2010. Any dose not administered at the recommended age should be administered at a subsequent visit, when indicated and feasible. The use of a combination vaccine generally is preferred over separate injections of its equivalent component vaccines. Considerations should include provider assessment, patient preference, and the potential for adverse events. Providers should consult the relevant Advisory Committee on Immunization Practices statement for detailed recommendations: **http://www.cdc.gov/vaccines/pubs/acip-list.htm**. Clinically significant adverse events that follow immunization should be reported to the Vaccine Adverse Event Reporting System (VAERS) at **http://www.vaers.hhs.gov** or by telephone, **800-822-7967**.

1. **Tetanus and diphtheria toxoids and acellular pertussis vaccine (Tdap).** (Minimum age: 10 years for Boostrix and 11 years for Adacel)
   - Persons aged 11 through 18 years who have not received Tdap should receive a dose followed by Td booster doses every 10 years thereafter.
   - Persons aged 7 through 10 years who are not fully immunized against pertussis (including those never vaccinated or with unknown pertussis vaccination status) should receive a single dose of Tdap. Refer to the catch-up schedule if additional doses of tetanus and diphtheria toxoid–containing vaccine are needed.
   - Tdap can be administered regardless of the interval since the last tetanus and diphtheria toxoid–containing vaccine.
2. **Human papillomavirus vaccine (HPV).** (Minimum age: 9 years)
   - Quadrivalent HPV vaccine (HPV4) or bivalent HPV vaccine (HPV2) is recommended for the prevention of cervical precancers and cancers in females.
   - HPV4 is recommended for prevention of cervical precancers, cancers, and genital warts in females.
   - HPV4 may be administered in a 3-dose series to males aged 9 through 18 years to reduce their likelihood of genital warts.
   - Administer the second dose 1 to 2 months after the first dose and the third dose 6 months after the first dose (at least 24 weeks after the first dose).
3. **Meningococcal conjugate vaccine, quadrivalent (MCV4).** (Minimum age: 2 years)
   - Administer MCV4 at age 11 through 12 years with a booster dose at age 16 years.
   - Administer 1 dose at age 13 through 18 years if not previously vaccinated.
   - Persons who received their first dose at age 13 through 15 years should receive a booster dose at age 16 through 18 years.
   - Administer 1 dose to previously unvaccinated college freshmen living in a dormitory.
   - Administer 2 doses at least 8 weeks apart to children aged 2 through 10 years with persistent complement component deficiency and anatomic or functional asplenia, and 1 dose every 5 years thereafter.
   - Persons with HIV infection who are vaccinated with MCV4 should receive 2 doses at least 8 weeks apart.
   - Administer 1 dose of MCV4 to children aged 2 through 10 years who travel to countries with highly endemic or epidemic disease and during outbreaks caused by a vaccine serogroup.
   - Administer MCV4 to children at continued risk for meningococcal disease who were previously vaccinated with MCV4 or meningococcal polysaccharide vaccine after 3 years (if first dose administered at age 2 through 6 years) or after 5 years (if first dose administered at age 7 years or older).
4. **Influenza vaccine (seasonal).**
   - For healthy nonpregnant persons aged 7 through 18 years (i.e., those who do not have underlying medical conditions that predispose them to influenza complications), either LAIV or TIV may be used.
   - Administer 2 doses (separated by at least 4 weeks) to children aged 6 months through 8 years who are receiving seasonal influenza vaccine for the first

time or who were vaccinated for the first time during the previous influenza season but only received 1 dose.
   - Children 6 months through 8 years of age who received no doses of monovalent 2009 H1N1 vaccine should receive 2 doses of 2010-2011 seasonal influenza vaccine. See *MMWR* 2010;59(No. RR-8):33–34.
5. **Pneumococcal vaccines.**
   - A single dose of 13-valent pneumococcal conjugate vaccine (PCV13) may be administered to children aged 6 through 18 years who have functional or anatomic asplenia, HIV infection or other immunocompromising condition, cochlear implant or CSF leak. See *MMWR* 2010;59(No. RR-11).
   - The dose of PCV13 should be administered at least 8 weeks after the previous dose of PCV7.
   - Administer pneumococcal polysaccharide vaccine at least 8 weeks after the last dose of PCV to children aged 2 years or older with certain underlying medical conditions, including a cochlear implant. A single revaccination should be administered after 5 years to children with functional or anatomic asplenia or an immunocompromising condition.
6. **Hepatitis A vaccine (HepA).**
   - Administer 2 doses at least 6 months apart.
   - HepA is recommended for children aged older than 23 months who live in areas where vaccination programs target older children, or who are at increased risk for infection, or for whom immunity against hepatitis A is desired.
7. **Hepatitis B vaccine (HepB).**
   - Administer the 3-dose series to those not previously vaccinated. For those with incomplete vaccination, follow the catch-up schedule.
   - A 2-dose series (separated by at least 4 months) of adult formulation Recombivax HB is licensed for children aged 11 through 15 years.
8. **Inactivated poliovirus vaccine (IPV).**
   - The final dose in the series should be administered on or after the fourth birthday and at least 6 months following the previous dose.
   - If both OPV and IPV were administered as part of a series, a total of 4 doses should be administered, regardless of the child's current age.
9. **Measles, mumps, and rubella vaccine (MMR).**
   - The minimum interval between the 2 doses of MMR is 4 weeks.
10. **Varicella vaccine.**
   - For persons aged 7 through 18 years without evidence of immunity (see *MMWR* 2007;56[No. RR-4]), administer 2 doses if not previously vaccinated or the second dose if only 1 dose has been administered.
   - For persons aged 7 through 12 years, the recommended minimum interval between doses is 3 months. However, if the second dose was administered at least 4 weeks after the first dose, it can be accepted as valid.
   - For persons aged 13 years and older, the minimum interval between doses is 4 weeks.

The Recommended Immunization Schedules for Persons Aged 0 Through 18 Years are approved by the Advisory Committee on Immunization Practices (**http://www.cdc.gov/vaccines/recs/acip**), the American Academy of Pediatrics (**http://www.aap.org**), and the American Academy of Family Physicians (**http://www.aafp.org**).
Department of Health and Human Services • Centers for Disease Control and Prevention

FIGURE 22-2, cont'd

Infants and children can be immunized against diphtheria, tetanus, pertussis, hepatitis B, *Haemophilus influenzae* type B, polio, measles, mumps, rubella, and varicella. These primary immunizations dramatically reduce the incidence of disease in a community and lower mortality and morbidity rates from diseases that were once fatal to many young children. Although most children in the United States have been immunized by the time they enter school, the United States lags behind many other countries in the percentage of children immunized at an early age. Children who are homeschooled often are not immunized. Thus these diseases continue to be widespread and to do damage, particularly when young children bring infections home to older individuals whose immunity may be impaired. We now know that some early immunizations lose their ability to provide long-term immunity. Thus some adults who were vaccinated when they were children may develop pertussis or other diseases to which they believed they were immune. Widespread failure of diphtheria-pertussis-tetanus immunizations led to high rates of pertussis in California recently and guidelines now suggest that all health care providers have pertussis booster immunizations to increase their own immunity.

Every year different immunizations are offered for seasonal flu. As epidemics develop for particular diseases, such as H1N1 influenza, a limited number of immunizations are available. Health care workers should take advantage of these immunizations to protect themselves and to limit exposing their families to these organisms.

Two widespread fallacies have led to the lowered rate of immunizations for children. The first is that immunizations should be withheld if the child is sick. In most cases, a child should be immunized even if they have a mild upper respiratory tract infection or other infection. The second is the fear created by the idea that vaccine immunization in children is linked to the development of autism. There have been no reputable scientific studies to suggest this connection. Licensed practical and vocational nurses should immunize their own children and educate those around them that the risks to children not being immunized is greater than getting an immunization.

USES

Vaccines and toxoids are the biologic agents used in the routine schedule of active immunizations for adults and children. Specific biologic agents are reserved for use in people who live in areas where specific diseases (e.g., yellow fever, cholera, typhoid) are endemic (common in the community), and there is a high risk of infection. Other vaccines (e.g., pneumococcal vaccine, influenza vaccine) are recommended for people at high risk for specific diseases such as pneumonia or flu.

An additional group of biologic agents (e.g., purified protein derivative [PPD], histoplasmin, coccidioidin) is used in screening procedures to identify people who have been exposed to a specific disease or who may have an active disease such as tuberculosis.

In special circumstances, certain biologic agents (e.g., gamma globulins) may be useful to modify a disease process in the previously unimmunized person.

ADVERSE REACTIONS

In general, mild adverse effects of vaccines and other immune agents are common and include localized pain and swelling that are typically mild and of short duration. Claims that immunizations are linked to other health problems have not been supported by scientific studies and data. Although it is true there are rare instances of more serious problems, the risk of complications from the disease far outweighs the risk of adverse effects for all biologic products. Adverse effects occasionally seen include altered levels of consciousness, headaches, lethargy (sleepiness), rash, urticaria (hives), vesiculation (blistering), diarrhea, increased respiratory rate, shortness of breath, arthralgia (joint pain), fever, lymphadenopathy, and malaise (weakness).

Most states have laws requiring infants and children to be properly immunized before starting school. To reduce the liability faced by pharmaceutical companies, a special fund, the National Vaccine Injury Compensation Program, has been established by the federal government to reimburse medical costs incurred if a patient has a serious adverse effect from required immunizations. A certain percentage of the fee paid by the patient for each immunization goes toward this fund, which is administered by the Public Health Service, a division of the U.S. Department of Health and Human Services.

 Clinical Goldmine

Immunization Schedule

The American Academy of Pediatrics, the Advisory Committee on Immunization Practices, and the American Academy of Family Physicians collaborate on immunization guidelines that are updated each January.

 Clinical Goldmine

Adverse Effects of Immunization

Although some parents have concerns about adverse effects of immunizations, their children are statistically more likely to have complications from the preventable disease than they are to experience serious problems from the immunization.

DRUG INTERACTIONS

When several vaccines are given at the same time—for example, when cholera, plague, and typhoid vaccines are given together—the potential for adverse effects is increased. Someone who has passive immunity to a disease (has received antibodies from a maternal or a vaccine source or through blood products) may not have an adequate active antibody response to the administration of a live, attenuated vaccine.

❖ NURSING IMPLICATIONS AND PATIENT TEACHING

▪ Assessment

Find out as much as possible about the patient's health history, including the patient's previous immunization status and reaction to biologic agents; history of allergy, especially to eggs or feathers; results of any known allergy testing; the presence of underlying disease or concurrent infections; the use of immunosuppressant drugs, immune serums, blood, or blood products; or the possibility of pregnancy.

The patient may have a history of exposure to a specific organism or might plan to travel to areas where disease may be common. Find out if the person is at risk for infection, as well as whether there are children who require primary immunizations. The U.S. State Department regularly issues travelers' warnings, and the nurse can call the embassy of a foreign government to see if certain immunizations are required for entry into that country.

▪ Diagnosis

Determine the patient's risk for infection. Has the patient or parent verbalized reservations about being able to return for scheduled immunizations? If so, the risk for noncompliance with the immunization schedule must be shared with the primary health care provider so that adjustments can be made. Enhancing the likelihood that immunizations will be completed involves the entire health care team.

▪ Planning

The best policy is that immunizations should not be given to patients with active infection, severe febrile illness, or a history of serious side effects from previous vaccinations. Live, attenuated vaccine is usually contraindicated in pregnancy. To be safe, clinicians often do not provide immunizations to children who are being seen for minor illnesses. However, because many children are taken to the health care provider only when they are ill, clinicians may have to give the immunizations then. Otherwise, they may lose a very valuable opportunity to provide increased protection to the child.

Many biologic agents are prepared with animal serum or in chick embryos. Thus people with known allergies may have sensitivity reactions to these preparations. Live, attenuated virus vaccine should not be given if there is a recent history of acquired passive antibodies (immune globulins).

Patients should be screened for current illness. There is an increased risk in using immunologic agents in any person with a compromised immune status (for example, neonates, older adult patients, patients on immunosuppressive therapy, patients with acquired immune deficiency syndrome, or patients with chronic disease).

All vaccines should be used with caution in women who are pregnant or breastfeeding.

▪ Implementation

It is important to follow specific protocols and schedules for administration. There are usually specialized storage instructions, modes of administration, sites, and site preparation techniques for each vaccine. It is also important to consult the package insert for each manufacturer's product information, because these products often differ in some way.

Figure 22-2 shows the dosage schedule recommended for primary immunization of infants, children, and adolescents.

Uncomfortable reactions to active vaccines are frequent and generally range from localized irritation and soreness to a systemic response with fever, malaise, and anorexia (lack of appetite). Specific biologic agents may predispose the patient to a variety of allergic reactions. These range from a localized rash, pruritus (itching), or urticaria to an anaphylactic (shock) reaction.

A record of the patient's immunizations should be kept, and the patient should be provided with a copy of the record to take home for their personal file.

Occasionally, determining antibody blood titers before vaccine administration is helpful to assess antibody development. This is particularly true for rubella.

Table 22-1 provides a summary of agents used for immunity.

▪ Evaluation

Patients receiving immune serums should be evaluated for suppression of the disease. Other patients should be monitored for adverse effects. Adverse effects may occur immediately or be delayed for some time after the preparation has been administered. At all visits, patients should be asked whether their immunizations are current. There has been a decrease in the number of children who are getting the recommended immunizations over the past few years. In addition, few adults obtain the booster immunizations they need unless they are in the military, travel to foreign countries, or work in the food industry.

▪ Patient and Family Teaching

Tell the patient and family the following:

- Localized discomfort may be relieved by treating the symptoms by using warm compresses on the area, taking acetaminophen, and resting. The health care provider may recommend antihistamines.
- The patient (or family member) should record the immunization in a personal health file.
- The patient should notify the health care provider immediately if fever, rash, itching, or difficulty breathing develops.
- Patients or family should periodically discuss immunizations with the health care provider to make certain that they have adequate immunity.

Get Ready for the NCLEX® Examination!

Key Points

- Immunologic agents provide active or passive immunity to specific diseases.
- Types of immunologic agents are vaccines, toxoids, and other serologic agents used to prevent or modify disease.
- Immunity can be either naturally acquired or artificially acquired.
- It is important to follow specific protocols and schedules for administering these products.
- Adults are commonly underimmunized because they do not realize that their immunity has expired.

Additional Learning Resources

SG Go to your Study Guide for additional learning activities to help you master this chapter content.

evolve Go to your Evolve website (http://evolve.elsevier.com/Edmunds/LPN/) for additional online resources.

Review Questions for the NCLEX® Examination

1. The nurse has administered a PPD injection to a patient. The nurse will interpret the area of induration as being positive if is:
    1. 9 mm or more
    2. 5-9 mm
    3. 3-5 mm
    4. <3 mm

2. The nurse is preparing to administer RespiGam. The nurse recognizes that the medication dosage will be based on the patient's:
    1. height
    2. age
    3. weight
    4. gender

3. The patient has been ordered a dose of black widow spider species antivenin. The most appropriate area for the patient to receive the injection is:
    1. deltoid
    2. anterolateral thigh
    3. ventrogluteal
    4. dorsogluteal

4. The nurse is preparing to administer the Hepatitis A vaccine. The nurse recognizes that the most appropriate area for the patient to receive the injection is:
    1. deltoid
    2. ventrogluteal
    3. dorsogluteal
    4. vastus lateralis

5. The nurse instructs the patient that after the initial injection of hepatitis A vaccine, he will need to return for a booster injection. This should occur:
    1. 1-3 months after the initial injection
    2. 3-6 months after the initial injection
    3. 6-12 months after the initial injection
    4. 12-15 months after the initial injection

Case Study

Mr. John Phillips, 53, a state highway patrol officer, discovered an injured dog along the highway. As he attempted to remove it from the road, the dog scratched and bit him. The dog was taken to the local animal control department, where it was discovered to be infected with rabies.

1. What treatment should Mr. Phillips receive?
2. Mr. Phillips tells the nurse he has had prophylactic rabies injections. Does this make a difference in the treatment?
3. Administering rabies vaccine to Mr. Phillips is an example of what type of immunity?
4. Which groups of people are commonly considered at high risk for rabies and thus should receive prophylactic therapy?

Get Ready for the NCLEX® Examination!—cont'd

Drug Calculation Review

1. Order: Immune globulin IV (IGIV) 14,000 mg IV over 2 hours. Supply: Immune globulin 14,000 mg in 100 mL of 5% dextrose in water (D_5W).
   Question: How many milliliters per hour should the IV infusion device be set for?
2. Order: Diphtheria antitoxin 20,000 units intramuscular. Supply: Diphtheria antitoxin 100,000 units/mL.
   Question: How many milliliters of diphtheria antitoxin are needed for each dose?
3. Order: Lymphocyte immune globulin 20 mg/kg/day.
   Question: How many milligrams of lymphocyte immune globulin are needed each day for a person weighing 65 kg?

Critical Thinking Questions

1. Outline the benefits versus the risks of immunizations and their potential adverse effects.
2. The nurse is asked to give immunizations to four children of various ages who are visiting the clinic this afternoon. Draw up a general list of assessment, planning, and implementation strategies that can be used for all four children.
3. Suggest appropriate actions the nurse and patient can take in response to hypersensitivity or allergic reactions commonly seen with immunologic agents.

4. Give examples of the process or development of each of the following types of immunity: (1) artificially acquired active immunity, (2) artificially acquired passive immunity, (3) naturally acquired active immunity, and (4) naturally acquired passive immunity.
5. Identify and suggest ways to counteract the most common side effects of immunologic agents.
6. After giving him an immunization, the nurse explains to Mr. Stavros that he will need a booster later. Mr. Stavros has never heard of a booster. Explain what a booster is, along with the rationale for getting one.
7. When might a patient exhibit extra sensitivity to an immunologic agent?
8. Why is it important to know if patients are allergic to eggs or feathers before immunizing them?
9. Alicia, who is 5 years old, comes to her appointment for her school physical with her mother. As the nurse is preparing to administer the immunizations for school entry, the nurse asks her mother if she has any concerns about Alicia starting school in a few months. Her mother tells the nurse, "Well, I am a little worried. Alicia is very close to my mother, you know. She's been sick with cancer, and Alicia has been spending a lot of time with her, keeping her company. I think my mother's going to be a little lonely when Alicia goes to school every day." Why is this information significant?

Topical Medications

Objectives

1. Identify major categories of medications used topically.
2. Describe specific administration techniques for topical products.

3. List at least three preparations used to treat eye, ear, and skin problems.

Key Terms

anorectal preparations (ā-nō-RĔK-tăl, p. 411)
antiglaucoma agents (ĂN-tĭ-glăw-KŌ-mă, p. 416)
antipsoriatics (ĂN-tĭ-SŌ-rē-ĂT-ĭks, p. 417)
antiseptics (ăn-tĭ-SĔP-tĭks, p. 412)

mydriasis (mĭ-DRĪ-ă-sĭs, p. 416)
pediculicides (pĕ-DĬK-ū-lĭ-sīdz, p. 417)
scabicides (SKĂB-ĭ-sīdz, p. 417)
vasoconstrictors (vās-ō-kŏn-STRĬK-tŏrz, p. 417)

OVERVIEW

This chapter presents a brief overview of the many products that may be used topically somewhere on the skin or mucous membranes. Many of these products are purchased over the counter (OTC). Because hundreds of preparations are available, and new products come onto the market very quickly, only a few selected examples of drugs in the major categories can be presented. The nurse may play a major role in teaching the patient the proper administration of these medications and precautions for their use. Side effects are usually local unless systemic sensitization (allergic reaction) develops or absorption systemically (throughout the body) occurs.

INTEGUMENTARY SYSTEM

The integumentary system is made up of the skin, hair, nails, and sweat glands (Figure 23-1). The skin provides the most important barrier to infection and protects the body, regulates temperature, prevents water loss, and produces the chemicals that develop into vitamin D.

The skin; mucous membranes; and surfaces of the eye, ear, nose, mouth, and vagina are often the sites of minor infections. Medications are frequently used to treat conditions in these areas. For medication to go deep within these tissues, special preparations and procedures are required.

TOPICAL MEDICATIONS

ANORECTAL PREPARATIONS

Action and Uses

Anorectal preparations include emollients, foams, and gels for topical anesthesia or healing of the rectal area. They are used for symptomatic relief of discomfort from hemorrhoids. They may be used on a long-term basis or briefly for hemorrhoids associated with pregnancy, prolonged sitting, or other temporary problems. Table 23-1 presents a summary of these preparations.

Adverse Reactions

The patient may have sensitization to the product.

MOUTH AND THROAT PREPARATIONS

Action and Uses

Miscellaneous products are used to soothe minor irritation in the mouth and throat. Some release oxygen to provide cleansing, whereas others contain an anesthetic property to reduce pain. These preparations are used for minor oral inflammation, such as canker sores, dental irritation, and pain after dental procedures; for relief of dryness of the mouth and throat; or for treatment of minor sore throat discomfort and control of cough caused by colds.

Products are available in mouthwashes, sprays, solutions, troches, lozenges, and disks. The patient should be taught the appropriate administration technique for the drug form being used. Patients should not take these products for longer than 3 or 4

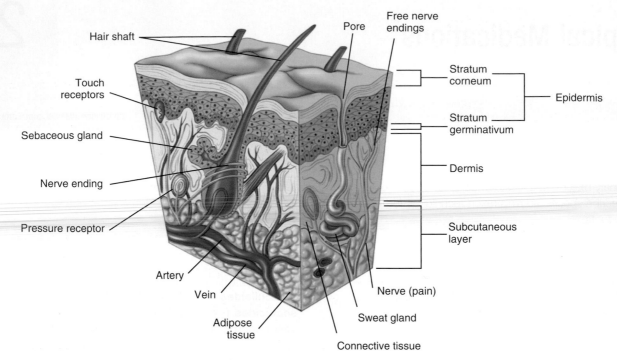

FIGURE 23-1   The integumentary system.

Table **23-1**	**Anorectal Preparations**	
GENERIC NAME	**TRADE NAME**	**COMMENTS**
dibucaine	Nupercainal (OTC)	Patient should apply ointment morning and night and after each bowel movement. For suppositories, one should be inserted after each bowel movement.
hydrocortisone acetate	Anusol-HC	Contains hydrocortisone.
zinc sulfate monohydrate	Anusol (OTC) Preparation H (OTC)	Suppository should be inserted in the morning and at bedtime for 3-6 days or until inflammation subsides; or cream may be applied to anal area and gently rubbed in 3 to 4 times daily for 3-6 days.
hydrocortisone foam	ProctoFoam-HC	Steroid used for antiinflammatory treatment of ulcerative proctitis and distal ulcerative colitis. Contains hydrocortisone. Patient should insert one applicator full in rectum daily or twice daily for 2-3 wk, then every other day, decreasing therapy gradually.

OTC, Over the counter.

days for normal therapy. Table 23-2 presents a summary of these products.

OPHTHALMIC DRUGS

Action and Uses

A wide variety of preparations are used for eye problems (Table 23-3). Local anesthetics are useful in procedures such as tonometry, gonioscopy, cataract surgery, and removal of foreign bodies from the cornea. Antiseptics are compounds capable of preventing infection. They are used for the prevention of gonorrheal ophthalmia neonatorum when babies are born or any time germicidal or astringent (tissue constricting) action is needed. Antiinfectives are used to treat common eye infections caused by bacteria, fungi, or

viruses. Artificial tears provide lubrication to relieve dry eyes, eye irritation secondary to wearing contact lenses, or deficient tear production caused by a wide variety of disorders. Diagnostic products include topical fluorescein stains, which are used to detect foreign bodies or scratches.

Increased intraocular pressure is a sign of the eye condition called *glaucoma*. This condition results from either excess production or reduced outflow of aqueous humor (ocular fluid). There are three major forms of glaucoma. *Primary glaucoma* includes narrow-angle glaucoma and wide-angle glaucoma. Patients with narrow-angle glaucoma have a shallow anterior chamber, possibly because of the anatomy or physiologic action they were born with. Drugs are used to

Table 23-2   Mouth and Throat Preparations

GENERIC NAME	TRADE NAME	COMMENTS
Oral Preparations		
carbamide peroxide	Orajel	Do not dilute. Apply directly to affected area 4 times daily, spit out after 2-3 min.
Lozenges and Troches		
—	Cepacol Cepastat Robitussin Sucrets	For mouth pain. Dissolve 1 lozenge in mouth up to every hour if needed. Take no more than 12 lozenges daily.
clotrimazole	Mycelex	For oral thrush. Take 1 troche 5 times/day for 14 days. Dissolve slowly in mouth.
Gargles, Gels, Mouthwashes, and Sprays		
—	Cepacol Chloraseptic	For mouth pain. Follow directions on bottle or package. Wide variation exists among products.
nystatin	Mycostatin	Antifungal; for oral thrush. Take 400,000-600,000 units for 10-14 days. Dissolve slowly in mouth.
Saliva Substitutes		
—	Salivart	Used to relieve dry mouth and throat; spray into mouth as needed.

Table 23-3   Ophthalmic Preparations

GENERIC NAME	TRADE NAME	COMMENTS
Local Anesthetics		
benoxinate	Fluress	Often used when suturing of eye is required. Use before eye procedures.
proparacaine	Alcaine	Use immediately before tonometry, 2-3 min before suture removal or removal of foreign body.
tetracaine	Pontocaine	Use drops or ointment to lower conjunctival area.
Antiseptic Ointments		
silver nitrate	Silver Nitrate	After birth, clean infant's eyes with cotton ball and use 2 gtt 1% solution once.
Ophthalmic Antiinfectives (Preparations Must be Labeled "Ophthalmic")		
Alpha$_2$-Adrenergic Agonist		
brimonidine	Alphagan P	Use 1 drop in the affected eye(s) q8h.
Antibiotics		
bacitracin	AK-Tracin	Apply sparingly into conjunctival sac 2 to 3 times daily.
chloramphenicol		Apply small amount of ointment to lower conjunctival sac, or use 2 drops of solution q3h for the first 48 hr, then PRN. Continue for at least 48 hr after the eye appears to be normal.
ciprofloxacin	Ciloxan	Put into conjunctival sac, close eyes, and apply light pressure over lacrimal sac for 1 minute.
erythromycin	Ilotycin	Apply to affected eye 3 times daily or more often, depending on severity of infection.
gentamicin	Garamycin Genoptic Gentacidin	Put drops into affected eye q4h. In severe infections, dosage may be increased to hourly. Apply ointment sparingly 2 to 3 times daily.
levofloxacin	Quixin Levaquin	Use drops in the affected eye(s) q2h while awake, up to 8 times/day for 2 days. Then use drops in affected eye(s) q4h while awake, up to 4 times/day for days 3 through 7.
norfloxacin	Noroxin	Put into conjunctival sac, close eyes, and apply light pressure over lacrimal sac for 1 min after.

Continued

Table 23-3 Ophthalmic Preparations—cont'd

GENERIC NAME	TRADE NAME	COMMENTS
ofloxacin	Ocuflox	Put into conjunctival sac, close eyes, and apply light pressure over lacrimal sac for 1 min after.
polymyxin B	polymyxin B	Use very hour PRN.
sulfacetamide sodium	AK-Sulf Sodium Sulamyd	Use drops q2-3h during day, less at night. May also apply ointment in lower conjunctival sac at night.
tobramycin	Tobrex AK-Tob	Use drops 4 to 6 times daily.
Antiviral Agents		
fomivirsen		Adults: Use a single intravitreal injection every other week for 2 doses followed by maintenance dose once every 4 wk in treatment of cytomegalovirus retinitis.
ganciclovir	Vitrasert	Used in treating cytomegalovirus retinitis in patients with AIDS. Provided as a 4.5-mg insert designed to release drug over a 5- to 8-mo period. May be repeated as needed.
trifluridine	Viroptic	Put onto ulcerated cornea of eye q2h while awake for a maximum of 9 drops/day. Continue until reepithelialization, then for 7 days give q4h while awake.
Artificial Tears		
—	Isopto Tears Liquifilm Forte Refresh Plus Systane Tearisol Tears Plus	Drops may be used in eyes 3 to 4 times daily or PRN. Some preparations, such as Tearisol, are not to be used with soft contact lenses. Keep solution free from contamination.
—	Lacrisert	Insert once a day into inferior cul-de-sac beneath base of tarsus.
Antiglaucoma Agents		
Sympathomimetics		
apraclonidine	Iopidine	Use solution before laser surgery.
dipivefrin	Propine	Put into eyes q12h.
epinephrine ★		Use drops into affected eyes daily to twice daily.
		Use daily or twice daily.
Beta Blockers		
betaxolol	Betoptic	Use drops twice daily.
carteolol	Ocupress	Use drops twice daily.
levobetaxolol	Betaxon	Use drops twice daily.
levobunolol	Betagan Liquifilm	Use drops daily.
metipranolol	OptiPranolol	Use drops twice daily.
timolol	Timoptic	Use drops twice daily.
Miotics, Direct-Acting		
acetylcholine Cl	Miochol-E	Use drops 3 times daily.
carbachol	Isopto-carbachol	Use drops up to 3 times daily.
pilocarpine	Pilocar Pilostat	Use drops up to 6 times daily.
pilocarpine ocular therapeutic system	Ocusert	The system is placed in and removed from the eye by the patient, according to instructions in the package. Releases 20 or 40 mcg pilocarpine per hour for 1 wk.
Miotics, Cholinesterase Inhibitors		
demecarium		Put drops into eyes daily.
echothiophate	Phospholine Iodide	Use drops daily.

Table 23-3   Ophthalmic Preparations—cont'd

GENERIC NAME	TRADE NAME	COMMENTS
Carbonic Anhydrase Inhibitors		
brinzolamide	Azopt	Use 3 times daily.
dorzolamide	Trusopt	Use 3 times daily.
Mydriatic-Cycloplegics		
atropine		Use solution daily to 3 times daily, or ointment daily to 3 times daily.
cyclopentolate	Cyclogyl	Use 1% or 2% solution; repeat in 5 min. Refraction can occur in 40-50 min.
homatropine	Isopto-Homatropine	Use 2% or 5% solution; repeat 2 to 5 times until desired results occur.
scopolamine	Isopto Hyoscine	Use 0.25% solution daily to 3 times daily.
tropicamide	Mydriacyl	Use 1% solution; repeat in 5 min.
Mydriatic		
phenylephrine	Neo-Synephrine	Mydriasis: Use 2.5%-10% solution topically on conjunctiva. Repeat in 5 min PRN. Mydriasis: Use 2.5%-10% solution topically on conjunctiva. Repeat in 5 min PRN. Conjunctivitis: Use qh until condition improves, and then 1 drop 3 to 4 times daily.
Other Ophthalmic Preparations		
Alpha-Adrenergic Blocking Agent		
dapiprazole		Use drops, followed 5 min later by additional drops.
Prostaglandin Agonists		
bimatoprost	Lumigan	Use daily in the evening to reduce IOP.
latanoprost	Xalatan	Use drop in affected eye(s) once daily in the evening. Do not exceed prescribed dose.
travoprost	Travatan	Use drop daily in the evening to reduce IOP.
unoprostone		Use drop twice daily. May be used with other drops if administered at least 5 min apart.
Antihistamines		
azelastine	Optivar	Use drops twice daily to reduce itching from allergic conjunctivitis.
emedastine	Emadine	Use drops in affected eye(s) 4 times daily. Do not use if patient is wearing contact lenses.
olopatadine	Patanol	Use drops twice daily at intervals of 6-8 hr.
Vasoconstrictors and Mydriatics		
hydroxyamphetamine		Use drops in conjunctival sac.
naphazoline		Use drops 2 to 3 times daily PRN to relieve irritation or redness. Mydriasis occurs within 1 hr, recedes within 6 hr of administration. NOTE: DO NOT GIVE TO PATIENTS WITH ANGLE-CLOSURE GLAUCOMA OR NARROW ANTERIOR ANGLE.
oxymetazoline		Use drops q6h.
tetrahydrozoline	Murine Tears Plus Visine	Use drops in each eye 2 to 3 times daily PRN. Mydriasis occurs in 1 hr, recedes within 6 hr. NOTE: DO NOT GIVE TO PATIENTS WITH NARROW-ANGLE GLAUCOMA.
Eye Diagnostic Products		
fluorescein	Fluor-I-Strip Ophthifluor Fluorescite AK-Fluor Ful-Glo	For examination of corneal and conjunctival epithelium, pour 1 drop sterile water on strip, touch to cornea, and close lid for 60 sec. Use Wood lamp to visualize. Add drops; patient should blink. Examine eye under fluorescing light, and areas of foreign body or abrasion should fluoresce bright green or yellow.

Continued

Table 23-3   Ophthalmic Preparations—cont'd

GENERIC NAME	TRADE NAME	COMMENTS
Nonsteroidal Antiinflammatory Drugs		
diclofenac	Voltaren	Use drops in affected eye 4 times daily beginning 24 hr after cataract surgery and continuing throughout first 2 wk of postoperative period.
flurbiprofen	Ocufen	For inhibition of intraoperative miosis, for inflammation after cataract, glaucoma, or laser surgery and uveitis syndromes: Use every 30 min beginning 2 hr before surgery.
ketorolac	Acular	For relief of ocular itching caused by seasonal allergic conjunctivitis and treatment of postoperative inflammation of postcataract extraction: 1 drop to affected eye(s) 4 times daily beginning 24 hr after cataract surgery and continuing for 2 wk.
suprofen	Profenal	For treatment of postoperative inflammation after cataract extraction: On day before surgery, put drops into conjunctival sac every 4 hr while awake; on day of surgery at 3 hr, 2 hr, and 1 hr before surgery.
Mast-Cell Stabilizers		
nedocromil	Alocril	Use drops in each eye twice daily to treat itching of allergic conjunctivitis.
pemirolast	Alamast	Use drops in each eye 4 times daily to prevent itching from allergic conjunctivitis.
Ophthalmic Decongestants		
cromolyn sodium	Crolom	Use drops 4 to 6 times daily.
lodoxamide	Alomide	For patients with vernal conjunctivitis or vernal keratitis: Use drops in each eye 4 times daily for up to 3 mo.
ketotifen	Zaditor	Use drops q8-12h to prevent itching of eye from allergic conjunctivitis.
levocabastine	Livostin	Use drops in affected eye(s) 4 times daily for up to 2 wk.
Ophthalmic Corticosteroids		
dexamethasone	AK-Dex Maxidex	Sol: Use drops qh during the day and q2h at night until symptoms reduce; then q4h.
fluorometholone	Flarex Fluor-Op	Suspension: Shake well and use drops in conjunctival sac 2 to 4 times daily. Ointment: Apply ribbon of medication into conjunctival sac 1 to 3 times daily.
loteprednol	Lotemax Alrex	Use drops 4 times daily. Shake well before using.
medrysone	HMS	Shake well and put drops into conjunctival sac up to every 4 hr.
prednisolone	AK-Pred Pred Forte Pred Mild Inflamase	Shake well and put drops in conjunctival sac 2 to 4 times daily.
rimexolone	Vexol	Put drops in affected eye 4 times daily beginning 24 hr after ocular surgery and for 2 wk.

AIDS, Acquired immune deficiency syndrome; *IOP,* intraocular pressure; *PRN,* as needed; *Sol,* solution.
★ Indicates "Must-Know Drugs," or the 35 drugs most prescribers use.

control the acute problem before there is a permanent surgical solution. Wide-angle glaucoma has a gradual onset, and its control depends on permanent drug therapy. *Secondary glaucoma* may result from other eye problems such as cataract extraction; it is treated with medication. *Congenital glaucoma* is a birth defect requiring surgical correction. Medications for treating glaucoma use a variety of mechanisms to increase outflow of aqueous humor.

Antiglaucoma agents make up a large class of medications with a variety of actions. Mydriatic-cycloplegics block the action of acetylcholine. The sphincter of the iris is paralyzed, causing **mydriasis,** or abnormal dilation (opening) of the pupil, and the ciliary muscles are paralyzed, blocking accommodation (the ability to switch from near to far vision and back), or adjustment of the focus of the eye. These agents are used in some tests for glaucoma. Atropine and scopolamine are long-acting agents that produce complete cycloplegia, or paralysis. Homatropine, cyclopentolate, and tropicamide have shorter durations of action and are most useful for diagnostic procedures. Long-acting cholinesterase inhibitors include miotic-antiglaucoma agents that inactivate acetylcholinesterase. This provides iris sphincter contraction, leading to miosis (small pupils), and ciliary muscle constriction, which leads to increased aqueous humor outflow. Parasympathomimetic or miotic drugs, such as carbachol, act as cholinergic agonists to reduce intraocular pressure by causing iris sphincter contraction, leading to miosis. This allows an increased outflow of aqueous humor by opening up the anterior chamber angle. Cholinesterase inhibitors such as physostigmine salicylate briefly inactivate acetylcholinesterase to allow acetylcholine to accumulate, which increases parasympathetic tone. This causes iris sphincter contraction, resulting in miosis, increased ciliary muscle constriction, and an increase in aqueous humor outflow. Timolol is a beta blocker that reduces intraocular pressure, probably by reducing the formation of aqueous humor. Sympathomimetic agents such as epinephrine produce vasoconstriction (narrowing of the blood vessels) and decreased intraocular pressure in open-angle glaucoma, probably as a result of decreased production of aqueous humor. Phenylephrine acts as a mydriatic, causing constriction of the dilator muscles of the pupil, leading to mydriasis and vasoconstriction of the arterioles of the conjunctiva. **Vasoconstrictors** such as naphazoline cause direct stimulation of the alpha receptors of vascular smooth muscle, leading to vasoconstriction. This action lasts for several hours.

 Clinical Goldmine

Ophthalmic Preparations

Ophthalmic preparations are the mildest chemicals used on the body. If something is safe enough to put in the eye, it should be safe enough for use anywhere else. Each of these preparations has numerous precautions, contraindications, and minor adverse effects. Check the package inserts for more detailed information and Table 23-3 for a summary.

Before administering any ophthalmic agent, it is especially important for the nurse to learn whether the patient has a history of glaucoma. Dilating the pupils of a patient who may have glaucoma could provoke angle closure and lead to a surgical emergency.

OTIC PREPARATIONS
Action and Uses
Topical antibiotics are used to control superficial infections of the ear through bactericidal or bacteriostatic mechanisms. Other products may be used for prophylaxis of infections in swimmers and for removing cerumen (earwax) plugs. There are also some steroid products available for ear problems. Check the package inserts of individual products for precautions, contraindications, and adverse effects. Table 23-4 presents a summary of otic preparations.

TOPICAL SKIN PREPARATIONS
Action and Uses
Topical preparations for the skin may include medicated bar soaps and foams, sulfur preparations, topical antibiotics, and medications used for acne. A wide variety of steroids are also available for topical use in a variety of dermatologic disorders. These preparations come in mild, intermediate, and strong concentrations. Fluorinated products should not be used on the face because they may cause thinning of the skin and leave scars. Steroids should not be used if there is strong indication of bacterial or fungal infection because the steroid may suppress the action of the antibiotic or antifungal and allow the infection to get worse.

Antipsoriatics accelerate scaling and healing of dry lesions in chronic psoriasis. Antiseborrheic shampoos promote shedding and softening of the horny cell layer and inhibit the growth of microorganisms in seborrhea and dandruff. There are now antiviral agents used to treat herpes simplex. These agents help reduce the severity of symptoms and lengthen the time between outbreaks. **Scabicides** are applied to the skin and in the hair to treat scabies, a condition caused by the microscopic mite *Sarcoptes scabiei*. **Pediculicides** are used to treat pediculosis, an infestation with lice seen mostly in children. There are also a variety of burn preparations, cauterizing agents, emollients, keratolytics, and wet dressings and soaks on the market. These agents all have their own individual precautions, adverse reactions, and drug interactions. The specific product information should be consulted. These preparations are summarized in Table 23-5. Any of the chemicals in these products may interact with other medications the patient may be taking.

COMPLEMENTARY AND ALTERNATIVE PRODUCTS

Patients use a wide variety of topical herbal products. The Complementary and Alternative Therapies box summarizes common herbal preparations and their potential for interactions with other medications.

Complementary and Alternative Therapies

Oral and Topical Products for Eye, Ear, and Skin Problems

PRODUCTS	COMMENTS
ACNE	
Chasteberry/Vitex	Potential interaction with hormonal replacements or oral contraceptives
Tea tree	No known interactions
Olive leaf	No known interactions
ATHLETE'S FOOT	
Cat's claw	Potential interaction with anticoagulants, aspirin, NSAIDs, antiplatelet agents
Tea tree	No reported interactions
Olive leaf	No reported interactions
Garlic	Potential interaction with anticoagulants, aspirin, NSAIDs, antiplatelet agents, hypolipidemics, antihypertensives
CONTACT DERMATITIS AND ECZEMA	
Milk thistle	No reported interactions
Evening primrose	Potential interactions with anticoagulants, aspirin, NSAIDs, antiplatelet agents
Grapefruit seed extract	Avoid terfenadine, astemizole, cisapride, or other medications metabolized by cytochrome P-450 3A4 subsystem
Olive leaf	No reported interactions
Artichoke	No reported interactions
Aloe	No known interactions
Calendula	No known interactions
Echinacea	No known interactions
GLAUCOMA	
Bilberry	Potential interaction with anticoagulants, aspirin, NSAIDs, antiplatelet agents
Grapeseed	Potential interaction with anticoagulants, aspirin, NSAIDs, antiplatelet agents, methotrexate
OTITIS MEDIA	
Echinacea	Potential interaction with therapeutic immunosuppressants and corticosteroids
Astragalus	May interact with immune stimulants or immunosuppressants
Olive leaf	No reported interactions
PSORIASIS	
Coleus (PO)	Potential interaction with anticoagulants, aspirin, NSAIDs, antiplatelet agents, antihistamines, decongestants, anticoagulants, antihypertensives
Milk thistle (PO)	No known interactions
Gotu kola	Application may cause dermatitis
Evening primrose	Potential interaction with anticoagulants, aspirin, NSAIDs, antiplatelet agents
ROSACEA	
Cat's claw	Potential interaction with anticoagulants, aspirin, NSAIDs, antiplatelet agents
Chasteberry/Vitex (PO)	Potential interaction with hormone replacements or oral contraceptives
Milk thistle (PO)	No known interactions
Grapefruit seed extract (PO)	Avoid terfenadine, astemizole, cisapride, or other medications metabolized by cytochrome P-450 3A4 subsystem
Evening primrose	Potential interaction with anticoagulants, aspirin, NSAIDs, antiplatelet agents
SUNBURN	
Aloe	No known interactions
Lavender	No known interactions
St. John's wort	No known interactions if used topically

Modified from Krinsky DL, LaValle JB, Hawkins EB, et al: *Natural therapeutics pocket guide,* ed 2, Hudson, Ohio, 2003, Lexi-Comp, Inc.
NSAIDs, Nonsteroidal antiinflammatory drugs; *PO,* by mouth.

Table 23-4   Otic Preparations

GENERIC NAME	TRADE NAME	COMMENTS
Otic Preparations (Preparations Must be Labeled "Otic")		
benzocaine	Americaine	Swab ear with solution; use 4-5 drops of warmed solution. Insert cotton pledget in meatus. Patient should remain on side for a few minutes.
carbamide peroxide	Debrox	To remove ear wax, use 5-10 drops, keeping head tilted so solution stays in. Maintain position for a few minutes. Repeat twice daily for 3-4 days. May use before irrigation with bulb syringe.
chloramphenicol		Effective against many gram-positive and gram-negative organisms. Adults and children: Put drops into ear 3 times daily.
desonide, acetic acid	Tridesilon	Useful in superficial infections of the external canal; put drops into affected ear 3 to 4 times daily.
triethanolamine polypeptide oleate-condensate		To remove cerumen. May be given as drops to loosen cerumen. Use patch test to check for sensitivity 24 hr before use. Tilt patient's head to 45-degree angle and fill ear canal with solution. Insert cotton plug for 30 min. Gently flush ear with warm water using a soft rubber syringe.
Otic Steroid and Antibiotic Combinations		
ciprofloxacin, hydrocortisone	Cipro HC Otic	Use drops 3 or 4 times daily.
hydrocortisone, neomycin	Cortisporin-TC Otic	Use drops 3 or 4 times daily.
hydrocortisone, neomycin, and polymyxin B		Use drops 3 or 4 times daily.

Table 23-5   Topical Skin Products

GENERIC NAME	TRADE NAME	COMMENTS
Acne Products		
adapalene	Differin	Wash face then apply a thin film of gel once daily to affected areas. An exacerbation of acne may initially be seen; therapeutic results usually seen in 8-12 wk.
azelaic	Azelex	Wash face and dry thoroughly. Then apply thin film twice daily to affected areas and gently massage into skin. Results usually seen in 4 wk.
benzoyl peroxide cream and soaps	Clearasil Desquam-X Oxy Oil-Free Acne Wash	Apply daily to affected areas after cleansing skin. After 3-4 days, if redness, dryness, and peeling do not occur, increase application to twice daily. Use instead of soap. These products promote drying of skin and provide a gentle abrasive action when applied. If undue skin irritation develops, stop use and contact nurse, physician, or other health care provider. Available OTC.
isotretinoin	Accutane ♣	This product must not be taken by women who are pregnant, because severe fetal abnormalities may be produced. Women in childbearing years should be protected by adequate contraception methods during the course of therapy. Cystic acne: Dosage may adjusted for individual weight and severity of disease.
sulfur preparations	Liquimat	Thin film of medication should be applied daily or twice daily to clean skin. Used to treat oily skin and mild acne.
tazarotene	Tazorac	Wash face and then apply a thin film to affected areas once daily.
tretinoin	Retin-A Vesanoid ♣	Wash face and apply to affected area daily at bedtime. Start with low doses; may irritate skin initially. Makes individuals more sensitive to the sun, necessitating sunscreen. Evidence suggests that this product restores skin collagen and turgor, reversing fine wrinkles. Not for use by pregnant women.

Continued

Table 23-5	Topical Skin Products—cont'd	
GENERIC NAME	**TRADE NAME**	**COMMENTS**
Topical Antiinfectives		
bacitracin	Baciguent	Apply small amount to infected area 3 times daily; comes as cream.
chloramphenicol	Chloromycetin	Apply small amount to infected area 3 times daily; comes as cream.
clindamycin	Cleocin T	Apply small amount to infected area twice daily.
erythromycin	Akne-Mycin	Apply small amount to infected area 3 times daily; comes as cream.
gentamicin		Apply small amount to infected area 3 times daily; comes as cream.
mupirocin	Bactroban	New topical antibiotic. Used to treat impetigo; may produce superinfection. Apply small amount to affected area 3 times daily. May cover with gauze. Must be reevaluated within 3 days.
neomycin sulfate		Apply small amount to infected area 3 times daily; comes as cream.
Combination Products		
polymyxin B, neomycin, and bacitracin	Neosporin	Apply small amount to infected area 3 times daily; comes as ointment.
polymyxin B	Polysporin	Apply small amount to infected area 3 times daily; comes as ointment.
Topical Corticosteroids		
alclometasone	Aclovate	For relief of inflammatory and pruritic manifestations of corticosteroid-responsive dermatoses. Apply sparingly to affected areas 2 to 4 times daily.
amcinonide	Cyclocort	Apply sparingly to affected areas 2 to 4 times daily.
betamethasone dipropionate	Diprolene	Fluorinated product, relatively expensive. Comes as cream, lotion, ointment, or topical aerosol. Use sparingly for dermatoses needing antiinflammatory medication.
betamethasone valerate	Beta-Val Valisone	Fluorinated product that may be used with occlusive dressings; comes as cream, lotion, or ointment. Apply sparingly daily to 3 times daily for adults.
desonide	Tridesilon	Gently rub in medication 2 to 4 times daily.
desoximetasone	Topicort	Do not use near eyes; apply sparingly daily to twice daily.
diflorasone	Maxiflor	Apply sparingly to affected areas 2 to 4 times daily.
fluocinolone acetonide	Synalar	Rub cream in gently, 2 to 4 times daily. Apply very sparingly; use less frequent applications for children.
fluocinonide	Lidex	Comes as cream, gel, or ointment; apply 3 to 4 times daily.
flurandrenolide	Cordran	Shake lotion well; protect from light, heat, and freezing. Also comes as a film tape. Apply sparingly 2 to 3 times daily.
halcinonide	Halog	Ointment, cream, solution; protect ointment from light. Apply sparingly 2 to 3 times daily.
hydrocortisone ★	Cortizone Hycort	One of the few steroids that can be used safely on the face, axilla, and groin, and under the breasts. Comes as ointment, cream, or lotion. Apply thin coat once daily to 4 times daily; increase strength as indicated by condition.
hydrocortisone acetate	Cortaid Lanacort 5	This form is more expensive. Apply thin coat of ointment or apply the cream gently and sparingly. Apply once daily to 4 times daily as needed by condition. The lowest doses are available without a prescription.
hydrocortisone plus antibiotics	Cortisporin	Comes with neomycin sulfate and polymyxin B. Apply to affected area 2 to 3 times daily; withdraw gradually if medication has been used for a long time.
methylprednisolone	Medrol	Very expensive; apply ointment once daily to 4 times daily.

Table 23-5   Topical Skin Products—cont'd

GENERIC NAME	TRADE NAME	COMMENTS
triamcinolone acetonide	Aristocort Kenalog	Fluorinated steroid, highest potency; has many precautions to use. Apply to affected area 2 to 4 times daily. Do not use on face.
triamcinolone plus antifungals	Mycolog II	Many precautions and warnings. Apply ointment to affected areas 2 to 3 times daily. Ototoxicity (damage to the ear) and nephrotoxicity (damage to the kidney) have been reported if preparation is overused.
Anesthetics for Mucous Membranes and Skin		
benzocaine	Solarcaine Babee Teething lotion	Used for sunburn, wounds, toothaches, mouth ulcers, and lesions of oral mucosa. Apply 20% aerosol or gel to affected areas 2 to 3 times daily.
dibucaine	Nupercainal	For abrasions, minor burns, sunburn, and hemorrhoids. Apply ointment or cream sparingly to affected area 2 to 3 times daily.
tetracaine	Pontocaine	Used in treating hemorrhoids and minor skin disorders. Apply sparingly 3 to 4 times daily.
Antipsoriatics		
acitretin	Soriatane	Systemic psoriasis therapy for severe disease.
anthralin	Anthra Forte	Apply thin layer of 0.1% ointment once to twice daily for 2 wk.
calcipotriene	Dovonex	Synthetic vitamin D_3 derivative indicated for topical treatment of moderate plaque psoriasis. Calcipotriene is similar to vitamin D_3 in its effects on keratinocyte proliferation and differentiation, yet it has a less potent effect on calcium metabolism. Also modifies immune activity of monocytes, macrophages, and T lymphocytes. In clinical trials, improvement in psoriasis noted within 2 wk of initiating topical therapy (twice-daily application). Approximately 70% of patients have shown marked improvement after 8 wk of therapy, with 10% showing complete clearing. Apply thin layer twice daily and rub in completely.
tazarotene	Tazorac	For topical treatment of patients with stable plaque psoriasis with approximately 20% body surface area involvement. The 0.1% gel also is indicated for mild to moderately severe facial acne vulgaris.
Antiseborrheic Products		
povidone-iodine	Betadine	Shampoo with 2 tsp to hair and scalp. Lather with warm water and rinse. Repeat application and allow to remain on scalp 5 min; rinse thoroughly. Use twice weekly until improvement, then once weekly.
selenium	Selsun Blue	Massage 1-2 tsp into wet scalp. Allow medicated shampoo to remain on scalp for 2-3 min; rinse thoroughly; repeat application and rinse. Use twice weekly for 2 wk, then weekly for 2 wk.
Antiviral Agents		
acyclovir	Zovirax	For treatment of herpes simplex. Cover all lesions q3h, 6 times per day for 6 days. Approximately ½-inch ribbon of ointment per 4 square inches of surface area should be used. Oral forms are available for treatment of herpes labialis (cold sores).
penciclovir	Denavir	Apply cream q2h while awake for 4 days. Start treatment as early as possible to reduce symptoms.
Burn Preparations		
mafenide	Sulfamylon	Apply once or twice daily to a thickness of approximately 1/16 inch. No dressing required.
nitrofurazone	Furacin	Soluble dressing: apply directly to lesions daily; topical cream: apply directly to lesion once daily or every few days.
silver nitrate	Silver Nitrate	Saturate dressing with warmed solution and apply to burn wound. Mold dressing to body surface and cover with dry dressing. Reapply solution q2h. Change dressing at least once daily.
silver sulfadiazine	Silvadene	Apply once or twice daily to a thickness of approximately 1 1/16 inch. No dressing required.

Continued

Table 23-5   Topical Skin Products—cont'd

GENERIC NAME	TRADE NAME	COMMENTS
Scabicides and Pediculicides		
crotamiton	Eurax	Used in scabies and very pruritic skin conditions. Massage into skin of the whole body; apply a second coating 24 hr later. Clothing and bed linen should be changed after 24 hr. Bath should be taken 48 hr after the last application.
malathion	Ovide	Apply to hair and let hair dry naturally. Wash after 8-12 hr and comb hair. Repeat in 7-9 days, if necessary.
permethrin	Elimite Nix Acticin	Massage into skin from scalp to soles of feet. Wash off after 8-14 hr. For pediculosis capitis in infants, wet hair, shampoo, and then apply medication to hairline, neck, scalp, temple, and forehead, and wash off after 10 min
Miscellaneous Skin Preparations		
Cauterizing Agents		
dichloroacetic acid	Bichloracetic Acid	Apply petrolatum to tissue surrounding area to be treated. Solution should then be carefully applied to lesion. A kit is provided with detailed instructions.
monochloroacetic acid	Mono-Chlor	Used for removing verrucae or warts. Do not drip solution on normal tissue or mucous membranes. Apply solution with cotton-tipped applicator or capillary tube. Cover with bandage and allow to remain in place for 4-6 days. May require more than one application.
podofilox	Condylox	Apply solution or gel to venereal warts morning and evening with a cotton-tipped applicator.
podophyllum resin	Podofin Podocon-25	Applied to venereal warts only by health care provider. Cleanse area and then apply sparingly to lesion. Leave on 30-40 min to check sensitivity, and no longer than 4 hr. Remove with alcohol or soap and water.
silver nitrate solution or sticks		Apply to local area as needed.
trichloroacetic acid	Tri-Chlor	Use on débrided skin to remove verruca. Apply to wart, then cover for 5-6 days. Peel off wart tissue.
Emollients		
colloidal baths	Alpha Keri Aveeno	Bath additives for treating widespread eruptions. Limit bath time to 30 min; patient should be aware that preparations often make tub slippery. Follow directions on packet or bottle.
dexpanthenol	Panthoderm	Stimulates epithelization and granulation. Aids in the healing of skin lesions and relieves pruritus. Apply directly to clean skin once to twice daily.
salicylic acid	Mediplast-Salacid Wart-Off	Use creams for corns and calluses. Apply directly to area daily for 2 wk. Cut out piece of plaster to fit callus or apply gels to well-hydrated skin. Check callus q24h; discontinue if irritation develops.
urea	Aquacare Nutraplus	Hydrates skin and aids in removing scales and crusts. Apply directly to clean skin 2 to 3 times daily, affected area only.
vitamin E	Vite E Cream Vitec	Apply cream or ointment to skin to hydrate.
Vitamins A, D, and E	Retinol Clocream	Apply cream or ointment to skin.
Smoking Cessation Products		
nicotine transdermal system	Nicoderm CQ Nicotrol	Used to decrease withdrawal symptoms as part of smoking cessation program. No serious side effects. In association with behavior modification programs, use patch daily. Use 2 wk at each of 3 strengths in decreasing order of strength.
nicotine gum	Nicorette	Use 2- or 4-mg gum to reduce cravings. Chew gum steadily, and then place gum against buccal membranes.

Table 23-5 Topical Skin Products—cont'd

GENERIC NAME	TRADE NAME	COMMENTS
nicotine inhalation system	Nicotrol Inhaler	4-mg inhaler. Used as part of withdrawal system.
nicotine nasal spray	Nicotrol NS	Spray 0.5 mg into nostril to reduce symptoms of withdrawal.
Wet Dressings and Soaks		
Burow's solution	Domeboro	Used for open wet dressings in inflammatory conditions of skin; cool and dry through evaporation, which causes local vasoconstriction. Moisten dressing and apply multiple layers to prevent rapid drying and cooling. Reapply every 15-30 min as indicated for 4-8 hr.

OTC, Over the counter.
★ Indicates "Must-Know Drugs," or the 35 drugs most prescribers use.

Get Ready for the NCLEX® Examination!

Key Points

- This chapter presents a brief overview of the wide variety of topical preparations available, many of which are OTC products.
- Even though the dose of medication in these products is usually small, they may still interact with other medications the patient is taking.
- The nurse's role in the use of these medications often is one of teaching the patient how to apply or administer the products.
- Review the material on topical drug administration in Chapter 10.
- Side effects are usually localized unless systemic sensitization develops.

Additional Learning Resources

SG Go to your Study Guide for additional learning activities to help you master this chapter content.

℮volve Go to your Evolve website (http://evolve.elsevier.com/Edmunds/LPN/) for additional online resources.

Review Questions for the NCLEX® Examination

1. The patient has been ordered to be treated with Nicoderm CQ. The nurse anticipates that in addition to the medication, the patient will also need to have an order for:
   1. group therapy
   2. behavior modification
   3. antianxiety medication
   4. methadone

2. The patient has been ordered to be treated with Domeboro soaks. The nurse anticipates that for the first 8 hours, the soaks will need to be changed:
   1. 15-30 minutes
   2. 30 minutes-1 hour
   3. 1-2 hours
   4. 3-4 hours

3. The nurse notes that the patient has an order to start acyclovir (Zovirax). The nurse expects to see on the admission history that the patient has been diagnosed with:
   1. pediculosis
   2. scabies
   3. psoriasis
   4. herpes simplex

4. The patient is scheduled to begin treatment with triamcinolone plus (Mycolog II). The nurse will need to contact the physician if the patient verbalizes having a history of:
   1. vision loss
   2. neurologic damage
   3. hearing loss
   4. taste and smell changes

5. The nurse notes that the patient is scheduled to begin treatment with isotretinoin (Accutane). The highest priority instruction that the nurse should give the patient is:
   1. use contraception throughout the course of the treatment
   2. wash face thoroughly before applying medication
   3. sunscreen should be used conscientiously
   4. expect the skin to be more sensitive during treatment

Get Ready for the NCLEX® Examination!—cont'd

Case Study

Jenny Hawkes has worn contacts for more than 30 years. She has ophthalmic examinations about every 2 years and has been relatively free of problems. During her last visit, the ophthalmologist told her she had a little conjunctivitis and ordered an antibiotic.

1. What are some topical antiinfectives that might be ordered?
2. On her yearly visits, the ophthalmologist measures the intraocular pressure and dilates her eyes to view the retina. This year, there is some evidence that Jenny is developing glaucoma. Is there any concern about dilating her eyes if she might be developing glaucoma?
3. Why are there different categories of drugs used in the treatment of glaucoma?
4. After several follow-up visits, Jenny is started on Timoptic. What kind of a medication is this, and what are some of the anticipated reactions to the drug?
5. What other antiglaucoma products might Jenny take?
6. Jenny wakes up one morning with sharp, scratchy pains in her left eye. Her eye is tearing, and she is unable to keep it open. The ophthalmologist puts fluorescein sodium in her eye. Why?
7. The ophthalmologist discovers a small foreign body lodged in the cornea. It is removed with a needle, Jenny's eye is patched, and she is sent home. What types of medications might be required?
8. Jenny has noticed lately that her eyes feel dry after she has been reading for a time. What would be of benefit for her to treat this condition?
9. Jenny has mentioned to the nurse that she heard about taking grape seed for glaucoma and wanted to know if there would be any problem doing that. What might the nurse tell her?

Drug Calculation Review

1. Order: Nystatin 500,000 units, swish and swallow 4 times per day. Supply: Nystatin 100,000 units/mL.
   Question: How many milliliters of nystatin are needed with each dose?
2. Order: Accutane 40 mg by mouth twice a day. Supply: Accutane 20 mg per tablet.
   Question: How many tablets of Accutane are needed with each dose?
3. Order: Wash hair daily with selenium 10 mL.
   Question: How many teaspoons of selenium are needed for each wash?

Critical Thinking Questions

1. Mr. Samms comes to the clinic for an eye examination. His pupils must be dilated first. Describe the precautions the nurse should take when the patient has his pupils dilated.
2. Mr. Samms' physician has recommended an OTC ophthalmic product for control of mild glaucoma. Explain glaucoma to Mr. Samms, along with the actions and effects of the antiglaucoma agents.
3. Mr. Samms asks the nurse about different medicines that might have to take for glaucoma. Name at least three types of medications that might be ordered for glaucoma.
4. Mr. Samms also has to take medication in the form of eye drops for 1 week for a separate, minor disorder. He has never needed eye drops until now. He tells the nurse that he is nervous about being able to self-administer these. What are the important concepts to stress in teaching the patient about putting in eye drops?
5. Think about and then explain why are there differences between administration of eye ointments and that of eye drops?
6. Mrs. Johnson and her 4-year-old son come into the clinic needing treatment for swimmer's ear. Why is the administration of ear drops different for each of these patients?
7. The nurse practitioner (NP) also discovers that Mrs. Johnson's ears are filled with wax. What medication is the NP most likely to order for this?
8. Conduct an informal investigation at a nearby pharmacy or drugstore: Compare administration instructions on the labels or (if available) the package inserts of several OTC skin products. Are some more specific in their instructions than others? Why might that be?
9. The school nurse in an elementary school sees Daniel, who is in the third grade, in her office office scratching his head and complaining his head "itches." Upon checking his scalp, the nurse realizes he has pediculosis, or head lice. What instructions should the nurse give to his parents?

Vitamins and Minerals

Objectives

1. Identify the actions and indications for vitamins and minerals.
2. List at least six products used to treat vitamin or mineral deficiencies.
3. Present a teaching plan for patients who require vitamin or mineral supplements.

Key Terms

ascorbic acid (ăs-KŎR-bĭk, p. 430)
minerals (MĬN-ĕr-ălz, p. 432)
niacin (NĪ-ă-sĭn, p. 427)
riboflavin (RĪ-bō-flā-vĭn, p. 427)

thiamine (THĪ-ă-mĭn, p. 426)
vitamin A (VĪ-tă-mĭn, p. 426)
vitamins (VĪ-tă-minz, p. 425)

 ## OVERVIEW

This chapter discusses the uses of vitamins and minerals. An overview of their actions, indications for use, and common adverse effects and drug interactions is presented. Vitamins are taken by people to maintain health and also by those who use medications to correct nutritional deficiencies. There may be drug interactions between vitamins and medications that affect both nutrient and drug absorption. Brief comments of importance for the nurse are included. Summaries of a sample of vitamin and mineral supplements available on the market are included in tables at the end of each major discussion. These over-the-counter (OTC) products change quickly, and the latest information should always be obtained for specific products. See Chapter 15 for additional related information about fluid and electrolyte products.

VITAMINS

OVERVIEW

Vitamins are chemical compounds found naturally in plant and animal tissues but most are not made in the human body. Some are available in their active form; others come from food as a "precursor" or "provitamin" that then is converted to the active form. Two vitamins, Vitamin K and biotin, are not from food at all but are synthesized by bacteria inside the intestinal tract. They are necessary for life and essential to normal metabolism. They can act as coenzymes to regulate the creation of compounds in the body. Vitamins are classified into two types. *Fat soluble* vitamins are found primarily in various plant and animal oils or fats and can be stored in the body so daily intake is not essential. These vitamins are transported through the body by the bloodstream and remain dissolved because of unique-carrier proteins. Deficiencies are slow to develop. *Water soluble* vitamins are readily excreted in the urine and not stored in the body. The vitamins are destroyed by heat and deficiencies are quickly seen in patients. Usually patients get enough vitamins from a well-balanced, nutritious diet, except when certain conditions prevent them from eating food (such as intravenous therapy when a patient is taking nothing by mouth) or when the vitamins are not absorbed or their action is blocked (as in disorders that block fat metabolism) or the metabolism is accelerated (with some types of thyroid disease or pregnancy). Such conditions may require a vitamin supplement until a normal diet can be resumed or the underlying problem corrected.

Although controversy exists over natural versus synthetic vitamin preparations, current research confirms that vitamins are still vitamins, and the least expensive vitamin preparation is most likely as good therapeutically as a more expensive version. There are still many mysteries about the action of various vitamins in the body, but research has consistently demonstrated that taking large amounts of vitamins is unnecessary, may be harmful, and should be avoided.

There is a lot of literature about antioxidant vitamins and nutritional supplements. The major antioxidants are vitamin E (alpha-tocopherol), beta-carotene (a precursor, or forerunner, to vitamin A), vitamin C (ascorbic acid), and the mineral selenium. All of these are found in fruits and vegetables. Many research studies are looking at the mechanism of action of antioxidants. Current research suggests that when low-density lipoprotein (LDL) cholesterol is oxidized, sometimes incomplete oxidation takes place, producing free radicals that lead to atherosclerotic plaques. (An analogy has been made to wood that burns incompletely in a fireplace and "pops," sending sparks against the screen.) It is thought that antioxidants retard or prevent LDL oxidation because they are oxidized in preference to LDL. This slows or eliminates the progression of atherosclerosis. It is also believed that antioxidants may slow the process that may cause cancer in cells. This has resulted in a large market for antioxidants to reduce the risk of cardiovascular disease and cancer.

Although many major research studies have looked at antioxidants after the fact and have suggested major benefits from increased use for many disease states, there are at present no intervention studies that support the role of antioxidants in cancer prevention. Epidemiologic evidence does indicate that those who eat fruits and vegetables regularly have a lower risk of cancer, although there is no conclusive evidence that this is the result of antioxidants. Therefore supplementation with vitamin antioxidants may be beneficial; however, in certain populations, such as smokers, research has found that it may actually be harmful. Nonetheless, the U.S. Department of Agriculture and the U.S. Department of Health and Human Services released new food guidelines in early 2011 based on what should be on a plate rather than the food pyramid. Today there is more emphasis than ever on eating fruits, vegetables, and whole-grain products, and on taking in fewer calories and getting more exercise to reverse widespread obesity in all age groups.

VITAMIN A

ACTION AND USES

Vitamin A is a fat-soluble, long-chain alcohol that comes in several isometric forms: retinol, retinene, carotene, and retinoic acid. Its best understood action is helping the eye adjust to changes from light to darkness. Less understood actions include: (1) helping to stabilize and maintain the cell membrane structure, especially epithelial cell membranes, thereby helping the body resist infection; (2) affecting the synthesis of protein, which affects growth of skeletal and soft tissue; and (3) playing an essential role in reproduction.

Vitamin A supplementation is used to treat deficiency that may be provoked by sprue, colitis, regional enteritis, biliary tract or pancreatic disease, or partial gastrectomy. It is also used for the treatment of specific eye diseases and night blindness.

ADVERSE REACTIONS

If vitamin A is given in high doses for a long time, the treatment should be stopped at times to avoid hypervitaminosis. Any patient receiving 25,000 International Units or more should be closely supervised. Pregnant women should not receive more than 6000 International Units daily, or they may risk fetal abnormalities.

DRUG INTERACTIONS

Women taking oral contraceptives often show elevated plasma vitamin A levels and should be closely monitored for hypervitaminosis. Mineral oil interferes with the absorption of fat-soluble vitamins. Certain antihyperlipidemic agents may also affect absorption of this product.

❖ NURSING IMPLICATIONS AND PATIENT TEACHING

One International Unit of vitamin A is equivalent to 0.6 mcg of beta-carotene or 0.3 mcg of retinol. This medication may be given orally, intravenously, or intramuscularly, depending on the rapidity of needed replacement.

Recommended daily allowances (RDAs) are as follows:

Children 0 to 9 years: 300 to 450 mcg/day
Children 9 to 18 years: 575 to 750 mcg/day
Adults 18 to 75 years and older: 750 mcg/day
Pregnant women (second and third trimesters): 750 mcg/day
Lactating women: 1200 mcg/day

Some foods rich in vitamin A are animal products such as dairy products; eggs; and organ meats (all contain preformed vitamin A); and deep orange, yellow, and green fruits and vegetables (these contain carotene). In addition, some fortified sources of vitamin A are infant formula, skim milk, margarine, and some cereals.

VITAMIN B₁ (THIAMINE)

ACTION AND USES

Vitamin B₁, or thiamine, is water soluble and functions as a coenzyme that is closely involved with carbohydrate metabolism. Thiamine is involved in 24 different reactions, including the citric acid cycle. It also has been thought to have a role in neurophysiologic function. Thiamine is excreted in the urine.

Vitamin B₁ is used to treat beriberi, which is rare but not unknown in the United States. Vitamin B deficiency is usually found in patients with alcoholism, gastric lesions, or hyperemesis of pregnancy. Symptoms include anorexia (lack of appetite), vomiting, fatigability, aching muscles, ataxia (poor coordination) of gait, and emotional disturbances such as moodiness, depression, or excess alcohol use.

ADVERSE REACTIONS

Adverse reactions to thiamine include sensitivity (allergy) reactions, particularly after parenteral administration, which can be severe, including anaphylaxis (shock). Fatalities may occur. Sensitivity tests should be done before the therapeutic dose is given. Intravenous (IV) doses should be given very slowly. Feelings of warmth, pruritus (itching), urticaria (hives), nausea, angioneurotic edema (abnormal collection of fluid in deep layers of skin, often with lip swelling and hives), pulmonary edema, sweating, tightness of the throat, malaise (weakness), and cyanosis (blue color to the skin) are also seen.

DRUG INTERACTIONS

Products that have neutral or alkaline solutions will produce poor stability of thiamine preparations.

❖ NURSING IMPLICATIONS AND PATIENT TEACHING

Thiamine is easily leached (lost) out of food and is destroyed when food is heated to more than 100° C, fried in hot pans, or cooked for a long time under pressure. There is some loss of thiamine during dehydration of vegetables. Thiamine is also sensitive to ultraviolet light. Foods rich in thiamine include pork, whole grains, enriched breads, cereals, and legumes. Satisfactory sources include green vegetables, fish, meats, fruits, and milk.

VITAMIN B₂ (RIBOFLAVIN)

ACTION AND USES

Vitamin B_2, or **riboflavin**, is water soluble and acts as a precursor of two essential enzymes that deal with metabolism of proteins, fats, and carbohydrates. It is related to the release of energy to the cells and is active in tissue respiratory systems. It is used for the prophylaxis or treatment of riboflavin deficiency with symptoms which include soreness and burning of the tongue, lips, and mouth; discomfort in eating and swallowing; and photophobia (sensitivity to light), lacrimation (excess tear production), burning and itching of the eyes, visual fatigue, and the loss of visual acuity.

DRUG INTERACTIONS

Riboflavin is only slightly soluble in water. Riboflavin levels in the body can be decreased by oral contraceptives, even in low doses. This loss has been shown through studies to be greater when patients have been taking oral contraceptives for at least 3 years.

❖ NURSING IMPLICATIONS AND PATIENT TEACHING

B_2 or riboflavin supplements should be protected from light by keeping it in a tightly closed, light-resistant container. The medication turns urine a yellow color.

Food sources naturally rich in riboflavin include milk; eggs; liver; kidney; heart; green, leafy vegetables; and enriched breads and cereals.

NIACIN

ACTION AND USES

Niacin, previously called vitamin B_3, is water soluble and an essential part of two coenzymes involved with intracellular respiration. These coenzymes convert lactic acid to pyruvic acid and function in energy release and in amino acid metabolism.

Niacin is used to prevent or treat deficiency states caused by a limited dietary intake of niacin, excessive dietary intake of leucine (which increases the daily need for niacin), general anorexia related to disease or other problems, or malabsorption syndrome. The deficiency state known as *pellagra* is rare but may be more prevalent in geographic regions where corn is the major staple food. Pellagra is usually found along with other vitamin deficiencies.

Pellagra symptoms are seen as changes in mucous membranes, skin, the gastrointestinal (GI) tract, and the central nervous system (CNS). Anorexia, irritability, anxiety, and mental changes such as hallucinations, lassitude (weariness), apprehension, and depression may be noticed.

GI symptoms include glossitis (swollen, beefy, red tongue), stomatitis (inflammation of the mouth), and diarrhea. Dermatitis of different body parts exposed to sun or trauma may develop, as well as lesions on the skin that result from sun, fire, or heat. Mental changes that are mild early in deficiency may progress to disorientation, loss of memory, confusion, hysteria, and, sometimes, manic outbursts.

ADVERSE REACTIONS

Adverse reactions to niacin include dry skin, pruritus, skin rash, GI disorders, allergies, feelings of warmth, headache, tingling of the skin, and transient flushing (red color in the face and neck).

DRUG INTERACTIONS

Sympathetic blocking agents (antihypertensives) may increase the vasodilatory effect of niacin, leading to postural hypotension (low blood pressure when a person suddenly stands up).

❖ NURSING IMPLICATIONS AND PATIENT TEACHING

Flushing is a frequent side effect of niacin. If patients feel weak or dizzy, they should lie down until they feel better. Usually this reaction does not require stopping the drug. The usual dose is 8 mg/1000 kcal for infants and 6.6 mg/1000 kcal for children and adolescents. Less than 8 mg/day should not be given. The recommended intake for adults is 13 mg/day for women and 18 mg/day for men.

Foods rich in niacin are lean meats, peanuts, yeast, and cereal (especially bran and wheat germ). Other good sources include eggs, liver, red meat, whole grains, and enriched bread.

PANTOTHENIC ACID

ACTION AND USES

Pantothenic acid, previously known as *vitamin B₅*, is essential for the synthesis of coenzyme A, which has a role in the release of energy in fats, proteins, and carbohydrates. This vitamin has been used to treat paralytic ileus after surgery, possibly acting to stimulate GI motility. Deficiency states are produced only in the laboratory.

❖ NURSING IMPLICATIONS AND PATIENT TEACHING

When food is cooked to more than the boiling point, considerable loss of pantothenic acid occurs. The loss is smaller when food is moderately cooked or baked.

This vitamin is available naturally in all plant and animal tissues. Much of the original vitamin content is lost from frozen meat in the liquid that drips off during thawing. Rich sources include yeast, liver, kidney, egg yolk, wheat bran, and fresh vegetables. Human milk contains 2.2 mg/L and cow's milk contains 3.4 mg/L.

VITAMIN B₆

ACTION AND USES

Vitamin B₆, or pyridoxine hydrochloride, is water soluble and functions as a coenzyme in the metabolism of protein, carbohydrates, and fat.

Pyridoxine is used to treat pyridoxine deficiency seen in patients with inborn errors of metabolism, such as vitamin B₆ dependency; vitamin B₆-responsive chronic anemia; and other rare vitamin problems.

Pyridoxine deficiency is most likely to develop in the older adult population and in women of childbearing age, especially those who are pregnant or breastfeeding. Women taking oral contraceptives, alcoholics, and those whose diets are of poor quality and quantity or are high in refined foods are also at risk.

Symptoms of deficiency include malaise, nervousness, irritability, and difficulty in walking. There may also be personality changes in adults, such as depression and a loss of sense of responsibility. High doses of pyridoxine may produce neurotoxicity—ataxia, numb feet, and clumsiness.

ADVERSE REACTIONS

Adverse effects are not commonly seen in patients taking pyridoxine. Pyridoxine dependency (a state of conditioned need) may develop in adults taking doses exceeding 200 mg/day for a month.

DRUG INTERACTIONS

Oral contraceptives may induce pyridoxine deficiency. Concurrent use with levodopa will neutralize CNS effects. Pyridoxine may prevent chloramphenicol-induced optic neuritis. Some drugs interfere with vitamin activity enough to block action and produce symptoms of deficiency.

❖ NURSING IMPLICATIONS AND PATIENT TEACHING

Pyridoxine should be kept in a tightly sealed, light-resistant container. Good food sources of vitamin B₆ include yeast, wheat, corn, egg yolk, liver, kidney, and muscle meats; limited amounts are available from milk and vegetables. It is also found in liver, whole-grain breads and cereals, and soybeans.

Appropriate food preparation is important in preserving this vitamin. Freezing of vegetables results in a 20% loss of pyridoxine, and the milling of wheat results in a 90% loss.

FOLIC ACID

ACTION AND USES

Folic acid (also known as *vitamin B₉*) is required for normal erythropoiesis, or red blood cell formation, and nucleoprotein synthesis. It is metabolized in the liver, where it is changed to its more active form. Folic acid is used to treat anemias caused by folic acid deficiency; it is also used in alcoholism, hepatic disease, hemolytic anemia, infancy (especially for infants receiving artificial formulas), lactation, oral contraceptive use, and pregnancy. Folic acid supplements may be needed in low-birth-weight infants, infants nursed by mothers deficient in folic acid, or infants with infections or prolonged diarrhea.

Recent guidelines have emphasized the importance of increased folic acid intake by all women of childbearing age, especially in those women intending to get pregnant and in early pregnancy to help prevent spinal cord malformations in the fetus (neural tube defects). The folic acid additives in commercial bread and grain products have been increased in an attempt to provide more adequate supplies of this important vitamin.

Research has suggested that concentrations of the amino acid homocysteine increases in the body with age and low levels of folate and vitamins B₆ and B₁₂. High homocysteine levels may be involved in the development of occlusive vascular disease (atherosclerosis), which may increase the risk of myocardial infarction. Therefore the level of folate in persons younger than 65 years of age should be measured.

ADVERSE REACTIONS

Folic acid is not toxic. An allergic reaction may produce bronchospasm, erythema (redness or irritation), malaise, pruritus, and rash; large amounts may discolor the urine.

DRUG INTERACTIONS

Chloramphenicol and methotrexate are folate antagonists, and they may cause decreased folic acid activity. *Para*-aminosalicylic acid and sulfasalazine may cause symptoms of folic acid deficiency. Use with many anticonvulsants may decrease the anticonvulsant effect, leading to increased seizure activity. Use of oral contraceptives may lead to folic acid deficiency.

❖ NURSING IMPLICATIONS AND PATENT TEACHING

The RDAs of folic acid are as follows:
Adult men: 0.15 to 0.2 mg/day
Adult women: 0.15 to 0.18 mg/day
Pregnant and lactating women: 0.4 mg/day
These RDAs are usually provided by an adequate diet.

Folic acid for parenteral use must be protected from light.

Proper nutrition is essential, and dietary measures are preferable to drug therapy. The patient should be counseled to eat foods high in folic acid to prevent a deficiency problem in the future.

Blood for hematologic laboratory tests should be drawn before beginning therapy. Drug therapy should improve the blood test results within 2 to 5 days.

Patient education should include the importance of remaining under medical supervision while receiving therapy. The patient may need to have the dose increased or decreased. Patients often fail to return for follow-up visits when they begin to feel better.

Diet is important in restoring proper folic acid levels and preventing deficiencies in the future. The patient should eat foods high in folate, including fresh, leafy green vegetables; other vegetables and fruits; yeast; and organ meats.

VITAMIN B$_{12}$

ACTION AND USES

Vitamin B$_{12}$ is water soluble and contains cobalt. It is produced by the bacterium *Streptomyces griseus*. It functions in many metabolic processes in protein, fat, and carbohydrate metabolism. The coenzymes of B$_{12}$ are also part of the erythrocyte-maturing factor of the liver and are required in the synthesis of deoxyribonucleic acid (DNA). Vitamin B$_{12}$ has a hemopoietic activity identical to the antianemia factor of the liver, and it is essential for growth, cell reproduction, and nucleoprotein and myelin synthesis. Intrinsic factor must be present in the stomach and small intestine to absorb B$_{12}$. Vitamin B$_{12}$ interacts with folate in metabolic functions, and a deficiency in B$_{12}$ makes folate useless in the body.

Vitamin B$_{12}$ is used to treat all B$_{12}$ deficiency conditions, including pernicious anemia (with or without neurologic symptoms), certain other anemias, malabsorption syndromes, hemorrhage, blind loop syndrome, chronic liver disease complicated by deficiency of vitamin B$_{12}$, malignancy, and pregnancy and thyrotoxicosis (in which deficiency is seen because of increased metabolic rate), and renal disorders. Vitamin B$_{12}$ is also used as the flushing dose in Schilling test (a specific test used for pernicious anemia). Symptoms of deficiency are rare, occurring mainly in people on strict vegetarian diets, because although vitamin B$_{12}$ is water soluble, it is found only in animal products. Symptoms include dyspepsia, sore tongue, breathlessness, and a characteristic stiff back, often dubbed a "poker" or "vegan" back. Most patients with Vitamin B$_{12}$ deficiency have a malabsorption problem in the GI tract, and the vitamin replacement is injected which bypasses the GI tract. Parenteral, nasal, or oral therapy may be used to maintain normal B$_{12}$ levels.

Nascobal is a vitamin B$_{12}$ nasal spray used as a maintenance drug for persons in remission after undergoing intramuscular (IM) therapy for pernicious anemia. The dose is usually 500 mcg intranasally once weekly. If the patient develops adverse effects such as infection, headache, glossitis, nausea, and rhinitis after taking the nasal spray, it is often necessary to start IM vitamin B$_{12}$ again.

ADVERSE REACTIONS

Allergy to vitamin B$_{12}$ is rare. The patient may report pruritus, a feeling of swelling of the entire body, or a severe anaphylactic reaction. A few patients may experience mild pain, localized skin irritation, or mild transient diarrhea after an injection of cyanocobalamin.

DRUG INTERACTIONS

Alcohol, colchicine, and *para*-aminosalicylic acid lower the absorption of vitamin B$_{12}$. Some antibiotics lower the response to vitamin B$_{12}$ therapy.

❖ NURSING IMPLICATIONS AND PATIENT TEACHING

Irreparable neurologic damage may occur if a deficiency state continues longer than 3 months or when treatment for pernicious anemia includes only folic acid. If colchicine, *para*-aminosalicylic acid, or excessive alcohol intake occurs for more than 2 weeks, malabsorption of vitamin B_{12} may occur.

The recommended daily intake of cyanocobalamin for adults is 3 mcg. The best food sources of B_{12} include organ meats; bivalves such as clams and oysters; nonfat dry milk; fermented cheese such as Camembert and Limburger; and seafood such as lobster, scallops, flounder, haddock, swordfish, and tuna.

VITAMIN C

ACTION AND USES

Vitamin C, or **ascorbic acid**, has multiple functions, some of which are understood better than others. Vitamin C functions in a number of enzyme systems and is involved in intracellular oxidation-reduction potentials. It aids in the change of folic acid and the metabolism of certain amino acids, assists the absorption of iron and calcium, and blocks the absorption of copper in the GI tract. Ascorbic acid protects vitamins A and E and polyunsaturated fatty acids. It is also necessary for the formation of the ground substance of bones, teeth, connective tissue, and capillaries and for the synthesis of collagen. Ascorbic acid aids in wound healing and may be involved in blood clotting.

Ascorbic acid is used to treat debilitated (weak) patients, especially after surgery in older adult patients with fractures, and as a supplement for burn victims or patients undergoing severe stress. Infection, smoking, chronic illness, and febrile states may increase the need for vitamin C. It is used along with iron therapy and in patients on prolonged IV therapy. Premature infants require relatively large doses. It is also used for the prophylaxis and treatment of scurvy, the deficiency state.

With modern refrigeration and processing methods of citrus fruits, scurvy is rarely seen in the United States, but it may be found when other vitamin deficiencies are present. Symptoms include tender, painful muscles, joints, and bones; muscle cramps; anorexia; fatigue; malaise; and sore gums. Wound healing is impaired, and hemorrhagic manifestations are demonstrated by subperiosteal bleeding and petechial hemorrhages. Vasomotor instability, bruising, faulty bone and tooth development, loosened teeth, and gingivitis also may develop.

ADVERSE REACTIONS

The patient may experience mild, brief soreness at injection sites if the medication is given intramuscularly or subcutaneously. Patients may also experience brief episodes of faintness or dizziness when IV injections are given too rapidly. Excessive doses are usually rapidly excreted into the urine. Doses in excess of 1 to 3 g daily may result in GI complaints, glycosuria, oxaluria, and development of renal stones, especially in patients prone to these problems. Patients who chronically overuse vitamins may develop dependency.

DRUG INTERACTIONS

Ascorbic acid may have varying effects on anticoagulants, blocking the action of some and prolonging the intensity and duration of others. Ascorbic acid increases the effect of salicylates through increased renal tubular reabsorption. There is also an increased chance of crystallization of sulfonamides in the urine when ascorbic acid is given at the same time. Ascorbic acid decreases the effect of tricyclic antidepressants by decreasing renal tubular reabsorption. Calcium ascorbate may cause cardiac dysrhythmias (irregular heartbeats) in patients receiving digitalis. Ascorbic acid is chemically incompatible with potassium penicillin G and should not be mixed in the same syringe. Smoking may lead to an increased need for vitamin C by decreasing ascorbic acid serum levels. Intermittent use of ascorbic acid in patients taking ethinyl estradiol may increase the risk of contraceptive failure. Large doses of vitamin C may interfere with urine testing in some diabetic testing methods.

❖ NURSING IMPLICATIONS AND PATIENT TEACHING

Vitamin C comes in three major forms that may be given orally or parenterally: ascorbic acid, sodium ascorbate, and calcium ascorbate. The recommended daily intake is 60 mg for adults.

Vitamin C is easily destroyed by air, heat, and light. This medication should be kept tightly capped in its own container. Foods high in vitamin C should not be boiled for long periods or left uncovered in the refrigerator.

Good food sources of vitamin C include oranges; grapefruit; strawberries; cauliflower; cantaloupe; beef liver; asparagus; green, leafy vegetables; and potatoes.

VITAMIN D

ACTION AND USES

"Vitamin D" is a label used for a group of fat-soluble, chemically similar sterols. The three main categories within this group are:

1. Ergocalciferol (vitamin D_2), which is very limited in nature in both distribution and concentration but can be artificially manufactured by ultraviolet irradiation on ergot and yeasts.
2. Cholecalciferol (vitamin D_3), which occurs naturally in fish liver oils and can be formed in animals and humans by ultraviolet irradiation on the skin.
3. Other lesser compounds (vitamins D_4, D_5, D_6, and D_7), which are formed by irradiation of sterols.

Therefore the term *vitamin D* has become rather ambiguous.

The main action of this group of sterols is the movement of calcium and phosphorus ions into three main sites: the small intestine (to promote absorption of calcium and phosphorus from the gut), the kidneys (to cause phosphate reabsorption in the proximal convoluted tubules and, to a lesser extent, to stimulate calcium and sodium reabsorption), and bone (to help increase the mineralization of newly formed bone). Vitamin D_3 has been shown to inhibit the spread of fibroblasts and keratinocytes in the skin and to promote epidermal keratinocyte differentiation. It is used in the treatment of some skin disorders.

Vitamin D preparations are used to treat childhood rickets and adult osteomalacia, hypoparathyroidism, and familial hypophosphatemia. In childhood, rickets may be diagnosed by complaints of excessive sweating and GI disturbances. These may be the first symptoms, appearing before any objective findings. In adult cases of osteomalacia, patients may complain of skeletal pain and progressive muscular weakness.

ADVERSE REACTIONS

Symptoms of vitamin D toxicity include anorexia, nausea, malaise, weight loss, vague aches and stiffness, constipation, diarrhea, convulsions, anemia, mild acidosis, and impairment of renal function. The renal effects are usually reversible. A variety of more serious systemic effects may be seen in adults. Dwarfism may be present in infants and children. Most toxic effects persist for several months in adults at doses of 100,000 International Units or more daily or in children at doses of 20,000 International Units or more daily. Reactions gradually disappear if treatment is discontinued at the first sign of symptoms.

DRUG INTERACTIONS

Mineral oil and some of the antihyperlipidemic agents may interfere with the absorption of fat-soluble vitamins. Thiazide diuretics and vitamin D together contribute to hypercalcemia. There is a possible connection between phenytoin (Dilantin) and phenobarbital use leading to hypocalcemia, which, in turn, may contribute to rickets or osteomalacia.

❖ NURSING IMPLICATIONS AND PATIENT TEACHING

The dosage of vitamin D must be planned for each patient and given under close supervision, because the range between the therapeutic and the toxic levels is narrow. Calcium intake should be enough to give a serum calcium level between 9 and 10 mg/dL. In rickets, 12,000 to 500,000 International Units/day can be taken. In hypoparathyroidism, the initial dose is typically 50,000 to 200,000 International Units/day, with a maintenance dosage of 50,000 to 400,000 International Units/day. Most people obtain all the vitamin D they need from the food in their diets. Natural sources of vitamin D are few, so the majority of vitamin D is obtained from fortified sources. Fortified foods high in this vitamin are milk, evaporated milk, infant formula, and powdered skim milk. Cereals, margarine, and diet foods also contain vitamin D supplements. Breast milk is usually already Vitamin D rich. Vitamin D should be protected from light in a light-resistant container.

VITAMIN E

ACTION AND USES

Vitamin E is fat soluble and consists of naturally occurring tocopherols. Vitamin E is considered an essential nutrient for humans, even though its specific functions are not yet understood. Vitamin E may function as an antioxidant to prevent damage to cell membranes. It stabilizes red-blood-cell walls and protects them from hemolysis or destruction. It may also increase vitamin A use and stop platelet aggregation.

Many suggested uses of vitamin E are controversial and unproved. The only established use is to prevent or treat vitamin E deficiency. Vitamin E has been touted as a powerful antioxidant. New evidence suggests that vitamin E supplements do not reduce the risk of cancer or major cardiovascular disease and may even increase the risk of heart failure. High intake of vitamin E from food as tocopherol may be inversely related to Alzheimer disease. Vitamin E in supplements is usually present as alpha-tocopherol and is less helpful in decreasing risk of Alzheimers.

ADVERSE REACTIONS AND DRUG INTERACTIONS

Vitamin E appears to be the least toxic of the fat-soluble vitamins. No signs and symptoms of toxicity or hypervitaminosis have been identified as yet in humans. However, results of a 2004 metaanalysis of research studies suggests that doses over 150 International Units/day increase the risk of all-cause mortality. The higher the dose taken, the higher the mortality rate. The most common marketed dose in the United States is 400 International Units. Many individuals take up to 2000 International Units/day.

❖ NURSING IMPLICATIONS AND PATIENT TEACHING

Food sources of vitamin E are primarily from plants. The highest amounts are found in vegetable oils such as soybean and corn and in nuts; wheat germ; rice germ; and green, leafy vegetables. Meat and dairy products provide less. An accurate assessment of tocopherol levels in food is difficult to obtain. The amount in the body depends on the initial concentration of vitamin E and the processing, storage, and preparation of the food. Vitamin E products should be stored in tightly closed, light-resistant containers.

VITAMIN K

ACTION AND USES

Vitamin K helps hepatic formation of active prothrombin (factor II), proconvertin (factor VII), plasma thromboplastin component (factor IX), and the Stuart factor (factor X), which are essential for normal blood clotting. The exact mechanism is unknown. Menadione (K_3) and phytonadione (K_1) are synthetic lipid-soluble forms of vitamin K. Menadiol sodium diphosphate (K_4) is changed in the body to menadione. Menadione is not commonly available now.

Vitamin K is used to treat or prevent various blood clotting disorders that result in damaged formation of factors II, VII, IX, and X. The American Academy of Pediatrics recommends routine phytonadione (K_1) injection at birth to prevent hemorrhagic disease of the newborn. Vitamin K does not counteract the anticoagulant activity of heparin, although it is helpful in reversing the effects of warfarin (Coumadin) overdosage.

ADVERSE REACTIONS

Specific adverse reactions to menadione (K_3)/menadiol sodium diphosphate (K_4) include headache, rash, urticaria, gastric upset, redness, and pain or swelling at injection site. Specific adverse reactions to phytonadione (K_1) include brief hypotension (low blood pressure), rapid and weak pulse, dizziness, flushing, sweating, unusual taste sensations, redness, and pain or swelling at injection site. Severe reactions, including fatalities, have occurred with the use of IV phytonadione, even when caution is used (dilution of drug, slow infusion).

DRUG INTERACTIONS

Concurrent use of vitamin K with oral anticoagulants may decrease the effects of the anticoagulant. Mineral oil and cholestyramine inhibit GI absorption of oral vitamin K.

❖ NURSING IMPLICATIONS AND PATIENT TEACHING

The preferred routes of administration of vitamin K are subcutaneous or IM. IV administration is not recommended because of the risk of anaphylaxis. Naturally occurring vitamin K is found in liver and green, leafy vegetables.

A summary of selected vitamin preparations on the market is presented in Table 24-1.

MINERALS

☀ OVERVIEW

There are 19 inorganic substances called **minerals** present in the body, at least 13 of which are essential to normal metabolism and function. These minerals are present as ions with positive and negative charges, leading to the formation of salts. They act as catalysts to speed up various biochemical reactions. Minerals are obtained from a diet that includes a variety of animal and vegetable products and meets the energy and protein needs of the body. The Food and Nutrition Board of the National Research Council has established recommended daily intakes for calcium and iron. Calcium, iron, and iodine are the three elements most frequently missing in the diet. Zinc, iron, copper, magnesium, and potassium are the five minerals most frequently involved in disturbances of metabolism. As electrolytes, these preparations are commonly infused to critically ill patients unable to take food orally.

CALCIUM

ACTION AND USES

Calcium is a major mineral in the body and is essential for muscular and neurologic activity, especially in the cardiac system. Calcium functions in the formation and repair of skeletal tissues (bones and teeth); activates several enzymes that influence cell membrane permeability and muscle contraction; aids in blood clotting by stimulating the release of thromboplastin and the conversion of fibrinogen to fibrin; activates pancreatic lipase; influences the intestinal absorption of cobalamin; and, in extracellular fluids, is involved in the transmission of neurotransmitters and in metabolic processes. Calcium is also involved in the regulation of lymphocyte and phagocyte function through interaction with calmodulin.

Calcium is used as a supplement when dietary levels of calcium are not adequate. Calcium requirements may be increased during adolescence, pregnancy, breastfeeding, and for postmenopausal women. Calcium is also used to treat neonatal hypocalcemia and to prevent and treat postmenopausal and senile osteoporosis. It may also be used as a supplement to parenterally administered vitamin D in cases of hypoparathyroidism, pseudohypoparathyroidism, rickets, and osteomalacia.

ADVERSE REACTIONS

Watch for symptoms of hypercalcemia, such as polyuria (excretion of a large amount of urine), constipation, abdominal pain, dryness of mouth, anorexia, nausea, and vomiting.

DRUG INTERACTIONS

Vitamin D is essential for the absorption of calcium in the body. Calcium status is affected by the calcium-to-phosphorus ratio in the body and by the level of protein in the diet. Phytic acid (found in bran and whole-grain cereals) and oxalic acid (found in spinach and rhubarb) may interfere with calcium absorption by combining with calcium to form insoluble salts in

Table 24-1 Vitamins

GENERIC NAME	TRADE NAME	COMMENTS AND DOSAGE
vitamin A	Aquasol A	Adults: Give 50,000-100,000 International Units/day for 3 days to 2 wk, followed by 10,000-20,000 International Units/day for 2 mo.
vitamin B$_1$	—	Medications may be given PO, IM, or IV. Daily average dose is 0.5 mg/1000 kcal intake, or usually 1-1.4 mg/day PO. Usual dosage is 50 mg IM for deficiency states, 5-10 mg PO.
vitamin B$_2$ (riboflavin)		Infants: Give 0.3-0.4 mg/day. Children: Give 0.5-0.9 mg/day. Adult Men: Give 1.3-1.6 mg/day. Adult Women: Give 1-1.1 mg/day. For deficiency states, usually 50 mg IM and 5-10 mg daily as dietary supplement for adults and children older than 12.
niacin (vitamin B$_3$) niacinamide (nicotinamide)	Niacor	May be given IM, subcutaneously, or IV; IV route with slow drip preferred when parenteral medication is necessary. Deficiency states: Give 50-100 mg daily. Pellagra: Give up to 500 mg/day. Adults: Give 500 mg PO daily, or 100-200 mg 1 to 5 times daily.
pantothenic acid (vitamin B$_5$)	Pantothenic 250	NOTE: A RECOMMENDED DAILY ALLOWANCE IS NOT ESTABLISHED. FOR SUPPLEMENTATION GIVE: Infants (0-1 yr): 1.7-1.8 mg/day PO. Children (1-13 yr): 2-4 mg/day PO. Adults and adolescents 14 yr or older: 5 mg/day PO. Adult or adolescent lactating and pregnant women: 6-7 mg/day PO.
vitamin B$_6$ (pyridoxine)	Neuro-K	Recommended daily allowances range from 2 to 2.2 mg. Preparation may be given PO, IM, or IV. Dietary deficiency: Give 10-20 mg/day for 3 wk, then 2-5 mg/day for several weeks. Vitamin B$_6$ dependency states: up to 600 mg/day initially, dropping to 50 mg/day for life.
folic acid and derivatives (vitamin B$_9$)	Folvite	Dietary supplement: 100 mcg (0.1 mg)/day (up to 1 mg/day in pregnancy); may be increased to 500 mcg (0.5 mg) to 1 mg daily or more if underlying condition causes increased requirements (for example, in tropical sprue, 3-15 mg daily may be needed). Treatment of deficiency: 250 mcg (0.25 mg) initially to 1 mg daily PO, IM, IV, or deep subcutaneous until hematologic response occurs; maintenance 400 mcg-1 mg/day.
vitamin B$_{12}$ (cyanocobalamin)	Crystamine	Nutritional deficiency: Give 100-250 mcg/day PO. Vitamin B$_{12}$ deficiency: PO: Give 1000 mcg/day. IM, subcutaneously: Give 15 mcg/day. If patients have normal GI absorption, give along with other multiple vitamins. In other cases, give 30 mcg daily for 5-10 days, and then 100-200 mcg monthly for life.
	Nascobal	Intranasal spray: Give 500 mcg once weekly.
vitamin C (ascorbic acid)	Cevi-Bid Cecon	Adults: Give 60 mg/day.
vitamin D	Calcifediol	Adults: Give 20-50 mcg/day or 100-200 mcg every other day.
	Calcijex	Adults: Give 300-350 mcg/wk administered daily or every other day.
	D-Tabs	Initial: Give 0.25 mcg/day, increased by 0.25 mcg/day at 2- to 4-wk intervals until satisfactory response obtained. Some patients may respond to doses of 0.25 mcg every other day. Patients undergoing hemodialysis may require doses of 0.5 to 1 mcg/day. Initial: Give 0.75-2.5 mg daily for several days.
	DHT	Maintenance: Give 0.2-1 mg daily, titrated by serum calcium levels. Average dose 0.6 mg.

Continued

Table 24-1 Vitamins—cont'd

GENERIC NAME	TRADE NAME	COMMENTS AND DOSAGE
ergocalciferol		Vitamin D–resistant rickets: Give 50,000-500,000
	Calciferol drops	International Units daily. Hypoparathyroidism: Give 50,000-400,000 International Units of vitamin D daily.
vitamin E	Aquavit-E	A range of 10-20 International Units of vitamin E should provide adequate levels.
vitamin K	AquaMEPHYTON	Anticoagulant-induced prothrombin deficiency: 2.5-10 mg or up to 25 mg initially. Frequency and dosage of subsequent therapy determined by prothrombin time response.

GI, gastrointestinal; *IM,* Intramuscular; *IV,* intravenous; *PO,* by mouth.

the intestine. Calcium compounds and calcium-rich substances such as milk interfere with the absorption of oral tetracycline, so their use together should be avoided. Use of corticosteroids may also decrease the absorption of calcium.

❖ NURSING IMPLICATIONS AND PATIENT TEACHING

In patients with low calcium levels, carpal spasm may be elicited by compressing the upper arm with a blood pressure cuff, causing ischemia (decreased blood supply) to the distal nerves. The patient may report a tingling sensation and may inadvertently flex the arm. Excessive amounts of calcium may lead to hypercalcemia and hypercalciuria, especially in hyperthyroid patients. Serum and renal calcium levels should be followed to detect the development of renal stones; calcium should not be given to patients who already have renal stones.

Calcium products come in combination with various other chemicals, with a concentration of between 6% and 40%. Preparations come in both parenteral and oral forms. OTC antacids containing calcium (i.e. Tums) are composed of calcium carbonate, the most elemental form of calcium. It is better absorbed than many calcium products and is a smaller tablet than many other calcium products, making administration easier.

The recommended daily intake of calcium is 1200 mg/day for adults and for adolescents, 800 mg/day for children, 360 to 540 mg/day for infants from birth to 1 year, and 1500 mg/day for nursing mothers. Milk and dairy products are the richest sources of calcium. Egg yolks and most dark green, leafy vegetables are also good sources.

FLUORIDE

ACTION AND USES

Fluoride is concentrated in bones and teeth and is present in soft tissues only in very small amounts. It is an essential trace element but has not been proven to be essential to life. Fluoride is taken into the surface enamel of teeth in higher concentrations than in deeper layers. This strengthening of the enamel provides greater resistance to damage by acids produced in dental plaque. Fluoride has therefore been found useful in reducing dental caries.

Fluoride is recommended for the prevention of dental caries in all age groups. It may be used topically or systemically. It is primarily administered in places without fluoride in the water supply or to individuals with a genetic tendency for dental caries.

ADVERSE REACTIONS

Gastric distress, headache, urticaria, and malaise may be seen in hypersensitive individuals. Excessive salivation, mottling of teeth, GI disturbances, and nausea are seen in acute overdosage.

DRUG INTERACTIONS

Fluoride in the water supply may produce calcium fluoride, a poorly absorbed product, when taken with dairy foods.

❖ NURSING IMPLICATIONS AND PATIENT TEACHING

Fluoride is available in gels, pastes, drops, tablets, capsules, and mouth rinses. The preparation and quantity chosen should be adjusted to the fluoride level of the local water supply. The county water commissioner may be contacted for this information. Fluoride products should be taken as ordered. Tablets and drops may be dissolved in water used for making infant formula or added to food or juices. Tablets may also be swallowed, chewed, or allowed to dissolve slowly in the mouth. Products are best taken after meals. For rinses and gels, teeth should be brushed thoroughly, and then the coating should be applied to clean teeth. The fluoride coating should not be swallowed. The patient should not rinse the mouth, eat, or drink for 30 minutes after treatment. Plastic containers should be used for diluting fluoride drops or rinses, and glass should be avoided. Milk may decrease absorption of oral fluoride products, so the patient should avoid taking fluoride with milk or dairy products.

IODINE

ACTION AND USES

Iodine is a trace mineral found in most parts of the body. Its presence is essential to the normal function of the thyroid gland. Goiter is the classic symptom of iodine deficiency and can appear after several months of inadequate iodine. This deficiency is prevalent in the US and has an increasing rate in pregnant women where the deficiency can be dangerous to a forming fetus. Potassium iodine was once commonly administered to patients with excessive bronchiolar mucus production but this indication has fallen into disfavor. It is used as an antithyroid agent in the treatment of hyperthyroidism and thyrotoxicosis and preoperatively to induce the shrinking of the thyroid. It has also been used in some dermatologic conditions. Because certain brands of these products can provide protection against radioactive iodine exposure, they have been approved by the FDA for use in case of a nuclear plant accident or 'dirty bomb' containing [131] I exposure.

ADVERSE REACTIONS

Gastric distress is common and includes nausea/vomiting and diarrhea. Acneiform rash may develop from prolonged use and may be fatal. Iodine toxicity, or iodism, symptoms include metallic taste; sore gums, teeth, and mouth; burning in the throat or mouth; ulcerated mucous membranes; acute rhinitis; sneezing; and irritation of the eyes with swelling of the eyelids. Severe headache, productive cough, pulmonary edema, and tenderness and swelling of the parotid and submaxillary glands may also occur. Hypersensitivity reactions may also be seen with symptoms suggestive of serum sickness.

DRUG INTERACTIONS

Potassium iodide should not be administered with the thyroid hormones due to their opposite effects. Potassium iodide should be given cautiously with any other drugs that contain potassium because of the problem of producing hyperkalemia.

❖ NURSING IMPLICATIONS AND PATIENT TEACHING

The RDAs of iodine are as follows:
Infants 0-6 months: 110 mcg/day
Infants 7-12 months: 130 mcg/day
Children 1-8 years: 90 mcg/day
Children 9-13 years: 120 mcg/day
Adults: 150 mcg/day
Pregnant women: 220 mcg/day
Lactating women: 290 mcg/day

In case of a nuclear reaction, the patient should stop taking any other medications or supplements that might interfere with the iodide uptake into thyroid tissue.

IRON

ACTION AND USES

Iron is an essential mineral for the synthesis of myoglobin and hemoglobin. It stimulates the hematopoietic system and increases hemoglobin to correct iron deficiency. Iron from cellular hemoglobin is recycled and most is used again. During pregnancy, the reabsorption of iron increases to 15% as the body's way of adapting to physiologic anemia.

Iron is used to treat symptomatic iron deficiency anemia only after the cause of the anemia has been identified, and it is used to prevent hypochromic anemia during infancy, childhood, pregnancy, and breastfeeding; in patients recovering from other anemias; and after some GI surgeries.

ADVERSE REACTIONS

Adverse reactions to iron supplements include constipation, cramping, diarrhea, epigastric or abdominal pain, GI irritation, and allergic reactions to any component of the iron preparation. Symptoms of overdosage may occur after 30 minutes to several hours and include lethargy (sleepiness), nausea, vomiting, abdominal pain, diarrhea, melena (blood in stools), and dyspnea (uncomfortable breathing). Coma and metabolic acidosis may occur, as well as symptoms of systemic absorption. Children who mistake vitamins for candy are particularly sensitive to large amounts of iron and may die from overdoses.

DRUG INTERACTIONS

Large iron doses may cause a false-positive test result for occult blood using the toluidine test (Hematest, Occultist, Clinistix). Absorption of oral iron is inhibited by tannic acid in tea, antacids (particularly magnesium trisilicate–containing antacids), milk, and eggs. Patients receiving chloramphenicol concurrently with iron may show a delayed response to iron therapy. Absorption of iron increases when given with ascorbic acid (Vitamin C) in doses of 200 mg per 30 mg of iron. Iron interferes with absorption of oral tetracycline. Vitamin E decreases the response to iron therapy. Many other medications may have interactions.

❖ NURSING IMPLICATIONS AND PATIENT TEACHING

The cause of the anemia must be identified and treated. Help collect stools for occult blood tests after the patient has been on a red meat–free diet for at least 3 days. Although dietary lack may contribute to iron deficiency, especially in those older than 75 years of age, blood loss is the primary cause. Heavy menstrual periods and multiple pregnancies may produce anemia in women. Hematologic laboratory values are often normally lower in older adults, leading to overprescribing of iron for geriatric patients. Liquid preparations can discolor teeth and should be taken through a straw after dilution with liquid.

Replacement of iron in iron deficiency anemia requires 90 to 300 mg of elemental iron daily in divided doses (6 mg/kg/day). Symptoms should go away within 2 weeks, and laboratory studies should be normal within 2 months, if diagnosis and treatment are adequate. Therapy for 4 to 6 months after the anemia has been corrected is advised to replenish iron stores. More iron is absorbed if the iron is taken on an empty stomach with water or in an acid environment, although taking it after meals can reduce stomach irritation. Taking iron after a meal can reduce the absorption by 40% to 50%. Different oral preparations vary in cost and percentage of elemental iron. Product selection must be based on how well it is absorbed, how well it is tolerated, and the individual needs of the patient. All simple oral iron preparations are available OTC. The absorption of iron taken orally or through dietary foods is generally about 10%. The body does have the capability to increase iron absorption during times of physiologic stress, such as pregnancy and severe blood loss.

The recommended daily intake of elemental iron in adult males is 10 mg; in adult women, 18 mg (with an additional 10 mg during pregnancy or lactation); and in children, 10 to 15 mg. A diet high in natural iron should be encouraged to meet these needs. Fish, red meat, spinach, and dried fruits are the best sources of dietary iron.

Iron supplements can cause dark green or black stools. The patient should report constipation, diarrhea, nausea, or abdominal pain to the health care provider.

MAGNESIUM

ACTION AND USES

Magnesium is an electrolyte that is essential to several enzyme systems. It is important in maintaining osmotic pressure, ion balance, bone structure, muscular contraction, and nerve conduction. This mineral has been determined to be especially important in cardiac function, and only slight deficiencies may prolong the Q-T interval and lead to a very dangerous form of ventricular tachycardia (rapid heartbeat) called *torsades de pointes.*

ADVERSE REACTIONS

Excessive magnesium intake may produce diarrhea.

❖ NURSING IMPLICATIONS AND PATIENT TEACHING

Magnesium deficiencies are seen primarily when malabsorption syndromes are present. Magnesium is usually used with other vitamins as a general dietary supplement when multiple deficiencies are suspected. Deficiency states have been associated with convulsions, slowing of growth, digestive disturbances, spasticity of muscles and nerves, accelerated heartbeat, dysrhythmias, nervous conditions, and vasodilation (opening of blood vessels). Magnesium is available in adequate quantities in meat, milk, fruits, and vegetables, and special dietary planning is unnecessary.

MANGANESE

ACTION AND USES

Manganese activates many enzymes, assists in normal skeletal and connective tissue development, helps in the initiation of protein synthesis, and plays a part in the synthesis of cholesterol and fatty acids. It is found throughout all body tissues and fluids. No precise RDA has been established.

Manganese is used in dietary supplements. Usually it is used with other vitamins when multiple deficiencies are suspected. Research subjects with manganese deficiency experienced weight loss, changes in beard and hair growth (usually slowing of growth), and occasional nausea and vomiting. There are no known adverse effects or drug interactions.

Nuts, whole-wheat cereals, and grains are the foods richest in manganese. Tea and cloves are exceptionally rich. Meat, fish, and dairy products have low amounts of manganese.

POTASSIUM

ACTION AND USES

Potassium is the principal intracellular cation of most body tissues, acting in the maintenance of normal renal function, contraction of muscle, and transmission of nerve impulses. It is found in the body within a very narrow range.

Potassium may be taken prophylactically (for prevention) when the patient has nephrotic syndrome, in hepatic cirrhosis with ascites, and in patients with hyperaldosteronism who have normal renal function. Potassium products are used prophylactically or to replace potassium that may be lost as a result of long-term diuretic therapy, digitalis intoxication, or low dietary intake of potassium. Supplementation may also be necessary for deficits resulting from vomiting and diarrhea, diabetic acidosis, metabolic alkalosis, corticosteroid therapy, or to counteract increased renal excretion of potassium because of acidosis, certain renal tubular disorders, or diseases that produce increased secretion of glucocorticoids or aldosterone.

ADVERSE REACTIONS

Either excess or deficit of potassium causes symptoms. Adverse reactions to potassium supplements include nausea, vomiting, diarrhea, abdominal discomfort, and GI bleeding. Potassium intoxication or hyperkalemia (increased potassium in the blood) may result from overdosage of potassium or from a change in the patient's underlying condition, which may make potassium buildup possible. Signs and symptoms of potassium intoxication include flaccid paralysis, paresthesias (numbness and tingling) of the hands and feet, mental confusion, restlessness, listlessness, malaise, and heaviness of the legs. Hypotension and cardiac dysrhythmias leading to heart block may also develop. Potentially fatal dysrhythmias may develop if potassium cannot be excreted (or if it is administered too rapidly IV). When it is detected, hyperkalemia requires immediate treatment because lethal levels of potassium may be reached in a few hours in untreated patients. Potentially lethal dysrhythmias may also occur with hypokalemia (decreased potassium in the blood).

DRUG INTERACTIONS

Potassium should not be used in patients receiving potassium-sparing agents such as aldosterone antagonists or triamterene, because overdosage may develop.

❖ NURSING IMPLICATIONS AND PATIENT TEACHING

All potassium supplements must be diluted properly or taken with plenty of liquid to avoid producing GI ulcers. The usual adult dietary intake of potassium ranges between 40 and 60 mEq/day. The loss of 200 or more mEq of potassium from the total body store is enough to produce hypokalemia.

The dosage must be titrated (increased or decreased slowly) based on the individual's needs and the patient should be closely watched during therapy, especially in the initial stages of therapy. For patients receiving diuretic therapy, 20 mEq/day is usually adequate for the prevention of hypokalemia. In cases of potassium depletion, 40 to 100 mEq/day or more may be required for replacement. Blood levels must be monitored closely.

Potassium comes in various salt combinations; potassium chloride is the form most frequently prescribed. It may be ordered either by percentage of potassium chloride or in milliequivalents of potassium chloride, with 10 mEq KCl per 15 mL equivalent to 5% KCl. Other salt combinations are potassium gluconate, potassium citrate, potassium acetate, and potassium bicarbonate. Potassium is also available in combination with vitamin C, ammonium chloride, citric acid, betaine HCl, and L-lysine monohydrochloride.

Many health care providers tell patients to eat a potassium-rich diet in addition to taking a potassium supplement. A potassium-rich diet includes foods such as bananas, citrus fruits (especially tomatoes and oranges), apricots, and dried fruits such as raisins, prunes, and dates. Fresh cantaloupe and watermelon, nuts, dried beans, beef, and fowl also contain ample quantities of potassium.

ZINC

ACTION AND USES

Zinc is a part of many enzymes and is essential for normal growth and tissue repair. Zinc functions in the mineralization of bone and in the detoxification and oxidation of methanol and ethylene glycol. It plays a role in the creation of DNA and the synthesis of protein from amino acids. It is important in wound healing and functions in moving vitamin A from liver stores.

Zinc supplements are used to prevent zinc deficiency and to treat delayed wound healing. There is some evidence to support the use of zinc OTC products in reducing the severity of symptoms of the common cold.

Patients taking zinc may complain of abnormalities of taste and smell, rough skin, and anorexia with profound disinterest in food. Patients who lack zinc may demonstrate sexual immaturity, delayed wound healing, and decreased absorption of dietary folate.

ADVERSE REACTIONS

Adverse reactions to zinc supplements include gastric ulceration, nausea, and vomiting. Doses in excess of 2 g produce emesis (vomiting). Acute zinc intoxication produces drowsiness, lethargy, light-headedness, staggering gait, restlessness, and vomiting leading to dehydration.

DRUG INTERACTIONS

Calcium competes with zinc for absorption. Phytates form insoluble complexes with zinc and interfere with its absorption. Zinc impairs the absorption of tetracycline derivatives.

❖ NURSING IMPLICATIONS AND PATIENT TEACHING

The RDAs for zinc are as follows:

Infant to 12 months: 3 to 5 mg/day
Children 1-10 years: 10 mg/day
Adolescents 11-18 years: 15 mg/day
Adults: 15 mg/day
Pregnant women: 20 mg/day
Lactating women: 25 mg/day

Seafood and meats are rich sources of natural zinc; cereals and legumes also have significant amounts of this mineral.

Table 24-2 presents a summary of minerals discussed as supplements plus phosphorus and sodium

Table 24-2   Minerals

GENERIC NAME	TRADE NAME	COMMENTS AND DOSAGE
Calcium		
calcium acetate	PhosLo	Has 25% calcium. Adults: Give 1200-1800 mg daily.
calcium carbonate	Os-Cal 500	Has 40% concentration of calcium, the largest of any calcium.
calcium citrate	Citracal	Has 21% calcium. Adults: Give 1200-1800 mg qd.
calcium glubionate	Calciquid	Oral preparation contains 6% calcium. Administer before meals to increase absorption. Adults: (including pregnant and breastfeeding women) and children 4 yr or older: Give 15 mL 3 times daily.
calcium gluconate	Calcium Gluconate	Comes in both oral and parenteral forms. IV infusion preferred over IM injection; used frequently in emergency situations. Check equivalency of all oral products, because they vary from preparation to preparation. In parenteral forms, 10 mL contains 90 mg (4.5 mEq) calcium.
calcium lactate	Calcium Lactate	Contains 13% calcium and is given orally. Available without prescription.
tricalcium phosphate	Posture	Has 39% calcium. Adults: Give 1200-1800 mg daily.
Fluoride		
fluoride (oral)	Fluoritab	Adjust dosage according to local water fluoride level. General oral dosages is 1 g daily.
fluoride (topical)	Fluorigard Fluorinse Prevident	Products used between professional dental fluoride treatments for patients who have excessive problems with tooth decay. After brushing, hold preparation in mouth for at least 1 min, then spit out. To obtain maximum benefit, do not swallow; do not eat, drink, smoke, or rinse mouth for at least 15-30 min after treatment to obtain maximum benefit.
Iodine		
potassium iodide	PI	Most products are off the market. The government has stockpiles of PI which they distribute to communities that have nuclear reactors to keep on hand in the event of a nuclear disaster.
Saturated solution potassium iodide	SSKI	Oral drops given to help relieve bronchial mucus. Now only rarely ordered.
Iron		
ferrous fumarate	Femiron	Few reported side effects with this product. Better tolerated than sulfate or gluconate. Contains 33% elemental iron.
ferrous gluconate	Fergon	Less corrosive than ferrous sulfate. Indicated for those who cannot tolerate sulfate because of gastric irritation. Contains 11.6% elemental iron. Adults: Give 320-640 mg PO 3 times daily. Children 6-12 yr: Give 100-300 mg PO 3 times daily.
ferrous sulfate	Feosol Fer-In-Sol	Ferrous sulfate is the standard preparation against which all other iron salts are compared. Optimal compound because it is the least expensive and contains 20% elemental iron. Timed-release capsules are more expensive and less well absorbed but reportedly have fewer side effects. Liquid Feosol cannot be mixed with juice.
ferrous sulfate	FeroSul Feratab	Product contains more elemental iron per milligram of compound than other products. More expensive than plain ferrous sulfate.

Table **24-2** Minerals—cont'd

GENERIC NAME	TRADE NAME	COMMENTS AND DOSAGE
iron dextran	DexFerrum INFeD Infurfer 🍁	Used when oral iron administration is impossible or unsatisfactory. Parenteral iron has caused fatal anaphylactic-type reactions and must be used with care. Test dose: Give 0.5 mL IV or IM 1 hr before the therapeutic dose (to rule out hypersensitivity). Calculate total dose required using the following formula: $$0.3 \times \text{Weight in lb} \times \left(\frac{100 - \text{hemoglobin g/dL} \times 100}{14.8} \right) = \text{mg iron}$$ For patients weighing less than 30 lb, reduce to 80% total calculated. The Z-track method should be used for injection into the gluteus maximus muscle only. Inject deeply using a 2- or 3-inch 19- or 20-gauge needle.
Magnesium		
magnesium gluconate	Magonate Magtrate	RDA for adult men is 350 mg; adult women, 330 mg. As a dietary supplement: 27-133 mg daily to 3 times daily
Manganese		
manganese sulfate	Mangimin	No RDA has been determined. Suggested daily intakes include 0.5-0.7 mg PO for infants, 2.5-5.0 mg PO for adolescents, and 3-7 mg PO for adults.
Potassium		
potassium chloride liquid powder	Cena-K Kaon K-Lor K-Lyte	Wide variation in concentration, price, flavor. Make certain medication is diluted with water or juice or is taken with adequate quantities of liquid. Titrate to individual requirements. Usual dosage is 20 mEq/day for prophylaxis and 40-100 mEq/day for treatment of potassium depletion.
Combinations of Potassium Gluconate, Potassium Citrate, Potassium Acetate, Potassium Bicarbonate		
effervescent tablets	Effer-K K-Lyte	These products, most of which require prescriptions, are used primarily in patients in whom chloride is restricted. Because some of these products do contain chloride, it is important to carefully choose the potassium salt desired. There is wide variability in the cost of these products, with most tending to be more expensive than potassium chloride products. Effervescent tablets must be dissolved completely in water before administration. Dosage should be titrated to individual needs. Usual dosage is 20 mEq/day for prophylaxis and 40-100 mEq/day for treatment of potassium depletion.
liquids	Cena-K Kaon Kaylixir	
powders	Klorvess Kolyum	
Zinc		
zinc sulfate	Orazinc	Adults: Give 15 mg daily.
Phosphorus		
phosphate (sodium, potassium)	Neutra-Phos	Adults: Give 800-1200 mg. May have mild laxative effect.
Sodium Chloride		
sodium chloride	Slo-Salt	Provide supplementation on rare occasions.

IM, Intramuscular; *IV*, intravenous; *PO*, by mouth; *qd*, every day; *RDA*, recommended daily allowance.

chloride that are occasionally included with other mineral preparations.

VITAMIN AND MINERAL DEFICIENCIES

☼ OVERVIEW

In accepting that many people in the United States eat poorly, the American Medical Association has for the first time recommended the use of a daily multiple vitamin supplement if patients do not eat a well-balanced diet and eat lots of high-fat or "empty calorie" foods. Supplements or vitamins cannot make up for a poor diet or other unhealthful lifestyle practices such as smoking or lack of exercise. If patients cannot tolerate certain foods such as dairy products, they may need to supplement their diet to ensure they are getting the nutrients provided by that food group.

A deficiency of one vitamin in a diet that is otherwise adequate is rare. Deficiency signs and symptoms in a patient may point to a lack of one vitamin, but usually a deficiency of several vitamins will be found. Because of the vast number of multiple-vitamin preparations that are easily available to consumers, as well as television and magazine advertisements, hypervitaminosis (excess amounts of several vitamins) is more likely to occur than are deficiencies of single vitamins.

❖ NURSING IMPLICATIONS AND PATIENT TEACHING

■ Assessment

Try to learn as much as possible about the patient's health history, including the presence of hypersensitivity, pregnancy, breastfeeding, underlying systemic disease, hereditary disorders, and use of other medications that may cause drug interactions. The patient should be assessed for symptoms of multiple deficiency or disease states.

■ Diagnosis

In addition to the medical problems resulting in the need for vitamin or mineral products, does the patient have financial, cultural, or nutritional problems or attitudes that contribute to the problem? Does the patient have a lack of knowledge about how to prepare, store, or use water- or fat-soluble vitamins? Does the patient do things that would interfere with getting vitamins from the food normally eaten? Does the patient try to make up for poor diet by taking vitamins or nutritional supplements?

■ Planning

Many vitamin and mineral supplementation regimens require baseline laboratory assessment before starting therapy so that progress may be monitored.

Make certain the medication or supplement is stored properly and protected from light and heat to avoid destruction of the essential nutrient.

■ Implementation

Confirm the route of administration for the medication before the product is given. Many products must be given very slowly or only by certain routes.

■ Evaluation

Watch for the therapeutic effect or to see if the patient has adverse effects. The nurse may need to help arrange for the patient to get follow-up laboratory studies to measure improvement.

■ Patient and Family Teaching

Tell the patient and family the following:
- The patient should take the vitamin or mineral supplement exactly as ordered. If a dose is missed, it should be taken as soon as remembered but not if it is almost time for the next dose. The doses should not be doubled. The nurse, physician, or other health care provider should be informed if doses of vitamin K are missed.
- The patient will need to make regular return visits to see the nurse, physician, or other health care provider while taking some vitamins. The patient should inform all physicians and dentists about vitamin and mineral products he or she is taking.
- The patient must not take other medications, including OTC drugs, without first discussing them with the nurse, physician, or other health care provider.
- Some forms of the drugs may cause unusual taste sensations, must be protected from light and heat, or have special storage instructions. The patient must be taught how to store and use the medications.
- The patient should avoid overdosage of vitamins and minerals. Taking too much is not helpful and may lead to toxicity or dependency or to waste when the excess vitamin/mineral passes into the urine.
- The patient should eat well-balanced meals. The nurse, physician, or other health care provider should teach the patient about foods that contain naturally occurring vitamins.
- Vitamin and mineral preparations should be kept out of the reach of children and all others for whom they are not prescribed.
- Vitamins and minerals sold as special products in health food stores may not demonstrate any nutritional superiority over less expensive products sold elsewhere.

Get Ready for the NCLEX® Examination!

Key Points

- Vitamins and minerals are essential for the body to function properly.
- They are often taken as supplements when dietary levels are inadequate.
- There is still much to be learned about the action of vitamins and minerals in the body.
- It is important to note that vitamin and mineral overdose can create as many problems as deficiency and should be avoided.

Additional Learning Resources

SG Go to your Study Guide for additional learning activities to help you master this chapter content.

evolve Go to your Evolve website (http://evolve.elsevier.com/Edmunds/LPN/) for additional online resources.

Review Questions for the NCLEX® Examination

1. The patient has been ordered to be treated with potassium chloride (K-Lor). The highest priority action on the part of the nurse regarding administration of the medication is:
   1. make certain that the medication is taken on an empty stomach
   2. make certain that the medication is taken with food
   3. make certain that the medication is diluted with water or juice
   4. make certain that the medication is taken undiluted

2. The patient is scheduled to receive a dose of DexFerrum. The nurse recognizes that the muscle that should be used when administering the medication by injection is the:
   1. vastus lateralis
   2. gluteus maximus
   3. deltoid
   4. ventrogluteal

3. The patient is being treated with Prevident. The nurse instructs the patient to brush his teeth using the preparation and then:
   1. rinse his mouth immediately and spit out
   2. hold the preparation in his mouth for at least a minute
   3. wait 5 minutes and then rinse out his mouth
   4. swallow the preparation immediately

4. The patient tells the nurse that she has been taking zinc supplements to prevent cold symptoms. She complains to the nurse that despite doubling the amount of the zinc that she is taking daily, she is experiencing exhaustion, dizziness, and vomiting. The nurse recognizes that the patient could be experiencing:
   1. anaphylactic reaction
   2. zinc deficiency
   3. expected side effect
   4. zinc intoxication

5. An appropriate dietary choice for a patient who needs to increase his amount of potassium in his diet is:
   1. chicken salad sandwich with tomatoes
   2. Caesar salad and ice cream
   3. turkey sandwich and oatmeal cookies
   4. bacon, eggs, and whole-wheat toast

Case Study

Mrs. Casper, 77, has been in a nursing home for several years. She suffers from a variety of chronic diseases. When she was recently admitted to the hospital for pneumonia, the physician discovered that she was mildly anemic. She was prescribed the following:

- Ferrous sulfate: 300 mg 3 times daily PO
- Vitamin C: 1000 mcg daily
- Ciprofloxacin: 750 mg PO q12h

1. Why is the ferrous sulfate ordered?
2. Why is vitamin C given?
3. Why is ciprofloxacin given?
4. After several days of therapy, the patient does not seem to be getting any better. What reason might account for this?
5. The nurse is preparing a diet plan to help Mrs. Casper incorporate more food with vitamin C in her diet. She tells the nurse that she does not like to eat fruit. What are some options that the nurse can offer her?

Drug Calculation Review

1. Order: Vitamin B_{12} 200 mcg IM every month. Supply: Vitamin B_{12} 1000 mcg/mL.
   Question: How many milliliters of vitamin B_{12} is needed with each dose?
2. Order: Iron dextran 100 mg IV over 6 hours. Supply: Iron dextran 100 mg/250 mL 0.9% normal saline.
   Question: How many milliliters per hour should the IV infusion device be set for? (Round to the nearest whole number.)
3. Order: Potassium chloride 60 mEq in 200 mL 0.9% normal saline. Facility's policy: Infuse potassium at a maximum rate of 10 mEq/hr.
   Question: How many milliliters per hour should the IV infusion device be set for? (Round to the nearest whole number.)

Get Ready for the NCLEX® Examination!—cont'd

Critical Thinking Questions

1. What are the two types of vitamins? Overall, how does each type react differently in the body?
2. What are two circumstances under which a patient may be unable to obtain sufficient amounts of vitamins, despite having a well-balanced, nutritious diet?
3. Explain the difference between vitamins and minerals.
4. Mr. Baker leads a very athletic life and is proud of his strict diet and voluminous intake of vitamins, which he says he "keeps on the kitchen counter so [he] won't forget them." He comes to the clinic feeling "a little under the weather." He is surprised and confused when he is told that he has developed hypervitaminosis. After listening to the nurse's explanation of hypervitaminosis, its causes, and its effects, Mr. Baker remains confused, insisting that "A vitamin is a vitamin, and more is better when it comes to vitamins . . . and minerals, too, as far as that goes." What would be an appropriate approach to use for educating Mr. Baker?
5. Create a nutrition chart to show Mr. Baker how he can get adequate amounts of vitamins and minerals by eating a well-balanced diet. Be prepared to counteract Mr. Baker's frequent protest: "A vitamin is a vitamin!"
6. What three minerals are most often missing from our diets? Why is that?
7. Ms. Mariani stops to talk to the nurse after seeing her doctor for a physical examination. She is upset because the doctor told her she has anemia, and "now I have to get a needle once a week. Why can't I just eat more red meat or liver to build up my blood?" What should the nurse tell her about her anemia?

Appendix A: Answers to NCLEX Review Questions

CHAPTER 1
1. 2
2. 3
3. 1
4. 4
5. 3

CHAPTER 2
1. 4
2. 3
3. 1
4. 2
5. 4

CHAPTER 3
1. 3
2. 4
3. 2
4. 2
5. 1

CHAPTER 4
1. 4
2. 1
3. 2
4. 4
5. 2

CHAPTER 5
1. 2
2. 1
3. 3
4. 4
5. 1

CHAPTER 6
1. 2
2. 4
3. 1
4. 3
5. 3

CHAPTER 7
1. 4
2. 2
3. 3
4. 1
5. 4

CHAPTER 8
1. 4
2. 2
3. 3
4. 1
5. 4

CHAPTER 9
1. 4
2. 1
3. 3
4. 2
5. 3

CHAPTER 10
1. 4
2. 4
3. 2
4. 1
5. 2

CHAPTER 11
1. 4
2. 2
3. 3
4. 2
5. 4

CHAPTER 12
1. 2
2. 1
3. 1
4. 3
5. 4

CHAPTER 13
1. 2
2. 3
3. 4
4. 1
5. 3

CHAPTER 14
1. 3
2. 4
3. 2
4. 1
5. 3

CHAPTER 15
1. 4
2. 1
3. 3
4. 4
5. 3

CHAPTER 16
1. 3
2. 2
3. 1
4. 4
5. 2

CHAPTER 17
1. 4
2. 4
3. 1
4. 2
5. 3

CHAPTER 18
1. 3
2. 4
3. 2
4. 3
5. 1

CHAPTER 19
1. 3
2. 2
3. 1
4. 4
5. 2

CHAPTER 20
1. 4
2. 1
3. 3
4. 2
5. 4

CHAPTER 21
1. 3
2. 2
3. 1
4. 1
5. 1

CHAPTER 22
1. 1
2. 3
3. 2
4. 1
5. 3

CHAPTER 23
1. 2
2. 1
3. 4
4. 3
5. 1

CHAPTER 24
1. 3
2. 2
3. 2
4. 4
5. 1

Be sure to visit the companion Evolve site at http://evolve.elsevier.com/Edmunds/LPN/ for rationales and page references.

CHAPTER 9: CALCULATING DRUG DOSAGES

1. $? \text{ days} = \dfrac{1 \text{ day}}{1 \text{ tablespoon}} \Bigg| \dfrac{1 \text{ tablespoon}}{3 \text{ teaspoons}} \Bigg| \dfrac{1 \text{ teaspoon}}{5 \text{ mL}} \Bigg| 500 \text{ mL} = \dfrac{500}{3(5)} = \dfrac{500}{15} = 33 \text{ days}$

2. $? \text{ mL} = \dfrac{1 \text{ mL}}{100 \text{ units}} \Bigg| 30 \text{ units} = \dfrac{3}{10} = 0.3 \text{ mL}$

3. $? \text{ mL} = \dfrac{1 \text{ mL}}{330 \text{ mg}} \Bigg| 500 \text{ mg} = \dfrac{50}{33} = 1.5 \text{ mL}$

4. $? \dfrac{\text{gtt}}{\text{min}} = \dfrac{10 \text{ gtt}}{1 \text{ mL}} \Bigg| \dfrac{2500 \text{ mL}}{24 \text{ hr}} \Bigg| \dfrac{1 \text{ hr}}{60 \text{ min}} = \dfrac{10(25)}{24(6)} = \dfrac{2500}{144} = 17 \text{ gtt/min}$

5. $? \dfrac{\text{mg}}{\text{kg/min}} = \dfrac{\overset{10}{500} \text{ mg}}{\underset{5}{250} \text{ mL}} \Bigg| \dfrac{1 \text{ mL}}{60 \text{ megtt}} \Bigg| \dfrac{\overset{3}{150} \text{ megtt}}{\underset{1}{50} \text{ kg/min}} = \dfrac{10(3)}{5(60)} = \dfrac{30}{300} = 0.1 \text{ mg/kg/min}$

6. $? \text{ mL} = \dfrac{1 \text{ mL}}{5000 \text{ units}} \Bigg| 7500 \text{ units} = \dfrac{75}{50} = 1.5 \text{ mL}$

7. $? \text{ mL} = \dfrac{1 \text{ mL}}{gr \dfrac{1}{150}} \Bigg| gr \dfrac{1}{300} = \dfrac{\dfrac{1}{300}}{\dfrac{1}{150}} = \dfrac{1}{300} \times \dfrac{150}{1} = \dfrac{150}{300} = 0.5 \text{ mL}$

8. $? \text{ tablets} = \dfrac{1 \text{ tablet}}{0.1 \, g} \Bigg| \dfrac{1 \, g}{\underset{20}{1000} \text{ mg}} \Bigg| \overset{1}{50} \text{ mg} = \dfrac{1}{0.1(20)} = \dfrac{1}{2} \text{ tablet}$

9. $? \text{ mL} = \dfrac{1 \text{ mL}}{\underset{1}{0.05} \text{ mg}} \Bigg| \overset{5}{0.25} \text{ mg} = \dfrac{5}{1} = 5 \text{ mL}$

10. $? \text{ tablets} = \dfrac{1 \text{ tablet}}{400 \text{ mg}} \Bigg| \dfrac{1000 \text{ mg}}{1 \, g} \Bigg| 1 \, g = \dfrac{10}{4} = 2.5 \text{ tablets}$

CHAPTER 11: ALLERGY AND RESPIRATORY MEDICATIONS

1. *Fraction*: $\dfrac{300 \text{ mg}}{100 \text{ mg}} \times 1 \text{ tablet} = \dfrac{300}{100} = 3 \text{ tablets}$

Ratio-proportion: 100 mg : 1 tablet :: 300 mg : x tablets

$100x = 300$

$$\frac{100x}{100} = \frac{300}{100} = 3$$

$x = 3$ tablets

Dimensional analysis: ? tablets $= \dfrac{1 \text{ tablet}}{100 \text{ mg}} \left| \dfrac{300 \text{ mg}}{1} \right. = \dfrac{3}{1} = 3$ tablets

2. *Fraction:* $\dfrac{4 \text{ mg}}{2 \text{ mg}} \times 1 \text{ tablet} = \dfrac{4}{2} = 2$ tablets

Ratio-proportion: 2 mg : 1 tablet :: 4 mg : x tablets

$2x = 4$

$$\frac{2x}{2} = \frac{4}{2} = 2$$

$x = 2$ tablets

Dimensional analysis: ? tablets $= \dfrac{1 \text{ tablet}}{2 \text{ mg}} \left| \dfrac{4 \text{ mg}}{1} \right. = \dfrac{4}{2} = 2$ tablets

3. *Fraction:* $\dfrac{25 \text{ mg}}{50 \text{ mg}} \times 1 \text{ mL} = \dfrac{25}{50} = \dfrac{1}{2} = 0.5 \text{ mL}$

Ratio-proportion: 50 mg : 1 mL :: 25 mg : x mL

$50x = 25$

$$\frac{50x}{50} = \frac{25}{50} = 0.5$$

$x = 0.5$ mL

Dimensional analysis: ? mL $= \dfrac{1 \text{ mL}}{\underset{2}{\cancel{50} \text{ mg}}} \left| \dfrac{\overset{1}{\cancel{25}} \text{ mg}}{} \right. = \dfrac{1}{2} = 0.5 \text{ mL}$

CHAPTER 12: ANTIINFECTIVE MEDICATIONS

1. *Fraction:* $\dfrac{600 \text{ mg}}{100 \text{ mg}} \times 1 \text{ mL} = \dfrac{600}{100} = 6 \text{ mL}$

Ratio-proportion: 100 mg : 1 mL :: 600 mg : x mL

$100x = 600$

$$\frac{100x}{100} = \frac{600}{100} = 6$$

$x = 6$ mL

A. ? mL $= \dfrac{1 \text{ mL}}{100 \text{ mg}} \left| \dfrac{600 \text{ mg}}{1} \right. = \dfrac{6}{1} = 6 \text{ mL}$

B. Dorsal or ventral gluteal

C. This injection needs to be divided into two doses of 3 mL each.

2. *Fraction:* $\dfrac{1,000,000 \text{ units}}{600,000 \text{ units}} \times 1 \text{ mL} = \dfrac{1,000,000}{600,000} = 1.67 \text{ mL}$

Ratio-proportion: 600,000 units : 1 mL :: 1,000,000 units : x mL

$600,000x = 1,000,000$

$$\frac{600,000x}{600,000} = \frac{1,000,000}{600,000} = 1.67 \text{ mL}$$

$x = 1.67$ mL

$$\textit{Dimensional analysis: } ?\,\text{mL} = \frac{1\,\text{mL}}{600,000\,\text{units}} \left| \frac{1,000,000\,\text{units}}{1} \right. = \frac{10}{6} = 1.67\,\text{mL}$$

3. *Fraction:* $\dfrac{1\,\text{g}}{1.5\,\text{g}} \times 150\,\text{mL/hr} = \dfrac{150}{1.5} = 100\,\text{mL/hr}$

   Ratio-proportion: 1.5 gm : 150 mL/hr = 1 gm : x mL/hr

   $1.5x = 150$

   $\dfrac{1.5x}{1.5} = \dfrac{150}{1.5} = 100$

   $x = 100\,\text{mL/hr}$

   Dimensional analysis: $?\,\text{mL/hr} = \dfrac{150\,\text{mL}}{1.5\,\text{gm}} \left| \dfrac{1\,\text{gm}}{1\,\text{hr}} \right. = \dfrac{150}{1.5} = 100\,\text{mL/hr}$

4. *Fraction:* $\dfrac{400\,\text{mg}}{500\,\text{mg}} \times 2.2\,\text{mL} = \dfrac{400(2.2)}{500} = \dfrac{880}{500} = 1.76\,\text{mL} = 1.8\,\text{mL}$

   Ratio-proportion: 500 mg : 2.2 mL :: 400 mg : x mL

   $500x = 2.2(400) = 880$

   $\dfrac{500x}{500} = \dfrac{880}{500} = 1.76$

   $x = 1.76$ or 1.8 mL

   Dimensional analysis: $?\,\text{mL} = \dfrac{2.2\,\text{mL}}{500\,\text{mg}} \left| \dfrac{400\,\text{mg}}{1} \right. = \dfrac{2.2(4)}{5} = \dfrac{8.8}{5} = 1.76\,\text{mL} = 1.8\,\text{mL}$

CHAPTER 13: ANTIVIRALS, ANTIRETROVIRALS, AND ANTIFUNGAL MEDICATIONS

1. *For fraction and ratio-proportion, first convert pounds to kilograms:*

   2.2 lbs : 1 kg :: 110 lbs : x kg

   $2.2x = 110$

   $\dfrac{2.2x}{2.2} = \dfrac{110}{2.2} = 50$

   $x = 50\,\text{kg}$

   Fraction: $\dfrac{50\,\text{kg}}{1\,\text{kg}} \times 10\,\text{mg} = \dfrac{50(10)}{1} = \dfrac{500}{1} = 500\,\text{mg}$

   Ratio-proportion: 1 kg : 10 mg :: 50 kg : x mg

   $1x = 10(50) = 500$

   $x = 500\,\text{mg}$

   Dimensional analysis: $?\,\text{mg} = \dfrac{10\,\text{mg}}{1\,\text{kg}} \left| \dfrac{1\,\text{kg}}{2.2\,\text{lbs}} \right| \dfrac{110\,\text{lbs}}{1} = \dfrac{10(110)}{2.2} = \dfrac{1100}{2.2} = 500\,\text{mg}$

2. *Fraction:* $\dfrac{60\,\text{min}}{30\,\text{min}} \times 100\,\text{mL/hr} = \dfrac{60(100)}{30} = \dfrac{6000}{30} = 200\,\text{mL/hr}$

   Ratio-proportion: 30 min : 100 mL/hr :: 60 min : x mL/hr

   $30x = 60(100) = 6000$

   $\dfrac{30x}{30} = \dfrac{6000}{30} = 200$

   $x = 200\,\text{mL/hr}$

   Dimensional analysis: $?\,\text{mL/hr} = \dfrac{100\,\text{mL}}{30\,\text{min}} \left| \dfrac{\overset{2}{60}\,\text{min}}{1\,\text{hr}} \right. = \dfrac{100(2)}{1} = \dfrac{200}{1} = 200\,\text{mL/hr}$

CHAPTER 14: ANTINEOPLASTIC MEDICATIONS

1. *Dimensional analysis*:* $? \dfrac{\text{gtt}}{\text{min}} = \dfrac{2\cancel{0}\ \text{gtt}}{1\ \cancel{\text{mL}}} \left| \dfrac{100\cancel{0}\ \text{mL}}{1\cancel{0}\ \cancel{\text{mg}}} \right| \dfrac{1.25\ \cancel{\text{mg}}}{1\ \cancel{\text{hr}}} \left| \dfrac{1\ \cancel{\text{hr}}}{6\cancel{0}\ \text{min}} \right. = \dfrac{2(100)(1.25)}{6} = \dfrac{250}{6} = 42\ \text{gtt/min}$

2. *Fraction:* $\dfrac{45\ \text{units}}{15\ \text{units}} \times 1\ \text{vial} = \dfrac{45}{15} = 3\ \text{vials}$

   Ratio-proportion: 15 units : 1 vial :: 45 units : x vials
   $15x = 45$

   $\dfrac{15x}{15} = \dfrac{45}{15} = 3$

   $x = 3$ vials
   Dimensional analysis: $?\ \text{vials} = \dfrac{1\ \text{vial}}{15\ \text{units}} \times \dfrac{45\ \text{units}}{1} = \dfrac{45}{15} = 3\ \text{vials}$

3. *Fraction:* $\dfrac{65\ \text{kg}}{1\ \text{kg}} \times 10\ \text{mg} = \dfrac{65(10)}{1} = \dfrac{650}{1} = 650\ \text{mg}$
   Ratio-proportion: 1 kg : 10 mg :: 65 kg : x mg
   $1x = 65(10) = 650$
   $x = 650$ mg
   Dimensional analysis: $?\ \text{mg} = \dfrac{10\ \text{mg}}{1\ \cancel{\text{kg}}} \times \dfrac{65\ \cancel{\text{kg}}}{1} = \dfrac{10(65)}{1} = 650\ \text{mg}$

4. *Fraction:* $\dfrac{3,000,000\ \text{IU}}{6,000,000\ \text{IU}} \times 1\ \text{mL} = \dfrac{3,000,000}{6,000,000} = 0.5\ \text{mL}$

   Ratio-proportion: 6,000,000 IU : 1 mL :: 3,000,000 IU : x mL
   $6,000,000x = 3,000,000$

   $\dfrac{6,000,000x}{6,000,000} = \dfrac{3,000,000}{6,000,000} = 0.5$

   $x = 0.5$ mL
   Dimensional analysis: $?\ \text{mL} = \dfrac{1\ \text{mL}}{\underset{2}{\cancel{6}}\ \cancel{\text{IU}}} \left| \dfrac{\overset{1}{\cancel{3}}\ \cancel{\text{IU}}}{1} \right. = \dfrac{1}{2} = 0.5\ \text{mL}$

CHAPTER 15: CARDIOVASCULAR AND RENAL MEDICATIONS

1. *For fraction and ratio-proportion, first convert grams to milligrams:*
   1 g : 1000 mg :: 0.1 g : x mg
   $1x = 1000(0.1) = 100$
   $x = 100$ mg
   Fraction: $\dfrac{100\ \text{mg}}{200\ \text{mg}} \times 1\ \text{mL} = 0.5\ \text{mL}$

   Ratio-proportion: 200 mg : 1 mL :: 100 mg : x mL
   $200x = 100$
   $\dfrac{200x}{200} = \dfrac{100}{200}$
   $x = 0.5$ mL

---

*Only dimensional analysis is shown because it is the most efficient method for solving this problem.

$$\text{Dimensional analysis: } ?\,\text{mL} = \frac{1\,\text{mL}}{\underset{1}{\cancel{200}\,\text{mg}}} \left| \frac{\overset{5}{\cancel{1000}}\,\text{mg}}{1\,\cancel{g}} \right| \frac{0.1\,\cancel{g}}{} = \frac{5(0.1)}{1} = \frac{0.5}{1} = 0.5\,\text{mL}$$

2. *Fraction:* $\dfrac{30\,\text{mg}}{20\,\text{mg}} \times 1\,\text{tablet} = \dfrac{30}{20} = 1.5\,\text{tablets}$

   Ratio-proportion: 20 mg:1 tablet :: 30 mg:x tablet
   $20x = 30$
   $\dfrac{20x}{20} = \dfrac{30}{20} = 1.5$
   $x = 1.5$ tablets

   $$\text{Dimensional analysis: } ?\,\text{tablets} = \frac{1\,\text{tablet}}{20\,\cancel{\text{mg}}} \left| \frac{30\,\cancel{\text{mg}}}{1} \right. = \frac{3}{2} = 1.5\,\text{tablets}$$

3. *Fraction:* $\dfrac{60\,\text{mg}}{20\,\text{mg}} \times 5\,\text{mL} = \dfrac{60(5)}{20} = \dfrac{300}{20} = 15\,\text{mL}$

   Ratio-proportion: 20 mg:5 mL :: 60 mg:x mL
   $20x = 5(60) = 300$
   $\dfrac{20x}{20} = \dfrac{300}{20}$
   $x = 15$ mL

   $$\text{Dimensional analysis: } ?\,\text{mL} = \frac{5\,\text{mL}}{\underset{1}{20\,\cancel{\text{mg}}}} \left| \frac{\overset{3}{\cancel{60}}\,\cancel{\text{mg}}}{1} \right. = \frac{5(3)}{1} = \frac{15}{1} = 15\,\text{mL}$$

CHAPTER 16: CENTRAL AND PERIPHERAL NERVOUS SYSTEM MEDICATIONS

1. *For fraction and ratio-proportion, first convert pounds to kilograms:*
   2.2 lb:1 kg :: 150 lbs:x kg
   $2.2x = 150$
   $\dfrac{2.2x}{2.2} \times \dfrac{150}{2.2} = 68.18$
   $x = 68.18$ kg

   Fraction: $\dfrac{15\,\text{mg}}{1\,\text{kg}} \times 68.18\,\text{kg} = \dfrac{15(68.18)}{1} = \dfrac{1023}{1} = 1023\,\text{mg}$

   Ratio-proportion: 1 kg:15 mg :: 68.18 kg:x mg
   $1x = 15(68.18) = 1023$
   $x = 1023$ mg

   $$\text{Dimensional analysis: } ?\,\text{mg} = \frac{15\,\text{mg}}{1\,\cancel{\text{kg}}} \left| \frac{1\,\cancel{\text{kg}}}{2.2\,\cancel{\text{lbs}}} \right| \frac{150\,\cancel{\text{lbs}}}{1} = \frac{15(150)}{2.2} = \frac{2250}{2.2} = 1023\,\text{mg}$$

2. *Fraction:* $\dfrac{200\,\text{mg}}{125\,\text{mg}} \times 5\,\text{mL} = \dfrac{200(5)}{125} = \dfrac{1000}{125} = 8\,\text{mL}$

   Ratio-proportion: 125 mg:5 mL :: 200 mg:x mL
   $125x = 5(200) = 1000$
   $\dfrac{125x}{125} = \dfrac{1000}{125} = 8$
   $x = 8$ mL

   $$\text{Dimensional analysis: } ?\,\text{mL} = \frac{\overset{1}{\cancel{5}}\,\text{mL}}{\underset{25}{125\,\cancel{\text{mg}}}} \left| \frac{200\,\cancel{\text{mg}}}{1} \right. = \frac{200}{25} = 8\,\text{mL}$$

3. *Fraction:* $\dfrac{0.5 \text{ mg}}{2 \text{ mg}} \times 1 \text{ mL} = \dfrac{0.5}{2} = 0.25 \text{ mL}$

Ratio-proportion: 2 mg : 1 mL :: 0.5 mg : x mL

$2x = 0.5$

$\dfrac{2x}{2} = \dfrac{0.5}{2} = 0.25$

$x = 0.25 \text{ mL}$

Dimensional analysis: $?\,\text{mL} = \dfrac{1 \text{ mL}}{2 \text{ mg}} \left| \dfrac{0.5 \text{ mg}}{1} \right. = \dfrac{0.5}{2} = 0.25 \text{ mL}$

CHAPTER 17: MEDICATIONS FOR PAIN MANAGEMENT

1. *Fraction:* $\dfrac{5 \text{ mg}}{10 \text{ mg}} = \dfrac{1}{2} = 0.5 \text{ mL}$

Ratio-proportion: 10 mg : 1 mL :: 5 mg : x mL

$\dfrac{1 \text{ mL}}{10} \times \dfrac{5 \text{ mg}}{10} = \dfrac{1}{2} = 0.5$

$x = 0.5 \text{ mL}$

Dimensional analysis: $?\,\text{mL} = \dfrac{1 \text{ mL}}{10 \text{ mg}} \left| \dfrac{5 \text{ mg}}{1} \right. = \dfrac{\overset{1}{\cancel{5}}}{\underset{2}{\cancel{10}}} = \dfrac{1}{2} = 0.5 \text{ mL}$

2. *Fraction:* $\dfrac{0.5 \text{ mg}}{20 \text{ mg}} \times 200 \text{ mL} = \dfrac{0.5(200)}{20} = \dfrac{100}{20} = 5 \text{ mL/hr}$

Ratio-proportion: 20 mg : 200 mL :: 0.5 mg : x mL

$20x = 200(0.5) = 100$

$\dfrac{20x}{20} = \dfrac{100}{20} = 5$

$x = 5 \text{ mL/hr}$

Dimensional analysis: $?\,\text{mL/hr} = \dfrac{\overset{10}{\cancel{200}} \text{ mL}}{\underset{1}{\cancel{20}} \text{ mg}} \left| \dfrac{0.5 \text{ mg}}{1 \text{ hr}} \right. = \dfrac{10(0.5)}{1} = \dfrac{5}{1} = 5 \text{ mL/hr}$

3. *Fraction:* $\dfrac{0.4 \text{ mg}}{0.2 \text{ mg}} \times 1 \text{ mL} = \dfrac{0.4}{0.2} = 2 \text{ mL}$

Ratio-proportion: 0.2 mg : 1 mL :: 0.4 mg : x mL

$0.2x = 0.4$

$\dfrac{0.2x}{0.2} = \dfrac{0.4}{0.2} = 2$

$x = 2 \text{ mL}$

Dimensional analysis: $?\,\text{mL} = \dfrac{1 \text{ mL}}{\underset{1}{\cancel{0.2}} \text{ mg}} \left| \dfrac{\overset{2}{\cancel{0.4}} \text{ mg}}{1} \right. = \dfrac{2}{1} = 2 \text{ mL}$

CHAPTER 18: GASTROINTESTINAL MEDICATIONS

1. *Fraction:* $\dfrac{20 \text{ mg}}{40 \text{ mg}} \times 5 \text{ mL} = \dfrac{20(5)}{40} = \dfrac{100}{40} = 2.5 \text{ mL}$

Ratio-proportion: 40 mg:5 mL :: 20 mg:x mL

$40x = 5(20) = 100$

$\dfrac{40x}{40} = \dfrac{100}{40} = 2.5$

$x = 2.5$ mL

Dimensional analysis: $?\,\text{mL} = \dfrac{5 \text{ mL}}{\overset{2}{\cancel{40 \text{ mg}}}} \left| \dfrac{\overset{1}{\cancel{20 \text{ mg}}}}{1} \right. = \dfrac{5}{2} = 2.5$ mL

2. *For fraction and ratio-proportion, first convert pounds to kilograms:*

2.2 lbs:1 kg :: 143 lbs:x kg

$2.2x = 143$

$\dfrac{2.2x}{2.2} = \dfrac{143}{2.2} = 65$

$x = 65$ kg

Fraction: $\dfrac{65 \text{ kg}}{1 \text{ kg}} \times 1.8 \text{ mg} = \dfrac{65(1.8)}{1} = 117$ mg

Ratio-proportion: 1 kg:1.8 mg :: 65 kg:x mg

$1x = 1.8(65) = 117$

$x = 117$ mg

Dimensional analysis: $?\,\text{mg} = \dfrac{1.8 \text{ mg}}{1 \cancel{\text{kg}}} \left| \dfrac{1 \cancel{\text{kg}}}{2.2 \cancel{\text{lbs}}} \right| \dfrac{143 \cancel{\text{lbs}}}{1} = \dfrac{1.8(143)}{2.2} = \dfrac{257.4}{2.2} = 117$ mg

3. *Fraction:* $\dfrac{1.5 \text{ g}}{1 \text{ g}} \times 10 \text{ mL} = \dfrac{1.5(10)}{1} = \dfrac{15}{1} = 15$ mL

Ratio-proportion: 1 g:10 mL :: 1.5 g:x mL

$1x = 10(1.5) = 15$

$x = 15$ mL

Dimensional analysis: $?\,\text{mL} = \dfrac{10 \text{ mL}}{1 \cancel{\text{gr}}} \left| \dfrac{1.5 \cancel{\text{gr}}}{1} \right. = \dfrac{10(1.5)}{1} = \dfrac{15}{1} = 15$ mL

CHAPTER 19: HEMATOLOGIC PRODUCTS

1. *Fraction:* $\dfrac{7500 \text{ units}}{20,000 \text{ units}} \times 1 \text{ mL} = \dfrac{7500}{20,000} = 0.375 \text{ or } 0.38$ mL

Ratio-proportion: 20,000 units:1 mL :: 7500 units:x mL

$20,000x = 7500$

$\dfrac{20,000x}{20,000} = \dfrac{7500}{20,000} = 0.375$

$x = 0.375 \text{ or } 0.38$ mL

Dimensional analysis: $?\,\text{mL} = \dfrac{1 \text{ mL}}{20,000 \cancel{\text{units}}} \left| \dfrac{7500 \cancel{\text{units}}}{1} \right. = \dfrac{75}{200} = 0.375 \text{ or } 0.38$ mL

2. *Dimensional anlysis*:* $?\,\text{mL/hr} = \dfrac{500 \text{ mL}}{24 \text{ hr}} = 20.8 \text{ or } 21$ mL/hr

*Only dimensional analysis is shown because it is the most efficient method for solving this problem.

3. *Fraction:* $\dfrac{30 \text{ mg}}{150 \text{ mg}} \times 1 \text{ mL} = \dfrac{30}{150} = 0.2 \text{ mL}$

Ratio-proportion: 150 mg:1 mL :: 30 mg:x mL

$150x = 30$

$\dfrac{150x}{150} = \dfrac{30}{150} = 0.2$

$x = 0.2 \text{ mL}$

Dimensional analysis: $? \text{ mL} = \dfrac{1 \text{ mL}}{\underset{5}{\cancel{150} \text{ mg}}} \left| \dfrac{\overset{1}{\cancel{30} \text{ mg}}}{} \right. = \dfrac{1}{5} = 0.2 \text{ mL}$

CHAPTER 20: HORMONES AND STEROIDS

1. *Fraction:* $\dfrac{6 \text{ mg}}{4 \text{ mg}} \times 1 \text{ mL} = \dfrac{6}{4} = 1.5 \text{ mL}$

Ratio-proportion: 4 mg:1 mL :: 6 mg:x mL

$4x = 6$

$\dfrac{4x}{4} = \dfrac{6}{4} = 1.5$

$x = 1.5 \text{ mL}$

Dimensional analysis: $? \text{ mL} = \dfrac{1 \text{ mL}}{\underset{2}{\cancel{4} \text{ mg}}} \left| \dfrac{\overset{3}{\cancel{6} \text{ mg}}}{1} \right. = \dfrac{3}{2} = 1.5 \text{ mL}$

2. *For fraction and ratio-proportion, first convert micrograms to milligrams:*

1000 mcg:1 mg :: 125 mcg:x mg

$1000x = 125$

$\dfrac{1000x}{1000} = \dfrac{125}{1000} = 0.125$

$x = 0.125 \text{ mg}$

Fraction: $\dfrac{0.125 \text{ mg}}{0.25 \text{ mg}} \times 1 \text{ tablet} = \dfrac{0.125}{0.25} = 0.5 \text{ tablet}$

Ratio-proportion: 0.25 mg:1 tablet :: 0.125 mg:x tablet

$0.25x = 0.125$

$\dfrac{0.25x}{0.25} = \dfrac{0.125}{0.25} = 0.5$

$x = 0.5 \text{ tablet}$

Dimensional analysis: $? \text{ tablets} = \dfrac{1 \text{ tablet}}{0.25 \text{ mg}} \left| \dfrac{125 \cancel{\text{ mcg}}}{1} \right| \dfrac{1 \cancel{\text{ mg}}}{1000 \cancel{\text{ mcg}}} = \dfrac{125}{0.25(1000)} = \dfrac{125}{250} = 0.5 \text{ tablet}$

3. *Fraction:* $\dfrac{60 \text{ mg}}{125 \text{ mg}} \times 1 \text{ mL} = \dfrac{60}{125} = 0.48 \text{ or } 0.5 \text{ mL}$

Ratio-proportion: 125 mg:1 mL :: 60 mg:x mL

$125x = 60$

$\dfrac{125x}{125} = \dfrac{60}{125} = 0.48$

$x = 0.48 \text{ or } 0.5 \text{ mL}$

Dimensional analysis: $? \text{ mL} = \dfrac{1 \text{ mL}}{125 \text{ mg}} \left| \dfrac{60 \text{ mg}}{1} \right. = \dfrac{60}{125} = 0.48 \text{ or } 0.5 \text{ mL}$

CHAPTER 21: IMMUNOLOGIC MEDICATIONS

1. *Dimensional analysis**: $?\,mL/hr = \dfrac{\overset{50}{\cancel{100}}\,\text{mL}}{\underset{1}{\cancel{2}}\,\text{hr}} = \dfrac{50}{1} = 50\,\text{mL/hr}$

2. *Fraction:* $\dfrac{20,000\ \text{units}}{100,000\ \text{units}} \times 1\,\text{mL} = \dfrac{20,000}{100,000} = 0.2\,\text{mL}$

   Ratio-proportion: 100,000 units : 1 mL :: 20,000 units : x mL
   $100,000x = 20,000$
   $\dfrac{100,000x}{100,000} = \dfrac{20,000}{100,000} = 0.2$
   $x = 0.2\,\text{mL}$

   Dimensional analysis: $?\,mL = \dfrac{1\,\text{mL}}{\underset{5}{\cancel{100,000}\ \text{units}}} \left|\ \dfrac{\overset{1}{\cancel{20,000}\ \text{units}}}{1}\right. = \dfrac{1}{5} = 0.2\,\text{mL}$

3. *Fraction:* $\dfrac{65\,\text{kg}}{1\,\text{kg}} \times 20\,\text{mg} = \dfrac{20(65)}{1} = 1300\,\text{mg}$

   Ratio-proportion: 1 kg : 20 mg :: 65 kg : x mg
   $1x = 1300$
   $x = 1300\,\text{mg}$

   Dimensional analysis: $?\,mg = \dfrac{20\,\text{mg}}{1\,\text{kg}} \left|\ \dfrac{65\,\cancel{\text{kg}}}{1}\right. = \dfrac{20(65)}{1} = 1300\,\text{mg}$

CHAPTER 22: ANTIINFLAMMATORY, MUSCULOSKELETAL, AND ANTIARTHRITIS MEDICATIONS

1. *Fraction:* $\dfrac{280\,\text{mg}}{80\,\text{mg}} \times 0.8\,\text{mL} = \dfrac{280(0.8)}{80} = \dfrac{224}{80} = 2.8\,\text{mL}$

   Ratio-proportion: 80 mg : 0.8 mL :: 280 mg : x mL
   $80x = 0.8(280) = 224$
   $\dfrac{80x}{80} = \dfrac{224}{80} = 2.8$
   $x = 2.8\,\text{mL}$

   Dimensional analysis: $?\,mL = \dfrac{0.8\,\text{mL}}{\underset{2}{\cancel{80}\ \text{mg}}} \left|\ \dfrac{\overset{7}{\cancel{280}\ \text{mg}}}{1}\right. = \dfrac{0.8(7)}{2} = \dfrac{5.6}{2} = 2.8\,\text{mL}$

2. *Fraction:* $\dfrac{15\,\text{mg}}{30\,\text{mg}} \times 1\,\text{mL} = \dfrac{15}{30} = 0.5\,\text{mL}$

   Ratio-proportion: 30 mg : 1 mL :: 15 mg : x mL
   $30x = 15$
   $\dfrac{30x}{30} = \dfrac{15}{30} = 0.5$
   $x = 0.5\,\text{mL}$

   Dimensional analysis: $?\,mL = \dfrac{1\,\text{mL}}{\underset{2}{\cancel{30}\ \text{mg}}} \left|\ \dfrac{\overset{1}{\cancel{15}\ \text{mg}}}{1}\right. = \dfrac{1}{2} = 0.5\,\text{mL}$

---

*Only dimensional analysis is shown because it is the most efficient method for solving this problem.

3. *Fraction:* $\dfrac{5\,\text{gr}}{1\,\text{gr}} \times 60\,\text{mg} = 300\,\text{mg} = 1\,\text{tablet}$

Ratio-proportion: 1 gr:60 mg :: 5 gr:x mg

$1x = 60(5) = 300$

$x = 300\,\text{mg} = 1\,\text{tablet}$

Dimensional analysis: $?\,\text{tablets} = \dfrac{1\,\text{tablet}}{300\,\text{mg}} \Bigg| \dfrac{60\,\text{mg}}{1\,\text{gr}} \Bigg| \dfrac{5\,\text{gr}}{1} = \dfrac{60(5)}{300} = \dfrac{300}{300} = 1\,\text{tablet}$

CHAPTER 23: TOPICAL PREPARATIONS

1. *Fraction:* $\dfrac{500,000\,\text{units}}{100,000\,\text{units}} \times 1\,\text{mL} = \dfrac{500,000}{100,000} = 5\,\text{mL}$

Ratio-proportion: 100,000 units:1 mL :: 500,000 units:x mL

$100,000x = 500,000$

$\dfrac{100,000x}{100,000} = \dfrac{500,000}{100,000} = 5$

$x = 5\,\text{mL}$

Dimensional analysis: $?\,\text{mL} = \dfrac{1\,\text{mL}}{100,000\,\text{units}} \Bigg| \dfrac{500,000\,\text{units}}{1} = \dfrac{5}{1} = 5\,\text{mL}$

2. *Fraction:* $\dfrac{40\,\text{mg}}{20\,\text{mg}} \times 1\,\text{tablet} = \dfrac{40}{20} = 2\,\text{tablets}$

Ratio-proportion: 20 mg:1 tablet :: 40 mg:x tablet

$20x = 40$

$\dfrac{20x}{20} = \dfrac{40}{20} = 2$

$x = 2\,\text{tablets}$

Dimensional analysis: $?\,\text{tablets} = \dfrac{1\,\text{tablet}}{\underset{1}{20\,\text{mg}}} \Bigg| \dfrac{\overset{2}{40\,\text{mg}}}{1} = \dfrac{2}{1} = 2\,\text{tablets}$

3. *Fraction:* $\dfrac{10\,\text{mL}}{5\,\text{mL}} \times 1\,\text{teaspoon} = \dfrac{10}{5} = 2\,\text{teaspoons}$

Ratio-proportion: 5 mL:1 teaspoon :: 10 mL:x teaspoons

$5x = 10$

$\dfrac{5x}{5} = \dfrac{10}{5} = 2$

$x = 2\,\text{teaspoons}$

Dimensional anlysis: $?\,\text{teaspoons} = \dfrac{1\,\text{teaspoon}}{\underset{1}{5\,\text{mL}}} \Bigg| \dfrac{\overset{2}{10\,\text{mL}}}{1} = \dfrac{2}{1} = 2\,\text{teaspoons}$

CHAPTER 24: VITAMINS AND MINERALS

1. *Fraction:* $\dfrac{200\,\text{mcg}}{1000\,\text{mcg}} \times 1\,\text{mL} = \dfrac{200}{1000} = 0.2\,\text{mL}$

Ratio-proportion: 1000 mcg:1 mL :: 200 mcg:x mL

$1000x = 200$

$\dfrac{1000x}{1000} = \dfrac{200}{1000} = 0.2$

$x = 0.2\,\text{mL}$

$$\textit{Dimensional analysis: } ?\,mL = \frac{1\,mL}{\underset{5}{\cancel{1000}}\;\cancel{mcg}}\;\bigg|\;\frac{\overset{1}{\cancel{200}}\;\cancel{mcg}}{1} = \frac{1}{5} = 0.2\,mL$$

2. *Dimensional anlysis*:* $?\,mL/hr = \dfrac{250\,mL}{6\,hr} = 41.66 \text{ or } 42\,mL/hr$

3. *Fraction:* $\dfrac{10\,mEq}{60\,mEq} \times 200\,mL = \dfrac{10(200)}{60} = \dfrac{2000}{60} = 33.3 \text{ or } 33\,mL/hr$

   Ratio-proportion: 60 mEq : 200 mL :: 10 mEq : x mL
   $60x = 200(10) = 2000$

   $\dfrac{60x}{60} \times \dfrac{2000}{60} = 33.3$

   $x = 33.3 \text{ or } 33\,mL/hr$

   $$\textit{Dimensional analysis: } ?\,mL/hr = \frac{200\,mL}{\cancel{60}\;\cancel{mEq}}\;\bigg|\;\frac{\cancel{10}\;\cancel{mEq}}{1\,hr} = \frac{200}{6} = 33.3 \text{ or } 33\,mL/hr$$

---

*Only dimensional analysis is shown because it is the most efficient method for solving this problem.

Bibliography

2011 ACCF/AHA/HRS (2011). Focused update on the management of patients with atrial fibrillation (update on dabigatran). American College of Cardiology Foundation/American Heart Association Task Force on Practice. *J Am Coll Cardiol* 57:1330-1337.

ALLHAT Officers and Coordinators for the ALLHAT Collaborative Research Group (2002). Major outcomes in high-risk hypertensive patients randomized to angiotensin converting enzyme inhibitor or calcium channel blocker vs diuretic: The Antihypertensive and Lipid-Lowering Treatment to Prevent Heart Attack Trial (ALLHAT). *JAMA* 288:2981-2997.

American Diabetes Association (2011). Clinical practice recommendations 2011. *Diabetes Care* 34:53. Available at http://care.diabetesjournals.org/content/34/Supplement_1.

American Psychiatric Association (2003). *Diagnostic and statistical manual of mental disorders*, 4th ed, Text Revision (DSM-IV-TR). Washington, DC: American Psychiatric Publishing.

American Psychiatric Association. *Treating Alzheimer's disease and other dementias of late life*. Available at http://www.psychiatryonline.com/pracGuide/pracGuideHome.aspx. Accessed May 5, 2011.

American Psychiatric Association (2004). *Practice guideline for the treatment of patients with acute stress disorder and post-traumatic stress disorder*. Arlington, VA: American Psychiatric Association. Available at http://www.psychiatryonline.com/pracGuide/pracGuideHome.aspx. Accessed May 5, 2011.

Bonow RO, Mann DL, Zipes DP, Libby P (2011). *Braunwald's heart disease: a textbook of cardiovascular medicine*, 9th ed. Philadelphia: Saunders.

Briggs GG, Freeman RK, Yaffe SJ (2011). *Drugs in pregnancy and lactation: A reference guide to fetal and neonatal risk*, 9th ed. Philadelphia: Lippincott Williams & Wilkins.

Brooks JT, Kaplan JE, Masur H (2009). What's new in the 2009 US guidelines for prevention and treatment of opportunistic infections among adults and adolescents with HIV? *Top HIV Med* 17(3):109-114.

Burton LL, Chabner B, Knollman B, Eds (2010). *Goodman & Gilman's the pharmacological basis of therapeutics*, 12th ed. New York: McGraw-Hill.

Centers for Disease Control and Prevention (2010). 2010 STD treatment guidelines. Available at http://www.cdc.gov/std/treatment/2010/default.htm. Accessed May 5, 2011.

Chessare JB (1998). Teaching clinical decision-making to pediatric residents in an era of managed care. *Pediatrics* 101(4, pt 2): 762-766.

Chobanian AV, Bakris GL, Black HR, Cushman WC (2003). The seventh report of the Joint National Committee on Prevention, Detection, Evaluation, and Treatment of High Blood Pressure: The JNC 7 Report. *JAMA* 289:2560.

Chou R, Huffman LH (2007). American Pain Society, American College of Physicians. Medications for acute and chronic low back pain: A review of the evidence for American Pain Society/American College of Physicians clinical practice guideline. *Ann Intern Med* 147(7):505-514.

Davis TM, Yeap B, Bruce DG, Davis WA (2007). *Lipid lowering therapy protects against peripheral sensory neuropathy in type 2 diabetes*, 67th scientific sessions (June 22-26, 2007). Abstract 0004-OR.

Drew RH (2007). Emerging options for treatment of invasive, multidrug-resistant *Staphylococcus aureus* infections. *Pharmacotherapy* 27(2):227-249.

Drug facts and comparisons. (2011). St Louis: Wolters Kluwer. Monthly update. Available online at http://www.factsandcomparions.com. Accessed May 5, 2011.

Feldman RD, Zou GY, Vandervoort MK et al (2009). A simplified approach to the treatment of uncomplicated hypertension. A cluster randomized controlled trial. *Hypertension* 53:646-653.

Folsom AR, Chambless LE, Ballantyne CM et al. (2006). An assessment of incremental coronary risk prediction using C-reactive protein and other novel risk markers: the Atherosclerosis Risk in Communities Study. *Arch Intern Med* 166:1368-1373.

Gilbert DN, Moellering RC, Eliopoulos GM, Sande MA (2011). *The Sanford guide to antimicrobial therapy*, 40th ed. Hyde Park, VT: Antimicrobial Therapy, Inc.

Glauser TA, Salinas GD, Roepke NL et al (2011). Management of mild-to-moderate osteoarthritis: A study of the primary care perspective. *Postgrad Med* 123(1):126-134.

Groves KEM, Flanagan PS, MacKinnon NJ (2002). Why physicians start or stop prescribing a drug: Literature review and formulary implications. *Formulary* 37:186-194.

Hammer SM, Norrby SR (2010). Principles of anti-infective therapy. In Cohen J, Powderly WG, Eds. *Infectious diseases*, 3rd ed. St Louis: Mosby.

Henderson RA, Timmis AD (2010). Almanac 2011: stable coronary artery disease. *Heart* 19:1552-1559.

Hopper DC (2005). Quinolones. In GL Mandell, JE Bennett, R Dolin, Eds. *Principles and practice of infectious diseases*, 6th ed. New York: Churchill Livingstone.

Hunt SA, Abraham WT, Chin MH et al (2009). ACC/AHA 2009 focused update: ACCF/AHA guidelines for the diagnosis and management of heart failure in adults. American College of Cardiology/American Heart Association Task Force on Practice Guidelines (Writing Committee to Update the 2001 Guidelines for the Evaluation and Management of Heart Failure): developed in collaboration with the American College of Chest Physicians and the International Society for Heart and Lung Transplantation. *J Am Coll Cardiol* 53(3):1343-1382. Available online at http://content.onlinejacc.org/cgi/content/full/53/15/1343. Accessed May 6, 2011.

Janssens JH, Janssen M, van de Lisdonk EH et al (2008). Use of oral prednisolone or naproxen for the treatment of gout arthritis: a double-blind, randomised equivalence trial. *Lancet* 371(9627):1854-1860.

Kaplan N, Rose BD (2011). Indications for use of specific antihypertensive drugs. In BD Rose, Ed, *UpToDate*. Waltham, MA: *UpToDate*. Accessed July 20, 2011.

Kaplan NM, Rose BD (2011). Choice of therapy in essential hypertension: Clinical trials. In BD Rose Ed, *UpToDate*. Waltham, MA: *UpToDate*. Accessed July 20, 2011.

Katzung BG, Masters S, Trevor A (2009). *Basic and clinical pharmacology*, 11th ed. New York: McGraw-Hill.

Kenred E, Nelson MD, Masters CF (2006). *Infectious disease epidemiology: Theory and practice*. New York: Jones and Bartlett.

Lazarou J, Pomeranz BH, Corey PN (1998). Incidence of adverse drug reactions in hospitalized patients: A meta-analysis of prospective studies. *JAMA* 279:1200-1205.

Lindenfield J, Albertt NM, Boehmer JP et al (2011) Executive summary. HFSA 2010 comprehensive heart failure practice guideline. *J Card Fail* 16(6):475-539. Available online at http://www.onlinejcf.com/article/S1071-9164(10)00174-0/fulltext. Accessed November 3 , 2011.

Long SS, Pickering LK, Prober CG (2009). *Principles and practice of pediatric infectious disease*, 3rd ed. New York: Churchill Livingstone.

Mandell GL, Bennett JE, Dolin R, eds. (2005). *Principles and practice of infectious diseases*, 6th ed. New York: Churchill Livingstone.

McKenry LM, Tessier E, Hogan MA et al (2006). *Mosby's pharmacology in nursing*, 22nd ed. St Louis: Mosby.

McPhee SJ, Papadakis MA, Tierney LM (2010). *Current medical diagnosis and treatment 2011*, 50th ed. New York: McGraw-Hill Medical.

National Institutes of Health, National Asthma Education and Prevention Program Expert Panel (2007). *Report 3: Guidelines for the diagnosis and management of asthma*, NIH Publication No. 08-4051. Washington, DC: US Government Printing Office. Available at http://www.nhlbi.nih.gov/guidelines/asthma/asthgdln.html2007.

National Center for Health Statistics, Advance Data Number 381 (December 12, 2006). *The state of childhood asthma, United States, 1980-2005*. Available at http://www.cdc.gov/nchs/data/ad/ad381.pdf.

National Center for Immunization and Respiratory Diseases (2011). General recommendations on immunization—recommendations of the Advisory Committee on Immunization Practices (ACIP). *MMWR Recomm Rep* 60(2):1-64.

National Headache Foundation (NHF). Press Release. *The NHF unveils migraine prevention consensus statement*. Available at http://www.headaches.org. Accessed April 30, 2007.

National Institute on Alcohol Abuse and Alcoholism (2005). *Helping patients who drink too much: A clinician's guide 2005 edition*. U.S. Department of Health & Human Services, National Institutes of Health, NIH Publication No. 05-3769. Available at http://pubs.niaaa.nih.gov/publications/Practi

tioner/CliniciansGuide2005/clinicians_guide.htm. Accessed January 25, 2007.

North American Menopause Society (2011). Estrogen and progestogen use in peri- and postmenopausal women: 2010 position statement of The North American Menopause Society. Available at http://www.menopause.org/aoubtmeno/consensus.aspx. Accessed May 5, 2011.

O'Gara PT, Oparil S (2007). Treatment of hypertension in the prevention and management of ischemic heart disease: A scientific statement from the American Heart Association Council for High Blood Pressure Research and the Councils on Clinical Cardiology and Epidemiology and Prevention. *Circulation* 115(21):2761-2788.

Paulsen RH, Katon W, Ciechanowski P (2011). Treatment of resistant depression in adults. In Rose BD, ed, *UpToDate*. Waltham, MA: *UpToDate*. Accessed July 20, 2011.

Ramakrishnan K, Salinas RC (2007). Recommendations for treating peptic ulcer disease. *Am Fam Physician* 76:1005-1012.

Saw JT, Bahari MDB, Ang HH, Lim YH (2006). Potential drug-herb interaction with antiplatelet/anticoagulant drugs. *Complement Ther Clin Pract* 12(4): 236-241.

Simoni-Wastila L, Stuart BC, Shaffer T (2006). Over-the-counter drug use by Medicare beneficiaries in nursing homes: Implications for practice and policy. *J Am Geriatr Soc* 54(10): 1543-1549.

Talley NJ (2005). American Gastroenterological Association medical position statement: Evaluation of dyspepsia. *Gastroenterology* 129(5):1753-1755.

Talley NJ (2007). Functional gastrointestinal disorders in 2007 and Rome III: Something new, something borrowed, something objective. *Rev Gastroenterol Disord* 7(2):97-105.

The Robert Wood Foundation Initiative on the Future of Nursing, at The Institute of Medicine. The Future of Nursing: Leading Change, Advancing Health. Released October 5, 2010. Available at: http://www.iom.edu/Reports/2010/The-Future-of-Nursing-Leading-Change-Advancing-Health/Report-Brief-Scope-of-Practice.aspx. Accessed May 8, 2011.

Yang YX, Lewis JD, Epstein S, Metz DC (2006). Long-term proton pump inhibitor therapy and risk of hip fracture. *JAMA* 296(24):2947-2953.

Zuckerbrot RA, Cheung AH, Jensen PS et al (2007). GLAD-PC Steering Group. Guidelines for adolescent depression in primary care (GLAD-PC): I. Identification, assessment, and initial management. *Pediatrics* 120(5):e1299-1312.

Illustration Credits

CHAPTER 5

Figure 5-1: From Moore KL, Persaud TVN (2007). *The developing human: clinically oriented embryology*, 8th ed. Philadelphia: WB Saunders.

CHAPTER 9

Figure 9-4: From Lilley LL, Rainforth Collins S, Harrington S, Snyder JS (2010). *Pharmacology and the nursing process*, 6th ed. St Louis: Elsevier; modified from data by Boyd E, West CD. In Behrman RE, Kleigman RM, Jensen HB (eds) (2007). *Nelson textbook of pediatrics*, 18th ed. Philadelphia: WB Saunders.

CHAPTER 10

Figure 10-7A, 10-27, 10-28: Copyright Baxter Healthcare Corporation, Deerfield, IL.

Figure 10-7B, 10-11: From Potter PA, Perry AG (2008). Fundamentals of nursing, 7th ed. St Louis: Elsevier.

Figure 10-26: Copyright 2011 Alaris, San Diego, CA.

Figure 10-28: Copyright Medtronic, Inc., Cincinnati, OH.

Figure 10-29: Copyright WalkMed Infusion, Englewood, CO.

Figure 10-30: From deWit S (2009). Fundamental Concepts and Skills for Nursing, 3rd ed. St. Louis: Elsevier.

CHAPTER 11

Figure 11-1: From Herlihy B (2006). *The human body in health and illness*, 3rd ed. Philadelphia: Elsevier.

Figure 11-2: From Thibodeau G (2009). *The human body in health and disease*, 5th ed. St. Louis: Elsevier.

CHAPTER 12

Figure 12-1, 12-2: From Wecker L (2009). *Brody's Human Pharmacology*, 5th ed. Philadelphia: Elsevier.

CHAPTER 13

Figure 13-1: Redrawn from McCance KL, Huether SE (1994). *Pathophysiology: the biological basis for disease in adults and children*, 2nd ed. St Louis: Mosby.

Figure 13-2: Redrawn from McCance KL, Huether SE (1994). *Pathophysiology: the biological basis for disease in adults and children*, 2nd ed. St Louis: Mosby; modified from Yarcoan R, Metsuya H, Broder S (1989). *AIDS therapies, the science of AIDS*, readings from Scientific American, New York: WH Freeman.

CHAPTER 14

Figure 14-1: From Brenner G, (2009). *Pharmacology* 3rd ed. Philadelphia: Elsevier.

CHAPTER 15

Figures 15-1, 15-2, 15-5A, 15-9, 15-10: From Herlihy B (2011). *The human body in health and illness*, 4th ed. Philadelphia: Elsevier.

Figure 15-3: From Thibodeau GA, Patton KT (2003). *Anatomy & physiology*, 5th ed. St Louis: Mosby.

Figure 15-5B: Modified from Herlihy B (2011). *The human body in health and illness*, 4th ed. Philadelphia: Elsevier.

Figure 15-7B: From Damjanov I, Linder J, (eds) (1996). *Anderson's pathology*, 10th ed. St Louis: Mosby.

Figure 15-12: From Brundage DJ (1992). *Renal disorders*, St Louis: Mosby.

Figure 15-13: Redrawn from McCance KL, Huether SE (1996). *Pathophysiology: the biological basis for disease in adults and children*, 2nd ed. St Louis: Mosby.

Figure 15-14: Redrawn from National Heart, Lung, and Blood Institute, National High Blood Pressure Education Program (2003). *The seventh report of the Joint National Committee on the Prevention, Detection, Evaluation and Treatment of High Blood Pressure*, Bethesda, MD: National Institutes of Health.

CHAPTER 16

Figure 16-2: From Wecker L (2009). *Brody's Human Pharmacology*, 5th ed. Philadelphia: Elsevier.

Figure 16-3: From Varcarolis E (2009). *Foundations of Psychiatric Mental Health Nursing*, 6th ed. St. Louis: Elsever.

Figure 16-4: From Lehne R (2009). *Pharmacology for nursing care*, 7th ed. Philadelphia: Elsevier.

CHAPTER 17

Figure 17-1: From Wecker L (2009). *Brody's Human Pharmacology*, 5th ed. Philadelphia: Elsevier.

Figure 17-2: From Black JM, Hawks JH (2009). *Medical-surgical nursing: clinical management for positive outcomes*, 8th ed. Philadelphia: Elsevier.

Figure 17-3: Hockenberry M, Wilson D (2011). *Wong's nursing care of infants and children*, 9th ed. St Louis: Copyright Elsevier, Inc. Reprinted with permission.

Figure 17-4A: Copyright Baxter Healthcare Corporation, Deerfield, IL.

Figure 17-4B: From deWit SC (2009). *Fundamental concepts and skills for nursing*, 3rd ed. Philadelphia: Elsevier.

CHAPTER 18

Figure 18-3: From Mckenry (2006). *Mosby's pharmacology in nursing*, 22nd ed. Philadelphia: Elsevier.

CHAPTER 19

Figure 19-1: Modified from Herlihy B (2011). *The human body in health and illness*, 4th ed. Philadelphia: Elsevier.

CHAPTER 21

Figures 21-1, 21-2: Modified from Herlihy B (2011). *The human body in health and illness*, 4th ed. Philadelphia: Elsevier.

Figure 21-3: From Harkreader H, Hogan MA, Thobaben M, (2007). *Fundamentals of nursing: caring and clinical judgment*, 3rd ed. Philadelphia: Elsevier.

CHAPTER 22

Figure 22-1: From Thibodeau GA, Patton KT (2011). *Anatomy & physiology*, 7th ed. St Louis: Elsevier.

Figure 22-2: From the U.S. Department of Health and Human Services. Centers for Disease Control and Prevention. *2011 Child and Adolescent Immunization Schedules.* Atlanta, GA, United States.

CHAPTER 23

Figure 23-1: From Herlihy B (2011). *The human body in health and illness*, 4th ed. Philadelphia: Elsevier.

A

abortifacients Drugs used to stimulate uterine contractions and cause the uterus to empty.

absorption The process by which a drug enters the body and passes into the body fluids and tissues; occurs through diffusion, filtration, or osmosis.

acetylcholine One of two major neurotransmitters in the body; acts on the parasympathetic nerves.

acquired immune deficiency syndrome (AIDS) A disease caused by the human immunodeficiency virus (HIV), which enters the body through mucous membranes or infected blood and produces a defect in the ability of the immune system to fight infection. AIDS is associated with a long course marked by increasing weakness and is manifested by various opportunistic infections.

action potential duration Length of time for one cell to electrically fire (depolarize) and recover (repolarize).

acute pain Pain related to an injury such as recent surgery, trauma, or infection; ends within an expected time.

addiction The desperate need to have and use a drug for a nonmedical reason.

additive effect When two drugs are given together, the combined effect of the drugs is equal to either that of the more active drug or the sum of the effects of the individual drugs.

adolescence The period in development between the onset of puberty and adulthood. For calculation of drug dosage, it generally refers to the ages between 12 and 16.

adrenergic blocking agents Agents that block the release of epinephrine and norepinephrine at the postganglionic nerve endings of the sympathetic nervous system, producing dilation of the blood vessels and a decrease in cardiac output.

adrenergic drugs Drugs that produce sympathetic nervous system effects; also called *sympathomimetics* or *catecholamines*.

adrenergic fibers Sympathetic nerve fibers that release epinephrine at a synapse when a nerve impulse passes.

adverse reactions Unexpected and undesirable symptoms or problems that arise because of a medication. The more severe reactions often require hospitalization and may cause death. Also called *adverse effects*.

agonists Drugs that bond well with receptor sites in the patient's body and activate the receptor, producing an action similar to that of the body's own chemicals.

alkylating agents Synthetic compounds that combine readily with other molecules and interfere with the normal process of cell division; used in chemotherapy.

allergy Acquired sensitivity or heightened immune response to a drug or a foreign substance (antigen).

alternative medicine Health practices that are either scientifically untested or lacking in supportive data. Some alternative therapies are herbal therapies, aromatherapy, chiropractic, acupuncture, massage, and homeotherapy.

ampoules Small, breakable glass containers that contain one dose of medication in each; used for intramuscular injections or intravenous infusions.

anaphylactic reaction Life-threatening allergic reaction to medication so severe that the patient has difficulty breathing and may have cardiovascular collapse.

androgens The male hormone testosterone and its related hormones; help develop and maintain the male sex organs at puberty and develop secondary sex characteristics in men.

anorectal preparations Emollients, foams, or gels used for topical anesthesia or healing of the rectal area; used for symptomatic relief of discomfort associated with hemorrhoids.

antacids Drugs that neutralize hydrochloric acid and increase gastric pH, thus inhibiting pepsin.

antagonistic effect When two drugs are given together, one drug interferes with the action of the other.

antagonists Agents that attach at a receptor site but then produce no new chemical reaction; prevent activation of the receptor, stopping other chemical reactions from occurring.

antibiotic preparations Antimicrobial agents used therapeutically, not for their antiinfective properties, but to delay or prevent cell division of malignant cells.

antibiotics Antimicrobial chemicals that are produced from other living microorganisms and are antagonistic to some other forms of life. Their actions are classified as *bactericidal* or *bacteriostatic*.

anticholinergics Agents that block the release of acetylcholine and inhibit cholinergic activity; they reduce gastrointestinal tract spasm and intestinal motility, acid production, and gastric motility, which reduces the associated pain.

anticoagulants Agents that inhibit the blood clotting mechanism and increase the time it takes for blood to clot.

antidiarrheals Agents that reduce the fluid content of the stool or decrease peristalsis and motility of the intestinal tract.

antiflatulents Agents that break up and prevent mucus-surrounded pockets of gas from forming in the intestine.

antifungal medications Medications used to treat mycotic infections.

antigen-antibody response Response that occurs when foreign substances (antigens) that invade the body cause the immune system to make proteins (antibodies) that react specifically with the foreign substances to help neutralize their effects. This response is seen in allergies and infectious disease.

antiglaucoma agents Medications used to reduce the secretion of aqueous humor in the eye, block the action of acetylcholine, produce complete paralysis, aid in diagnostic procedures, provide iris sphincter contraction, and act as cholinergic agonists to reduce intraocular pressure.

antihistamines Drugs given to relieve the effects of histamine on body organs and structures. Histamine is responsible for the signs and symptoms of allergic reactions.

antimetabolites Agents that disrupt normal cell functions by interfering with various metabolic functions of the cells.

antimicrobials Chemicals that kill or damage pathogenic organisms.

antipsoriatics Agents that accelerate scaling and healing of dry lesions in chronic psoriasis.

antiretrovirals Drugs used to slow growth or prevent duplication of retroviruses (for example, human immunodeficiency virus).

antiseptics Compounds that are capable of preventing infection.

antiserums Serums made up of concentrated antibodies (immune globulins) obtained from humans or animals that have developed these antibodies in response to a specific antigen.

antitussives Drugs used to relieve coughing.

apothecaries' system System used in England for measuring and weighing drugs and solutions. Uses whole numbers and fractions; basic units are grains for solids and minims for liquids.

arthritis Painful, swollen, and stiffened joints caused by more than 100 types of joint disease in which destruction or inflammation is present.

artificially acquired active immunity Resistance to disease that is developed in individuals by giving them laboratory-produced vaccines that contain either live, attenuated (weakened) or killed antigens.

ascorbic acid An essential vitamin found in fresh fruits and vegetables, especially citrus fruits; also called *vitamin C*. Has multiple functions and is important in wound healing and for increasing resistance to disease.

asepsis Freedom from contaminated or infectious material; prevention of infection.

assessment Process of gathering information about the patient, the patient's problem, and any factors that may influence the choice of drug to be given.

auscultation One of the four standard physical assessment techniques; generally involves using a stethoscope to listen to heart, lung, or bowel sounds.

B

bactericidal Drug that kills bacteria.

bacteriostatic Drug that limits or slows the growth of bacteria.

barbiturates Primary category of anticonvulsants used for their sedative effect on the brain.

barrel Portion of a syringe that is the container for holding medication; it is marked by calibrations (printed numbers) to indicate the volume of medication inside it.

bioequivalent Products that are chemically identical and so are interchangeable.

biotransformation Metabolic process by which medication is gradually broken down, primarily in the liver, through complex chemical reactions until it becomes chemically inactive.

body surface area (BSA) A formula used to calculate the total tissue area; used to determine pediatric dosages of medication. It is calculated in square meters by using charts constructed from height and weight data.

broad-spectrum drugs Antiinfective medications that are effective against a wide variety of organisms.

bronchodilators Drugs used in patients with asthma or chronic obstructive pulmonary disease to open the bronchi and allow air to pass out more freely.

bronchospasm A narrowing or collapse of bronchial airways, often associated with increased mucus production. Irritation of the reduced airway often causes the patient to cough.

buccal administration Applying medication directly against the buccal or mucous membranes of the cheek, where it is rapidly absorbed into the bloodstream, bypassing the liver.

C

capsules Gelatin containers that hold powder or liquid medicine.

catecholamines Drugs that produce effects in the body similar to those produced by norepinephrine; also called *adrenergic* or *sympathomimetic* drugs.

celsius Scale that measures temperature; boiling point is 100° and freezing point is 0°.

central nervous system (CNS) The portion of the nervous system consisting of the brain and spinal cord.

chemical name The name for a drug that describes the chemical composition and the atomic or molecular structure.

chemotherapeutic agents Drugs used to treat malignant diseases by slowing cell growth or delaying the spread of the malignant cells throughout the body.

cholinergic drugs Agents whose action is similar to acetylcholine; also called *parasympathomimetics*.

cholinergic fibers Parasympathetic nerve fibers that release acetylcholine at a synapse when a nerve impulse passes.

chronic heart failure (CHF) A syndrome of weak or inadequate heart action caused by many different factors. Signs and symptoms include a decrease in cardiac output, less effective removal of waste products by the kidneys, and pooling of fluid between the cells or organs or in other dependent tissues.

chronic pain Any pain that continues beyond the usual course of an acute injury process.

chronotropic Affects the rate of rhythmic movements, such as the heartbeat.

Clark's rule A method for determining the pediatric dosage of medication based on the child's body weight; calculated by ratios and proportions.

common denominator A denominator (the bottom number of a fraction) that is the same number for each fraction used in a calculation. Needed when the calculation involves fractions with different denominators; can be found by multiplying the denominators of each fraction by one another.

compelling indications Other diseases for which a specific class of drugs that was developed for a disease has been shown to improve the patient's condition.

complementary medicine Alternative (nontraditional) therapies used in addition to standard medical care.

complex fraction A fraction that contains a fraction in its numerator (top number in the fraction), its denominator (bottom number in the fraction), or both.

compliant Term that describes a patient who follows a prescribed plan of care.

concordance Partnership between the nurse, patient, family, and pharmacist in which all work together to reduce problems with taking drugs.

contraindications Factors that rule out the use of a particular drug or class of drugs to treat a medical condition.

controlled substances Category of drugs that are most heavily regulated by U.S. federal legislation because of their high potential for abuse; includes major pain killers (narcotics) and some sedatives or tranquilizers.

corticosteroids Substances manufactured by the adrenal cortex that influence many organs, structures, and life processes of the body; composed of glucocorticoids and mineralocorticoids.

culture The shared values, beliefs, customs, and behavior of the members of a specific group; learned through both formal teaching and informal life experiences.

D

database Combined information about a patient's level of health, health care practices, past and present illnesses, and physical examination that serves as the basis for the plan of care.

dehydration Loss of a large amount of water from the body tissues, along with loss of electrolytes.

delegation When the responsibility for performing a task is passed from one person to another, but the accountability for what happens, or the outcome, remains with the original person.

denominator Number in the bottom part of a fraction, below the line.

dependence A state in which the body shows withdrawal symptoms when the drug is stopped or a reversing drug (antagonist) is given.

depolarization The movement of electrolytes into and out of the cell as it prepares to send another electrical message.

desired action The expected response of a medication.

diabetes mellitus Disorder of carbohydrate metabolism that may result from a relative lack of insulin or an insensitivity of the body to the available insulin. Abnormalities in fat and protein metabolism also result from serious carbohydrate metabolism disruptions.

diagnosis Conclusion about what the patient's problems are; made by the health care team after critically assessing the patient's condition through history, physical examination, and laboratory testing.

digestive enzymes Substances that promote digestion by acting as replacement therapy when the body's natural pancreatic enzymes are lacking, not secreted, or not properly absorbed.

digitalis toxicity A life-threatening condition in which a patient shows gradual onset of uncomfortable and harmful reactions to digitalis. High concentration of medication results in gradual poisoning of tissues.

digitalizing dose Frequent, high doses of digitalis given when a patient begins taking digitalis; done so that a specific level of medication can be quickly achieved in the blood to improve cardiac function or control dysrhythmias or other adverse conditions.

dimensional analysis A mathematical procedure often used in biology, physics, chemistry, and pharmacology to solve problems by using a grid to establish proportional relationships; reduces the chance of errors in conversion of units.

displacement When two drugs are given together, one drug replaces another at the drug receptor site, increasing the effect of the first drug.

distribution The extent to which drugs have moved from circulating body fluids to their sites of action in the body.

disulfiram reaction Immediate and severe nausea, vomiting, and diarrhea, as well as many other adverse reactions, caused when a patient mixes disulfiram with alcohol. Some medications, such as metronidazole (Flagyl; used to treat vaginal infections), can produce a similar reaction.

dromotropic Influences the speed of passage of an electrical impulse in nerve or cardiac muscle fibers.

drop factor The number of drops per milliliter of liquid in an intravenous solution; determined by the size of the drops.

drug interaction A change in the effect of a drug when it is administered with food or another drug; may increase or decrease the action of the drug.

dysrhythmia Irregular beating of the heart.

E

ectopic beats Irregular or premature beats of the heart caused by increased sensitivity of electrical cells.

edema Abnormal pooling of fluid in the spaces between cells or organs or in other dependent tissues.

effective refractory period Period during which the muscle cells cannot discharge their electrical activity.

electrocardiogram (ECG) A graphic record of the electrical activity of the heart produced by an electrocardiograph.

elixirs Clear liquid made up of drugs dissolved in alcohol and water; may have coloring and flavoring agents added.

emetics Drugs used in emergency situations to cause vomiting so as to remove poisons from the stomach before they can be absorbed.

emulsions Solutions that have small droplets of water and medication dispersed in oil, or oil and medication dispersed in water.

end-organ damage Damage to the vascular tissues of the heart, kidneys, brain, eyes, and other organs; caused by a continuing increase in systolic and diastolic blood pressure.

engineering controls Safety features built into equipment to reduce risk of infection and other hazards in health care institutions.

enteral (route) Administration of drug directly into the gastrointestinal tract through the mouth, nasogastric tube, or rectum.

estrogen Principal female sex hormone, manufactured in the ovaries; responsible for development of the female reproductive organs and secondary sex characteristics and involved with ovulation, pregnancy, and menstruation.

evaluation Process of looking at the results when a plan is implemented and determining if the results are what is intended. The plan is modified until the desired results are obtained.

excretion Process by which inactive chemicals, chemical by-products, and waste are removed from the body. The kidney is the most important organ of excretion, but feces, tears, and the respiratory tract are also locations of excretion.

expectorants Agents that decrease the thickness of respiratory secretions and aid in their removal.

F

Fahrenheit Scale that measures temperature; boiling point is 212° and freezing point is 32°.

fibrin A netlike substance in the blood that traps red and white blood cells and platelets and forms the matrix of a blood clot.

fibrinogen A protein found in the blood plasma that is converted to fibrin by the action of thrombin; also known as *clotting factor I.*

first-pass (effect) The percentage of medication that is inactivated after it goes through the liver the first time.

flow rate The rate at which intravenous fluids are given; measured in drops per minute.

fluid and electrolyte mixtures Solutions of water and calories in the form of carbohydrates, with minerals and electrolytes such as sodium, potassium, chloride, calcium, and phosphorus. These are given when oral food intake has been stopped or to prevent dehydration.

fraction One or more equal parts of a unit; written as two numbers separated by a line, such as 1/2.

G

generation Term used to describe a group of drugs based on their development from other similar medications. Later generations of drugs are often more specific in action but may also have more adverse effects.

generic name Assigned name for a drug; not licensed and can be used by any manufacturer.

geriatric Pertaining to the physiology of aging and the diagnosis and treatment of diseases affecting the older adult population; also refers to older adults.

glucometers Handheld machines used to measure the blood glucose level.

gout A form of arthritis caused by overproduction or underexcretion of uric acid.

gram Unit of weight used in the metric system of measurement.

H

half-life The time it takes to remove 50% of a drug from the body.

health disparity When the inability to read and write puts a person at higher risk for disease and disability.

health literacy The ability to understand and use information important in keeping oneself healthy.

health promotion Performing specific activities intended to maintain or improve one's health and well-being.

helminthiasis Infestation by worms.

hepatotoxic Having the potential to damage the liver.

herbal Compounds made from plant sources used in alternative or complementary medical practice to relieve symptoms. Often prepared as teas, poultices, or wraps.

histamine Chemical responsible for the inflammatory response in the body. When the body is injured or sensitized to an allergen, histamine is released.

histamine H$_2$-receptor antagonists Agents that promote healing of ulcers and act with antacids to produce more alkaline conditions in the gastrointestinal tract.

hormones Chemicals made in an organ or gland and carried through the bloodstream to another part of the body, where they stimulate that part of the body to increase its activity or secretion.

human immunodeficiency virus (HIV) A type of retrovirus that causes acquired immune deficiency syndrome (AIDS). It is transmitted through contact with an infected individual's blood, semen, cervical secretions, cerebrospinal fluid, or synovial fluid. It produces defects in cellular immunity.

hydration The amount of fluid in body tissue.

hyperglycemia Condition seen with fasting blood glucose levels greater than 150 mg/dL. Signs include glycosuria, ketonuria, Kussmaul respiration, tachycardia, and acetone breath. People may have hyperglycemia for a variety of reasons; chronic high blood glucose levels are usually associated with diabetes mellitus.

hyperlipidemia An increase in levels of one or more of the types of lipoproteins in the blood. This may mean that there are high amounts of cholesterol, triglycerides, or both.

hyperlipoproteinemia An increase in the lipoprotein concentration in the blood, usually caused by defects in lipoprotein transport or metabolism.

hypersensitivity Increased reaction to a drug; often used to describe an allergy.

hyperthyroidism Overproduction of thyroid hormone. Symptoms include weight loss, decreased or absent menstruation, rapid or pounding heart, heat intolerance, nervousness, irritability, diarrhea, sweaty skin, inability to fall asleep, fever, and chest pain.

hypnotic agent Drug that produces sleep, relaxation, or loss of memory in a patient.

hypoglycemia Condition in which serum glucose levels are less than 60 mg/dL. Produces sudden onset of nervousness; hunger; weakness; cold, clammy, skin; lethargy; no urine glucose or acetone; pallor; diaphoresis; change in level of consciousness; and shallow respirations. May be caused by excessive doses of insulin.

hypothyroidism Condition in which there is a decrease in production of thyroid hormone. Symptoms include fatigue, weakness, lethargy, moderate weight gain with minimal appetite, cold intolerance, menorrhagia, dry skin, coarse hair, hoarseness, impaired memory, and constipation.

I

idiopathic Of an unknown cause; for example, most hypertension is idiopathic in origin.

idiosyncratic response Strange, unique, or unpredicted response to a drug.

immunity Resistance to invading proteins and diseases produced by either having a disease and recovering from it or being immunized to prevent getting the disease.

implementation Performance of the nursing care plan; involves administering therapeutic agents, helping with feeding or activities of daily living, providing dressing changes, or giving teaching and counseling.

improper fraction Fraction that has a numerator (top number in the fraction) the same as, or larger, than the denominator (bottom number in the fraction).

incompatibility When two drugs do not mix well chemically; an attempt to combine them in a syringe causes a chemical reaction so that neither can be used.

infants Children from the first month after birth to approximately 12 months of age, when babies are able to assume an erect posture; some extend the period to 24 months of age.

initial insomnia Difficulty falling asleep.

inspection One of the four traditional physical assessment techniques; involves the nurse looking closely for physical findings or observing the patient.

insulin Hormone necessary for the metabolism and use of glucose in the body; produced by the beta cells of the pancreas.

insulin-dependent diabetes mellitus (IDDM) Former name for type 1 diabetes.

integrative practices Health care using both alternative (nontraditional) and traditional practices and products.

interference When two drugs are given together, one drug promotes the rapid excretion of the other drug, thus reducing its activity.

intermittent insomnia Inability to stay asleep.

intramuscular (IM) injections Injections that deposit medication past the dermis and subcutaneous tissue, deep into the muscle mass where the rich blood supply allows for rapid and complete absorption.

intravenous (IV) route Route used to administer a drug directly into the bloodstream via a needle.

L

laxatives Drugs that help draw fluid into the intestine to promote fecal softening, speed the passage of feces through the colon, or increase peristalsis to aid in the elimination of stool from the rectum.

legal responsibility A nurse's authority as clearly defined by the nurse practice act of each state. Involves a nurse's judgment and actions while performing professional duties. Because of the variability of practice in different states, it is mandatory that each nurse learn what is legally authorized with regard to medications and ensure that the rules are clearly followed.

leukotriene receptor inhibitors Drugs that block receptors for the leukotriene bronchoconstrictors; used in the treatment of asthma.

lipodystrophy Shrinkage and loss of the fatty tissue when medication, particularly insulin, is given in the same spot too frequently.

liter Unit of volume used in the metric system of measurement.

literacy The ability to read, write, and speak in English; to do math; and to solve problems at the level necessary to function on the job and in society.

lozenges Medicine mixed with a sugar base to produce small, hard preparations of various sizes or shapes. They are sucked to obtain the medication.

M

male or female hormones Chemicals produced by sex glands that are responsible for secondary sex characteristics, fertility, and reproduction.

malignancy Refers to rapid and uncontrolled growth of abnormal or cancerous cells that can travel throughout the body, spread into other areas, occupy space, and rob tissues of the nutrients required to maintain normal health.

metastasis Movement of uncontrolled, rapidly growing cells from their point of origin (primary site) into other tissues adjacent to or far removed from the primary site (for example, a lung tumor that metastasizes to the brain).

meter Unit of length used in the metric system of measurement.

metric system System of measurement developed in France and based on the decimal system. Built on multiples of 10, basic units are *meter* for length, *liter* for volume, and *gram* for weight.

minerals Inorganic elements essential to normal metabolism and function because of their role in speeding up biochemical reactions.

miosis Constriction of the pupil of the eye.

mitotic inhibitors Group of medications that interfere with or stop cell division directly.

mixed number A number that consists of a whole number and a proper fraction.

Mix-o-vial A two-compartment vial that contains a sterile solution in one compartment and medication powder in the other, separated by a rubber stopper. Solution and powder are mixed together immediately before use.

motility Spontaneous, unconscious, or involuntary movement; may apply to food moving through the gastrointestinal tract or to muscular activity.

mycotic infections Yeastlike or moldlike diseases in humans that are produced by a fungus.

mydriasis Abnormal dilation of the pupil.

myocardial infarction Death of cardiac muscle cells resulting from decreased blood supply through the coronary artery, as in coronary thrombosis.

myocardium Middle layer of the heart wall; made up of special muscle cells.

myxedema Severe form of hypothyroidism. Skin changes include nonpitting edema; doughy skin; puffy face; large tongue; decreased body hair; and cool, dry skin. May lead to coma and death.

N

narcotic Any substance that produces stupor associated with analgesia.

narrow-spectrum drugs Antiinfective medications useful against only a few organisms.

nasogastric (NG) tube An enteral route for medication; tube that goes through the nose and opens directly into the stomach.

naturally acquired active immunity Immunity obtained by the development of antibodies when a person gets an infectious disease.

needle Instrument used with a syringe to deliver medication; made up of the hub, which attaches to the syringe; the shaft, which is the hollow part through which the medication passes; and the beveled tip, which pierces the skin.

neonates The newborn or initial stage of life from birth to 1 month of age.

neoplasms Tumors or abnormal growths; may be benign or malignant.

nephrotoxic Having the potential to damage the kidney.

neurotransmitters Chemical messengers released at the nerve synapse; take part in the transmission of impulses from one nerve ending to another and convey information from the brain to other body parts, producing physiologic responses.

niacin Water-soluble and essential B complex vitamin that is a component of two coenzymes that transfer hydrogen in intracellular respiration.

nomogram Chart that displays relationships between two types of data; used so that complex mathematical calculations are not necessary. In pharmacology, an example is a chart used to calculate body surface area.

noncompliance A decision or action on the part of the patient not to adhere to a therapeutic suggestion. This may be because of a health belief, a cultural or spiritual value, misunderstanding, failure to appreciate risk, or a problem in the relationship between the provider of the recommendation and the patient. Also refers to the inappropriate use of medications.

noncompliant Term used to describe a patient who does not follow a prescribed plan of care.

non–insulin-dependent diabetes mellitus (NIDDM) Former name for type 2 diabetes.

nonsteroidal antiinflammatory drugs (NSAIDs) Agents that have analgesic, antiinflammatory, and antipyretic effects; used in treating rheumatic diseases, degenerative joint disease, osteoarthritis, and acute musculoskeletal problems.

norepinephrine One of two major neurotransmitters in the body; acts on the sympathetic nerves.

normal sinus rhythm The regular beating of the heart using the usual path of electrical communication throughout the heart. The electrical stimuli in the cardiac muscle originate in the sinoatrial node, pass through the atrium to the atrioventricular node, through the bundle of His, through the right and left bundle branches, and out through the Purkinje fibers of the myocardium. The heart will then contract, forcing blood out into the arteries. Then the cycle begins again.

numerator Number in the top part of a fraction, above the line.

nurse practice act State law passed to license practical nurses, registered nurses, nurse practitioners, nurse-midwives, and nurse anesthetists. Describes minimal requirements the individual must have that will protect the public safety. Provides title protection to those who can document their educational preparation and show willingness to accept professional responsibility. Describes what functions the nurse is authorized to perform, including drug prescription or administration.

nursing process Plan developed over the years that organizes and coordinates the nurse's activities. Its five major parts are assessment, diagnosis, planning, implementation, and evaluation.

O

objective data Information obtained from documentation that patients may bring with them, such as electrocardiogram results or x-ray examinations, or information that can be directly observed during a physical examination or obtained from laboratory tests and diagnostic procedures.

official name Name given to a drug by the Food and Drug Administration; may be similar to the brand or trade name.

opioids Narcotics used for treating severe pain.

opportunistic infections Infections caused by normally nonpathogenic organisms in a person whose resistance has been decreased by such disorders as diabetes mellitus, acquired immune deficiency syndrome (AIDS), or cancer; by a surgical procedure such as a cerebrospinal fluid shunt or a cardiac or urinary tract catheterization; or by immunosuppressive drugs.

oral hypoglycemics Products that stimulate insulin release by the beta cells of the pancreas.

osteoarthritis Common form of arthritis with localized joint destruction, particularly in weight-bearing joints or stressed joints, resulting gradually from overuse and increasing age.

ototoxic Drug that may damage hearing.

over-the-counter (OTC) medications Category of drugs identified by federal legislation as having low risk to patients and that may be purchased without a prescription; have low risk for abuse and are safe if directions are followed.

oxytocic agents Drugs that cause the uterus to contract, produce narrowing of the blood vessels, and stimulate the flow of breast milk; used to help labor move on to delivery.

P

pacemaker Special group of nerve fibers located in the sinoatrial node that starts the spread of electrical impulses throughout the other muscle cells in the heart, causing the heart to pump.

pain An unpleasant sensation or emotion that produces or might produce tissue damage.

palpation One of the four standard physical assessment techniques; involves use of the hands and the sense of touch to gather data about the patient's physical condition.

parenteral route Administration of drug by injection directly into dermal, subcutaneous, or intramuscular tissue; epidurally into the cerebrospinal fluid; or through intravenous injection into the bloodstream.

Parkinson disease Paralysis agitans; a chronic disorder of the central nervous system that is thought to involve an imbalance or relative decrease in chemical neurotransmitters within the brain.

partial agonists Drugs that attach at the receptor site but produce only a small chemical response.

passive immunity Short-term resistance to invading proteins and diseases that is produced in two ways: (1) by taking immune globulins from a person who has had a specific antigen-antibody response and giving them to another person who has not had this response to protect that individual from a specific disease, or (2) when antibodies pass from the mother to the fetus through the placenta or to the nursing infant through the breast milk.

pathogen An organism that produces infection.

pediatric Pertaining to preventive and primary health care and treatment of children and the study of childhood diseases; also refers to children from infancy to adolescence.

pediculicides Agents used to treat pediculosis, an infection of the dermis seen mostly in children.

percent Parts per hundred units; symbol: %.

percussion One of the four traditional physical assessment techniques. Uses tapping of tissues overlying various body organs and structures to produce vibration and sound to detect underlying abnormalities.

percutaneous (route) Administration of drug through topical (skin), sublingual (under the tongue), buccal (against the cheek), or inhalation (breathing) methods.

perennial allergic rhinitis (PAR) Inflammation of the nasal mucous membranes caused by reaction to indoor allergens (for example, animal dander and dust mites).

erennial nonallergic rhinitis (PNAR) Inflammation of the nasal mucous membranes caused by conditions other than allergies.

peripheral nervous system The portion of the nervous system that consists of the nerves connecting the brain and spinal cord to other parts of the body.

pharmacodynamics The effects of drugs on functions of the body.

pharmacokinetics The action of drugs in the body.

pharmacotherapeutics The use of drugs in the treatment of disease.

physical dependence Physiologic need for a medication to relieve shaking, pain, or other symptoms.

piggyback infusion A second intravenous infusion added to allow administration of medication while the original infusion is clamped off. Patient requires only one needle for both infusions.

pill Oral, solid medication; may be a tablet or capsule.

plunger Inner portion of a syringe that fits into the barrel. When the plunger is pushed into the barrel, the medication is forced out through the needle.

positive inotropic action Drug effect that increases the strength of each heartbeat and, in turn, increases cardiac output.

precautions Factors that indicate that a particular drug or class of drugs should be used with great care to treat a medical condition.

prescription, or legend, drugs Category of drugs regulated by federal legislation because they are dangerous, and their use must be controlled; may be purchased only when prescribed by an authorized prescriber. Examples are antibiotics and oral birth control pills.

primary hypertension Hypertension (elevation of a patient's blood pressure above normal values for the patient's age) with unknown causes; accounts for 80% to 90% of all cases of high blood pressure. Also called *essential hypertension*.

problem-oriented medical record (POMR) A format for patient charts developed by Lawrence Weed in 1969. It uses a list of numbered patient problems as an index to the chart and includes a summary sheet, history and physical examination, problem list, physician's orders, progress notes, graphic record, laboratory tests, and consultations.

professional responsibility The obligation of nurses to act appropriately, ethically, and to the best of their abilities as health care providers.

progesterone Sex steroid hormone produced by the ovaries, by the placenta, and in small amounts by the adrenal cortex; helps prepare the uterus for implantation. Along with estrogen, it helps maintain normal uterine and mammary gland function.

proper fraction Part of a whole number, or numbers less than 1. Numerator (top number) is less than denominator (bottom number) in these fractions.

prophylaxis Prevention of or protection against disease.

proportion A way of expressing a relationship of equality between two ratios. When written, the two ratios are separated by a double colon.

psychologic dependence Feeling of anxiety, stress, or tension if a patient does not have a medication.

R

ratio A way of expressing the relationship of one number to another number, or of expressing a part of a whole number. When written, the numbers are separated by a colon. Term is often used along with *proportion.*

rebound effect Increase in symptoms that you are trying to stop; frequently caused by taking too much medication or when medication is suddenly stopped.

rebound vasodilation Condition in which a drug that was given to constrict the veins causes them to become dilated instead because of its action on both types of receptors; causes an increase in blood flow that may lead to further symptoms.

receptor A structure that acts as a "lock" for a specific chemical ("key") that must fit into the receptor before an action can be produced.

receptor site A specific site in the body where a medication bonds chemically.

refractoriness Lack of response to a drug that a patient has used before with good effectiveness.

regimen A specific medication plan or a therapeutic plan such as a diet or exercise schedule.

retrovirus A virus that contains ribonucleic acid (RNA) rather than deoxyribonucleic acid (DNA) as its genetic material. Retroviruses produce the enzyme reverse transcriptase, which allows transcription of the viral genome onto the DNA of the host cell.

rheumatoid arthritis A systemic disease that involves an autoimmune response caused by failure of the body to recognize its own tissue, resulting in destruction of the joint.

riboflavin Water-soluble vitamin (B_2) that functions as a precursor of two essential enzymes that deal with metabolism of proteins, fats, and carbohydrates.

roman numeral system System of numbers commonly used as units of the apothecaries' system of weights and measures in writing prescriptions. Consists of seven basic numerals in different combinations: I = 1, V = 5, X = 10, L = 50, C = 100, D = 500, and M = 1000.

S

salicylates Agents used to treat mild to moderate pain and reduce fever. They have analgesic, antipyretic, and antiinflammatory effects.

scabicides Agents applied to skin and in hair to kill scabies.

scheduled drugs Controlled substances that are highly regulated because they are commonly abused.

seasonal allergic rhinitis (SAR) Inflammation of the nasal mucous membranes caused by reaction to outdoor allergens (for example, pollen); also called *hay fever.*

secondary hypertension Hypertension resulting from a known disease or other problem, such as coarctation of the aorta.

sedative agent Medication that relaxes the patient and allows the patient to sleep.

seizures Sudden muscle contractions that happen without conscious control; a symptom of abnormal and excessive discharge of electrical impulses in the brain.

sex hormones Substances that influence many organs, structures, and life processes of the body as they prepare the body to reproduce. Produced in the adrenal cortex and gonads and include androgens and estrogens.

side effects Any unintended reactions or consequences that result from a medication; usually mild and may be beneficial or annoying.

six "rights" of medication administration Six points to check when administering a drug. These include five points to check before administering medication (the right drug, the right time, the right dose, the right patient, and the right route) and one point to check after administration (the right documentation).

skeletal muscle relaxants Drugs used to decrease muscle tone and involuntary movement without loss of voluntary motor function. They inhibit the transmission of impulses in the motor pathways at the level of the spinal cord and the brainstem or interfere with the mechanism that shortens the skeletal muscle fibers so they contract.

slow-acting antirheumatic drugs (SAARDs) Agents used in limiting joint destruction in significant cases of rheumatoid arthritis.

solubility The ability of a medication to dissolve.

Somogyi effect Rebound increase in glucose levels that is caused by hypoglycemia.

spectrum The variety or number of organisms against which a medication is effective.

status epilepticus A condition in which a series of severe grand mal seizures occur one after another without stopping.

steroids A group of hormones that have powerful effects on cell sensitization, healing, and development. May be associated with adverse effects, particularly in patients who must take them chronically.

subcutaneous injections Injections that place no more than 2 mL of fluid into the loose connective tissue between the dermis of the skin and the muscle layer.

subjective data Information supplied by the patient or family. It may be felt or known only by the patient and not detectable to anyone else.

sublingual administration Applying medication to mucous membranes under the tongue.

superinfection Overgrowth of other organisms not sensitive to a prescribed antiinfective medication when the medication kills sensitive organisms that would have kept them under control. Common adverse reaction seen when antibiotics kill all the bacteria in a patient and allow overgrowth of yeast.

suspensions Liquids with solid, insoluble drug particles dispersed throughout. Must be shaken before pouring because solids tend to settle out in layers.

sympathomimetics Beta-adrenergic agents that dilate the bronchi through their action on beta-adrenergic receptors.

synergistic effect When two drugs are given together, the effect is greater than the sum of the effects of each drug given alone.

syringes Calibrated containers used for injecting liquids into the body. May be plastic or glass and are available in 1-, 3-, 5-, 10-, 20-, and 50-mL sizes.

syrups Liquids with high sugar content designed to disguise the bitter taste of a drug; often used in pediatric patients.

systemic acidosis A condition in which the basic fluid and electrolyte balance of the body is disturbed, and the blood pH is decreased. Symptoms include nausea, vomiting, and changes in level of consciousness.

T

tablet Dried, powdered drugs compressed into shapes small enough to be swallowed whole; may contain coating to increase solubility or absorption.

teratogenic Likely to produce malformations or damage in the embryo or fetus.

terminal insomnia Early awakening with an inability to return to sleep.

therapeutic effects Occur when a drug produces the intended reaction and the therapeutic goal is met.

thiamine Water-soluble vitamin (B_1) that functions as a coenzyme and is closely involved with carbohydrate metabolism.

thrombi Blood clots made of fibrin, platelets, and cholesterol; often found in large veins. Pieces known as emboli may break off and travel to the heart, brain, or lung, causing strokes or death.

thromboplastin A complex substance that initiates the clotting process by converting prothrombin to thrombin in the presence of calcium ion. Found in most tissue cells, red cells, and leukocytes; functions as factor III in blood coagulation.

tip Portion of a syringe that holds the needle. The needle either screws onto the tip or fits tightly so it does not fall off.

tocolytics Agents that stop uterine contractions during labor.

tolerance A state in which the same amount of drug produces less effect over time.

topical medications Drugs applied directly to the area of skin requiring treatment; most common forms are creams, lotions, and ointments.

toxoid A toxin that is attenuated, or weakened.

trade name Brand name of a drug; licensed to a certain manufacturer and cannot be used by other manufacturers.

type 1 diabetes Insulin-dependent diabetes mellitus or juvenile diabetes; patient usually has little or no production of insulin by the pancreas.

type 2 diabetes Non–insulin-dependent diabetes mellitus or late-onset diabetes; patient usually has a functioning pancreas that can be encouraged by medication to produce more insulin.

U

uric acid A metabolite of protein present in the blood within a very specific range. Increased levels may precipitate as crystals in tissues, causing the condition known as *gout*.

uricosuric agents Drugs that increase the excretion of urate salts by blocking their renal tubular reabsorption. Also used to decrease the amount of circulating urate and the deposition of urate and promote reabsorption of urate deposits.

uterine relaxants Agents that act on the beta-adrenergic receptors to stop uterine smooth muscle contractions; used in the management of preterm or premature labor.

V

vaccines Substances containing weakened or dead antigens given to allow an individual to develop immunity to the antigen.

vasoconstrictors Agents that cause direct stimulation of the alpha receptors of vascular smooth muscle, leading to a narrowing of the blood vessels.

vials Small single- or multiple-dose glass containers of medication.

virions Rudimentary virus particles with a central nucleoid surrounded by a protein sheath or capsid. The complete nucleocapsid with a nucleic acid core may constitute a complete virus, or it may be surrounded by an envelope.

vitamin A Fat-soluble, long-chain alcohol that comes in several isometric forms; helps the eye adjust to changes from light to darkness.

vitamins Chemical compounds found naturally in plant and animal tissues but not made in the human body; necessary for life and essential to normal metabolism.

W

wheezing A musical respiratory sound heard during respiratory expiration when a patient with asthma begins to breathe faster or has a lot of bronchoconstriction.

withdrawal symptoms Changes in the body or mind, such as nausea or anxiety, that occur when a drug is stopped or reduced after regular use.

X

xanthines Bronchodilators that act directly to relax the smooth muscle cells of the bronchi, thereby dilating the bronchi.

Index

Note: Page numbers followed by f, t, and b indicate figures, tables, and boxes, respectively.

Lactulose, 346t
Lamictal. *See* Lamotrigine
Lamisil. *See* Terbinafine HCl
Lamivudine (3TC), 194t-195t
Lamotrigine, 260t, 265t
Lampit. *See* Nifurtimox
Lanoxin. *See* Digoxin
Lansoprazole, 339t-340t
Lantus. *See* Glargine
Lariam. *See* Mefloquine
Larodopa. *See* Levodopa
Lasix. *See* Furosemide
Latanoprost, 413t-416t
Latent-onset diabetes, 366-367
Lavender, 418b
Laws. *See* Legal issues
Laxatives, 341-347, 346t
 food/alcohol/drug interactions
  with, 38t-41t
 for geriatric patients, 345b
 hyperosmolar, 346t
Learning. *See also* Patient teaching
 evaluation of, 15
Lee-White coagulation time, 356
Leflunomide, 325t, 327
Legal issues, 17-30
 Canadian laws, 20-21
 controlled substances, 17-19, 18t,
  24-26
 delegation, 4
 documentation, 7, 22-24
 drug distribution systems, 24,
  25b
 federal laws, 17-20, 18t, 29
 health care worker safety, 29
 herbal product regulation, 61
 liability, 21
 licensure, 21
 medication errors, 7, 27-29
 state laws, 21-27
Legend drugs. *See* Prescription
 drugs
Lennox-Gastaut syndrome, 261
Lescol. *See* Fluvastatin
Letrozole, 204t-207t
Leukeran. *See* Chlorambucil
Leukotriene receptor inhibitors,
 148t-149t, 150-151
Leuprolide, 204t-207t
Leustatin. *See* Cladribine
Levamisole, 204t-207t
Levaquin. *See* Levofloxacin
Levarterenol. *See* Norepinephrine
Levemir. *See* Glargine
Levetiracetam, 260t
Levobetaxolol, 413t-416t
Levobunolol, 413t-416t
Levocabastine, 413t-416t
Levodopa, 270, 271t, 272
Levo-Dromoran. *See* Levorphanol
Levofloxacin, 170t-172t, 413t-416t
Levonorgestrel, estradiol and, 391
Levonorgestrel intrauterine system,
 392t
Levophed. *See* Norepinephrine
Levorphanol, 299t, 304t-305t
Levothroid. *See* Levothyroxine

Levothyroxine, 395t
Levsin. *See* l-hyoscyamine
Lexapro. *See* Escitalopram
Lexiva. *See* Fosamprenavir
Librax. *See* Clidinium
Librium. *See* Chlordiazepoxide
Lice, 417
Licensed practical/vocational
 nurses. *See* LPNs/LVNs
Licensure, 21
Licorice, 62, 65t, 158b
Lidex. *See* Fluocinonide
Lidocaine, 223t-224t, 309t
Lincocin. *See* Lincomycin
Lincoject. *See* Lincomycin
Lincomycin, 170t-172t
 adverse reactions to, 174t
 uses of, 173t
Lincosamides, 170t-172t
Lioresal. *See* Baclofen
Liothyronine (T$_3$), 395t
Liotrix, 395t
Lipid(s), 222-224
 metabolism of, 224, 225f
Lipid-lowering drugs, 52, 222-229,
 226t, 228t
 food/alcohol/drug interactions
  with, 38t-41t
 for geriatric patients, 228b
Lipitor. *See* Atorvastatin Ca
Lipodystrophy, 369
Lipofen. *See* Fenofibrate
Liquid dilution, 86-89
Liquids, dosage calculation for,
 85-86
Liquifilm. *See* Levobunolol
Liquifilm Forte, 413t-416t
Liquimat. *See* Sulfur preparations
Lisinopril, 238t
Literacy, 10-11
 health, 11, 54
Lithane. *See* Lithium
Lithium, 289-291, 290t
 adverse reactions to, 289, 291
 for geriatric patients, 290b
 for pediatric patients, 283
 serum levels of, 291
Lithium carbonate, food/alcohol/
 drug interactions with, 38t-41t
Lithonate. *See* Lithium
Liver function, in geriatric patients,
 drug metabolism and, 47
Livostin. *See* Levocabastine
Lobelia, 65t
Local anesthetics, 309t
 ophthalmic, 412, 413t-416t
 in OTC drugs, 60t
 skin and mucous membrane,
  419t-423t
Lodosyn. *See* Carbidopa
Lodoxamide, 413t-416t
Loestrin. *See* Estrogen and
 progestin combinations
Logen. *See* Diphenoxylate and
 atropine sulfate
Lomotil. *See* Diphenoxylate and
 atropine sulfate

Loniten. *See* Minoxidil
Loop diuretics, 235, 238t
Lo/Ovral. *See* Estrogen and
 progestin combinations
Loperamide, 342t-343t
Lopid. *See* Gemfibrozil
Lopinavir/ritonavir, 194t-195t
Lopressor. *See* Metoprolol
Loratadine, 141t
Lorazepam, 260t, 274t, 295t
Losartan, 238t
Losec. *See* Omeprazole
Losopan. *See* Magaldrate
Lotemax Altrex. *See* Loteprednol
Lotensin. *See* Benazepril
Loteprednol, 413t-416t
Lotions, 129
Lovastatin, 228t
Lovenox. *See* Enoxaparin
Low-density lipoproteins (LDLs),
 222-224
Loxapine, 284
Loxapine succinate, 286t
Loxitane. *See* Loxapine succinate
Lozenges, 94b, 413t
Lozol. *See* Indapamide
LPNs/LVNs
 demand for, 1
 protective equipment for, 102b
 substance abuse by, 19
 tasks and responsibilities of, 1-8.
  See also Nursing process
 delegation and, 21-22
 nurse practice acts and, 21-27
Lubricant laxatives, 343, 346t. *See
 also* Laxatives
Lufyllin. *See* Dyphylline
Lugol's Iodine. *See* Iodine products
Lumigan. *See* Bimatoprost
Luminal. *See* Phenobarbital
Lunelle. *See* Estrogen and progestin
 combinations
Lunesta. *See* Eszopiclone
Lungs, 137f, 139
Lupron. *See* Leuprolide
Luteinizing hormone, 378
Luvox CR. *See* Fluvoxamine
Lyme disease vaccine, 401t-403t
Lymphatic system, 400, 404f
Lymphocyte immune globulin,
 401t-403t
Lysodren. *See* Mitotane

M

Maalox. *See* Aluminum hydroxide
 and magnesium hydroxide
Macrolides, 165-167, 170t-172t
 food/alcohol/drug interactions
  with, 38t-41t
Mafenide, 419t-423t
Magaldrate, 339t-340t
Magnesium (magnesium citrate,
 milk of magnesia), 346t
Magnesium gluconate, 438t-439t
Magnesium hydroxide, 339t-340t
Magnesium oxide, 339t-340t
Magnesium salicylate, 317t

FDA PREGNANCY RISK CATEGORIES

CATEGORY	DESCRIPTION
A	Adequate, well-controlled studies in pregnant women have not shown an increased risk of fetal abnormalities.
B	Animal studies have revealed no evidence of harm to the fetus; however, there are no adequate and well-controlled studies in pregnant women. OR Animal studies have shown an adverse effect, but adequate and well-controlled studies in pregnant women have failed to demonstrate a risk to the fetus.
C	Animal studies have shown an adverse effect, but there are no adequate and well-controlled studies in pregnant women. OR No animal studies have been conducted, and there are no adequate and well-controlled studies in pregnant women.
D	Adequate, well-controlled, or observational studies in pregnant women have demonstrated a risk to the fetus. However, the benefits of therapy may outweigh the potential risk.
X	Adequate, well-controlled, or observational studies in animals or pregnant women have demonstrated positive evidence of fetal abnormalities. The use of the product is contraindicated in women who are or may become pregnant.

Modified from Meadows M: Pregnancy and the drug dilemma, *FDA Consumer Magazine,* 2001. Available at: www.fda.gov/fdac/features/2001/301_preg.html. Accessed September 16, 2008.

HALE'S LACTATION RISK CATEGORIES

L1: SAFEST

This drug has been taken by a large number of breastfeeding mothers without any observed increase in adverse effects in the infant. Controlled studies in breastfeeding women fail to demonstrate a risk to the infant, **and** the possibility of harm to the breastfeeding infant is remote, or the product is not orally bioavailable in an infant.

L2: SAFER

This drug has been studied in a limited number of breastfeeding women without an increase in adverse effects in the infant, **and/or** the evidence of a demonstrated risk that is likely to follow use of this medication in a breastfeeding woman is remote.

L3: MODERATELY SAFE

There are no controlled studies in breastfeeding women, but the risk of untoward effects to a breastfed infant is possible, **or** controlled studies show only minimal nonthreatening adverse effects. Drugs should be given only if the potential benefit justifies the potential risk to the infant.

L4: POSSIBLY HAZARDOUS

There is positive evidence of risk to the breastfed infant or to breast milk production, but the benefits from use in breastfeeding mothers may be acceptable despite the risk to the infant (for example, if the drug is needed in a life-threatening situation or for a serious disease for which safer drugs cannot be used or are ineffective).

L5: CONTRAINDICATED

Studies in breastfeeding mothers have demonstrated that there is significant and documented risk to the infant based on human experience, **or** it is a medication that has a high risk of causing significant damage to an infant. The risk of using the drug in breastfeeding women clearly outweighs any possible benefit. The drug is contraindicated in women who are breastfeeding an infant.

Modified from Hale TH: *Medications and mother's milk*, Amarillo, TX, 2002, 2008, Hale Publishing. More information available at Dr. Hale's website: neonatal.ttuhsc.edu/lact. Accessed September 16, 2008.